Fundamental Pharmacology
for Pharmacy Technicians, Second Edition

Jahangir Moini, MD, MPH, CPhT

Professor of Science and Health,
Eastern Florida State College, Palm Bay, Florida
and Former Professor and Director of Allied Health,
Everest University, Melbourne, Florida

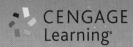
CENGAGE
Learning

Australia • Brazil • Mexico • Singapore • United Kingdom • United States

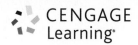

Fundamental Pharmacology for Pharmacy Technicians, Second Edition
Jahangir Moini

SVP, GM Skills & Global Product Management: Dawn Gerrain

Product Director: Matthew Seeley

Senior Director, Development: Marah Bellegarde

Senior Product Development Manager: Juliet Steiner

Product Manager: Steven Smith

Senior Content Developer: Darcy M. Scelsi

Product Assistant: Courtney Cozzy

Vice President, Marketing Services: Jennifer Ann Baker

Marketing Manager: Jonathan Sheehan

Senior Production Director: Wendy Troeger

Production Director: Andrew Crouth

Senior Content Project Manager: Kenneth McGrath

Senior Art Director: Jack Pendleton

Cover image(s): © stevecoleimages/iStock.com

Library of Congress Control Number: 2015943200

Book-only ISBN: 978-1-305-08735-4

Cengage Learning
20 Channel Center Street
Boston, MA 02210
USA

Cengage Learning is a leading provider of customized learning solutions with employees residing in nearly 40 different countries and sales in more than 125 countries around the world. Find your local representative at
www.cengage.com

Cengage Learning products are represented in Canada by Nelson Education, Ltd.

To learn more about Cengage Learning, visit **www.cengage.com**

Purchase any of our products at your local college store or at our preferred online store **www.cengagebrain.com**

Notice to the Reader

Printed in the United States of America.

Print Number: 01   Print Year: 2015

Dedication

This book is dedicated to

my wife Hengameh,

my daughters Mahkameh and Morvarid,

and my precious granddaughters Laila and Anabelle.

Table of Contents

Section I GENERAL ASPECTS OF PHARMACOLOGY

Section II PHARMACOLOGY RELATED TO SPECIFIC BODY SYSTEMS AND DISORDERS

Section III PHARMACOLOGY FOR DISORDERS AFFECTING MULTI-BODY SYSTEMS

Section IV PHARMACOLOGY FOR SPECIFIC POPULATIONS

Appendices

Preface

INTRODUCTION

Pharmacology is one of the most challenging aspects of study for pharmacy technicians. The study of pharmacology requires thorough knowledge of anatomy and physiology, chemistry, pathology, psychology, and sociology. This book clearly connects pharmacology with pathophysiology in order to foster a complete understanding of these sciences. Though pharmacology is a difficult topic, the approach of this book illuminates its key principles as well as the more complex points that must also be mastered.

In today's health care environment, drug therapy is of the utmost importance but is also a complicated area of understanding. The field of pharmacology is always changing. Pharmacy technicians who deal with pharmacology must continually improve in their knowledge with regular review and updating of the latest advancements.

ORGANIZATION OF CONTENT

This book is organized into four sections comprising 28 chapters that focus on various aspects of pharmacology. The first section introduces general concepts related to pharmacology. The middle sections of the book consist of chapters organized by body system and related disorders. The final section looks at pharmacology for specific populations. The book concludes with appendices, a glossary, and an index. In each chapter, drugs are discussed in terms of their mechanisms of action, indications, adverse effects, contraindications, precautions, and drug interactions. At the end of the book are 30 additional case studies with multiple questions (Appendix A).

The classification of drugs according to their related body systems allows the text to easily reference tables, figures, and other supportive content so that the intended effects of each drug may be related to the pertinent parts of the body. Terminology that is new to each chapter is highlighted in "Medical Terminology Review" margin notes that help the student to better understand and break down new terms into their component parts. Additionally, "Key Concept" margin notes highlight specific subjects that students must remember.

FEATURES

Each chapter contains an outline of the key topics, a glossary of important terms (set in bold type in the chapter text), and objectives that the student must be able to meet upon completion of the reading. Overview and anatomy review segments introduce the student to the key concepts of the chapter as well as related anatomical structures and functions. Figures serve to accurately illustrate chapter principles, organs, drug functions, and related information. Numerous helpful and accurate summary tables focus on key drugs and related topics that must be fully understood in order to master each chapter's content. The chapters conclude with a summary of information, followed by "Exploring the Web," which lists pertinent websites for additional study. Finally, unique varieties of review questions with an accompanying answer key are provided. Included in the review questions are short scenarios with "Critical Thinking" questions.

CURRENT DRUG INFORMATION

All of the included drug information was current and up to date at the time of the writing of this book. It is important to remember that drug information changes frequently and should always be verified before any preparation, compounding, or administration occurs. You should always consult a current edition of the *Physician's Desk Reference, Facts and Comparisons,* or the package inserts accompanying a drug. Pharmacists and physicians may also be able to provide current drug information.

NEW TO THIS EDITION

Chapter 1

- Added discussion of the Kefauver–Harris Amendment of 1963, the Omnibus Budget Reconciliation Act of 1990, the Health Insurance Portability and Accountability Act (HIPAA) of 1996, the FDA Modernization Act of 1997, the Medicare Prescription Drug, Improvement, and Modernization Act of 2003, and the Isotretinoin (Accutane) Safety and Risk Management Act (Proposal Only) of 2005.

Chapter 2

- Added discussion of the advantages and disadvantages of some common dosage forms of drugs.

Chapter 3

- Expanded and clarified discussion of the various processes involved in pharmacokinetics, including distribution, metabolism, and excretion.
- Expanded discussion of drug interactions.

Chapter 4

- New chapter focusing on medication orders and prescriptions.

Chapter 5

- Formerly Chapter 4.
- Drug tables have been revised and updated. They include relevant Black Box Warnings.

Chapter 6

- Updated drug tables include schedule classification, pronunciations, and relevant Black Box Warnings.

Chapter 10

- Updated drug tables include schedule classification, pronunciations, and relevant Black Box Warnings.

Chapter 11

- Updated drug tables include schedule classification, pronunciations, and relevant Black Box Warnings.

Chapter 12

- Updated drug tables include schedule classification, pronunciations, and relevant Black Box Warnings.

Chapter 13

- Updated drug tables include schedule classification, pronunciations, and relevant Black Box Warnings.

Chapter 14

- Formerly Chapter 18.
- Updated drug tables include schedule classification, pronunciations, and relevant Black Box Warnings.

Chapter 15

- Formerly Chapter 13.
- Added discussion of hemophilia drugs.
- Updated drug tables include schedule classification, pronunciations, and relevant Black Box Warnings.

Chapter 16

- Formerly Chapter 14.
- Updated drug tables include schedule classification, pronunciations, and relevant Black Box Warnings.

Chapter 17

- Formerly Chapter 15.
- Added discussion of prostaglandin E_1 analog.
- Updated drug tables include schedule classification, pronunciations, and relevant Black Box Warnings.

Chapter 18

- Formerly Chapter 16.
- Updated drug tables include schedule classification, pronunciations, and relevant Black Box Warnings.

Chapter 19

- Formerly Chapter 17.
- Updated drug tables include schedule classification, pronunciations, and relevant Black Box Warnings.

Chapter 20

- Formerly Chapter 19.
- Updated drug tables include schedule classification, pronunciations, and relevant Black Box Warnings.

Chapter 21

- Formerly Chapter 20.
- Updated drug tables include schedule classification, pronunciations, and relevant Black Box Warnings.

Chapter 22

- Formerly Chapter 21.
- Updated drug tables include schedule classification, pronunciations, and relevant Black Box Warnings.

Chapter 23

- Formerly Chapter 22.
- Added discussion of methicillin-resistant *Staphylococcus aureus* (MRSA).
- Expanded discussion of cephalosporins and aminoglycosides.
- Expanded drug tables include schedule classification, pronunciations, and relevant Black Box Warnings.

Chapter 24

- Formerly Chapter 23.
- Updated drug tables include schedule classification, pronunciations, and relevant Black Box Warnings.

Chapter 25

- Formerly Chapter 24.
- Updated drug tables include schedule classification, pronunciations, and relevant Black Box Warnings.

Chapter 26

- Formerly Chapter 25.
- Expanded discussion of childhood respiratory diseases to include sudden infant death syndrome (SIDS).
- Updated drug tables include schedule classification, pronunciations, and relevant Black Box Warnings.

Chapter 27

- Formerly Chapter 26.
- Added discussion of the Beers List.

Chapter 28

- New chapter covering misused, abused, and addictive drugs.

RESOURCES

Workbook to Accompany Fundamental Pharmacology for Pharmacy Technicians, *Second Edition*

The *Student Workbook* contains additional practice materials for review of the chapter content. Various question types are provided, including multiple choice, true/false, matching, and short answer.

Instructor Resources

This book is accompanied by an Instructor Companion Website, which contains an Instructor's Manual, PowerPoint slides for all chapters, and a test bank of additional questions. A student workbook is also available for additional practice.

To set up your account:

- Go to **www.cengagebrain.com/login**.
- Choose **Create a New Faculty Account**.
- Next you will need to select your **Institution**.
- Complete your personal **Account Information**.
- Accept the **License Agreement**.
- Choose **Register**.
- Your account will be pending validation—you will receive an e-mail notification when the validation process is complete.
- If you are unable to find your Institution; complete an **Account Request Form**.

Once you're account is set up or if you already have an account:

- Go to www.cengagebrain.com/login.
- Enter your e-mail address and password and select **Sign In**.
- Search for your book by author, title, or ISBN.
- Select the book and click **Continue**.
- You will receive a list of available resources for the title you selected.
- Choose the resources you would like and click **Add to My Bookshelf**.

Acknowledgments

The author would like to acknowledge the following individuals for their time and efforts in aiding him in the reviewing and editing of the book.

Maggie Daley, PharmD
Pharmacist Consultant
Melbourne, Florida

Mahkameh Moini, DMD
Dental Practitioner
West Palm Beach, Florida

Norman Tomaka, CRPh, LHRM
Consultant Pharmacy Services and
President, Florida Pharmacy Association
Melbourne, Florida

Greg Vadimsky
Pharmacy Technician and Editorial Assistant
Melbourne, Florida

REVIEWERS OF THE FIRST AND SECOND EDITIONS

Lisa Barnes, MBA, BPharm
Assistant Professor, Pharmacy Practice
Skaggs School of Pharmacy at the University of Montana
Missoula, Montana

Jesse Diaz, MS Ed, CPhT, CA-RPhT

Jennifer Dietz, CPhT
Pharmacy Technician Program Manager
Heritage College
Columbus, Ohio

Stephanie Garthrite, CPhT, AA, AS
Pharmacy Technician Instructor
Polaris Career Center
Middleburg Heights, Ohio

Sandra J. Johnson, CPhT, CCMA
Program Director
Virginia College
Montgomery, Alabama

Barbara Lacher, BS, RPhTech, CPhT
Assistant Program Director, Associate Professor
Pharmacy Technician Program
North Dakota State College of Science
Wahpeton, North Dakota

Paula Lambert, BS, CPhT
Pharmacy Technology Instructor North Idaho College
Coeur d'Alene, Idaho

Ashanti LaRoche, AS, CPhT, CTS, EMR
Pharmacy Program Instructor
Delgado Community College
New Orleans, Louisiana

Linh M. Lim, RPh, BS
Pharmacy Technician Program Instructor
Virginia College
Pensacola, Florida

Michelle McCranie, CPhT
Pharmacy Technology Instructor
Ogeechee Technical College
Statesboro, Georgia

Laurisa McKissack, BS, AAS, CPhT, RPT
Pharmacy Technician Program Instructor
Virginia College
Pensacola, Florida

James Mizner, RPh, MBA
Pharmacy Technician Program Director
Applied Career Training
Arlington, Virginia

Phillip Penrod, BS, AA, AA, CPhT
Medical Department Chair
Florida Metropolitan University
Tampa, Florida

Heather Pierce, PharmD
Adjunct Faculty
Rasmussen College
Romeoville, Illinois

Diana Rangaves, PharmD, RPh
Pharmacy Technician Program, Lead Instructor
Santa Rosa Junior College
Santa Rosa, California

Mohamed M. Tlass, BS, CPhT, PhTR
Professor
Houston Community College
Houston, Texas

Howard D. Turner, CPhT
Pharmacy Technician Program Manager
Heritage College
Oklahoma City, Oklahoma

Tammy Wilder, RN, MSN, CMSRN, BC
Adjunct Faculty
Ivy Tech Community College
Evansville, Indiana

About the Author

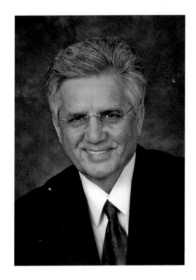

Dr. Moini was assistant professor at Tehran University School of Medicine for nine years teaching medical and allied health students. The author is a professor and former director (for 15 years) of allied health programs at Everest University. Dr. Moini established the associate degree program for pharmacy technicians in 2000 at EU's Melbourne campus. For five years, he was the director of the pharmacy technician program. He also established several other new allied health programs for EU. As a physician and instructor for the past 35 years, he believes that pharmacy technicians must be knowledgeable about pharmacology and have confidence in their duties and responsibilities in order to prevent medication errors.

Dr. Moini is actively involved in teaching and helping students to prepare for service in various health professions, including the roles of pharmacy technicians, medical assistants, and nurses. He worked with the Brevard County Health Department as an epidemiologist and health educator consultant for 18 years, offering continuing education courses and keeping nurses up to date on the latest developments related to pharmacology, medications errors, immunizations, and other important topics. Dr. Moini is currently a professor of science and health at Eastern Florida State College's Palm Bay campus. He has been an internationally published author of various allied health books since 1999.

General Aspects of Pharmacology

Introduction to Pharmacology, Drug Legislation, and Regulation

OUTLINE

OBJECTIVES

After completing this chapter, the reader should be able to:

1. Define the key terms.

2. Explain the four stages of drug product development.

3. Explain the differences between the DEA and the FDA.

4. Name the first drug act passed in the United States for consumer safety, and give the year it was passed.

5. Distinguish between legend drugs, over-the-counter drugs, and controlled substances.

6. Summarize the provisions of the Controlled Substances Act of 1970, and define the C-I to C-V schedules.

7. Describe the purpose of HIPAA.

8. Define OBRA-90 and explain its basic framework.

GLOSSARY

Clinical pharmacology – an area of medicine devoted to the evaluation of drugs used for human benefit

Controlled substance – any drug regulated under the Controlled Substances Act, which regulates the prescribing and dispensing of psychoactive drugs, including narcotics, hallucinogens, depressants, and stimulants

Drug Enforcement Administration (DEA) – the government agency concerned with controlled substances that enforces laws against drug activities, including illegal drug use, dealing, and manufacturing

Food and Drug Administration (FDA) – the branch of the U.S. Department of Health and Human Services that is responsible for the regulation of foods, drugs, cosmetics, and medical devices

Genetic engineering – techniques wherein genes from one organism are spliced into the chromosomes of another organism; also known as *recombinant DNA technology*

Investigational new drug (IND) application – an application for human drug testing that is submitted to the FDA once enough data have been collected on a new drug

Legend drug – a medication available through a written prescription from a physician or other authorized prescriber; a prescription drug

Narcotics – drugs that produce a sedative or pain-relieving affect

Over-the-counter (OTC) drug – a medication sold directly to a consumer that does not require a prescription from a health care professional; a nonprescription drug

Pharmacology – the science concerned with drugs and their sources, appearance, chemistry, actions, and uses

Recombinant DNA technology – techniques wherein genes from one organism are spliced into the chromosomes of another organism; also known as *genetic engineering*

OVERVIEW

Pharmacology is defined as the study of the sources, appearance, chemistry, actions, uses, and manufacturing of drugs and medications. This chapter presents a basic overview of the history of pharmacology, drug development, and drug legislation affecting the dispensing and use of medications.

THE HISTORY OF PHARMACOLOGY

Historical records show that drug use has long been a part of human culture worldwide. A historical timeline showing major pharmacological developments provides a continuum that may be divided into three distinct periods: the age of natural substances, the age of synthetic substances, and the age of biotechnology.

The Age of Natural Substances

The age of natural substances is characterized by the use of plant derivatives (e.g., morphine, which is derived from opium). The use of natural substances evolved in China and Egypt. One of the earliest records of medicinal uses of plants, known as the Ebers Papyrus (after George Ebers, who discovered it in 1875) was written in Egypt around 1500 BC. It contained formulas for more than 800 remedies. About 2000 BC, the Chinese began developing an interest in herbs as having value in the cure of diseases. Theophrastus, an early Greek philosopher and scientist (about 300 BC), compiled observations on the classification of plants by their various parts.

The Age of Synthetic Substances

The age of synthetic substances was characterized by the mass production of synthetic medicines and drug screening techniques (e.g., antibiotics and insulin). In the period from AD 1350 to 1650 (late Middle Ages through the Renaissance), rapid societal changes swept across Europe. During this period, Swiss-born physician Theophrastus Phillippus Aureolus Bombastus von Hohenheim, also known as Paracelsus, began to emphasize a chemical rather than a botanical orientation to medicine. He believed that disease was a chemical manifestation and should be treated chemically.

The production of synthetic substances for medicinal uses continued into the twentieth century. It was at this time that synthetic drugs began to be mass produced relatively cheaply in pharmaceutical laboratories. Once the

Medical Terminology Review

pharmacology
pharmac/o = drugs, medicine
-logy = the study of
the study of drugs or medicine

molecular structure of a natural drug is identified, it may be more convenient to synthesize it wholly in the laboratory instead of extracting it in its natural form, or else modify it chemically for better absorption, greater effectiveness, or fewer side effects.

The Age of Biotechnology

Biotechnology is defined as the use of proteins from cells and tissues from humans, animals, and plants to produce medicines and therapeutic treatments. These proteins are highly complex compounds, the functional characteristics of which are determined by subtle chemical bonds and structural arrangements. Biotechnological techniques involve the manipulation of these bonds and structural arrangements from microbial and human genetic material. A human gene can be inserted into one bacterium or fungal cell, which in turn divides to produce a colony in which each microbe contains the gene. This process is referred to as **recombinant DNA technology** or **genetic engineering** and was put into practice in the early 1970s. Clinical examples of this process include substances used in hormone replacement therapy (e.g., insulin and growth hormone).

DRUG PRODUCT DEVELOPMENT

In the United States, the development of new drugs and drug therapies can take anywhere from 7 to 15 years. The **Food and Drug Administration (FDA)**, a branch of the U.S. Department of Health and Human Services, is responsible for the regulation of foods, drugs, cosmetics, and medical devices. The FDA oversees the approval of new drugs, over-the-counter and prescription drug labeling, and standards related to the manufacture of drugs. The FDA considers a new chemical entity as an active pharmaceutical ingredient that has not been approved for marketing in the United States. Before a drug is approved for sale, it must go through several phases of drug product development.

Preclinical Investigation (Stage 1)

Animal pharmacology and toxicology data are obtained to determine the safety and effectiveness of the drug. It takes about one to three years, with the average being approximately 18 months. An **investigational new drug (IND) application** for human testing is submitted to the FDA once enough data have been collected on the new drug.

Clinical Investigation (Stage 2)

Clinical testing on humans takes place in three different phases called clinical phase trials. This is the longest part of the drug approval process and involves **clinical pharmacology**, an area of medicine devoted to the evaluation of drugs used for human benefit. Clinical phase trials are essential because responses among patients vary. If a drug appears to be effective without causing serious side effects, approval for marketing may be accelerated, or the drug may be used for treatment immediately in special cases, with careful monitoring. In any case, an IND must be submitted before a drug is allowed to proceed to the next stage of the approval process. During the clinical phase trials, healthy volunteers are used in large groups of selected patients to determine drug toxicity and tolerance. The trial phase takes between 2 and 10 years, with the average being five years.

Investigational New Drug (IND) Review (Stage 3)

A review of the IND is the third stage of drug approval. During this stage, the final phase of clinical trials and testing may continue, depending on the results obtained from preclinical testing. If the IND is approved, the process continues to the final stage. If the IND is rejected, the process stops until concerns are addressed. This stage takes from two months to seven years. The average is 24 months.

Postmarketing Studies (Stage 4)

Postmarketing surveillance is the fourth stage of the drug approval process. It takes place after clinical trials and the IND review process have been completed. Testing in humans is continued to check for any new side effects in larger and more diverse populations. Some adverse effects take longer to appear and are not identified until a drug is used by large numbers of patients.

REMOVAL OF A DRUG FROM THE MARKET

The FDA holds annual public meetings to hear comments from patients and professional and pharmaceutical organizations about the effectiveness and safety of new drug therapies. If the FDA discovers a serious problem, it will require that a drug be withdrawn from the market and its use discontinued.

PRESCRIPTION DRUGS

A prescription drug is a medication that can only be legally dispensed to a patient with a written order (prescription) from a physician or another individual licensed to prescribe medications. Most prescription drugs are so designated by the FDA; however, states can also designate specific drugs or devices as prescription items. Prescription drugs may only be dispensed by a pharmacist, pharmacy technician under direction of a pharmacist, or by the prescriber. A prescription drug is also called a **legend drug**.

NONPRESCRIPTION DRUGS

When drugs are used over long periods of time and demonstrate "wide" margins of safety, prescription drugs may become nonprescription or **over-the-counter (OTC) drugs**. Unlike prescription drugs, OTC drugs do not require a physician's order. Patients may treat themselves safely if they carefully follow the instructions included with these drugs. If patients do not follow these guidelines, OTC drugs can have serious side effects.

CONTROLLED SUBSTANCES

A **controlled substance** is a medicinal product that has a high potential for abuse and is regulated by the **Drug Enforcement Administration (DEA)**, a part of the U.S. Department of Justice. The DEA is tasked with the enforcement of laws regulating drug activities, illegal drug use, illegal drug dealing and sale, and illegal manufacture of drugs. A controlled substance can only legally be obtained with a physician's prescription. Many **narcotics**, drugs producing sedative or pain-relieving affects, are classified as controlled substances.

FEDERAL DRUG LEGISLATION

Many laws and regulations have been enacted during the past century regulating pharmacy practice. Some of these laws include the Pure Food and Drug Act; the Harrison Narcotic Act; the Pure Food, Drug, and Cosmetic Act; and the Comprehensive Drug Abuse Prevention and Control Act. These laws have been passed to control the use of prescription drugs, nonprescription drugs, and controlled substances.

Pure Food and Drug Act of 1906

The Pure Food and Drug Act was the government's first attempt to control and regulate the manufacture, distribution, and sale of drugs. Before this law, the purity and potency of many drugs were questionable, and some of these agents were even dangerous for human consumption.

Harrison Narcotic Act of 1914

The Harrison Narcotic Act regulated the importation, manufacture, sale, and use of opium, codeine, and their derivations and compounds. Before this law, any narcotic could be purchased without a prescription. In 1970, the Harrison Narcotic Act was replaced by the Comprehensive Drug Abuse Prevention and Control Act.

Pure Food, Drug, and Cosmetic Act of 1938

In 1938, further amendments were made to the Pure Food and Drug Act of 1906, resulting in the Pure Food, Drug, and Cosmetic Act, which created the FDA. The FDA provided additional control over the manufacture and sale of cosmetics. Under this act, manufacturers must be concerned with the purity, strength, effectiveness, safety, and packaging of drugs. Foods and cosmetics are also regulated. The provisions of this act give the FDA the power to approve or deny new drug applications and even to conduct inspections to ensure compliance. The FDA approves the investigational use of drugs on humans and ensures that all approved drugs are safe and effective.

Key Concept

The FDA is concerned with general safety standards in the production of drugs, foods, and cosmetics. It is responsible for the approval and removal from the market of many products.

Kefauver-Harris Amendment of 1963

The Kefauver-Harris Amendment of 1963 further strengthened the federal regulation of food, drugs, and cosmetics. It required that both prescription and nonprescription drug products be pure, effective, and safe. It placed prescription drug advertising under FDA supervision, and established reviews of the qualifications of drug investigators. Actually consisting of several amendments, Kefauver-Harris provided for manufacturer registration, manufacturing site inspections, and a much higher level of manufacturer accountability.

Comprehensive Drug Abuse Prevention and Control Act of 1970

The Comprehensive Drug Abuse Prevention and Control Act, also called the Controlled Substances Act (CSA), regulates the manufacture, distribution, and dispensation of drugs with a potential for abuse. This law deals with control and enforcement of pharmaceuticals and places this control and enforcement under the jurisdiction of the DEA.

The CSA classifies drugs with the potential for abuse into five schedules designated by the letter C and a Roman numeral (I–V) to indicate their level of control (Table 1-1). Drugs in Schedule I have the highest potential for abuse and addiction. Those in Schedule V have the least potential for abuse. Records must be kept on the transactions of all pharmaceuticals that are classified as controlled substances. This area is also regulated by the DEA.

Key Concept

The DEA is concerned with controlled substances only, and enforces laws against drug activities, including illegal drug use, dealing, and manufacturing.

Drugs are frequently added, deleted, or moved to one schedule or another. The DEA determines if a drug should be moved from one schedule to another.

Omnibus Budget Reconciliation Act of 1990

Also known as *OBRA-90*, the Omnibus Budget Reconciliation Act of 1990 amended both Medicare and Medicaid in significant ways. Its primary goal was to reduce Medicaid costs by reducing inappropriate drug use by Medicaid recipients. It imposed a cap on taxable income, which was $113,700 as of 2013. OBRA-90 is administered by the Centers for Medicare and Medicaid Services. It required Medicaid pharmacy providers to obtain,

TABLE 1-1	Schedules of Controlled Substances			
Schedule	Manufacturer's Label	Abuse Potential	Prescription Requirement	Examples
I	C-I	high; no accepted medical use	no prescription permitted	heroin, LSD (lysergic acid diethylamide), marijuana, mescaline, and peyote
II	C-II	high; accepted medical use	prescription required; no refills permitted without a new written prescription	codeine, fentanyl, methadone hydrochloride, methamphetamine, methylphenidate, morphine, and opium (deodorized)
III	C-III	moderate; accepted medical use	prescription required; 5 refills permitted in 6 months	certain drugs compounded with small quantities of narcotics; also other drugs with strong potential for abuse (e.g., Tylenol® with codeine), and certain barbiturates
IV	C-IV	low; accepted medical use	prescription required; 5 refills permitted in 6 months	barbital, chloral hydrate, chlordiazepoxide, diazepam, and pentazocine hydrochloride
V	C-V	low; accepted medical use	no prescription required for individuals 18 years of age or older unless quantities are greater than 4 fluid ounces	cough syrups with codeine, diphenoxylate hydrochloride with atropine sulfate, and kaolin/pectin/opium

record, and maintain basic patient information, including disease history. It also expanded drug product rules to ensure more safety and effective drug therapy, which basically prohibited unapproved uses of prescription drugs. OBRA-90 was designed to save patients money, and expanded on OBRA-87, which included the Nursing Home Reform Act of 1987.

Under OBRA-90, pharmacists in every state must offer to counsel all patients and review medications that they are taking. It also required that manufacturers provide the lowest prices to Medicaid patients by rebating to every state Medicaid agency the difference between the average price and the lowest available price. Each state had to establish a drug use review board to stop fraud or inappropriate care by physicians and pharmacists.

Health Insurance Portability and Accountability Act (HIPAA) of 1996

This act was designed to improve health insurance continuity and portability, reduce fraud, establish medical savings accounts, improve long-term health care access, and simplify health care administration. It was designed to improve the storage and sharing of private health information. HIPAA provided health care coverage for people who lose or change their jobs. It also created national provider identifiers (NPIs) for health care providers, employers, and health insurance plans. These identifying numbers are unique for covered health care providers, consisting of 10 digits and no other characters such as letters. NPIs are free and very easy to obtain, as well as highly important for providers utilizing Medicare billing.

The three sections of HIPAA include privacy regulations, security regulations, and transaction standards. The privacy regulations concern patient access to their own records, information disclosure tracking, hospital privacy, changes to records, communication of health information, and the use and disclosure of health information. The security regulations ensure confidentiality. The transaction standards require unique health identifiers as well as common code sets and electronic claims standards.

FDA Modernization Act of 1997

The focus of the FDA Modernization Act of 1997 was to reform regulations concerning medical products, foods, and cosmetics. Patient access to medical devices and experimental drugs was increased, and manufacturers received incentives, via 6-month extensions, on new pediatric drugs being tested. This act required risk assessment reviews of all drugs and foods in the United States that contained mercury. It required the "R_x" symbol to be included on the packaging of all legend drugs. It also established Medicare Part D in order to subsidize prescription drug costs for people on Medicare using a Medicare Advantage plan or a prescription drug plan. However, Medicare Part D does not cover drugs that have not received FDA approval, those being used for nonapproved conditions, those not allowed to be prescribed within the United States, those already covered by parts A or B of Medicare, and those excluded from coverage by Medicaid.

Medicare Prescription Drug, Improvement, and Modernization Act of 2003

This act, also known as the Medicare Modernization Act (MMA), widely revised the Medicare program, introducing tax breaks and subsidies for prescription drugs. New Medicare Advantage plans were authorized by this act, offering improved choices about health care, providers, other coverages, and federal reimbursements. As a result, Medicare became partially privatized. Pretax medical savings accounts were established, and wealthier senior citizens were required to pay certain fees that less-wealthy individuals were not required to pay.

Isotretinoin (Accutane) Safety and Risk Management Act (Proposal Only) of 2005

Though not passed, this proposed act was designed to establish restrictions on drugs containing isotretinoin, which is sold under the trade name Accutane®. Because of potential adverse effects, the drug's distribution would have been restricted. Isotretinoin, which is prescribed for acne, has caused severe birth defects in babies born to women taking the drug, as well as spontaneous abortions. The failure to pass this act led the FDA to implement the System to Management Accutane-Related Teratogenicity (SMART) program, but this effort has not greatly reduced harm caused by the drug.

SUMMARY

Pharmacology deals with the discovery, chemistry, effects, uses, and manufacturing of drugs. History shows that drug use has long been a part of human culture worldwide. Three distinct periods in the development of pharmacology have included the age of natural substances, the age of synthetic substances, and the age of biotechnology.

The development of a new drug is controlled by the FDA and consists of several phases. Drug product development is a long and difficult process, taking anywhere from 7 to 15 years.

In the past century, Congress has passed many laws to control and regulate the importation, manufacture, sale, and use of drugs. Any new drug that is developed must be safe and effective for the human body.

EXPLORING THE WEB

Visit **www.drugs.com**

- Look for information on drugs that are currently undergoing trials for FDA approval. Choose one drug and review the study and approval process from start to finish.

Visit **www.fda.gov**

- Search using the term *drug development*. Review documents and articles that provide details about the process of developing new drugs.

- Search using the term *pulled drugs*. Review articles discussing why drugs may be pulled off the market and how this decision is determined.

Visit **www.napra.ca**

- Under "Pharmacy Practice & Regulatory Resources," click on "Federal Drug Legislation." Review the information on the Controlled Drugs and Substances Act and regulations as well as the Food and Drugs Act and regulations.

REVIEW QUESTIONS

Short Answer

1. What types of drugs are listed in the C-II and C-V schedules?

2. Define the role of the DEA.

3. List three responsibilities of the FDA.

4. In what year was the first major U.S. drug act passed, and what was it called?

5. Define the following:

    a. The Controlled Substances Act (CSA)

    _____

    b. The Pure Food and Drug Act of 1906

    _____

    c. The Harrison Narcotic Act of 1914

    _____

    d. Legend drugs

    _____

Multiple Choice

1. The drugs with the highest potential for abuse and addiction, which are not accepted for medical use, are classified as which of the following schedules?

    A. I

    B. II

    C. IV

    D. V

2. Which of the following agencies oversees controlled substances and prosecutes individuals who illegally distribute them?

    A. FDA

    B. CDC

    C. DHHS

    D. DEA

3. Which of the following was the first period of historical drug development?

    A. synthetic substances

    B. natural substances

    C. biotechnical substances

    D. genetic engineering

4. The FDA is a branch of which department that controls all drugs for legal use?

    A. U.S. Department of Health

    B. U.S. Department of Health and Human Services

    C. U.S. Department of Agriculture

    D. U.S. Department of Labor

5. The best clinical example of a genetically engineered substance is which of the following?

    A. insulin

    B. penicillin

    C. aspirin

    D. vitamin A

6. Which of the following types of drugs has a high potential for abuse but is currently accepted for medical treatment in the United States?

    A. Schedule I

    B. Schedule II

    C. Schedule III

    D. Schedule IV

7. Into which of the following drug schedules are heroin, LSD, and marijuana placed?

    A. Schedule IV

    B. Schedule III

    C. Schedule II

    D. Schedule I

8. Stage 1 of drug product development may take:

    A. 2-7 months

    B. 18-24 months

    C. 1-3 years

    D. 2-10 years

9. Which of the following phases of drug product development may be improved as a result of equipment, regulatory, supply, or market demands?

A. Stage 1

B. Stage 2

C. Stage 3

D. Stage 4

10. Which of the following laws was the first to regulate the importation, manufacture, sale, and use of narcotic drugs?

A. Harrison Narcotic Act

B. Pure Food, Drug, and Cosmetic Act

C. Controlled Substances Act

D. Pure Food and Drug Act

11. An investigational new drug application for human testing is submitted to which of the following?

A. DEA

B. DHHS

C. FDA

D. The Joint Commission

12. Which of the following federal laws may control the use of prescription drugs, nonprescription drugs, and controlled substances?

A. Harrison Narcotic Act

B. Comprehensive Drug Abuse Prevention and Control Act

C. Pure Food and Drug Act

D. all of the above

13. Which of the following acts was intended to reduce Medicaid costs by reducing inappropriate drug use by Medicaid recipients?

A. Kefauver-Harris Amendment

B. Omnibus Budget Reconciliation Act

C. Harrison Narcotic Act

D. Medicare Prescription Drug Act

14. Which of the following acts required risk assessment reviews of all drugs and foods in the United States that contained mercury?

A. Accutane Safety and Risk Management Act

B. Omnibus Budget Reconciliation Act

C. Medicare Prescription Drug, Improvement, and Modernization Act

D. FDA Modernization Act

15. Which of the following acts created national provider identifiers for health care providers?

A. FDA Modernization Act

B. Pure Food and Drug Act

C. Health Insurance Portability and Accountability Act

D. Omnibus Budget Reconciliation Act

Matching

_____ 1. Schedule C-I

_____ 2. Schedule C-II

_____ 3. Schedule C-III

_____ 4. Schedule C-V

A. low abuse potential; accepted medical use

B. moderate abuse potential; accepted medical use

C. high abuse potential; accepted medical use

D. high abuse potential; no accepted medical use

Critical Thinking

Tom is a student in the pharmacy technician program who is taking the final exam for law and ethics. Many of his questions are related to federal drug acts.

1. What would be the correct name of the act that regulates the importation, manufacturing, sale, and use of opium, codeine, and their derivations and compounds?

2. Which agency has the power to approve or deny new drug applications?

3. What was the first federal drug act Congress passed in 1906?

Drug Sources and Dosage Forms

OBJECTIVES

After completing this chapter, the reader should be able to:

1. Differentiate between the chemical name, generic name, and trade name of drugs.

2. Explain the classification of drug sources.

3. Name three animal sources of drugs.

4. Distinguish between engineered and synthetic drug sources.

5. Describe the various dosage forms of drugs.

6. Distinguish between syrups and elixirs.

7. Distinguish between gelcaps, caplets, and capsules.

8. Explain advantages of granules.

GLOSSARY

Aromatic water – a mixture of distilled water with an aromatic volatile oil

Buffered tablet – a type of tablet manufactured to prevent irritation of the stomach

Caplet – a tablet shaped like a capsule

Capsule – a solid dosage form in which the drug is enclosed in either a hard or soft shell of soluble material

Chemical name – a drug's full name, which refers to its complete chemical makeup

Cream – a semisolid emulsion of either the oil-in-water or the water-in-oil type, ordinarily intended for topical use

Elixir – a clear, sweetened, flavored, hydroalcoholic liquid medication intended for oral use

Emulsion – a preparation containing two liquids that ordinarily cannot be mixed together in which one is dispersed in the form of very small globules throughout the other

Enteric-coated tablet – a tablet covered in a special coating to protect it from stomach acid, allowing the drug to dissolve in the intestines

Fluidextract – a pharmacopeial liquid preparation of vegetable drugs, made by filtration, containing alcohol as a solvent or as a preservative, or both

Gel – a jelly or the solid or semisolid phase of a colloidal solution

Gelcap – an oil-based medication that is enclosed in a soft gelatin capsule

Generic name – a drug not protected by a trademark, but regulated by the FDA; also called the *official* or *nonproprietary name*

Granule – a very small pill, usually gelatin- or sugar-coated, containing a drug to be given in a small dose

Liniment – a liquid preparation for external use, usually applied by friction to the skin

Lozenge – a small, disk-shaped tablet composed of solidifying paste containing an astringent, an antiseptic, or an oil-based drug used for local treatment of the mouth or throat; it is held in the mouth until dissolved; also known as a *troche*

Mixture – a mutual incorporation of two or more substances, without chemical union, in which the physical characteristics of each of the components are retained; also called a *suspension*

Ointment – a semisolid preparation usually containing medicinal substances and intended for external application

Pill – a small, globular mass of soluble material containing a medicinal substance to be swallowed

Plaster – a solid preparation that can be spread when heated and then becomes adhesive at the temperature of the body

Powder – a dry mass of minute separate particles of any substance

Solution – a liquid dosage form in which active ingredients are dissolved in a liquid vehicle

Spirit – an alcoholic or hydroalcoholic solution of volatile substances; also known as an *essence*

Suppository – a small, solid body shaped for ready introduction into one of the orifices of the body other than the oral cavity (e.g., rectum, urethra, or vagina), made of a substance, usually medicated, that is solid at ordinary temperature but melts at body temperature

Suspension – a liquid dosage form that contains solid drug particles floating in a liquid medium; also called a *mixture*

Sustained-release (SR) capsule – a capsule that provides a controlled release of the dosage over a special period of time

Syrup – a liquid preparation in a concentrated aqueous solution of a sugar, used for medicinal purposes or to add flavor to a substance

Tablet – a solid dosage form containing medicinal substances with or without suitable diluents

Tincture – an alcoholic solution prepared from vegetable materials or from chemical substances, used as a skin disinfectant

Trade name – a brand name given to a drug by its manufacturer (such drugs are marked with the registered symbol, ®); also called the *proprietary* or *brand name*

Troche – a small, disk-shaped tablet composed of solidifying paste containing an astringent, antiseptic, or oil-based drug used for local treatment of the mouth or throat; it is held in the mouth until dissolved; also known as a *lozenge*

OVERVIEW

The pharmacy technician must be familiar with many different forms of medication. There are various sources from which drugs are derived and forms in which drugs are prepared. A working knowledge of these sources and forms will aid the pharmacy technician in understanding how drugs are used and administered.

DRUG NAMES

It is not unusual for each drug entity to be known by several designations. Usually, a single drug may have up to three names: chemical, generic, and trade. The first type of name, usually applied to compounds of known composition, is the **chemical name**. For substances of plant or animal origin that cannot be classified as pure chemical compounds, scientific identification is given in terms of precise biochemical or zoological names. Chemical names are generally not useful to the physician, pharmacist, or other users of the drug.

When a new drug is proven to be useful through successive research stages to the point at which it appears that it may become a marketable product, a **trade name** is developed by the manufacturer. Properly registered trade names become the legal property of their owners, are protected by copyright laws, and cannot be used freely in the public domain. These two types of names do not fulfill the need for a single, simple, informative designation available for unrestricted public use. The nonproprietary name is the only name intended to function in this capacity.

The nonproprietary name often is referred to as the **generic name**. A generic name is the official name of the drug. This name is much simpler than the chemical name, and it is not protected by copyright. The use of generic names is encouraged over trade names to avoid confusion. Generic drugs are cheaper than brand name drugs. They are usually easier to remember and less complicated. A formulation of a drug is considered to

Medical Terminology Review

biochemical
bio = life; living systems
chemical = drug; agent
drug created from a living system

be *generically equivalent* (bioequivalent) to another formulation when the *active ingredients* are identical. If the levels of a generic and a trade name drug in the bloodstream are identical, the drugs should work the same. However, generic drug formulations may include *inert ingredients* that differ somewhat from those of brand-name equivalents. These differences may alter the ability of the drug to reach target cells and produce an effect. For these reasons, pharmacists should always verify with the prescribing physician whether a generic equivalent can be substituted for a trade-name drug specified in a prescription.

DRUG SOURCES

There are basically five sources of drugs: plants, animals (including humans), minerals or mineral products, synthetic (chemical substances), and engineered drugs (investigational drugs). Today, chemicals and even human tissues such as those used in stem-cell therapy can be manipulated to create new drug sources.

Plant Sources

Plant sources are grouped by their physical and chemical properties. Alkaloids are organic compounds that have been combined with acids to make a salt. Nicotine, morphine sulfate, and atropine sulfate are examples of these chemical compounds. An important cardiac glycoside is digoxin. Digoxin is made from digitalis, a derivative of the foxglove plant.

Animal Sources

Animal sources, such as the body fluids and glands of animals, can act as drugs. The drugs obtained from animal sources include enzymes such as pancreatin and pepsin. Hormones such as thyroid and insulin are also derived from animal sources.

Mineral Sources

Minerals from the earth and soil are used to provide inorganic materials unavailable from plants and animals. They are used as they occur in nature. Examples include iron, potassium, silver, and gold, which are used to prepare medications. Sodium chloride (table salt) is one of the best-known examples in this category. Gold is sometimes used to control severe rheumatoid arthritis, and coal tar is used to treat seborrheic dermatitis and psoriasis.

Synthetic Sources

New drugs may be created from the application of chemistry, biology, and computer technology to previously identified substances from living organisms (organic substances) or nonliving materials (inorganic substances). These drugs are called synthetic or manufactured drugs because they are not found naturally in this state but rather are created artificially through the application of chemistry and biology. Common examples of synthetic drugs include meperidine (Demerol®), sulfonamides, and oral contraceptives. Certain organic drugs such as penicillin are semisynthetic and are made by altering their natural compounds or elements. Some drugs are both organic and inorganic, such as propylthiouracil, which is an antithyroid hormone.

Engineered Sources

The newest area of drug origin is gene splicing or genetic engineering. The newer forms of insulin for use in humans have been produced with this technique. Other engineered drugs include tissue plasminogen activator, growth hormones, cancer drugs, and drugs that combat HIV. The replacement of missing or nonfunctional genes is an emerging area of genetic engineering.

DOSAGE FORMS OF DRUGS

Pharmaceutical principles are the underlying physiochemical principles that allow a drug to be incorporated in a pharmaceutical dosage form such as tablets and solutions. These principles apply whether the drug is extemporaneously compounded by the pharmacist or manufactured for commercial distribution as a drug product. Drug dosage forms are classified according to their physical state and chemical composition. They may include gases, liquids, solids, and semisolids. Some substances can undergo a change of state or phase, from solid to liquid states (melting) or from liquid to gaseous states (vaporization). Certain drugs are soluble in water, some are soluble in alcohol, and others are soluble in a mixture of liquids.

Solid Drugs

Intermolecular forces of attraction are stronger in solids than in liquids or gases. Solid drugs include tablets, pills, plasters, capsules, caplets, gelcaps, powders, granules, troches, or lozenges (Figure 2-1).

Tablet

A **tablet** is a pharmaceutical preparation made by compressing the powdered form of a drug and bulk filling material under high pressure (see Figure 2-1). Tablets are sometimes erroneously called pills, but that term more properly refers to a specific formulation, as explained below. Most tablets are intended to be swallowed whole for dissolution and absorption from the gastrointestinal tract. Some are intended to be dissolved in the mouth or in water. Tablets come in various sizes, shapes, and colors, and

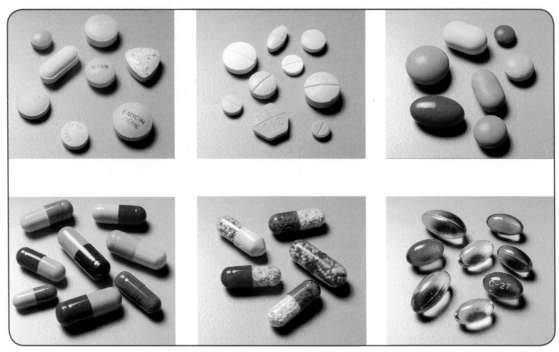

Figure 2-1 Examples of solid dosage forms.

also vary in composition. The various forms of tablets include chewable, sublingual, buccal, enteric-coated, and buffered tablets. An advantage of tablets is that almost all drug molecules can be formulated into a tablet since the manufacturing process is relatively simple. A disadvantage is that they may not be swallowed easily by children and some adults.

Chewable tablets must be chewed. They contain a flavored or sugar base. Chewable tablets are commonly used for antacids and antiflatulents, and are often recommended for children who cannot swallow other forms of medication. Sublingual tablets must be dissolved under the tongue for rapid absorption. An example is nitroglycerin for angina pectoris. Buccal tablets are placed between the cheek and the gum until they are dissolved and absorbed. An **enteric-coated tablet** has a special coating to protect against stomach acid, allowing the drug to dissolve in the alkaline environment of the intestines. A **buffered tablet** contains antacids that have been added to reduce irritation to the stomach by active ingredients, thus preventing ulceration or severe irritation of the stomach wall. Antacids and some other tablets are coated with a volatile liquid that is meant to dissolve in the mouth.

Pill

A single-dose unit of medicine made by mixing the powdered drug with a liquid, such as syrup, and rolling it into a round or oval shape is called a **pill**.

Plaster

Any composition of a liquid and a powder that hardens when it dries is called a **plaster**. Plasters may be solid or semisolid. An example is the salicylic

Medical Terminology Review

nitroglycerin
nitro = nitrate; nitrogen
glycerin = preparation obtained from fats and oils
drug preparation containing nitrogen

acid plaster used to remove corns. Advantages of plasters are that they are relatively easy to use, safe, and effective. A disadvantage is that long-term storage in unfavorable conditions may result in mixing of the medication with the adhesive used to adhere the plaster to the skin.

Capsule

A **capsule** is a medication dosage form in which the drug is contained in an external shell (see Figure 2-1). Capsule shells are usually made of hard cylindrical gelatin and enclose or encapsulate powder, granules, liquids, or some combinations of these. Liquids such as vitamin E and cod liver oil may be placed in soft gelatin capsules. Capsules are often used when medications have an unpleasant odor or taste. They can be pulled apart, and the entire contents can be added as powder to food for individuals who have difficulty swallowing. Some forms of capsules come with a controlled-release dosage and are used over a defined period of time. These are called **sustained-release (SR)** or timed-release capsules. These drugs should never be crushed or dissolved, because this would negate their timed-release action.

Caplet

A **caplet** is shaped like a capsule but has the form of a tablet. The shape and film-coated covering make swallowing easier.

Gelcap

A **gelcap** is an oil-based medication that is enclosed in a soft gelatin capsule (see Figure 2-1). Advantages of gelcaps are that they are easy to swallow, release contents very quickly, can mask odors and unpleasant tastes, may enhance bioavailability of active ingredients, and are tamper resistant. Among their disadvantages are that water-soluble materials are difficult to incorporate, high sensitivity to heat and humidity means they can become degraded if kept in a warm or moist environment (such as a bathroom medicine cabinet), they cannot contain materials that will degrade their shells, they cost more to manufacture, and they may not be appropriate for people with certain dietary restrictions since the gelatin they contain is usually made from animal bones and skins.

Powder

A drug that is dried and ground into fine particles is called a **powder**. An example is potassium chloride powder (Kato powder). Powders have several advantages: they are the easiest drug form to prescribe, compound, and administer; dosages are easily adjusted; they are very stable, are rapidly dissolved and absorbed, may be mixed with various types of drinks, and have a low manufacturing cost. Disadvantages include dose inaccuracy, limited applicability for some drug types; and a possibly bitter or unpleasant taste if taken with water.

Medical Terminology Review

chloride
chlor = chlorine
ide = compound substance containing chlorine

Granule

A small pill, usually accompanied by many others most commonly encased within a gelatin capsule, is called a **granule**. In most cases, granules within capsules are specially coated to gradually release medication over a period of up to 12 hours (see Figure 2-1). Advantages of granules are the ability to control the amount of dust when compounding, ease of compressibility, high stability, ease of use in solutions, and uniformity of particle size. There are no documented disadvantages to the use of granules.

Troche or Lozenge

A hard or semisolid dosage form containing a medication intended for local application in the mouth or throat is called a **troche** or **lozenge**. These are flattened disks. Typically, a troche is placed on the tongue or between the cheek and gum and left in place until it dissolves. The medications most commonly administered by means of troches include cough suppressants and treatments for sore throat. Advantages of troches or lozenges are their ability to be quickly dissolved and absorbed. A disadvantage is that they may be perceived as candy by children, leading to overdosage.

Semisolid Drugs

Semisolid drugs are often used as topical applications. These drugs are soft and pliable. Semisolid drugs include suppositories, ointments, and gels.

Suppository

A bullet-shaped dosage form intended to be inserted into a body orifice is called a **suppository**. Suppositories contain medication usually intended for a local effect at the site of insertion. Suppositories maintain their shape at room temperature but melt or dissolve when inserted. The most common sites of administration for suppositories are the rectum, vagina, and urethra. Advantages of suppositories are their ease of use and ready absorption. Disadvantages include unpleasant side effects, allergic reactions, and differences in absorption rates among patients; children may also resist their use.

Ointment

An **ointment** is a semisolid, greasy medication intended for external application, usually by rubbing (Figure 2-2). Medications that may be administered in ointment form include anti-inflammatory drugs, topical anesthetics, and antibiotics. Examples are zinc oxide ointment and Ben-Gay® ointment. Advantages of ointments include their ability to seal in moisture effectively and ease of use. Disadvantages are side effects involving the skin, including blocked pores, and excessive greasiness.

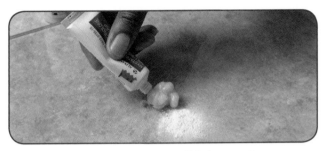

Figure 2-2 Example of a semisolid dosage form.

Cream

A **cream** is a semisolid preparation that is usually white and nongreasy; it has a water base. It is applied externally to the skin or administered via an applicator intravaginally. Advantages of creams are that they are less greasy than ointments. A disadvantage is that they do not stay on the skin as well as ointments.

Gel

A **gel** is a jelly-like substance that may be used for topical medication. Some gels have a high alcohol content and can cause stinging if applied to broken skin. Advantages of gels are that they are nongreasy, may be rubbed in quickly, and may produce a cooling sensation. Gels have no significant disadvantages.

Liquid Drugs

Liquid preparations include drugs that have been dissolved or suspended. Examples of liquid drugs are syrups, spirits, elixirs, tinctures, fluidextracts, liniments, emulsions, solutions, mixtures, suspensions, aromatic waters, sprays, and aerosols (Figure 2-3). They are also classified by site or route of administration, such as local (topical) on or through the skin, through the mouth, through the eye (ophthalmic), through the ear (otic), or through the rectum, urethra, or vagina. Liquid drugs may also be administered systemically by mouth or by injection throughout the body.

Syrup

A drug dosage form that consists of a high concentration of a sugar in water is called a **syrup**. It may or may not have medicinal substances added (e.g., simple syrup, ipecac syrup). An advantage of syrups is their quick absorption. Disadvantages include strong or unpleasant taste and a high sugar content, which may not be appropriate for all patients.

Solution

A **solution** is a drug or drugs dissolved in an appropriate solvent. An example of a solution is normal saline, which is salt (sodium chloride) dissolved in water. Advantages of solutions are their quick absorption, dosing

Key Concept

Liquid drugs are very popular for use in children because other oral forms, such as tablets and capsules, are harder to swallow. Children have far less difficulty in taking liquid drugs.

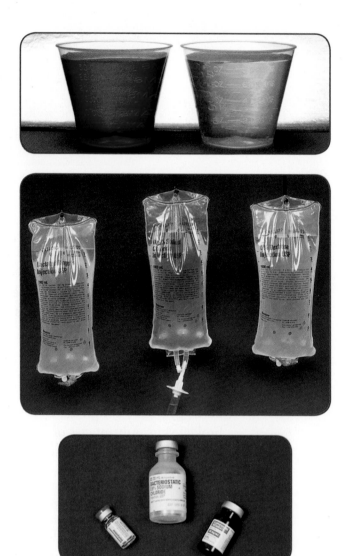

Figure 2-3 Examples of liquid dosage forms.

flexibility, utility with multiple administration routes, good dispersion of particles throughout, and ease in swallowing. Disadvantages include dosing inaccuracy, instability, strong or unpleasant taste, difficulties in transporting without breakage, variances in solubility, and the need for measuring devices when preparing or administering this drug form.

Spirit

An alcohol-containing liquid that may be used pharmaceutically as a solvent is called a **spirit**. It is also known as an essence (e.g., essence of peppermint, camphor spirit). An advantage of spirits is their ability to dissolve substances that are less soluble in water. A disadvantage is their contraindication in certain patients, such as alcoholics.

Elixir

A drug vehicle that consists of water, alcohol, and sugar is known as an **elixir**. It may or may not be aromatic and may or may not have active medicinal properties. The alcohol content of elixirs makes them convenient liquid dosage forms for many drugs that are only slightly soluble in water. In these cases, the drug is first dissolved in alcohol, and then the other elixir components are added. All elixirs contain alcohol (e.g., terpin hydrate elixir, phenobarbital elixir). Elixirs differ from tinctures in that they are sweetened. They should be used with caution in patients with diabetes or a history of alcohol abuse.

Tincture

A **tincture** is an alcoholic preparation of a soluble drug, usually from plant sources. In some cases, the solution may also contain water (e.g., iodine tincture, digitalis tincture). An advantage of tinctures is their ability to dissolve substances that are less soluble in water. A disadvantage is that the alcohol content may denature medicinal ingredients.

Fluidextract

A concentrated solution of a drug removed from a plant source by mixing ground parts of the plant with a suitable solvent, usually alcohol, and then separating the plant residue from the solvent is called a **fluidextract**. Typically, 1 mL (1 cc) contains 1 g of the drug. Fluidextracts are not intended to be administered directly to a patient. Instead, they are used to provide a source of drug in the manufacture of final dosage forms. Only vegetable drugs are used (e.g., glycyrrhiza fluidextract). An advantage is that fluidextracts are highly concentrated. A disadvantage is that they may be too strong for certain patients.

Liniment

A **liniment** is a mixture of drugs with oil, soap, water, or alcohol, that is intended for external application by rubbing. Most liniments are counterirritants intended to treat muscle or joint pain (e.g., camphor liniment, chloroform liniment). Advantages are that liniments are less viscous than ointments or creams and they contain counterirritant components. A disadvantage is that they cannot be used on broken skin.

Emulsion

A pharmaceutical preparation containing two agents that cannot ordinarily be combined or mixed is called an **emulsion**. In the typical emulsion, oil is dispersed inside water; however, water can also be dispersed inside oil. Most creams and lotions are emulsions (e.g., Petrogalar Plain®). An advantage is that emulsions may be used in many different dosage forms. Disadvantages include their lack of stability and sometimes short shelf life.

Mixtures and Suspensions

In a **mixture** or a **suspension**, an agent is mixed with a liquid but not dissolved. These preparations must be shaken before the patient takes them.

An example is Milk of Magnesia®. Advantages of this dosage form are the ability to mask unpleasant tastes, utility for medicines with low solubility, better control on rate of drug availability, and may have prolonged drug action. Disadvantages include lack of stability, the need to shake well before every use, and potentially short shelf life.

Aromatic Water

In pharmacy, a mixture of distilled water with an aromatic volatile oil is called an **aromatic water**. Aromatic waters may be used for medicinal purposes (e.g., peppermint water, camphor water). An advantage is their utility for a wide variety of conditions in patients of all ages. Among their disadvantages are the possibility that they may contain synthetic or adulterated ingredients, or alcohol.

Gaseous Drugs

Pharmaceutical gases include the anesthetic gases such as nitrous oxide and halothane. Compressed gases include oxygen for therapy (Figure 2-4) or carbon dioxide. Advantages of gaseous forms are targeted drug action and quickness of drug effects. Disadvantages include volatility and potential for overdosage.

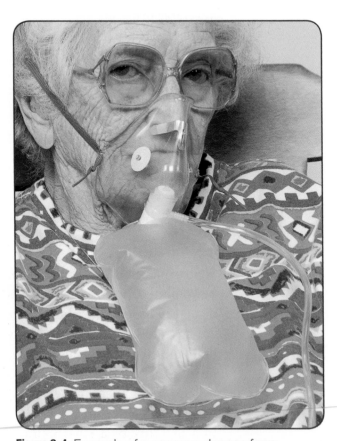

Figure 2-4 Example of a gaseous dosage form.

SUMMARY

A single drug may have up to three names: chemical, generic, and trade. There is only one chemical name and one generic name for each drug, whereas a drug may have several trade names, with similar ingredients in each marketed drug product.

Drug sources may include plants, animals (including humans), minerals, synthetics (chemical substances), and engineered drugs (investigational drugs). Drug dosage forms are classified according to their physical state and chemical composition. They may include solids, semisolids, liquids, and gases. Some substances may change from solid to liquid states (melting) or from liquid to gaseous states (vaporization). Certain drugs are water soluble, some are soluble in alcohol, and others are soluble in a mixture of liquids.

EXPLORING THE WEB

Visit **www.fda.gov**

- Search using the phrase *dosage form definitions*. Review information that outlines the characteristics of the dosage forms.

- Search for the various drug sources and review information related to the drugs derived from those sources.

Visit **www.ismp.org**

- Click on "Tools" and review information listed under the link "Medication Safety Tools and Resources." Discover the common types of errors that can occur with drugs and what strategies can be used to avoid them.

Visit **www.mapharm.com**

- Click on "Types of Drugs" and then "Medical Drug Sources." What additional information can you find here on the various forms of medications available?

REVIEW QUESTIONS

Multiple Choice

1. Which of the following is an important cardiac glycoside?

   A. nicotine

   B. digoxin

   C. morphine sulfate

   D. atropine sulfate

2. Tablets are often mistakenly called:

   A. pills

   B. powders

   C. buffered

   D. gelcaps

3. Which of the following is an example of a semi-solid drug?

   A. caplet

   B. gelcap

   C. gel

   D. granule

4. Which of the following is an example of a plant drug source?

   A. insulin

   B. pepsin

   C. meperidine

   D. morphine

5. Any composition of a liquid and a powder that hardens when it dries is called a:

   A. capsule

   B. plaster

   C. gelcap

   D. granule

6. Which of the following is an example of spirits?

   A. phenobarbital liquids

   B. peppermint and camphor liquids

   C. iodine and digitalis liquids

   D. Milk of Magnesia®

7. A preparation that can be used rectally is called a:

   A. powder

   B. gel

   C. pill

   D. suppository

8. A solution containing alcohol is called a(n):

   A. emulsion

   B. solution

   C. syrup

   D. elixir

9. A small, disk-shaped medication, which is composed of a solidifying paste and used for local treatment is called a(n):

   A. lozenge

   B. liniment

   C. ointment

   D. gelcap

10. Nicotine, morphine sulfate, and atropine sulfate are examples of which of the following types of compounds?

    A. engineered sources (investigational drugs)

    B. animal or human sources

    C. plant sources

    D. synthetic sources

11. Which of the following is an advantage of generic drugs over equivalent trade-name drugs?

    A. less toxic

    B. absorbed more slowly

    C. taste better

    D. cheaper

12. A dry mass of minute separate particles of any substance is called a:

    A. powder

    B. plaster

    C. pill

    D. granule

13. An example of a drug that is available in a plaster form is:

    A. potassium chloride

    B. zinc oxide

    C. glycyrrhiza

    D. salicylic acid

14. A disadvantage of a suppository is:

    A. an unpleasant feeling

    B. its varied absorption rate

    C. potential for overdosage

    D. its cooling sensation

15. An example of a drug that comes from an animal source is:

    A. meperidine

    B. morphine

    C. digitalis

    D. insulin

Matching

_____ 1. Not intended to be administered directly to a patient

_____ 2. A bullet-shaped dosage form intended to be inserted into a body orifice

_____ 3. A drug or drugs dissolved in an appropriate solvent

_____ 4. Can prevent ulceration or severe irritation of the stomach wall

_____ 5. An alcoholic preparation of a soluble drug, usually from plant sources

_____ 6. A semisolid, greasy medication intended for external application, usually by rubbing

_____ 7. Placed between the cheek and the gum until dissolved

_____ 8. A mixture of distilled water with a volatile oil

_____ 9. Shells usually made of hard cylindrical gelatin

_____ 10. Most creams and lotions

A. emulsion

B. aromatic water

C. ointment

D. buccal tablet

E. buffered tablet

F. tincture

G. capsule

H. solution

I. suppository

J. fluidextract

Critical Thinking

A pharmacist decides to switch from a trade-name drug that was ordered by a physician to a generic-equivalent drug instead.

1. What advantages does this substitution have for the patient?

2. What disadvantages might the switch cause?

3. What must the pharmacist do before switching from a trade-name drug to a generic-equivalent drug?

Biopharmaceutics

OBJECTIVES

After completing this chapter, the reader should be able to:

1. Describe the mechanisms of drug action and define pharmacokinetics and pharmacodynamics.
2. Explain the importance of the first-pass effect.
3. Explain the significance of the blood-brain barrier to drug therapy.
4. Identify the major processes by which drugs are eliminated from the body.
5. Describe the process of filtration, secretion, and reabsorption for renal excretion of drugs.
6. Describe factors affecting drug action.
7. Explain how rate of elimination and plasma half-life ($t_{1/2}$) are related to the duration of drug action.
8. Define idiosyncratic and anaphylactic reactions.

GLOSSARY

Absorption – the movement of a drug from its site of administration into the bloodstream

Active transport – a process that moves particles in fluid through membranes from a region of lower concentration to a region of high concentration

Agonist – a drug that produces a functional change in a cell

Anaphylactic reaction – a severe, life-threatening allergic reaction to a drug

Antagonist – a drug that blocks a functional change in the cell

Antimetabolite – a substance produced during drug metabolism, altering the actions of liver enzymes

Bioavailability – measurement of the rate of absorption and total amount of drug that reaches the systemic circulation

Biotransformation –conversion of a drug within the body; also known as *metabolism*

Diffusion – the process in which particles in a fluid move from an area of higher concentration to an area of lower concentration, resulting in an even distribution of the particles in the fluid

Dose-effect relationship – the relationship between drug dose and blood (or other biological fluid) concentrations

Drug clearance – elimination rate over time divided by the drug's concentration

Excretion – the process whereby waste products of metabolism are eliminated, material is removed to regulate composition of body fluids and tissues, or substances are expelled; in pharmacokinetics, the final step in which the drug is removed from the body

Filtration – in the kidney, the movement of water and dissolved substances from the glomerulus to the Bowman's capsule

First-pass effect – the process of partial metabolism that occurs when a drug reaches the liver, which reduces its concentration before being sent to the body

Glomerular filtration rate (GFR) – the rate of filtration in the kidneys

Half-life – the time it takes for the plasma concentration (e.g., of a drug) to be reduced by 50%

Hepatic portal circulation – the circulation of blood through the liver

Idiosyncratic reaction – experience of a unique, strange, or unpredicted reaction to a drug

Lipid solubility – the ability to dissolve in a fatty medium

Metabolism – the conversion of a drug within the body; also known as *biotransformation*

Passive transport – the most common and important mode of traversal of drugs through membranes; diffusion

Pharmacodynamics – the study of the biochemical and physiological effects of drugs

Pharmacokinetics – the study of the absorption, distribution, metabolism, and excretion of drugs; these processes are abbreviated as "ADME"

Placebo – an inert substance given to a patient instead of an active medication; often in the form of a sugar pill or sterile water

Reabsorption – in the kidney, the movement of water and selected substances from the tubules to the peritubular capillaries

Target sites – the areas where a drug's greatest action takes place at the cellular level

Tolerance – reduced responsiveness of a drug because of adaptation to it

Tubular secretion – in the kidney, the active secretion of substances such as potassium from the peritubular capillaries into the tubules

OVERVIEW

Drugs differ widely in their biochemical and physiological properties, as well as their mechanisms of action. In clinical applications, a drug must be absorbed, transported to the target tissue or organ, and then it must penetrate into the cell membranes, their organelles, and alter the ongoing processes. The drug may be distributed to a number of tissues, bound or stored, then metabolized to inactive or active products. Then it must be excreted. The usual route of drug administration, distribution, and elimination are factors in the effectiveness of a drug's ability to produce a desired outcome. The principles explaining the manner in which drugs act within the body are explained in this chapter.

PHARMACOKINETICS

Pharmacokinetics is the study of the action and movement of drugs within the body, including the mechanisms of absorption, distribution, metabolism, and excretion of drugs. These mechanisms are also collectively referred to under the acronym "ADME." It defines the processes by which the body ingests a drug, breaks down the drug, distributes it throughout the body, uses it, and then excretes the waste products of the drug. This may be simplified by the definition "drug concentration in the blood or plasma over time."

Drug Absorption

The movement of a drug from its site of administration into the bloodstream is **absorption**. In most cases, this is the first step the body takes to begin processing a drug. For absorption to occur, a drug must be transported across one or more biological membranes to reach the blood circulation. This process can take place via passive (diffusion) or active transport. Drugs given intravenously go directly into the blood, thus bypassing absorption to allow an almost immediate effect.

Passive Transport

The most common and important mode of traversal of drugs through membranes is **passive transport** or diffusion. **Diffusion** is the process in

Medical Terminology Review

pharmacokinetics
pharmac/o = drugs, medicine
-kinet- = movement
-ic = pertaining to
the movement of drugs through the body

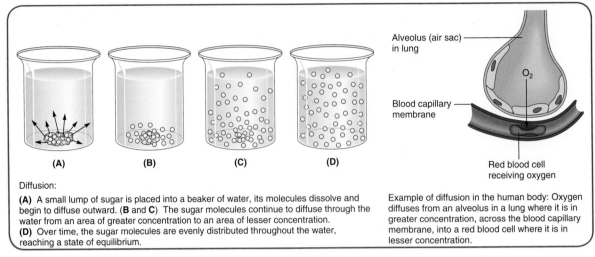

Diffusion:

(A) A small lump of sugar is placed into a beaker of water, its molecules dissolve and begin to diffuse outward. **(B** and **C)** The sugar molecules continue to diffuse through the water from an area of greater concentration to an area of lesser concentration. **(D)** Over time, the sugar molecules are evenly distributed throughout the water, reaching a state of equilibrium.

Example of diffusion in the human body: Oxygen diffuses from an alveolus in a lung where it is in greater concentration, across the blood capillary membrane, into a red blood cell where it is in lesser concentration.

Figure 3-1 The process of diffusion.

which particles in a fluid move from an area of higher concentration to an area of lower concentration, resulting in an even distribution of the particles in the fluid (Figure 3-1). This mechanism requires little or no energy. In the body, diffusion depends upon **lipid solubility** (ability to be dissolved in a fatty substance) of the drug. Cell membranes consist of a fatty bi-layer through which drugs must pass for diffusion to occur. Agents that are relatively lipid soluble diffuse more rapidly than less lipid-soluble drugs.

Active Transport

Active transport is a process that moves particles in fluid through membranes from a region of lower concentration to a region of high concentration. It uses specific carrier molecules (proteins) in the cell membranes and requires energy (Figure 3-2).

Absorption of Medications Through the Digestive System

Oral administration of drugs is the most convenient, economical, and common route of administration. Absorption of most drugs administered orally takes place through the digestive system. Drugs given orally are usually absorbed across the stomach or upper intestinal wall and enter blood vessels of the **hepatic portal circulation** (Figure 3-3). The **hepatic portal circulation** carries blood directly to the liver, where it is exposed to metabolism by the liver enzymes before reaching the systemic circulation. This exposure is called the **first-pass effect**; thus, upon reaching the liver the drug undergoes partial metabolism before being sent to the body, where it has systemic effects. Drugs that are administered parenterally or sublingually do not undergo a first-pass effect. Therefore, parenteral medications are often given in lower doses than those given orally.

Key Concept

In the stomach, a water-soluble drug will be dissolved well, but a lipid-soluble drug will be absorbed even better. Therefore, drugs are usually formulated as weak acids or weak bases so that they readily dissolve and are absorbed. For example, potassium penicillin and morphine sulfate are drugs formulated as salts, so that they dissolve and are absorbed easily.

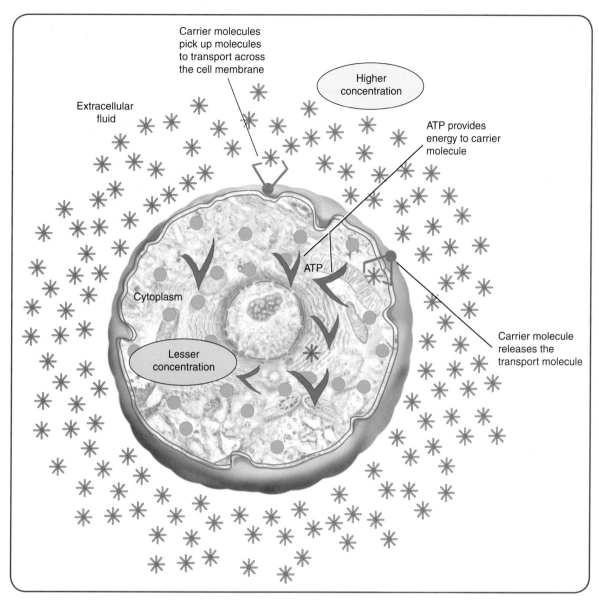

Figure 3-2 Active transport moves molecules from a lesser concentration area to a higher concentration area.

Factors Influencing Absorption

There are many factors that may alter the rate of absorption of drugs into the body. Such factors to consider are the acidity of the stomach, presence of food in the stomach, dosage of drugs, bioavailability, and the routes of administration.

Acidity of the Stomach

Drugs with an acidic pH, such as aspirin, are easily absorbed in the acid environment of the stomach, whereas alkaline medications are more readily absorbed in the alkaline environment of the small intestine. Milk products

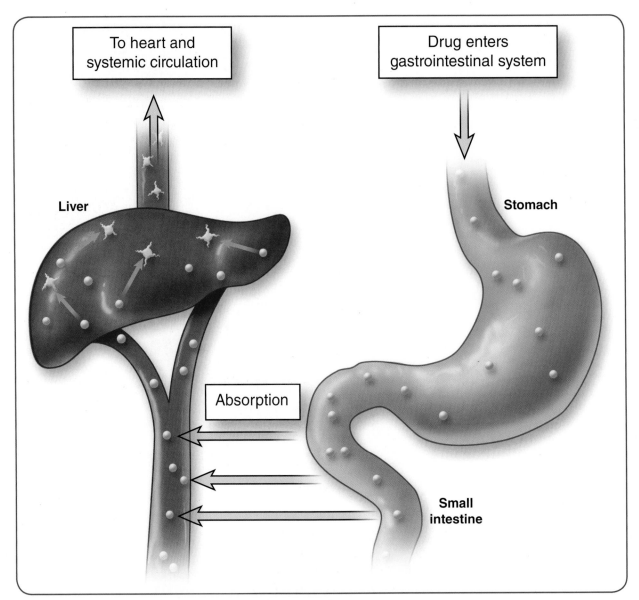

Figure 3-3 First-pass effect. Drugs are absorbed from the small intestine into the portal vein. From the portal vein, the drugs travel to the liver where they are metabolized into inactive forms. The drugs then leave the liver to be distributed through general circulation.

and antacids tend to change the pH of the stomach. Therefore, some drugs are not absorbed properly. The infant who is taking formula or milk may need to take medications on an empty stomach because the regular feedings will change the stomach acid level.

Presence of Food in the Stomach

The presence of food in the stomach or intestine can have a profound influence on the rate and extent of drug absorption. Food in the stomach decreases the absorption rate of medications, while an empty stomach increases the rate. Sometimes the drug must be put into effect quickly, requiring the stomach to be empty. If the medication causes irritation of the stomach, food should be eaten to serve as a buffer and decrease irritation.

Dosage of Drugs

Drugs administered in high concentrations tend to be more rapidly absorbed than those administered in low concentrations. The relationship between drug dose and blood (or other biological fluid) concentrations is called the **dose-effect relationship**.

Drug Bioavailability

Bioavailability is a term that indicates measurement of both the rate of drug absorption and total amount of drug that reaches the systemic blood circulation from an administered dosage form. The route of drug administration in this matter is essential. If a drug is administered by intravenous injection, all the dose enters the blood circulation. This is not true for drugs administered by other routes, especially for drugs given orally. Solid drugs such as tablets and capsules must dissolve. This is a major source of difference in drug bioavailability. Poor solubility of a drug or incomplete absorption of a drug in the gastrointestinal tract, and rapid metabolism of a drug during its first pass through the liver, are other factors that influence bioavailability.

Routes of Administration

Absorption will vary based upon the route of administration. Some oral drugs are administered sublingually (under the tongue) or buccally (inner lining of cheek); these drugs are absorbed through the mucous membranes directly into the bloodstream to protect the drug from decomposition and deterioration in the stomach or liver. Topical drugs may be absorbed through several layers of skin for local absorption. For example, nitroglycerin commonly is applied to the skin in the form of an ointment or transdermal patches; it is absorbed rapidly, and provides sustained blood levels. When the drug is injected directly into the bloodstream (vein or artery) and distributes throughout the body, it acts rapidly; the process of absorption is bypassed. The drug may be injected deeply into a skeletal muscle. The rate of absorption depends on the vascularity of the muscle site, and the lipid solubility of the drug. If it is injected beneath the skin, drug absorption is less rapid, because the subcutaneous region is less vascular than the muscle tissues.

Drug Distribution

The process by which drug molecules leave the bloodstream and enter the tissues of the body is called distribution. When a drug reaches the bloodstream, it is ready to travel through blood, lymphatics, and other fluids to its site of action. Drugs interact with specific receptors. Some drugs are frequently bound to plasma proteins (albumin) in the blood. If these drugs

---

Medical Terminology Review

sublingual
sub- = under
lingu/o = tongue
-al = pertaining to
under the tongue

buccal
bucc/o = cheek
-al = pertaining to
related to the cheek

subcutaneous
sub- = under
cutaneous = of the skin
under the skin

Key Concept

Nitroglycerin decomposes very easily and is also prone to sticking to plastic containers. Therefore, it must be stored in dark glass containers.

are bound to albumin, they are known as inactive drugs, while those that are unbound are called pharmacologically active drugs. If binding is extensive and firm, it will have a considerable impact on the distribution and excretion of the drug in the body. Only when the protein molecules release the drug can it diffuse into the tissues, interact with receptors, and produce a therapeutic effect.

The brain and placenta possess special anatomical barriers that prevent many chemicals and drugs from entering. These barriers are referred to as the blood-brain barrier and fetal-placental barrier. Drug distribution varies, based on lipid solubility and blood flow to specific tissues. The liver, heart, and kidneys are examples of organs with higher blood flow, meaning that they receive increased amounts of a drug more quickly than areas of less blood flow such as fatty, muscle, and peripheral tissues. Plasma and tissue protein binding also greatly affects drug distribution. Drugs bind to albumin, and other plasma proteins, in various amounts. When competition for these sites occurs between two drugs, there may be high concentrations of unbound, pharmacologically active drugs. An example is the use of the two antiseizure drugs phenytoin and valproic acid, in which the more pharmacologically active phenytoin may require a reduced dose.

Drug Metabolism

Drug **metabolism** is a chemical reaction in which a drug is converted into compounds, and then easily removed from the body. It occurs once the drug reaches the liver, before the drug reaches its intended site within the body. Most drugs are acted upon by one or more enzymes in the body, and are converted to metabolic derivatives during **metabolism**. The process of conversion is called **biotransformation**.

The liver is the major site of biotransformation, and its actions are classified as either phase I or phase II metabolism. In phase I metabolism, chemical reactions occur that result in a metabolite, which is a different molecule from a parent drug. The simpler phase II metabolism involves the conjoining of a drug or phase I metabolite with a molecule produced by the body. Examples of these molecules include glucuronides, glutathiones, and sulfates. Aspirin undergoes a phase I metabolism to salicylic acid, which is then conjugated in a phase II metabolism with a glucuronide.

Many biotransformations in the liver occur in the smooth endoplasmic reticulum of the hepatocytes. Cytochrome P-450 enzymes are the major drug-metabolizing enzymes and are present in the highest concentrations in the liver and intestines. There are more than 50 cytochrome P-450 enzymes, but only six are significantly related to drug-drug interactions. The type most commonly involved in these reactions is called *CYP3A4*. Drugs that induce production of more enzyme are called inducers. They act to decrease the effect of the substrate drug, which is the drug metabolized by the enzyme.

Medical Terminology Review

lymphatic
lymph/o = lymph
-ic = pertaining to related to the lymph

Key Concept

Sedatives, antianxiety drugs, and anticonvulsants readily cross the blood-brain barrier to produce their actions on the central nervous system.

Alcohol, cocaine, caffeine, nicotine, and certain prescription drugs easily cross the placental barrier and can potentially harm the fetus.

People with low enzyme activity levels cannot metabolize drugs as efficiently as others. This condition is often inherited.

Liver enzymes react with drugs, creating metabolites. The majority of these metabolites are inactive and toxic. The two major pathways of drug elimination are metabolism by liver enzymes and excretion by the kidneys. Drug metabolism influences drug action, such as duration of drug action, drug interactions, drug activation, and toxicity or side effects. In most cases, biotransformation can terminate the pharmacological action of the drug and increase removal of the drug from the body. Drugs that are water soluble are most easily excreted, and these include both ionized and hydrophilic drugs.

Drug Excretion

The final step of pharmacokinetics is **excretion**, which is the removal of drugs from the body. Drugs may be excreted from the body by many routes, including urine, feces (unabsorbed drugs, and those secreted in the bile), saliva, sweat, breast milk, lungs (alcohols and anesthetics), and tears. Any route may be important for a given drug, but the kidney is the major site of excretion for most drugs. Unchanged drugs or drug metabolites can be eliminated by the kidneys, which are the most important organs for drug excretion. The main role of the kidney is to remove all foreign and harmful agents in the bloodstream while keeping a balance of other natural substances. Kidney impairment can significantly prolong drug action and cause drug toxicity. Renal excretion of drugs and their metabolites may undergo three processes: (1) filtration, (2) secretion, and (3) reabsorption.

Drug Filtration

Urine formation begins in the glomerulus and Bowman's capsule in the kidneys. **Filtration** causes water and dissolved substances to move from the glomerulus into Bowman's capsule. Filtration occurs when the pressure on one side of a membrane is greater than the pressure on the opposite side. Small substances such as water, sodium, potassium, chloride, glucose, uric acid, and creatinine move through the wall of the glomerulus very easily. These substances are filtered in proportion to their plasma concentration.

In other words, if the concentration of a particular substance or drug in the plasma is high, many of these substances are filtered (Figure 3-4). Approximately one-fifth of the plasma reaching the kidney is filtered. The rate of filtration is referred to as the **glomerular filtration rate (GFR)** and is normally 125 to 130 milliliters per minute (mL/min). Together, glomerular filtration and tubular secretion remove drugs from the body. Drugs such as nonsteroidal anti-inflammatory drugs can reduce the glomerular filtration rate, slowing drug excretion via the kidneys. In elderly people, after age 70, approximately 30% of the nephrons are reduced because of exposure to various drugs and chemical substances. Therefore, it is very important that

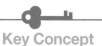

Medical Terminology Review

hepatocyte
hepat/o = liver
-cyt = cell
liver cell

Key Concept

Patients with liver disease may require lower dosages of a drug, or a drug that does not undergo biotransformation in the liver.

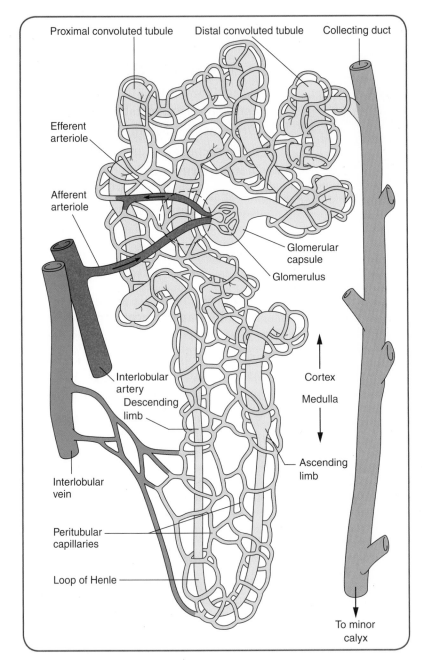

Proximal convoluted tubule

Distal convoluted tubule

Collecting duct

Efferent arteriole

Afferent arteriole

Glomerular capsule

Glomerulus

Interlobular artery

Descending limb

Cortex

Medulla

Ascending limb

Interlobular vein

Peritubular capillaries

Loop of Henle

To minor calyx

Figure 3-4 Structure of a nephron.

elderly people receive appropriate dosage of drugs since their filtration rate is less, and toxicity is more common.

Drug Secretion

Although most of the water and dissolved substances enter the tubules of the kidneys as a result of filtration across the glomerulus, a second process moves very small amounts of substances from the blood into the tubules. This is called **tubular secretion**. It involves the active secretion of substances such as potassium ions (K^+), hydrogen ions (H^+), uric acid, the ammonium ion, and drugs from the peritubular capillaries into the tubules. Secretion occurs primarily in the proximal convoluted tubule (see Figure 3-4). This is an active process mediated by two carrier systems, one specific for organic acids and one specific for organic bases.

Therefore, the pH of the urine may affect the rate of drug excretion by changing the chemical form of a drug to one that can be more readily excreted or to one that can be reabsorbed. Penicillins or barbiturates are weak acids, and available as sodium or potassium salts. These agents can be better excreted if the urine pH is less acidic. Also, drugs can compete with each other for secretion. For example, when a patient who takes probenecid to manage gout is given oral penicillin for an infection, the probenecid competes with the penicillin, causing more penicillin to be retained in the body.

Conversely, any drug that is available as sulfate, hydrochloride, or nitrate salts, such as atropine or morphine, can be better excreted if the urine is more acidic. By altering the pH of urine, increased elimination of certain drugs can be facilitated, thus preventing prolonged action or overdosage of a toxic compound. Another technique to alter the rate of excretion of a drug is to produce a competitively blocking effect. Thus, as in the earlier example, probenecid may be used to block the renal excretion of penicillin. This prolongs the effect of the antibiotic by maintaining a higher therapeutic plasma level. Secretions of drugs are active transport systems. They require energy and may become saturated.

Drug Reabsorption

Reabsorption may occur throughout the tubules of the nephrons (see Figure 3-4). It causes water and selected substances to move from the tubules into the peritubular capillaries. The mechanism is passive diffusion; therefore, only the non-ionized form of a drug is reabsorbed. Reabsorption of the drug is dependent on its lipid solubility, with non-ionized and lipophilic drugs being reabsorbed from the glomerular filtrate back into the blood. Conversely, ionized and hypophilic drugs are not reabsorbed, and are subsequently excreted.

The kidneys selectively reabsorb substances such as glucose, proteins, and sodium, which they have already secreted into the renal tubules. These reabsorbed substances return to the blood. Tubular reabsorption, therefore, prevents certain drugs from being excreted into the urine. Drug reabsorption is also affected by cellular transporters and the pH of the urine.

DRUG CLEARANCE

Drug clearance describes drug elimination (excretion plus metabolism). It is defined as elimination rate over time divided by the drug's concentration. Drug clearance can also be described as being equal to the volume of fluid completely cleared of a drug per a unit of time. It is usually expressed in milliliters per minute (mL/min) or liters per hour (L/hour). Plasma clearance divided by blood clearance equals blood concentration divided by plasma concentration. Total clearance equals the sum of clearances of individual body processes. The eliminated drug amount is proportional to the clearance of the respective elimination process. Drug clearance can be altered by changing urine pH, with weakly acidic drugs being more ionized when the urine is alkaline. For example, if a patient has taken an overdose of aspirin, sodium bicarbonate is given intravenously to alkalinize the urine. This means that the aspirin, a weak acid, will remain ionized so that it cannot be reabsorbed. Its toxic levels are then reduced.

PHARMACODYNAMICS

Pharmacodynamics is the study of the biochemical and physiological effects of drugs. It is also defined as the study of a drug's mechanism of action. After administration, most drugs enter the blood circulation, and expose almost all body tissues to their possible effects. All drugs produce more than one effect in the body. The primary effect of a drug is the desired or therapeutic effect. Secondary effects are all other effects, whether desirable or undesirable (causing harmful effects), produced by the drug. Most drugs have an affinity for certain organs or tissues and exert their greatest action at the cellular level in those specific areas, which are called **target sites**.

Most often, there are links between pharmacokinetics and pharmacodynamics that demonstrate the relationship between drug dose and blood (or other biological fluid) concentration. The pharmacological response by itself does not provide information about some very important determinants of that response; for example, dose, and drug concentration in plasma or at the site of action. Pharmacokinetic and pharmacodynamics can determine the dose-effect relationship (Figure 3-5).

DRUG ACTION

Drugs produce their effects by altering the normal function of the cells and tissues of the body. They do not create new cellular functions. Instead, they change existing cellular functions. Drug action is generally described relative to a physiological state that was in existence when a drug was administered. Some drugs accumulate in specific tissues because they have an affinity for a tissue component. The most common way that drugs exert their action is by forming chemical bonds with certain receptors in the body. This usually occurs only if the drug and its receptor have a compatible chemical shape. Drugs with molecules that fit precisely into a given receptor elicit a comparable drug response and are known as **agonists**. Those that do not fit perfectly produce only a weak response or no response at all (Figure 3-6).

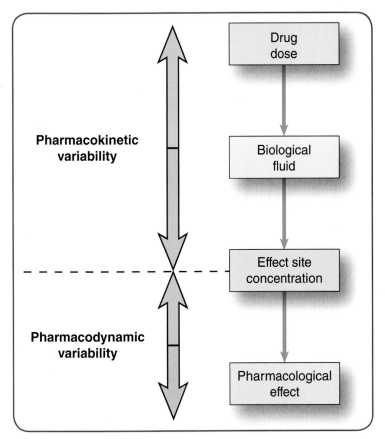

Figure 3-5 The dose-effect relationship.

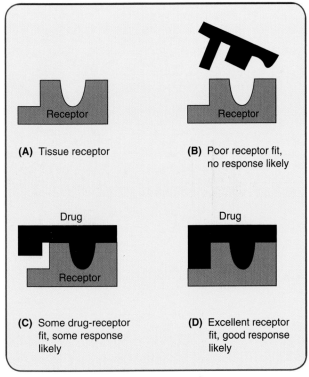

Figure 3-6 Drug-receptor interaction. Binding with specific receptors occurs only when the drug and its receptors have a compatible chemical shape.

Not all drugs that bind to specific cells cause a functional change in the cell. These drugs act as **antagonists** to the natural process and work by blocking a sequence of biochemical events.

Some drugs may act by affecting the enzyme functions of the body. When drugs are metabolized in the liver, they produce **antimetabolites**. These antimetabolites interrupt or inhibit the actions of particular enzymes, thus enabling a desired therapeutic effect to occur.

Factors Affecting Drug Action

There are various factors that are important in determining the correct drugs for a patient, such as drug half-life, age, sex, body weight, time of day administered (e.g., a.m. or p.m.) presence of illnesses, psychological factors, tolerance, toxicity of drugs, idiosyncratic reactions, and drug interactions.

Drug Half-Life

The **half-life** of a drug is a related measurement used to ensure that maximum therapeutic dosages are given. The half-life of a drug is the time it takes for the concentration of the drug in plasma to be reduced by one-half (50%). It is an indication of how long a medication will produce its effect in the body. The larger the half-life value, the longer it takes for a drug to be eliminated. This is one of the most common methods used to explain drug actions. The half-life of each drug may be different: for example, a drug with a short half-life, such as 2 or 3 hours, will need to be administered more often than one with a long half-life, such as 8 hours. Another method of describing drug action is by the use of graphic depiction of the plasma concentration of the drug versus time (Figure 3-7).

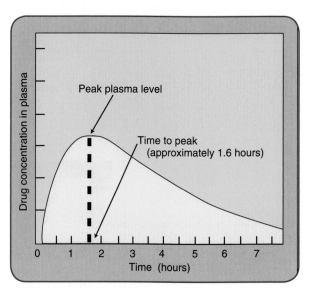

Figure 3-7 Plot of drug concentration in plasma versus time after single oral administration of a drug.

Age

Newborns and elderly individuals show the greatest effects of a drug's actions. Because of their ages and either immature or impaired body systems, they are more sensitive to medications that affect the central nervous system and are at risk for developing toxic drug levels. Calculations of drug dosages for these two groups must be carefully measured, and treatment usually starts with very small doses. These factors are discussed in greater depth in Chapter 26 (pediatrics) and Chapter 27 (geriatrics).

Sex

Men and women respond to drugs differently. Men absorb intramuscular drugs more quickly than women. These drugs remain in women's tissues longer because of their higher body fat content. Women and men differ in the way they are affected by other types of drugs as well.

A pregnant woman is at risk when taking some medications because of their ability to damage the developing fetus. In addition, certain drugs may have side effects that can stimulate uterine contractions, causing premature labor and delivery. The effects of drugs on pregnant and lactating women are addressed more thoroughly in Chapter 25.

Body Weight

Basically, the same dosage has less effect on an individual who weighs more than the normal range for his or her height, and a greater effect on one who weighs less. This is because body weight is an important factor for drug action, and some medication doses must be adjusted based on body weight. Pediatric medications are designed for the body weight or body surface of children. If adult medications are used for children, the correct dosage must be calculated and adjusted for the child's body weight.

Diurnal Body Rhythms

Diurnal (during the day) body rhythms play an important part in the effects of some drugs, because they can affect the intensity of a person's response to a drug. For example, sedatives given in the morning will not be as effective as when administered before bedtime. On the other hand, corticosteroid administration is preferred in the morning, because this best mimics the body's natural pattern of corticosteroid production and elimination.

Presence of Illnesses

Patients with liver or kidney disease may respond to drugs differently, because the body is not able to detoxify and excrete chemicals properly. The liver and kidneys are the major sites of elimination of chemical substances. Other illnesses that affect the physical health of the liver and kidneys must also be considered.

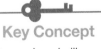

Key Concept

Acute or chronic illnesses of the liver in elderly patients may cause severe toxicity. For example, diazepam may cause coma in severely liver-damaged patients when given in average doses.

Psychological Factors

Psychological factors involve how patients feel about the drug(s) they are prescribed, and the different ways they respond to them. If an individual believes in the therapy, even a **placebo** (an inert substance given to a patient instead of an active medication, often in the form of a sugar pill or sterile water) may help to bring about relief. Some patients cooperate in following the directions for a specific drug, and a patient's mental attitude can reduce or increase an expected response to a drug.

Tolerance

Tolerance is the phenomenon of reduced responsiveness to a drug. It occurs when the body becomes so adapted to the presence of a drug that it cannot function properly without it. The only way to prevent drug tolerance from occurring is to avoid the repeated use of the drug. An increase in the amount of a drug required by the body to achieve the desired effects is a sign of drug tolerance. Certain drugs that stimulate or depress the central nervous system are prone to causing drug tolerance.

Drug Toxicity

Almost all drugs are capable of producing toxic effects. There is a range between the therapeutic dose of a drug and its toxic dose. This range is measurable by the therapeutic index, which is used to explain the safety of a drug. The therapeutic index is expressed in the form of a ratio:

$$\text{Therapeutic Index (TI)} = \frac{\text{Median lethal dose (LD}_{50})}{\text{Median effective dose (ED}_{50})}$$

The larger the difference between the two doses, the greater the therapeutic index. For example, if the therapeutic index is 3 (such as 30 mg, 10 mg), it means that three times the dose of a drug will be lethal to a patient.

Idiosyncratic Reactions

When a patient has experienced a unique, strange, or unpredicted reaction to a drug, this is termed an **idiosyncratic reaction**. Idiosyncratic reactions may be caused by underlying enzyme deficiencies from genetic or hormonal variation.

Drug Interactions

Drug interactions are defined as effects of medications taken together, which may be different from the anticipated effects of two or more drugs given separately. When two or more drugs are prescribed together, this generally results in one of the following:

1. The drugs have no effects on each other's action.

2. The drugs increase each other's effect, which can result in patient harm.

3. The drugs decrease each other's effect, which can decrease their therapeutic benefits.

Some drug interactions are beneficial and can be used therapeutically. An example is the use of a local anesthetic along with epinephrine; the local anesthetic has prolonged effects since epinephrine constricts blood vessels in the area in which it is used. Another example is the use of naloxone or other reversing agents to counteract the effects of narcotics used during surgery. A third example is the administration of probenecid with penicillin to increase the absorption of penicillin.

While most drugs do not have significant interactions with other drugs, some interactions have the potential to be life threatening. This is true because two drugs may compete for binding sites on protein molecules. Drug interactions may lead to elevated concentrations of drugs by displacement of protein-bound drugs or by reduced rates of drug disposition. This can result in toxic drug concentrations. The reverse is also true, causing two drugs to have a less-than-intended effect. In some cases, drug levels may fall more rapidly, with plasma concentrations decreasing to below minimum effective values. For example, some antibiotics make birth control pills less effective.

The term *drug interactions* includes not only interactions between drugs, but also drug-condition interactions, drug-food interactions, and drug-supplement interactions. One example of a drug-condition interaction occurs when sedatives are used in elderly people, since advanced age is a condition that increases the risk of drug interaction. Sedatives have a stronger effect in these patients, increasing their risk for falling. Another example is the need to use lower dosages of the anticoagulant warfarin, which has an increased risk of bleeding in the elderly. Older patients also require lower doses of narcotics.

Drug-food interactions occur when a drug's anticipated effect is altered by a certain food. Grapefruit juice increases the effects of some antihypertensive medications. Milk decreases absorption of antibiotics such as tetracycline and ciprofloxacin. Drug-supplement interactions include reduced absorption of thyroid supplements when taken with calcium, and increased effects of anticoagulants when taken with ginkgo biloba.

Additive Drug-Drug Interactions (DDIs) Additive drug-drug interactions occur when two drugs cause a greater effect than the effect of each of them used alone (1 + 1 = 2). A good example is the use of sleep medications combined with alcohol, which causes a much greater degree of drowsiness than either agent used alone. Another example is the use of aspirin (an antiplatelet drug) and heparin (an anticoagulant). This combination may increase the risks of bleeding. However, an additive DDI may be used therapeutically, as when two or more antihypertensives are used to lower blood pressure with more success than the single medications can do on their own.

Antagonistic Drug-Drug Interactions (DDIs) Antagonistic drug-drug interactions occur when a drug reduces or eliminates another drug's effects (1 − 1 = 0). These interactions are the basis for the use of antidotes to treat cases of poisoning. They may occur at the receptor level, which is how beta-blockers work, or in other ways. The toxic effects of acetaminophen overdose upon the liver may be treated with acetylcysteine, which eliminates the toxic metabolites of acetaminophen that actually cause the damage. Other examples of antagonistic DDIs include the reduced effect of sleep medications when taken with caffeine, and the reduced effects of anti-hypertensives when taken with a variety of herbal supplements designed for weight loss.

Synergistic Drug-Drug Interactions (DDIs) Synergistic drug-drug interactions occur when two drugs combine to produce effects that exceed either drug on its own (1 + 1 = 3). Often, two or more analgesics are used to achieve greater pain relief than is possible when a single drug is used. Other examples include the use of several antibiotics simultaneously, and the combination of aminoglycosides with penicillins to treat serious infections. However, unwanted synergistic DDIs also occur. For example, nitrates should not be used with erectile dysfunction drugs since together they may cause a potentially life-threatening drop in blood pressure.

Side Effects and Adverse Effects of Drugs

Side effects are different than adverse effects in that side effects are expected and well-known reactions to a drug that cause little or no change in treatment. Examples of side effects include nausea that is caused by chemotherapy and drowsiness that is caused by an antihistamine. An adverse effect is also known as an *adverse drug event* or *adverse drug reaction*, and is defined as any unexpected, undesired, unintended, or excessive response to a drug that results in the drug being discontinued, modified in its dosage, or replaced by another drug. Adverse effects may also cause hospitalization or increased length of hospital stays. They often require supportive treatment, complicate diagnoses, and negatively affect prognoses, and may even lead to significant patient harm, disability, or death.

Hypersensitivity or Allergy

Allergies or hypersensitivity reactions are another unpredictable reaction that some drugs such as aspirin, penicillin, or sulfa products may cause in some patients. Hypersensitivity reactions generally occur when a patient has received a drug and the body has developed antibodies against it. After this process of antibody production, if the patient is reexposed to the drug, the antigen-antibody reaction produces itching, rash, swelling of the skin, or hives (urticaria; Figure 3-8). This is a common type of allergic reaction.

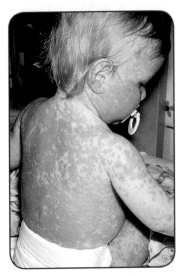

Figure 3-8 Allergic or hypersensitivity reaction to a drug.

Anaphylactic Reaction

An **anaphylactic reaction** to a drug is a severe form of allergic reaction that is life threatening. The patient develops severe shortness of breath, and may even have cardiac collapse. An anaphylactic reaction is a medical emergency because the patient may suffer paralysis of the diaphragm, swelling of the oropharynx, and an inability to breathe.

SUMMARY

A biological response is induced within a living organism when a drug is administered to that organism. This chapter reviews the study of the absorption, distribution, metabolism, and excretion (ADME) of drugs. It also reviews the study of the biochemical and physiological effects of drugs. The mechanisms of drug action depend on several factors that affect pharmaceutical, pharmacokinetic, and pharmacodynamic phases. Drug interaction is another major consideration. Multiple-drug therapy should never be employed without a convincing indication that each drug is beneficial and less harmful. In addition, drugs may induce side effects or adverse reactions. An adverse drug effect is more serious and its effect is unintended, undesirable, and often unpredictable.

EXPLORING THE WEB

Visit **www.aafp.org**

- Search using the term *drug interactions*. What common foods may interfere with the actions of some drugs? What drugs when taken together may cause adverse effects?

- Search using the term *adverse drug reactions*. What information can you find related to identifying and reducing these reactions?

Visit **www.fda.gov**

- Search using the following terms: *drug absorption, drug distribution, drug metabolism, drug excretion*. What additional information can you find to help reinforce your understanding of these concepts?

Visit **www.medscape.com**

- Click on the link "Pharmacists." Review the resources available on this page.

Visit **www.nlm.nih.gov/medlineplus**

- Become familiar with the resources and information available at this site.

REVIEW QUESTIONS

Multiple Choice

1. For action to occur, a drug must be transported to tissues or organs, penetrate cell membranes, and must be:

   A. filtered

   B. secreted

   C. absorbed

   D. therapeutic

2. The study of the action of drugs within the body is known as:

   A. metabolism

   B. pharmacokinetics

   C. pharmacology

   D. pharmacodynamics

3. The most common and important mode of traversal of drugs through membranes is:

   A. filtration

   B. transportation

   C. diffusion

   D. transaction

4. Idiosyncratic reactions may be caused by which of the following factors?

A. genetics

B. obesity

C. gender

D. age

5. The process by which drug molecules leave the bloodstream and enter the tissues of the body is called:

A. solubility

B. distribution

C. suitability

D. concentration

6. The process of converting drugs to metabolic derivatives during metabolism is known as:

A. ionization

B. binding

C. excretion

D. biotransformation

7. The major site or sites of excretion for most drugs:

A. is the spleen

B. are the sweat glands

C. is the gall bladder

D. are the kidneys

8. A second process that moves very small amounts of substances such as potassium and hydrogen from the blood into the renal tubules is known as:

A. tubular secretion

B. pH alteration

C. increased elimination

D. blocking effect

9. Which of the following is the study of the biochemical and physiological effects of drugs?

A. pathophysiology

B. pharmacology

C. pharmacodynamics

D. pharmacokinetics

10. A drug that has a specific affinity for a particular cell receptor is known as the:

A. antagonist

B. agonist

C. blocker

D. biochemical event

11. Which of the following pharmacokinetic phases may cause a major problem in patients with liver impairment?

A. excretion

B. distribution

C. absorption

D. metabolism

12. Tubular secretion occurs primarily in the:

A. proximal convoluted tubule

B. distal convoluted tubule

C. glomerulus

D. collecting duct

13. Sedatives given in the morning will not be as effective as when they are administered before bedtime. This is due to the effect of:

A. diurnal (during the day) body rhythms

B. nocturnal (during the night) body rhythms

C. corticosteroids

D. placebos

14. The phenomenon of reduced responsiveness to a drug is known as:

A. adaptation

B. toxicity

C. tolerance

D. therapeutic index

15. When a patient has experienced a unique, strange, or unpredicted reaction to a drug, this reaction is called:

A. hormonal

B. idiosyncratic

C. hypersensitive

D. biologic

Fill in the Blank

1. A mechanism whereby drugs are absorbed across the intestinal wall and enter into blood vessels known as the hepatic portal circulation is called _____.

2. The elimination rate of a drug over time divided by the drug's concentration is known as _____.

3. The study of how the body responds to drugs and natural substances is called _____.

4. The rate of filtration in the kidney is referred to as the _____.

5. Lipid-soluble drugs enter the central nervous system _____.

6. _____and elderly individuals show the greatest effects of a drug.

7. Sugar pills or sterile water that are thought to be a drug are referred to as a _____.

Critical Thinking

A 75-year-old man was diagnosed with a urinary tract infection and a high fever. After obtaining the results of a urine culture, his physician ordered intravenous (IV) gentamicin at a 2 mg/kg loading dose, followed by 3–5 mg/kg/day in divided doses. Consider the nephrotoxicity of this agent to elderly patients, and answer the following questions.

1. What formula should be used to calculate drug toxicity?

2. Since the patient is 75 years old, what must the physician consider for calculating the correct dosage?

3. Why are elderly people more susceptible to nephrotoxicity because of certain drugs?

Ordering Medications

OUTLINE

OBJECTIVES

After completing this chapter, the reader should be able to:

1. Describe the components of a prescription.
2. Explain approved as well as nonapproved abbreviations.
3. Define a verbal order and explain its disadvantages.
4. List a few examples of standard protocol.
5. Describe prescription refills and why Schedule II drugs are not allowed to be refilled.
6. Describe hospital drug charts.
7. Describe the meaning of the abbreviations "ac", "bin", "ad", "noct", and "NPO".
8. List five abbreviations that are on the "Do Not Use" list.

GLOSSARY

Inscription – the portion of a prescription that indicates the medication prescribed

Legend drug –a medication available through a written prescription from a physician or other authorized prescriber; a prescription drug

Medication administration record (MAR) – the report of drugs administered to a patient in a hospital; it becomes part of the patient's permanent record in the medical chart

Prescription – an official instruction by a physician or other authorized prescriber to use a medicine, therapy, or medical device

Refills – second or additional fillings of medical prescriptions

Signa – the portion of a prescription indicating the directions for the patient

Standard protocol – a signed set of orders to be used with specific procedures

Standing orders – standard medication orders that are used in specific circumstances, such as a certain antipyretic to be used for a child with a fever prior to being seen by a physician

Subscription – the portion of a prescription indicating the dispensing instructions to the pharmacist

Superscription – the portion of a prescription containing the R_x symbol

Verbal order – an instruction from a physician to an allied health care professional or pharmacy technician to prepare a medication order for a patient; verbal orders must be documented in writing as soon as possible after they are given

OVERVIEW

Medications are ordered by physicians and other authorized prescribers from both community and hospital pharmacies. Pharmacy technicians must be familiar with abbreviations used in medication orders, as well as the structures of prescriptions. They use drug knowledge and each patient's information to maximize the therapeutic effects of drugs, and minimize their adverse effects. Pharmacy technicians must understand the principles of drug actions for both prescription and nonprescription drugs. They should be familiar with drug references, classifications, routes, and the various drug forms. Though most prescriptions are handwritten or typed, verbal orders are also sometimes given, which must be put into writing as quickly as possible. Prescriptions should be refilled only after being approved by their prescribers. Medication orders in health care facilities will often be communicated electronically; however, some may still be transmitted on paper. The pharmacy technician must be familiar with all forms of communication related to medication orders.

COMMON ABBREVIATIONS USED IN MEDICATION ORDERS

The pharmacy technician should be familiar with common abbreviations in order to dispense prescriptions safely. Common abbreviations that are used in medication orders originate from Greek or Latin words. They are used as "shorthand" for directions in prescriptions on a daily basis. Aside from these abbreviations, there are also abbreviations that must be avoided in order to prevent medication errors. It is vital for pharmacy technicians to understand both approved and nonapproved abbreviations so that medication errors can be minimized to the greatest possible extent.

Only standard abbreviations should be used as shorthand so that they can be understood correctly by other health care professionals. Prescriptions are legal documents, and abbreviations that are misunderstood may result in lawsuits. Any abbreviation that is not universally accepted should be avoided. Appropriate abbreviations provide clarity and conciseness for prescriptions. Commonly used abbreviations found in prescriptions and medication orders are listed in Table 4-1. Abbreviations and numbering (involving incorrect use of decimals) that must be avoided are listed in Table 4-2.

TABLE 4-1	Common Abbreviations Used in Medication Orders		
Abbreviation	Meaning	Abbreviation	Meaning
aa, aā	of each	per	through or by
ac	before meals	p.m., PM	afternoon
ad	to, up to	po, PO	by mouth
ad lib	as desired	PR	through the rectum
a.m., AM	morning	prn, PRN	as needed
amt	amount	pulv, PULV	Powder
aq	water	q	Every
bid, BID	twice a day	q2h	every 2 hours
bin	twice a night	qh	every hour
c	with	qid, QID	four times a day
cap, caps	capsule	QN	every night
comp	compound	qs, qv	as much as you wish (sufficient quantity)
d	day	s	without (*sine*)
dil	dilute	sig	write on label
disp	dispense	sol	solution
elix	elixir	sos	if necessary
hr, h	hour	sp	spirits
h.s.	before sleep, at bedtime	stat	immediately
IM	intramuscular	supp	suppository
inj, INJ	inject	syr	syrup
IV	intravenous	tab	tablet
Liq	liquid	tid, TID	three times a day
mixt	mixture	top	topically
noct, noc	at night	tr, tinct	tincture
non rep	do not repeat, no refills	vo, V/O	verbal order
NPO	nothing by mouth (*nulla per os*)	×	multiplied by
oint	ointment		
pc	after meals		

TABLE 4-2	"Do Not Use" Abbreviations and Decimals
Do Not Use	**Use Instead**
U	Write out "unit"
IU	Write out "international unit"
Q.D., QD, q.d., qd	Write out "daily"
Q.O.D., QOD, q.o.d., qod	Write out "every other day"
MS, MSO_4	Write out "morphine sulfate"
Trailing zeroes such as the amount "1.0 mg"	Write "1 mg" for this amount instead
Decimals that require a leading zero when no leading zero appears, such as the amount ".1 mg"	Write "0.1 mg" for this amount instead

Key Concept

Medication errors are common causes of morbidity and preventable death. The goal of every health care facility should be to reduce medication errors to the least possible amount.

DISPENSING DRUGS

The two methods of dispensing drugs are over-the-counter (OTC) and by **prescription**. Over-the-counter drugs are available without a prescription. Pharmacy technicians should have a thorough understanding of OTC drugs. Patients generally like to make informed choices about the OTC drugs they purchase, and this requires them to have access to factual information. If used as directed on their packaging, most OTC drugs are very safe. Some OTC drugs are requested on prescriptions, but this is often for insurance reasons since some insurers require them to be listed on a prescription for reimbursement purposes.

Prescription or legend drugs require actual prescription orders from authorized and licensed health care providers, which may include physicians, dentists, and in certain states, nurse practitioners and pharmacists. A prescription drug is one that the U.S. federal government lists as dangerous, powerful, or habit forming. Prescription drugs are illegal to use except under a prescriber's order. A prescription may include compounding, dispensing, or administration instructions. Each prescription must be signed by the authorized prescriber or it cannot be filled. Prescription drugs bear the legend *"Caution: Federal Law prohibits dispensing without a prescription."* This legend is printed on each prescribed medication's label. In certain circumstances, prescriptions can be sent to a pharmacy by means of fax machines, computers, or telephone.

Verbal Orders

A **verbal order** occurs when a physician tells an allied health professional or pharmacy technician which medications to administer to a patient. It is intended for one specific patient, and describes the exact medication, its dose

Medical Terminology Review

prescription
pre- = before
script = written
-ion = action
a previously written order for various forms of treatment

and form, and the time and route of administration. Verbal orders should be avoided as much as possible, since they involve a higher chance of errors and confusion. Anyone receiving a verbal order should write it down and read it back to the prescriber. Medication names should always be spelled out to avoid confusion with sound-alike medications.

Documentation of all verbal orders must be completed as soon as possible to avoid administration errors. The written order should include the abbreviation "V/O" to indicate that it came from a verbal order. According to the law, *any order that is not documented has not been performed.* For correctness, the documentation should be signed by the prescriber as soon as possible. If there are any questions about the verbal order, you must ask for clarification from the prescriber before medications are administered, or before the order is sent to another health care professional.

Standing Orders

Standing orders are standard medication orders that are used in specific circumstances. An example of a standing order is the use of a certain antipyretic medication, such as acetaminophen, for any child with a high fever who is waiting for consultation by the physician. Similarly, a **standard protocol** involves a signed set of orders to be used with specific procedures. An example of a standard protocol is the use of an enema, laxative, or suppository before a colonoscopy. In the patient's medical record, an allied health care professional may write "standard protocol" to designate that he or she knows what the physician will have intended, and that he or she has performed the administration exactly as documented in the office's policies and procedures manual.

For a standard protocol or standing order, health care professionals should always make certain that medications used are in fact appropriate, accurate, and will not conflict with a patient's health status, age-appropriate dosage, or any known allergies. This is also true for patients being transferred to other health facilities. It must be ascertained that the patient has no health condition that would cause adverse reactions. All standing orders and standard protocols should be kept in one designated place. They must always be signed by the prescribing physician, since failure to do so may result in future legal outcomes. They must be signed by the prescribing physician. Always, immediate documentation of performance of related drug administration or procedures must be made in the medical record.

Other Medication Orders

There are a few other types of medication orders used today. Some medication orders are called "PRN orders," meaning that they are given on an as-necessary or when-needed basis, in a certain time frame. An order that is given only one time is known as a *single order*. An order for a medication that must be administered immediately is known as a *stat order*. These are very common in emergency situations.

Electronic orders utilize fax machines or computers and are transmitted by an authorized prescriber, or his or her authorized agent. They must include the authorized agent's full name and title. The fax machines or computers used to receive facsimile orders must be kept inside the pharmacy prescription area and not where the public has access to them. The sender's electronic/facsimile identification number must appear on each medication order, along with the date and time of the transmission. The pharmacy should have safeguards in place to protect all electronic orders from being accessed, modified, or otherwise changed. If anything is suspicious, incomplete, or not understood by the pharmacist, he or she should call the prescriber and confirm the electronic order over the phone.

Prescriptions

Prescriptions indicate medications required and directions for correctly using the medication and meeting patient needs. Prescriptions are made after a patient's symptoms have been evaluated by a physician or another qualified health care professional. In certain states, these include nurse practitioners and physician's assistants. Once a diagnosis has been made, a prescription is written for medications required for treatment.

A prescription pad may be used to write a prescription for the patient, identifying instructions concerning compounding, dispensing, or administration of medications. All prescriptions must be recorded in the patient's medical record. Only licensed health care professionals may sign prescriptions. However, an allied health professional or pharmacy technician may be instructed to complete the prescription form for the prescriber to sign. Ultimately, the prescriber has the responsibility of checking all information contained in the prescription for accuracy prior to signing.

Components of Prescriptions

All prescriptions must be clear, concise, and correct (Figure 4-1). The components of a prescription relate to five of the seven rights of medication administration. These include the patient's name and address *(right patient)*, generic or trade name of the drug *(right drug)*, the strength and dosage of the drug *(right dose)*, the route of administration *(right route)*, and dosage instructions or the frequency of administration *(right time)*. The other information included on a prescription includes the date it was written; the prescriber's name, office address, and signature; any refill or special labeling information; and the prescriber's license number or Drug Enforcement Administration (DEA) number.

The Latin terms used for various components of a prescription include:

- The **inscription** – the medication prescribed
- The **superscription** – the **R**$_x$ symbol
- The **subscription** – the dispensing instructions to the pharmacist
- The **signa** – the directions for the patient

Interpreting Prescriptions

Pharmacy technicians must understand how to interpret the language of prescriptions. Even a small mistake in interpreting a prescription can cause a medication error to occur. Therefore, pharmacy technicians must be sure that they understand the prescriber's handwriting and all information contained in the prescription. Following are several examples (Figures 4-2 through 4-11) that you can use to practice interpreting information included on prescriptions.

Electronic Prescriptions

Today, computer software is commonly used to create and sign prescriptions online. This is known as *electronic prescribing* or *e-prescribing*. It allows physicians, other prescribers, and pharmacies to communicate electronically regarding new prescriptions, refills, changes, cancelations, and patient compliance. The use of faxed prescriptions or printed paper prescriptions is not considered part of electronic prescribing. E-prescribing allows

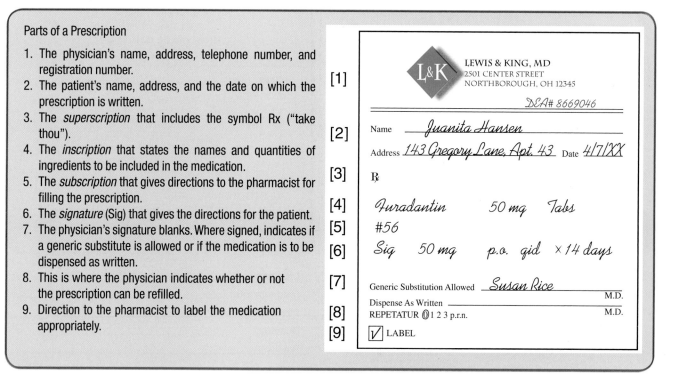

Parts of a Prescription

1. The physician's name, address, telephone number, and registration number.
2. The patient's name, address, and the date on which the prescription is written.
3. The *superscription* that includes the symbol Rx ("take thou").
4. The *inscription* that states the names and quantities of ingredients to be included in the medication.
5. The *subscription* that gives directions to the pharmacist for filling the prescription.
6. The *signature* (Sig) that gives the directions for the patient.
7. The physician's signature blanks. Where signed, indicates if a generic substitute is allowed or if the medication is to be dispensed as written.
8. This is where the physician indicates whether or not the prescription can be refilled.
9. Direction to the pharmacist to label the medication appropriately.

[1]

LEWIS & KING, MD
2501 CENTER STREET
NORTHBOROUGH, OH 12345
DEA# 8669046

[2] Name _Juanita Hansen_
Address _143 Gregory Lane, Apt. 43_ Date _4/7/XX_

[3] R

[4] _Furadantin   50 mg   Tabs_

[5] _#56_

[6] _Sig   50 mg   p.o.   qid   × 14 days_

[7] Generic Substitution Allowed _Susan Rice_
_____ M.D.
Dispense As Written _____ M.D.

[8] REPETATUR ⓪ 1 2 3 p.r.n.

[9] ☑ LABEL

Figure 4-1 Prescriptions are written legal documents that must contain specific elements.

Jane Doe M.D.
123 Suspension Road
West Palm Beach, FL, USA
DEA# AS2345678

NAME ___Zack Hefron___ DATE __0 9/08/00__
ADDRESS __Oceanview Terrace, West Palm Beach, FL__

Rx   Lipitor 20 mg

Sig: i tab po daily
        #90

SUBSTITUTION ALLOWED_____No_____
LABEL
Refill __3__.   _____D.O.
                    (signature)

Drug name: _____
Drug strength: _____
Directions (signa): _____
Quantity: _____
Refills: _____

Figure 4-2 Sample prescription. Practice your interpretation in the space provided.

Terry Jones M.D.
987 Wellness Street
Fort Lauderdale, FL, USA
DEA# AS9876543

NAME ___Julia Phelps___ DATE __0 9/08/00__
ADDRESS __120 Century Dr., Ft. Lauderdale, FL__

Rx   Glucophage XR 500 mg

Sig: ii tab po with evening meal
        #60

SUBSTITUTION ALLOWED_____No_____
LABEL
Refill __2__.   _____D.O.
DISPENSE AS WRITTEN   (signature)

Drug name: _____
Drug strength: _____
Directions (signa): _____
Quantity: _____
Refills: _____

Figure 4-3 Sample prescription. Practice your interpretation in the space provided.

Terry Jones M.D.
987 Wellness Street
Fort Lauderdale, FL, USA
DEA# AS9876543

NAME ___Joe Knapp___ DATE __0 9/08/00__
ADDRESS __1730 Bleaker St., West Palm Beach, FL__

Rx   Advair 250/50
            #1 month
Sig: i BID

SUBSTITUTION ALLOWED_____No_____
LABEL
Refill __12__.   _____D.O.
                    (signature)

Drug name: _____
Drug strength: _____
Directions (signa): _____
Quantity: _____
Refills: _____

Figure 4-4 Sample prescription. Practice your interpretation in the space provided.

John Smith M.D.
201 Tablet Lane
Melbourne, FL, 32901 USA
DEA# AS1234567

NAME ___Wendy Tubman___ DATE __0 9/08/00__
ADDRESS __42 Manatee Way, Melbourne, FL__

Rx   Nitro-DUR 0.2
            Apply 8am.
            Remove @ hs
            #30

SUBSTITUTION ALLOWED_____Yes_____
LABEL
Refill __XI__.   _____D.O.
                    (signature)

Drug name: _____
Drug strength: _____
Directions (signa): _____
Quantity: _____
Refills: _____

Figure 4-5 Sample prescription. Practice your interpretation in the space provided.

John Smith M.D.
201 Tablet Lane
Melbourne, FL, 32901 USA
DEA# AS1234567

NAME _Cathy Davis_   DATE _0 9/08/00_
ADDRESS _1616 Seabend Dr., Melbourne, FL_

Rx   _Tegretol 200 mg_
         _#210_
Sig: _tid_

SUBSTITUTION ALLOWED_____ _No_ _____
LABEL
Refill _0_ .   _____ D.O.
                    (signature)

Drug name: _____
Drug strength: _____
Directions (signa): _____
Quantity: _____
Refills: _____

Figure 4-6 Sample prescription. Practice your interpretation in the space provided.

Jane Doe M.D.
123 Suspension Road
West Palm Beach, FL USA
DEA# AS2345678

NAME _Joshua Allen_   DATE _0 9/08/00_
ADDRESS _591 Crestview Ctr., West Palm Beach, FL_

Rx   _Lamictal 100 mg_
         _#80_
Sig: _bid_

SUBSTITUTION ALLOWED_____
LABEL
Refill _0_ .   _____ D.O.
                    (signature)

Drug name: _____
Drug strength: _____
Directions (signa): _____
Quantity: _____
Refills: _____

Figure 4-7 Sample prescription. Practice your interpretation in the space provided.

Terry Jones M.D.
987 Wellness Street
Fort Lauderdale, FL, USA
DEA# AS9876543

NAME _Barbara Bruno_   DATE _0 9/08/00_
ADDRESS _23 Sea Island Rd., Ft. Lauderdale, FL_

Rx   _Aceon 4 mg_
         _#30_
Sig: _po once daily_

SUBSTITUTION ALLOWED_____ _Yes_ _____
LABEL
Refill _0_ .   _____ D.O.
                    (signature)

Drug name: _____
Drug strength: _____
Directions (signa): _____
Quantity: _____
Refills: _____

Figure 4-8 Sample prescription. Practice your interpretation in the space provided.

Jane Doe M.D.
123 Suspension Road
West Palm Beach, FL, USA
DEA# AS2345678

NAME _Matthew Sanders_   DATE _0 9/08/00_
ADDRESS _634 Lighthouse Way, West Palm Beach, FL_

Rx   _Lodine 400 mg_
         _#45_
Sig: _bid_

SUBSTITUTION ALLOWED_____ _No_ _____
LABEL
Refill _1_ .   _____ D.O.
                    (signature)

Drug name: _____
Drug strength: _____
Directions (signa): _____
Quantity: _____
Refills: _____

Figure 4-9 Sample prescription. Practice your interpretation in the space provided.

Greg Marass M.D.
69 Elizabeth Court
Palm Bay, FL, USA
DEA# AS9659493

NAME _Frances Bara_ DATE _0 9/08/00_
ADDRESS _10101 Brunette Pkwy., Palm Bay, FL_

Rx _Paracetamol 500 mg_
_#30_
Sig: _1 tab po tid_

SUBSTITUTION ALLOWED_____ _Yes_ _____
LABEL
Refill _0_ . _____D.O.
(signature)

Drug name: _____
Drug strength: _____
Directions (signa): _____
Quantity: _____
Refills: _____

Figure 4-10 Sample prescription. Practice your interpretation in the space provided.

Judy Anheir M.D.
888 Chestnut Drive
Rockledge, FL, USA
DEA# AS1928374

NAME _Etta Dyner_ DATE _0 9/08/00_
ADDRESS _210 Shatterwind Place, Rockledge, FL_

Rx _Sodium sulfacyl oint. 20%_
_10g_
Sig: _Apply to eye bid_

SUBSTITUTION ALLOWED_____ _No_ _____
LABEL
Refill _2_ . _____D.O.
(signature)

Drug name: _____
Drug strength: _____
Directions (signa): _____
Quantity: _____
Refills: _____

Figure 4-11 Sample prescription. Practice your interpretation in the space provided.

information to be shared among various health care organizations, streamlining drug formularies, medication histories, patient eligibility, and many other factors.

Approximately three out of four physicians today utilize e-prescribing, which improves safety, increases efficiency, reduces medication errors, and allows for automated drug safety checks. Prescribers can easily verify information about patient allergies, drug interactions, duplicate therapies, correct dosages, and insurance coverage (Figure 4-12). Electronic medical record or electronic health record software is able to store thousands of drug names and a variety of other information, making e-prescribing fast, accurate, and simple to use.

Prescription Safety

Prescriptions must be secured so that only authorized individuals have access to them. Forged prescriptions are a serious problem and have been implicated in many legal cases throughout history. Prescription pads are not allowed to be used for anything other than their legal purposes. They should never be left anywhere in the medical office where patients could easily remove individual prescriptions from them. Physicians should only use one prescription pad at a time, and each pad should be numbered as well as printed in colored, nonreproducible ink. Except for the single pad in use, other prescription pads should be stored in locked drawers or cabinets. When filling out a prescription, the actual amount of the medication should be written out and

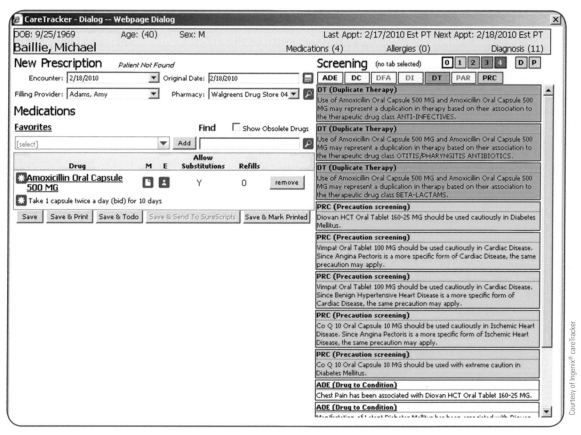

Figure 4-12 An electronic prescription software sample, showing medication information.

also expressed in numerical form. This helps to ensure that another person cannot change the amount that has been prescribed. Prescribers should never sign a prescription until actually ready to give it to the patient.

Prescription Refills

On an initial prescription of a medication, the prescriber must indicate the number of allowed **refills**, if any. Many prescription refills may be ordered from a pharmacy in writing, electronically, or over the phone. However, Schedule II medications cannot be refilled except in emergencies, and then only in 72-hour supplies. They must be followed up by a new written, signed prescription available for the pharmacy within 72 hours of emergency dispensing.

Patients may phone in refill requests to allied health personnel or pharmacy technicians. In these situations, specific information needed by the prescriber includes:

- The date and time of the phone call
- The pharmacy that will handle the refill, the correct store (if part of a chain pharmacy), and their phone number
- The desired medication, its strength, and the last time the prescription was filled
- The route of administration and instructions for the patient

- The patient's telephone number
- The signature of the allied health professional or pharmacy technician receiving the refill request

The prescriber must decide whether a refill is permitted based on the information discussed during the phone call. Pharmacists are also permitted to call with refill requests. Regardless of the person who calls, the patient's medical record must be obtained so that the prescriber can evaluate the request. Verbal orders for refills must be added into the medical record immediately. The prescriber must confirm all the patient's current prescriptions prior to the refill being phoned in to the pharmacy.

The allied health professional who takes a patient's phone call about a refill should tell the patient an *approximate time* when the request, if approved, will be phoned in to the pharmacy for dispensing. Patients should always be encouraged to call in refill requests one to two days before they will actually be needed. This 24- to 48-hour period allows the medical office enough time to notify the patient about anything concerning his or her refill request. The allied health professional or pharmacy technician handling the refill request should always verify any patient allergies and adverse reactions.

Once a prescriber approves a request, he or she may signify approval on the request form or may document the refill in the medical record. If the prescriber forgets to do this, the allied health professional who calls in the refill should document it immediately. He or she should also make sure that the related prescription(s) have been sent to the pharmacy before refiling the medical record. The refill request should be sent to the pharmacy before the end of the workday.

When a refill request is denied, the patient should be informed by the allied health professional or pharmacy technician and then given instructions about follow-up visits, or told why the prescriber denied the request. The allied health professional can also schedule an appointment if required.

For mail-order pharmacies, two prescriptions are required for refills. One is sent to a local pharmacy to order enough medication until the mail-order pharmacy can refill the entire requested amount, and the second goes to the mail-order pharmacy itself. Patients must be instructed to allow sufficient time for shipments from the mail-order pharmacy so that they do not run out of their medications.

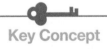

Key Concept

Pharmacy technicians must examine each prescription if there is any suspicious alteration to quantities, drug name, or strength

HOSPITAL DRUG CHARTS

In hospitals, prescription orders are usually written on drug charts or physician order forms (Figure 4-13). They are then transcribed onto a **medication administration record (MAR)**, an example of which is shown in Figure 4-14. Each MAR, which is part of a patient's medical record,

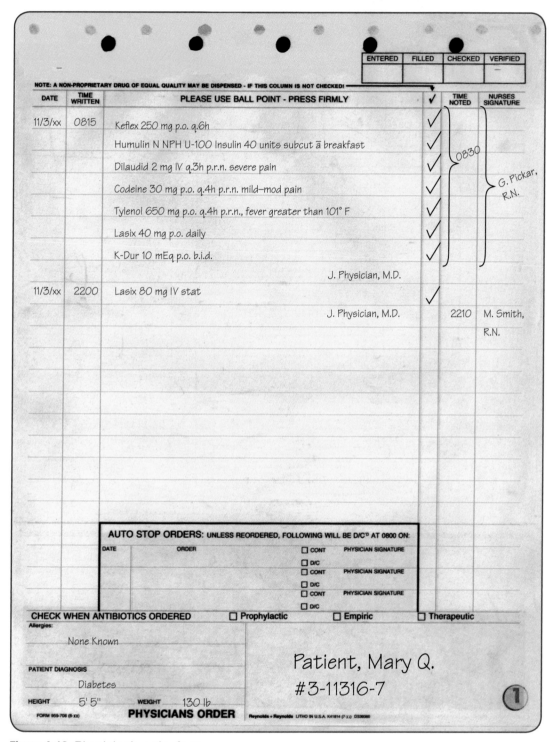

Figure 4-13 Physician's order form.

may expand to many pages. This is because hospitalized patients are often prescribed between 10 and 15 different medications during a single stay. Most hospitals now use computerized charting rather than paper charts. The MAR instructs all health professionals who enter information to do the following:

- Use approved drug names
- Avoid altering existing drug orders

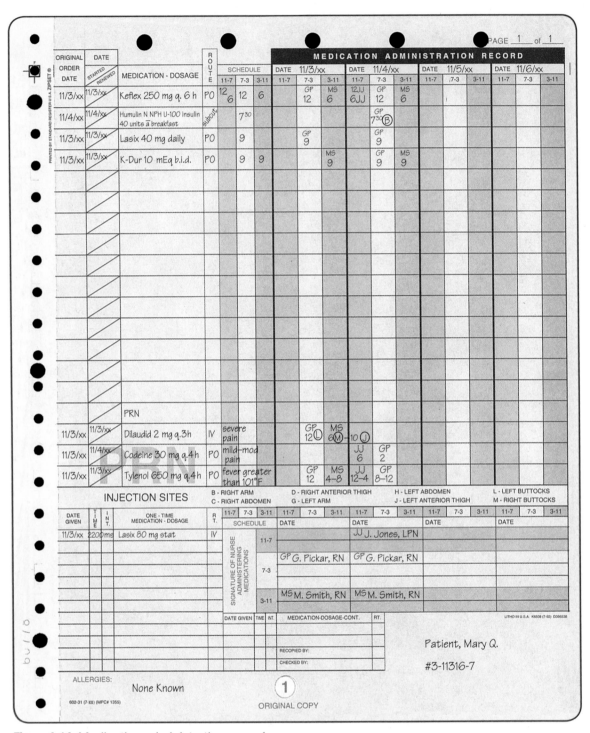

Figure 4-14 Medication administration record.

- Record all drug administrations or reasons why drugs were not administered
- Record intravenous (IV) fluid orders on a separate IV order chart
- Have any therapy initiated by nurses countersigned by the appropriate physician; such therapies may include antacids, laxatives, and mild analgesics

SUMMARY

The correct methods of ordering medications to meet patient needs help to ensure accuracy and reduce medication errors. There are literally thousands of drugs on the market, and many have the potential to interact with each other to cause patient harm or even death. Therefore, it is the goal of pharmacists and pharmacy technicians to ensure that all medication orders are correct and appropriate for each patient. Pharmacy technicians must be extremely knowledgeable about the effects of many medications so that they can effectively implement the prescriber's goals and assist the pharmacist in providing adequate patient care.

EXPLORING THE WEB

Visit **www.abbreviations.com**

- Under "Medical," click on "Prescription" to see many different abbreviations used in prescriptions, along with their definitions.

Visit **www.nccmerp.org**

- This is the official site for the National Coordinating Council for Medication
- Error Reporting and Prevention.

Visit **www.rxlist.com**

- Click on "Pill Identifier" to familiarize yourself with as many different medications as you like.

Visit **www.deadiversion.usdoj.gov**

- Click on "Registration" to read about DEA registration and DEA numbers.

REVIEW QUESTIONS

Multiple Choice

1. Verbal orders should be avoided as much as possible because they involve a higher chance of:

   A. contamination during drug dispensing

   B. infringement of patient privacy

   C. poor ethics

   D. errors and confusion

2. The dispensing instructions to the pharmacist are collectively referred to as the:

   A. subscription

   B. superscription

   C. inscription

   D. signa

3. Schedule II medications cannot be refilled except in emergencies. These refills should be supplied only for:

   A. 24 hours

   B. 48 hours

   C. 72 hours

   D. 96 hours

4. The physician's instructions on a prescription read as follows: "prn qid." This medication should be administered:

   A. every 4 hours

   B. as needed, four times per day

   C. as needed, every hour

   D. immediately every 4 hours

5. The physician ordered Zinacef® 250 mg q12h for 10 days. How many tablets should be dispensed?

   A. 10 tablets

   B. 20 tablets

   C. 30 tablets

   D. 40 tablets

6. The physician ordered Nexium® 20 mg/d PO for 8 weeks. Each tablet contains 20 mg of the medication. How many tablets should be dispensed?

   A. 16 tablets

   B. 28 tablets

   C. 36 tablets

   D. 56 tablets

7. A prescription commonly contains all of the following information, *except:*

   A. the physician's name

   B. the signa

   C. the patient's age

   D. the quantities of the ingredients

8. The physician ordered morphine sulfate 15 mg IV stat, which means:

   A. 15 mg, intravenous, as needed

   B. 15 mg, intravenous, immediately

   C. 15 mg, intravenous, as desired

   D. 15 mg, intravenous, before meals

9. The abbreviation "ac" means:

   A. before meals

   B. before bed

   C. by mouth

   D. if necessary

10. Prescription drugs are also called:

    A. over-the-counter drugs

    B. controlled substances

    C. legend drugs

    D. standard protocol

Fill in the Blank

1. The inscription signifies the _____ _____.

2. The superscription is the _____ _____.

3. The report of drugs administered to a patient in a hospital that becomes part of the patient's permanent record is called a(n) _____.

4. All _____ orders should be kept in one designated place.

5. The abbreviation "qn" means _____ _____.

Critical Thinking

A hospital pediatrician ordered ".4 mg of morphine prn" for a 4-month-old baby following surgery. The pharmacy technician dispensed "4 mg" of morphine. The pharmacist corrected the pharmacy technician's error concerning the amount of medication.

1. What was the pediatrician's error in writing the order?

2. What was the mistake of the pharmacy technician?

SECTION II

Pharmacology Related to Specific Body Systems and Disorders

CHAPTER 5

Drug Therapy for the Nervous System: Antipsychotic and Antidepressant Drugs

OUTLINE

OBJECTIVES

After completing this chapter, the reader should be able to:

1. List the main parts of the brain.

2. Describe the principal functions of the cerebrum and hypothalamus.

3. List the major chemical transmitters of the central nervous system (CNS).

4. Describe the major role of acetylcholine in the CNS.

5. Explain the role of dopamine in the brain.

6. Define schizophrenia, bipolar disorder, and depression.

7. List major groups of drugs that are used for schizophrenia.

8. Identify the drugs used for bipolar disorder.

9. List three major groups of drugs used to treat depression.

10. Describe the major adverse effects of monoamine oxidase inhibitors (MAOIs).

GLOSSARY

Acetylcholine – a neurotransmitter that plays a major role in cognitive function and memory formation as well as motor control

Anorexia nervosa – an eating disorder characterized by a psychological fear of being overweight; view of body image is distorted

Antidepressants – drugs used to treat depression

Antipsychotic drugs – the major therapeutic modality for psychotic disorders; also known as *neuroleptic drugs*

Bipolar disorder – a type of mental illness characterized by periods of extreme excitation, or mania, and deep depression.

Bulimia nervosa – an eating disorder characterized by recurrent (at least twice a week) episodes of binge eating, during which the patient consumes large amounts of food and feels unable to stop eating; then makes an effort to purge the food after the binge

Dementia – a chronic deterioration of intellectual function and other cognitive skills severe enough to interfere with the ability to perform activities of daily living

Depression – a mood disorder

Dopamine – a neurotransmitter that is naturally produced in the brain, affecting motor control, memory, attention span, the ability to problem solve, motivation, pleasure, and creative thought

Extrapyramidal – nerves in the brain that control movement

Gamma-aminobutyric acid (GABA) – a neurotransmitter distributed throughout the brain and spinal cord; now considered to be the major inhibitory neurotransmitter in the CNS, acting to modulate the activity of excitatory pathways

Glutamate – an amino acid that acts as a neurotransmitter and is a key molecule in cellular metabolism, playing an important role in the body's disposal of excess or waste nitrogen

Hallucinations – false or distorted sensory experiences that appear to be real perceptions

Mania – a severe medical condition characterized by extremely elevated mood, energy, and unusual thought patterns; a characteristic of bipolar disorder

Mental illness – any disturbance of emotional equilibrium, as manifested in maladaptive behavior and impaired functioning of behavior or personality

Monoamine oxidase inhibitor (MAOI) – a class of drug used in the treatment of depression

Neuroleptic drugs – the major therapeutic modality for psychotic disorders; also known as *antipsychotic drugs*

Neurotransmitter – a biochemical that is formed in and released from a neuron in order to stimulate or inhibit the actions of another cell

Nocturnal enuresis – nighttime bedwetting

Norepinephrine (noradrenaline) – released from the medulla of the adrenal glands, and is also a central nervous system and sympathetic nervous system neurotransmitter; regulates appetite, sleep, arousal, mood, temperature, and hormone release

Schizophrenia – a mental illness characterized by distortion of reality, disorganized thought patterns, social withdrawal, hallucinations, and poor judgment

Selective serotonin reuptake inhibitor (SSRI) – a class of drugs used as antidepressants; they block resorption of serotonin in nerve cells in the brain

Serotonin – a neurotransmitter that regulates appetite, sleep, arousal, mood, temperature, and hormone release

Serotonin syndrome – a rare condition resulting from intentional self-poisoning with serotonin, use of the drug therapeutically, or from inadvertent drug interactions characterized by progressively worsening symptoms such as mental confusion, shivering or muscle twitching, sweating or fever, hallucinations, hypertension, tachycardia, headache, tremor, nausea, diarrhea, coma, and death; also known as *serotonin toxicity*

Serotonin toxicity – same as serotonin syndrome

Tricyclic antidepressant (TCA) – a class of antidepressants; they inhibit reabsorption of serotonin, norepinephrine, and dopamine in the brain

OVERVIEW

The human brain is an extremely complex organ. It is responsible for all affective (emotional) and cognitive (thinking) processes, and is as capable of coordinating bodily functions (eating, sleeping, walking, talking) as it is of pursuing abstract thought. Sometimes imbalances in mental functioning occur that can result in one of a number of brain disturbances, producing disorders such as schizophrenia, depression, anxiety, or parkinsonism. The onset of such conditions can make normal functioning within society difficult, if not impossible. The use of psychopharmacology in the treatment of these conditions may be a necessary part of the reintegration of affected individuals in the community.

Mental health problems involve significant dysfunction in the areas of behavior or personality that interfere with a person's ability to function. Biochemical and structural abnormalities in the brain appear to contribute to the pathologies. Many disorders have a genetic component. Stressors may play a role in the development of mental illness. Psychotic illnesses include the more serious disorders such as schizophrenia, delusional disorders, and some affective or mood disorders. Many patients with psychotic disorders receive large doses of drugs with significant adverse effects. Other common mental disorders include anxiety, insomnia, and panic disorders, which are less severe but nevertheless disruptive.

ANATOMY REVIEW

The nervous system is composed of the brain, spinal cord, and nerves (Figures 5-1 and 5-2).

- The nervous system has two divisions: the central nervous system (CNS) and the peripheral nervous system (PNS).

- The brain and spinal cord make up the CNS. The nerves make up the PNS.

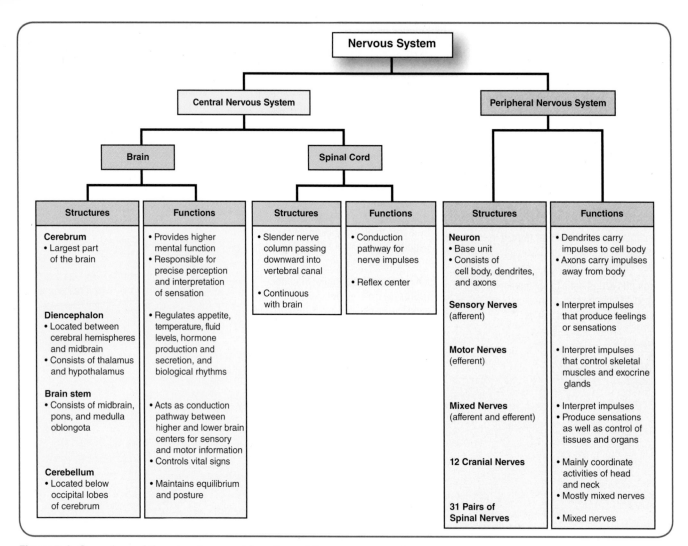

Figure 5-1 Overview of the structure and function of the nervous system.

- The brain is divided into specific regions; each region is responsible for the performance of specific functions within the body (Figures 5-3A and 5-3B).

- The brain consists of four parts: the cerebrum, diencephalon (thalamus and hypothalamus), cerebellum, and brain stem.

- The main functions of the cerebrum include the control of consciousness, memory, emotions, sensations, and voluntary movements.

- The thalamus receives sensory stimuli (except the sense of smell), relaying them to the cerebral cortex.

- The hypothalamus (located just below the thalamus) activates, controls, and integrates the peripheral autonomic nervous system.

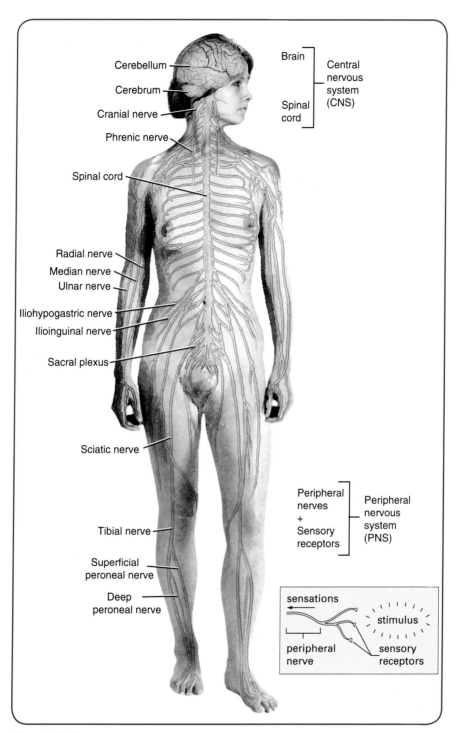

Figure 5-2 The nervous system.

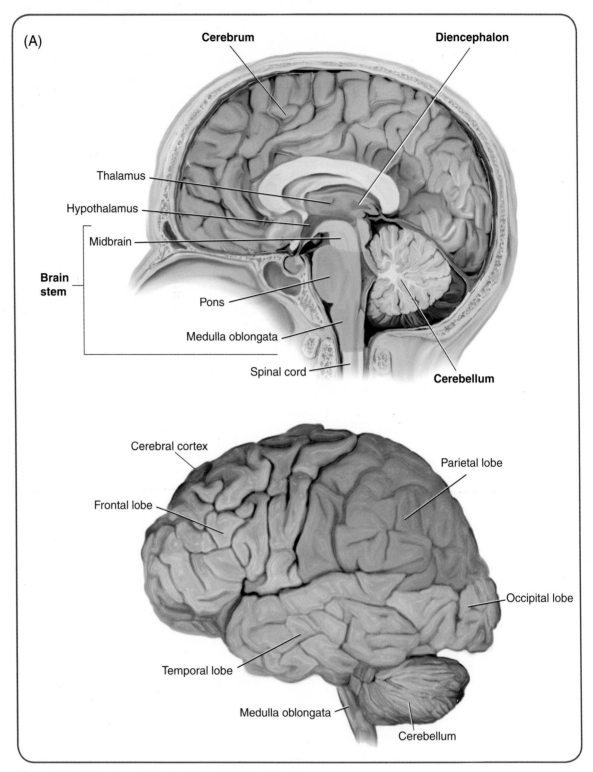

Figure 5-3A Divisions of the brain and related functions.

It also controls endocrine system processes, body temperature, appetite, sleep, and other sensory functions.

- The cerebellum, attached to the brain stem, maintains muscle tone and coordinates balance and movement.

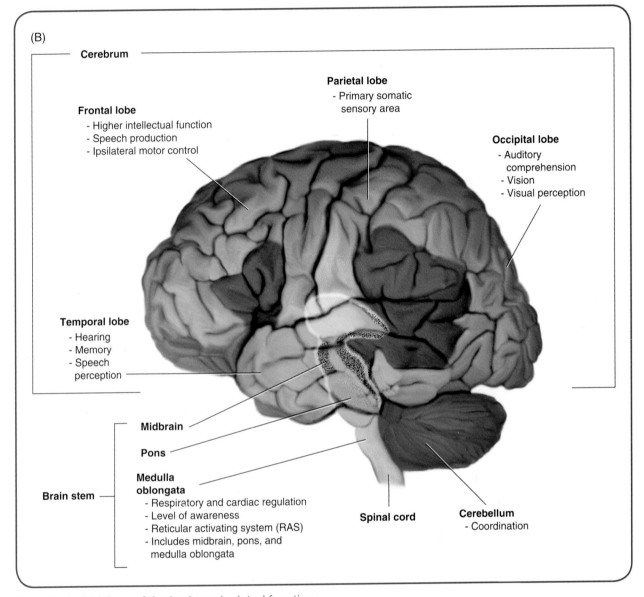

(B)

Cerebrum

Parietal lobe
- Primary somatic
  sensory area

Frontal lobe
- Higher intellectual function
- Speech production
- Ipsilateral motor control

Occipital lobe
- Auditory
  comprehension
- Vision
- Visual perception

Temporal lobe
- Hearing
- Memory
- Speech
  perception

Midbrain

Pons

**Medulla
oblongata**
- Respiratory and cardiac regulation
- Level of awareness
- Reticular activating system (RAS)
- Includes midbrain, pons, and
  medulla oblongata

Brain stem

Spinal cord

Cerebellum
- Coordination

Figure 5-3B Divisions of the brain and related functions.

- The brain stem controls blood pressure, respiration, pulse, and other body functions; it connects the hypothalamus with the spinal cord.
- The basic functional unit of the nervous system is the neuron (Figure 5-4).
- There are three types of nerves: sensory nerves transmit information that produces sensation and feelings, motor nerves transmit information that produces movement and function, and mixed nerves transmit information that produces both sensation and movement.
- The spinal cord provides a two-way communication system between the brain and body parts outside of the nervous system (Figure 5-5).

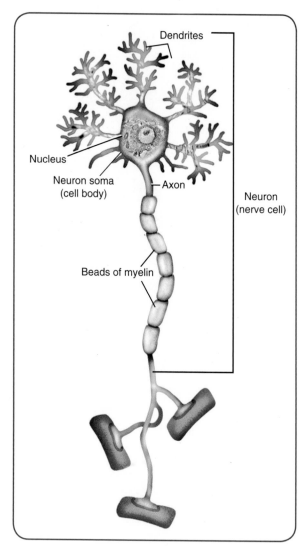

Figure 5-4 The neuron.

NEUROTRANSMITTERS

The term **neurotransmitter** refers to a biochemical that is formed in and released from a neuron in order to stimulate or inhibit the actions of another cell. Examples of neurotransmitters include acetylcholine, dopamine, noradrenaline, serotonin, glutamate, and gamma-aminobutyric acid (GABA). Disorders in the production and function of neurotransmitters may contribute to psychiatric illnesses.

Acetylcholine

Acetylcholine plays a major role in cognitive function and memory formation as well as motor control. It was the first neurotransmitter to be identified. Acetylcholine allows neurons to communicate with each other. This neurotransmitter is released by the axon terminals in response to a

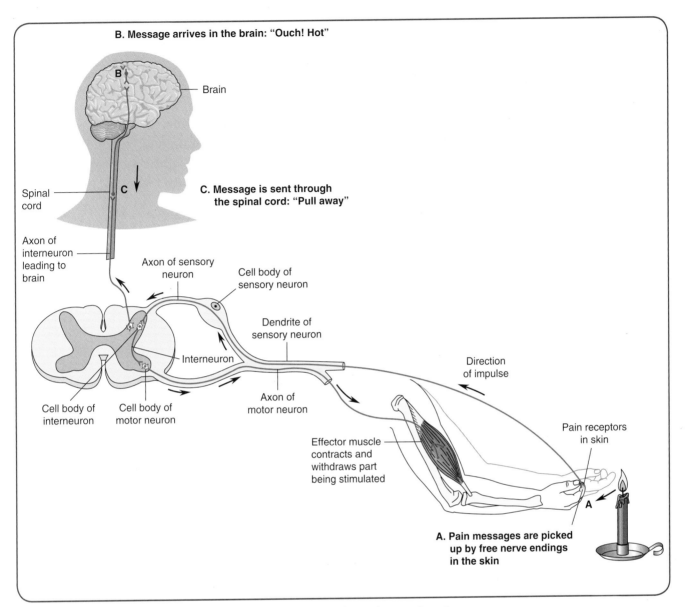

B. Message arrives in the brain: "Ouch! Hot"

Brain

C. Message is sent through the spinal cord: "Pull away"

Spinal cord

Axon of interneuron leading to brain

Axon of sensory neuron

Cell body of sensory neuron

Dendrite of sensory neuron

Interneuron

Direction of impulse

Axon of motor neuron

Cell body of interneuron

Cell body of motor neuron

Pain receptors in skin

Effector muscle contracts and withdraws part being stimulated

A. Pain messages are picked up by free nerve endings in the skin

Figure 5-5 The two-way communication system of the brain and nerve function.

nerve impulse. In relation to motor function, the release of acetylcholine will cause a change in the muscle cell and elicit a contraction of the muscle, producing movement.

Dopamine

Dopamine is a naturally produced agent that, in the brain, functions as a neurotransmitter. Dopamine release and dopamine levels within the brain affect motor control, memory, attention span, the ability to problem solve, motivation, pleasure, and creative thought. Alterations in dopamine production and secretion play a role in disorders such as Parkinson's disease (see Chapter 8), attention deficit disorder, and schizophrenia. It is also believed to play a role in addiction to drugs.

Norepinephrine and Serotonin

Both **norepinephrine** and **serotonin** seem to be involved in similar functions within the brain: regulation of appetite, sleep, arousal, mood, temperature, and hormone release.

Norepinephrine is also known as noradrenaline. As a stress hormone, it affects parts of the human brain where attention and responding actions are controlled. It is released from the medulla of the adrenal glands as a hormone into the blood, but is also a central and sympathetic nervous system neurotransmitter.

Serotonin is a neurotransmitter synthesized in the CNS as well as the gastrointestinal tract. It is believed to play an important role in regulating anger, aggression, body temperature, mood, sleep, vomiting, sexuality, and appetite. It was initially identified as a vasoconstrictor present in blood serum, and it was from here that its name was derived. Serotonin (also known as 5-hydroxytryptamine or 5-HT) may also have a role in pain perception and behavior. It acts as an inhibitory neurotransmitter.

Serotonin syndrome, also known as **serotonin toxicity**, is a rare condition that can result from intentional self-poisoning with serotonin, use of the drug therapeutically, or from inadvertent drug interactions. This condition includes progressively worsening symptoms such as mental confusion, shivering or muscle twitching, sweating or fever, **hallucinations**, hypertension, tachycardia, headache, tremor, nausea, diarrhea, coma, and death.

Glutamate

Glutamate is an amino acid, however, not one of the essential amino acids. It is a key molecule in cellular metabolism. Glutamate plays an important role in the body's disposal of excess or waste nitrogen. It is important for the ability to perceive taste sensations.

Glutamate is distributed throughout the CNS. It is considered the major excitatory CNS neurotransmitter. It can stimulate a number of receptor types in the brain and spinal cord. Glutamate is involved in the facilitation of learning and memory. The brain is very vulnerable to glutamate-mediated over-excitation. This results in excitotoxicity, which causes cell integrity to be disrupted and nerve cells to die. Excitotoxicity has been demonstrated in strokes and some neurodegenerative diseases. Glutamate has also been implicated in the development of epilepsy (see Chapter 9).

Gamma-Aminobutyric Acid

Gamma-aminobutyric acid (GABA) is distributed throughout the brain and spinal cord. It is now considered to be the major inhibitory neurotransmitter in the CNS and it acts to modulate the activity of excitatory pathways.

Medical Terminology Review

glutamate
glutam = glutamic acid
-ate = salt or ester
a salt containing glutamic acid

It is formed from the excitatory neurotransmitter glutamate. Motor control, consciousness, levels of arousal, and memory formation are all inhibited by GABA.

GABA has mostly excitatory effects during early development. It has been purported to increase the amounts of human growth hormone. It is unknown if GABA can cross the blood-brain barrier.

MENTAL DISORDERS

Mental illness is defined as any disturbance of emotional equilibrium, as manifested in maladaptive behavior and impaired functioning of behavior or personality. Biochemical and structural abnormalities in the brain appear to contribute to these disorders. Some of these disorders have a genetic component. Stressors may play a role in the development of these types of illnesses. Psychotic illnesses include the more serious disorders such as schizophrenia, bipolar disorder, and depression. Other common mental disorders including dementia and eating disorders (discussed here), as well as anxiety and sleep disorders (discussed in Chapter 6), are less severe but nevertheless disruptive.

Schizophrenia

Schizophrenia is a mental illness characterized by distortion of reality, disorganized thought patterns, social withdrawal, **hallucinations**, and poor judgment. Schizophrenia is one of the most devastating forms of mental illnesses. It occurs in approximately 1% of the population.

Schizophrenia includes a variety of syndromes, which present differently in each individual. Although the cause of this disorder has not been fully determined, some common changes do occur in the brains of patients suffering from schizophrenia, including reduction of the cortex (outer portion) of the temporal lobes, enlargement of the third and lateral ventricles, excessive dopamine secretion, and decreased blood flow to the front of the brain.

Schizophrenia appears to have no single cause but may involve a combination of genetic and other factors, including fetal brain damage caused by perinatal complications or viral infections in the mother during pregnancy. Onset is usually between the ages of 15 and 25 years in men, and between 25 and 35 in women. Stressful events appear to initiate the onset and recurrence of the disorder.

Bipolar Disorder

Bipolar disorder is a mental illness characterized by periods of extreme excitation or **mania**, and deep depression. It is not commonly understood why it takes months to move from one of these extremes to the other. Some patients have predominantly manic episodes or predominantly depressive episodes. Few patients experience the classic swing from mania to depression and back. Bipolar disorder is also called manic-depressive illness.

Depression

Depression is classified as a mood disorder, of which there are several subgroups. Major depression, or unipolar disorder, is a chemical deficit within the brain, and a precise diagnosis is based on biological factors or personal characteristics. The causes of depression include genetic and psychosocial stressors. Depression may also occur as a reactive episode, a response to a life event, or secondarily to many systemic disorders (including cancer, diabetes, heart failure, and AIDS). This condition is a common problem, and many patients with milder forms may be misdiagnosed and not receive treatment.

Eating Disorders

Anorexia nervosa is classified as an eating disorder. This complex psychological state is characterized by the fear of being overweight. Often, patients' perceptions are distorted to the extent that they believe they are overweight despite appearing emaciated to others. Without proper treatment, anorexia nervosa may be fatal.

Bulimia nervosa is an eating disorder that is characterized by recurrent (at least twice a week) episodes of binge eating, during which the patient consumes large amounts of food and feels unable to stop eating. This is followed by inappropriate compensatory effects to avoid weight gain, such as self-induced vomiting, laxative or diuretic abuse, vigorous exercise, or fasting.

Dementia

Dementia is a chronic deterioration of intellectual function and other cognitive skills severe enough to interfere with the ability to perform activities of daily living. Dementia may occur at any age and can affect young people as the result of injury or hypoxia. However, it is mostly a disease of the elderly.

ANTIPSYCHOTIC DRUGS

Antipsychotic drugs, also called neuroleptic drugs, are a major therapeutic modality for psychotic disorders, often in conjunction with psychotherapy and psychosocial rehabilitation. The antipsychotic drugs (conventional and atypical agents) are listed in Table 5-1.

TABLE 5-1   Antipsychotic Drugs*

Generic Name	Trade Name	Route of Administration	Average Adult Dosage
Conventional Agents			
chlorpromazine (klor-PRO-ma-zeen)	Thorazine®	PO, IM, IV, PR (suppository)	50–400 mg/day
fluphenazine (floo-FEN-ah-zeen)	Prolixin®	PO, IM	2.5–10 mg/day, in divided doses at 6–8 hour intervals
haloperidol (ha-lo-PAIR-ih-doll)	Haldol®	PO, IM	1–50 mg/day, highly individualized for patient needs – *Black Box Warning 1*
lithium (LITH-ee-um)	Eskalith®	PO	Immediate-release: 600 mg tid; extended-release: 900 mg bid.
loxapine (LOK-sa-peen)	Loxapine®	PO	10–100 mg/day
perphenazine (per-FEN-ah-zeen)	Perphenazine Tablets®	PO	4–16 mg/day bid–qid
pimozide (PIH-mo-zyd)	Orap®	PO	1–10 mg/day in divided doses
prochlorperazine (pro-klor-PAIR-ah-zeen)	Prochlorperazine Maleate Tablets®	PO	5–20 mg/day
thioridazine (thy-oh-RIH-da-zeen)	Mellaril®	PO	50–100 mg tid – *Black Box Warning 2*
thiothixene (thy-oh-THIK-zeen)	Navane®	PO	2–15 mg/day – *Black Box Warning 1*
trifluoperazine (try-floo-oh-PAIR-ah-zeen)	Stelazine®	PO, IM	1–5 mg bid
Atypical Agents			
aripiprazole (ah-rih-PIH-pra-zol)	Abilify®	PO	10–30 mg/day – *Black Box Warning 3*
arsenapine (ar-SEN-ah-peen)	Saphris®	PO	5 mg bid – *Black Box Warning 1*
clozapine (KLO-za-peen)	Clozaril®, Fazaclo®	PO	12.5 mg once or twice daily, increasing up to 300–450 mg/day within 2 weeks – *Black Box Warning 4*
iloperidone (eye-lo-PAIR-ih-dohn)	Fanapt®	PO	1 mg bid, increasing slowly up to 6–12 mg bid – *Black Box Warning 1*

continued on next page

Table 5-1 continued

lurasidone (loo-RAH-sih-dohn)	Latuda®	PO	40–160 mg/day – *Black Box Warning 2*
olanzapine (oh-LAN-za-peen)	Zyprexa®, Zyprexa Zydis®	PO, IM	PO: 5–20 mg/day; IM: 2.5–5 mg/injection – *Black Box Warning 1*
quetiapine (kweh-TY-ah-peen)	Seroquel®	PO	150–800 mg/day – *Black Box Warning 2*
risperidone (ris-PAIR-ih-dohn)	Risperdal®	PO	1–16 mg/day – *Black Box Warning 1*
ziprasidone (zih-PRAH-sih-dohn)	Geodon®	PO	40–160 mg/day – *Black Box Warning 1*

*NOTE that the following black box warnings apply to the indicated drugs above:

Black Box Warning 1 – Increased mortality in elderly patients with dementiarelated psychosis

Black Box Warning 2 – Increased mortality in elderly patients with dementiarelated psychosis; and suicidal thoughts and behaviors

Black Box Warning 3 – Increased mortality in elderly patients with dementiarelated psychosis and suicidality and antidepressant drugs

Black Box Warning 4 – Agranulocytosis; orthostatic hypotension, bradycardia, and syncope; seizure; myocarditis and cardiomyopathy; increased mortality in elderly patients with dementia-related psychosis

Medical Terminology Review

antipsychotic
anti = against
psych/o = mind
-tic = pertaining to
against the mind

neuroleptic
neuro = nerve
lep = seizure, attack
-tic = pertaining to
attack of the nerves

Key Concept

Antipsychotic drugs do not alter the underlying pathology of schizophrenia. Therefore, treatment is not curative.

Mechanism of Action

Antipsychotic drugs act by blocking receptors for dopamine, acetylcholine, histamine, and norepinephrine. The current suggestions are that conventional antipsychotic drugs suppress symptoms of psychosis by blocking dopamine receptors in the brain.

Indications

Schizophrenia is the primary indication for antipsychotic drugs. These agents effectively suppress symptoms during acute psychotic episodes and, when taken chronically, can greatly decrease the risk of relapse. Selection among these drugs is based primarily on their adverse effect profiles, rather than on therapeutic effects.

In addition to their antipsychotic properties, some of these drugs, such as prochlorperazine, are also used as antiemetics. Chlorpromazine is used for treating hiccups and lithium for managing bipolar disorders. Small doses of neuroleptics can be effective in controlling acute agitation in the elderly.

Adverse Effects

Antipsychotic drugs frequently cause a wide variety of adverse effects, which include dry mouth, blurred vision, urinary retention, orthostatic hypotension, tachycardia, sedation, headache, and behavior changes. These drugs may also produce agitation, confusion, lethargy, and paranoid reactions. Antipsychotic agents commonly cause adverse effects related to excessive **extrapyramidal** activity (involving nerves in the brain that control movement), or parkinsonian signs. Involuntary muscle spasms in the face, neck, arms, or legs (dystonia) may be present. Tardive dyskinesia may be present, such as chewing or grimacing, repetitive jerky or writhing movements of the limbs, tremors, or a shuffling gait. Extrapyramidal effects usually diminish with a decreased dosage of the antipsychotic medication.

Contraindications and Precautions

Antipsychotic drugs are contraindicated in patients with a known hypersensitivity, severe depression, blood dyscrasias, liver dysfunction, severe hypotension or hypertension, or Parkinson's disease.

Safe use of antipsychotic drugs during pregnancy and lactation has not been established. These agents are classified as pregnancy category C (except for clozapine, which is category B).

Antipsychotic agents should be used with caution in patients with glaucoma, asthma, epilepsy, prostatic hypertrophy, peptic ulcer, or renal dysfunction, and in those who have been exposed to extreme heat.

Drug Interactions

Antipsychotic medications may have drug interactions with antihistamines, alcohol, tranquilizers, narcotics, and barbiturates. They may result in additive CNS depression.

MOOD-ALTERING DRUGS

According to the National Institutes of Health, more than 5.7 million Americans suffer from bipolar disorder, formerly known as manic-depressive illness. This disease is a chronic condition that requires treatment for life.

Bipolar disorder is treated with three major groups of drugs: mood stabilizers, antipsychotics, and antidepressants. The mainstays of therapy are lithium and valproic acid, drugs with the ability to stabilize mood. In addition, benzodiazepines are commonly used for sedation. Antipsychotic drugs were discussed earlier and antidepressants will be discussed later in this chapter. This section focuses on mood stabilizers.

The principal mood stabilizers are lithium and two drugs originally developed for epilepsy: valproic acid and carbamazepine (see Chapter 9). Lithium has a low therapeutic index. As a result, toxicity can occur at blood levels only slightly greater than therapeutic levels. Accordingly, monitoring of lithium levels is mandatory.

Mechanism of Action

The precise mechanism of action of lithium is unknown. The lithium ion behaves in the body much like the sodium ion, but its exact mechanism of

Key Concept

Lithium is not a true antipsychotic drug, but it is used in regulating the severe fluctuations of the manic phase of bipolar disorder.

action is unclear. Lithium competes with various physiologically important cations: Na^+, K^+, Ca^{2+}, and Mg^{2+}. At the synapse, it accelerates catecholamine destruction, inhibits the release of neurotransmitters, and decreases sensitivity of postsynaptic receptors.

Indications

Lithium is a drug of choice for controlling acute manic episodes in patients with bipolar disorder, and for long-term prophylaxis against recurrence of mania or depression. In manic patients, lithium reduces euphoria, hyperactivity, and other symptoms, but does not cause sedation. Anti-manic effects begin five to seven days after the onset of treatment, but full benefits may not develop for two to three weeks.

Adverse Effects

Adverse effects of lithium, such as nausea, diarrhea, abdominal bloating, and anorexia, are common but transient. The other adverse effects include fatigue, muscle weakness, headache, confusion, memory impairment, polyuria, and thirst. Lithium-induced tremors can be augmented by stress and fatigue.

Contraindications and Precautions

Lithium is contraindicated in patients with known hypersensitivity, in those with significant cardiovascular or kidney disease, brain damage, dehydration, or sodium debilitation. Lithium is also contraindicated in pregnancy, especially during the first trimester (category D), in lactation, and in children younger than 12 years of age.

Lithium should be used with caution in older adults and in patients suffering from thyroid disease, epilepsy, cardiac disease, dehydration, diarrhea, renal impairment, and seizure disorders.

Drug Interactions

Diuretics promote sodium loss and can thereby increase the risk of lithium toxicity. Nonsteroidal anti-inflammatory drugs can increase lithium levels and increase renal reabsorption of lithium. Anticholinergics can cause urinary hesitancy coupled with lithium-induced polyuria.

ANTIDEPRESSANTS

As previously mentioned in this chapter, depression is classified as a mood disorder with several subgroups. Severe depression, or unipolar disorder, is endogenous (originating from within), and a precise diagnosis is based on biological factors or personal characteristics. Etiological factors include genetic, developmental, and psychosocial stressors. Bipolar disorder involves alternating periods of depression and mania. Depression may also occur as an exogenous or reactive episode, a response to a life event, or secondarily to many systemic disorders, including cancer, diabetes, heart failure, and systemic lupus erythematosus.

Antidepressants are commonly viewed in the context of nerve physiology within the brain. Five major drug classifications are used to treat depression: tricyclic antidepressants (TCAs), selective serotonin reuptake inhibitors (SSRIs), monoamine oxidase inhibitors (MAOIs), serotonin-norepinephrine reuptake inhibitors (SNRIs), and atypical antidepressant drugs (Table 5-2).

TABLE 5-2	Drugs Used to Treat Depression*		
Generic Name	**Trade Name**	**Route of Administration**	**Average Adult Dose**
Tricyclic Antidepressants (TCAs)			
amitriptyline (ah-mih-TRIP-tih-leen)	Elavil®	PO	75–100 mg/day (max: 150–300 mg/day)
amoxapine (ah-MOK-sah-peen)	Asendin®	PO	200–400 mg/day
desipramine (deh-SIP-rah-meen)	Norpramin®	PO	75–100 mg/day (max: 300 mg/day)
doxepin (DOK-sah-pin)	Sinequan®	PO	30–150 mg/day h.s. (max: 300 mg/day)
imipramine (ih-MIP-rah-meen)	Tofranil®	PO	75–100 mg/day (max: 300 mg/day)
maprotiline (mah-PRO-tih-leen)	Ludiomil®	PO	25–150 mg/day
nortriptyline (nor-TRIP-tih-leen)	Aventyl®	PO	25 mg tid–qid (max: 150 mg /day)
protriptyline (pro-TRIP-tih-leen)	Vivactil®	PO	15–40 mg/day in 3–4 divided doses (max: 60 mg/day)
trimipramine (try-MIP-rah-meen)	Surmontil®	PO	75–100 mg/day (max: 300 mg/day)
Selective Serotonin Reuptake Inhibitors (SSRIs)			
citalopram (sy-TAH-loh-pram)	Celexa®	PO	Start at 20 mg/day (max: 40 mg/day)
escitalopram (ee-sih-TAH-loh-pram)	Lexapro®	PO	10 mg/day (max: 20 mg/day after 1 wk)
fluoxetine (floo-OK-seh-teen)	Prozac®	PO	20 mg/day in a.m. (max: 80 mg/day)
fluvoxamine (floo-VOK-sah-meen)	Luvox®	PO	Start at 50 mg/day (max: 300 mg/day)

continued on next page

Table 5-2 continued

paroxetine (pah-ROK-seh-teen)	Paxil®	PO	10–50 mg/day (max: 60 mg/day)
sertraline (SER-trah-leen)	Zoloft®	PO	Start at 50 mg /day (max: 200 mg/day)
Monoamine Oxidase Inhibitors (MAOIs)			
isocarboxazid (eye-soh-kar-BOK-sah-zid)	Marplan®	PO	10–30 mg/day (max: 30 mg/day)
phenelzine (FEH-nel-zeen)	Nardil®	PO	15 mg tid (max: 90 mg/day)
tranylcypromine (trah-nil-SY-pro-meen)	Parnate®	PO	30 mg/day (20 mg in a.m. and 10 mg in p.m.) (max: 60 mg/day)
Serotonin-Norepinephrine Reuptake Inhibitors (SNRIs)			
desvenlafaxine (des-ven-lah-FAK-seen)	Pristiq®	PO	50 mg/day – *Black Box Warning 1*
duloxetine (doo-LOK-seh-teen)	Cymbalta®	PO	20–60 mg/day, usually in divided doses – *Black Box Warning 1*
nefazodone (neh-FAH-zoh-dohn)	Serzone®	PO	50–100 mg bid (max: 600 mg/day)
venlafaxine (ven-lah-FAK-seen)	Effexor®	PO	25–125 mg tid – *Black Box Warning 1*
Norepinephrine-Dopamine Reuptake Inhibitor (NDRI)			
bupropion (byoo-PRO-pee-on)	Wellbutrin®	PO	75–100 mg tid (max: 450 mg/day)
Noradrenergic and Specific Serotonergic Antidepressant (NaSSA)			
mirtazapine (mir-TAH-zah-peen)	Remeron®	PO	15 mg/day h.s. (max: 45 mg/day)
Serotonin Antagonist/Reuptake Inhibitor (SARI)			
trazodone (TRAY-zoh-dohn)	Desyrel®	PO	150 mg/day (max: 600 mg/day)

*NOTE that all antidepressants carry Black Box Warnings for increased risk of suicidal thoughts and behavior in children, adolescents, and young adults.

Medical Terminology Review

unipolar
uni = one
-polar = pole; mood
one mood

Tricyclic Antidepressants

Historically, **tricyclic antidepressants (TCAs)** were the first choice in the treatment of depression, until SSRIs entered the market. The term *tricyclic* derives from the common three-ringed structure of the drug molecule itself.

Mechanism of Action

Tricyclic antidepressants inhibit the reuptake of serotonin and noradrenaline into nerve terminals (Figure 5-6).

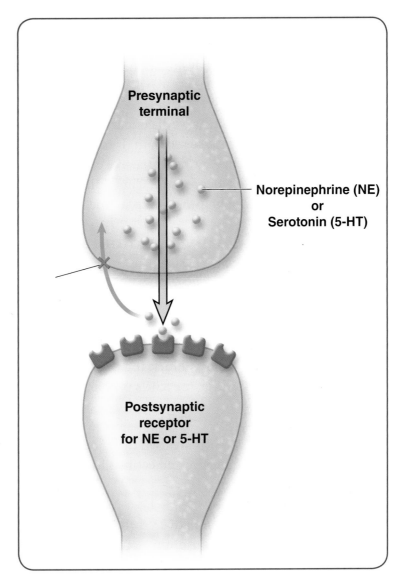

Figure 5-6 Mechanism of action for tricyclic antidepressants.

Key Concept

Antidepressant effects may not be observed for up to four weeks after treatment begins.

Medical Terminology Review

tricyclic
tri = three
-cyclic = related to cycles, circles, rings
three cycles

Indications

These drugs are mainly used for major depression, and imipramine may be used for the treatment of **nocturnal enuresis** (nighttime bedwetting) in children.

Adverse Effects

Common adverse effects of TCAs include dry mouth, blurred vision, postural hypotension, constipation, and urinary retention. Other adverse effects may include sedation, drowsiness, cardiovascular symptoms (such as dysrhythmias), and extreme hypertension.

Contraindications and Precautions

The TCAs are contraindicated in patients with known hypersensitivity to these drugs. They are also contraindicated in patients with glaucoma, hypertrophy of prostate gland, and during pregnancy or lactation.

Like other antidepressants, the tricyclics should be used with caution in patients who have heart disease (angina or paroxysmal tachycardia), hepatic or renal dysfunction, or a history of seizures.

Drug Interactions

The TCAs, with concurrent use of other CNS depressants, including alcohol, may cause sedation. If taking clonidine, patients may experience a decrease in the antihypertensive effects of the drug and are at an increased risk for CNS depression. Cimetidine (a histamine blocking agent) may prevent the metabolism of imipramine, leading to increased serum levels and toxicity.

Selective Serotonin Reuptake Inhibitors

Selective serotonin reuptake inhibitors (SSRIs) are antidepressants that have had a tremendous impact on prescribing patterns. They are now considered the first-line drugs in the treatment of major depression.

Mechanism of Action

The SSRIs block the presynaptic amine reuptake pump, as do the TCAs. However, the SSRIs primarily affect serotonin reuptake (Figure 5-7).

Indications

The SSRIs are used in major depression and may be prescribed for obsessive-compulsive and eating disorders.

Adverse Effects

Common adverse effects of SSRIs include headache, vomiting, diarrhea, nausea, insomnia, and nervousness. Generally, the adverse effects of SSRIs are relatively mild, of short duration, and cease as treatment continues. Cardiac toxicity and the risk of death after overdose are less likely than with the TCAs. However, in 2004 the FDA issued a Black Box Warning for increased suicidality in pediatric patients taking SSRIs. In 2006, this warning was extended to include young adults. Therefore, a medication guide must be dispensed with all SSRIs.

Contraindications and Precautions

The SSRIs are contraindicated in patients with known hypersensitivity to these agents and during pregnancy. They should be used with caution in patients with hepatic or renal dysfunction, diabetes mellitus, and during lactation.

Drug Interactions

Concurrent use of SSRIs with benzodiazepines may cause increased adverse CNS effects. Beta-blockers may cause decreased elimination of SSRIs, resulting in hypotension or bradycardia. Clozapine, phenytoin, and theophylline may interact with SSRIs and decrease their elimination and their toxicity.

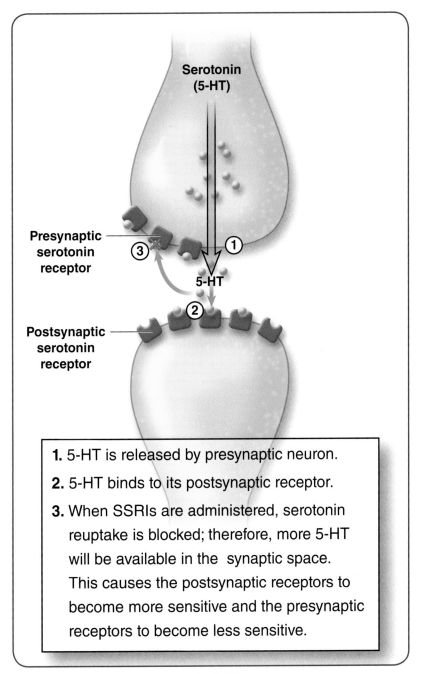

1. 5-HT is released by presynaptic neuron.

2. 5-HT binds to its postsynaptic receptor.

3. When SSRIs are administered, serotonin reuptake is blocked; therefore, more 5-HT will be available in the synaptic space. This causes the postsynaptic receptors to become more sensitive and the presynaptic receptors to become less sensitive.

Figure 5-7 Mechanism of action for SSRIs.

Monoamine Oxidase Inhibitors

Monoamine oxidase inhibitors (MAOIs) were the first drugs approved for the treatment of depression.

Mechanism of Action

These drugs inhibit monoamine oxidase (an enzyme) that stops the actions of dopamine, norepinephrine, epinephrine, and serotonin. Therefore, MAOIs intensify the effects of norepinephrine in adrenergic synapses.

Indications

The MAOIs are used to manage symptoms of depression that are not responsive to other types of pharmacotherapy. The effect of these drugs may continue for two to three weeks after therapy is discontinued.

Adverse Effects

Common adverse effects of the MAOIs include dizziness, vertigo, dry mouth, nausea, diarrhea or constipation, loss of appetite, orthostatic hypotension, and insomnia. Hypertensive crisis (severe hypertension) may occur if foods containing tyramine are ingested while taking MAOIs. Table 5-3 lists foods that contain tyramine.

Contraindications and Precautions

The MAOIs are contraindicated in patients with known hypersensitivity to these drugs; in patients with hepatic or renal disease, hypertension, congestive heart failure, cerebrovascular disease, and in the elderly. These drugs should be used with caution in patients with liver dysfunction, diabetes, hyperthyroidism, and history of seizures.

Drug Interactions

The MAOIs may interact with other antidepressant drugs such as SSRIs and TCAs, resulting in elevation of body temperature and seizures. Meperidine should be avoided with MAOIs due to increased risk of respiratory failure or hypertensive crisis.

Serotonin-Norepinephrine Reuptake Inhibitors

Serotonin-norepinephrine reuptake inhibitors (SNRIs) are newer forms of antidepressants. They are frequently prescribed to alleviate symptoms of depression for patients with bipolar disorder and are chemically unrelated

TABLE 5-3	Foods That Contain Tyramine
Type of Food	**Tyramine-Containing Foods**
alcohol	beer, wines (especially red wines and Chianti)
dairy products	cheese (except for cottage cheese), sour cream, yogurt
fruits	avocados, bananas, canned figs, papaya products (including meat tenderizers), raisins
meats	beef or chicken liver, bologna/hot dogs, meat extracts, pate, pepperoni, pickled or kippered herring, salami, sausage
other	chocolate
sauces	soy sauce
vegetables	pods of broad beans (fava beans)
yeast	all yeast or yeast extracts

to other antidepressants. The SNRIs include desvenlafaxine, duloxetine, nefazodone, and venlafaxine.

Mechanism of Action

The SNRIs inhibit the reabsorption of serotonin and norepinephrine. They elevate mood by increasing the levels of dopamine, serotonin, and norepinephrine in the CNS.

Indications

The SNRIs are indicated for mental depression. Venlafaxine (Effexor®) is also used for generalized anxiety disorder and social anxiety disorder.

Adverse Effects

Common adverse effects of the SNRIs include dry mouth, blurred vision, dizziness, headache, nausea, vomiting, orthostatic hypotension, increased appetite, and insomnia.

Contraindications and Precautions

The SNRIs are contraindicated in patients with known hypersensitivity to these agents. These drugs should be avoided in patients with hepatic diseases, pregnancy (category C), lactation, suicidal thoughts, and in children younger than eight years of age.

The SNRIs must be used cautiously in patients with renal failure, hepatic impairment, history of mania, acute closed-angle glaucoma, cardiac disorders, hypertension, hyperthyroidism, and history of seizures or seizure disorders.

Drug Interactions

The SNRIs may increase metabolism of carbamazepine, cimetidine, phenytoin, and phenobarbital. They may increase incidence of adverse effects of levodopa and MAOIs. They may cause additive cognitive and motor impairment with alcohol or benzodiazepines, and increase the risk of hypertensive crisis with MAOIs. Antihypertensive agents may potentiate their hypotensive effects. Levels of digoxin or phenytoin may be increased if used concurrently. Levels and toxicity of ketoconazole, indinavir, and ritonavir may be increased with concurrent use.

Miscellaneous Antidepressants

There are other agents that are considered miscellaneous antidepressants. These have different classifications from each other, with a single drug as an example, as follows:

- Norepinephrine-dopamine reuptake inhibitor (NDRI) – bupropion
- Noradrenergic and specific serotonergic antidepressant (NaSSA) – mirtazapine
- Serotonin antagonist/reuptake inhibitor (SARI) – trazodone

These agents are also listed in Table 5-2.

SUMMARY

The nervous system is composed of two divisions: the CNS (brain and spinal cord) and the peripheral nervous system (nerves). The major parts of the human brain are the cerebrum, diencephalon, brain stem, and cerebellum. The cerebrum is involved in motor and sensory function, and is the seat of intellect. The diencephalon comprises the thalamus, which acts as an information sorting area, and the hypothalamus, which is an integration area for visceral functioning. The brain stem contains control centers for heart rate, respiratory rate, and blood pressure. The cerebellum controls muscle tone and posture, and facilitates smooth and coordinated muscle movements. Acetylcholine, dopamine, noradrenaline, serotonin, and GABA are key neurotransmitters in the brain.

Antipsychotics are used in the treatment of psychoses such as schizophrenia, dementia, and restlessness. All antipsychotics exert their effect on dopamine receptors and antagonize dopaminergic activity in the CNS. Antipsychotics have a diverse and potentially debilitating adverse effect profile.

Depression is a state of profound sadness. It can be reactive, in response to a life event, or endogenous, without an apparent trigger. Antidepressant drugs act by raising the levels of one or both of these neurotransmitters. This is achieved by blocking a subtype of postsynaptic serotonin receptors (selective serotonin receptor blockers) or MAOIs.

EXPLORING THE WEB

Visit **www.fda.gov**

- Search using the term *antipsychotics*. Look for drug information sheets for patients. You can also search for information on specific drug names for additional information on specific drugs.

Visit **www.mentalhealth.com**

- Click on the link "Disorders." Choose one of the disorders discussed in the text and research what is known about the disorder and the treatments that are used to address it.

Visit **www.nimh.nih.gov**

- Choose one of the disorders discussed in the text and research what is known about the disorder and the treatments that are used to address it.

Visit **www.nlm.nih.gov/medlineplus**

- Choose one of the types of drugs discussed in the chapter and research the uses, mechanisms of action, adverse effects, contraindications and precautions, and drug interactions to further your understanding of the drug. Make index cards with the pertinent information to help you review and study.

Visit **www.rxlist.com**

- Bookmark this site to be used as a reference. It is one of several drug information sites available on the Web. What additional websites are available for drug information? Make sure the sites are reputable.

REVIEW QUESTIONS

Multiple Choice

1. Which of the following parts of the brain is responsible for the perception and interpretation of sensation?

   A. cerebellum

   B. cerebrum

   C. diencephalon

   D. brain stem

2. Which of the following disorders is the primary indication for antipsychotic drugs?

   A. insomnia

   B. anxiety

   C. manic-depressive illness

   D. schizophrenia

3. Lithium is a drug of choice for controlling which of the following mental disorders?

   A. schizophrenia

   B. restlessness

   C. acute manic episodes

   D. brain injury

4. Which of the following antidepressants have relatively mild adverse effects, and are the newest of these drugs?

   A. monoamine oxidase inhibitors

   B. tricyclic antidepressants

   C. atypical antidepressants

   D. selective serotonin reuptake inhibitors

5. Which of the following neurotransmitters is distributed throughout the central nervous system?

   A. GABA

   B. dopamine

   C. acetylcholine

   D. serotonin

6. Which of the following is the largest part of the brain?

   A. hypothalamus

   B. cerebellum

   C. brain stem

   D. cerebrum

7. Which of the following neurotransmitters is involved in hormone release, motor control, behavior, and emesis?

   A. serotonin

   B. dopamine

   C. acetylcholine

   D. GABA

8. Of the following neurotransmitters, which has functions within the brain similar to those of norepinephrine ?

   A. dopamine

   B. GABA

   C. serotonin

   D. acetylcholine

9. Bipolar disorder involves alternating periods of which of the following?

   A. depression and insomnia

   B. depression and mania

   C. depression and anxiety attacks

   D. insomnia and anxiety

10. Which of the following is the cure for schizophrenia?

    A. lithium

    B. chlorpromazine

    C. benzodiazepine

    D. no cure

Matching

_____1. Involved in the facilitation of learning and memory

_____2. Plays a major role in cognitive function and memory function

_____3. Involved in behavior and emesis

_____4. Formed from the excitatory neurotransmitter glutamate

_____5. Principally involved in the regulation of sleep

A. dopamine

B. serotonin

C. GABA

D. acetylcholine

E. glutamate

Fill in the Blank

1. Serotonin is also known as 5-hydroxytryptamine or _____.

2. Antipsychotic drugs are also called _____drugs.

3. Schizophrenia is one of the most devastating forms of _____.

4. Lithium is used for managing _____disorders.

5. Bipolar disorder was formerly known as _____illness.

6. The principal mood stabilizer is _____.

7. SSRIs are now considered the first-line drugs in the treatment of_____.

Critical Thinking

A 45-year-old woman has been diagnosed with major depression based on biological factors and personal characteristics. Her physician has several options for prescribing the best drugs to treat her. These are TCAs, SSRIs, MAOIs, and atypical antidepressants.

1. Which of these classes of antidepressants is the drug of choice?

2. Which of these classes of drugs are the newest types of antidepressants?

3. If the patient is taking MAOIs, which type of foods would be contraindicated?

Drug Therapy for the Nervous System: Antianxiety and Hypnotic Drugs

OBJECTIVES

After completing this chapter, the reader should be able to:

1. Identify the major classifications of anxiety disorders.
2. Describe the difference between a sedative or anxiolytic and a hypnotic.
3. Identify the various types of anxiolytics and hypnotics.
4. Explain the problems associated with anxiolytics and hypnotics.
5. List four benzodiazepine-like drugs and their mechanisms of action.
6. Discuss the therapeutic effects and adverse effects of the major barbiturates.
7. Explain miscellaneous drugs that are used for insomnia.
8. Differentiate between obsessive-compulsive disorder and social anxiety disorder.

GLOSSARY

Antianxiety agents – drugs that relieve anxiety; also known as *anxiolytics*

Anxiety – a state of apprehension and autonomic nervous system activation resulting from exposure to a nonspecific or unknown cause

Anxiolytics – drugs that relieve anxiety; also known as *antianxiety agents*

Compulsion – a ritualized behavior or mental act that a patient is driven to perform in response to his or her obsessions

Barbiturates – drugs that depress multiple aspects of central nervous system function and can be used for sleep, seizures, and general anesthesia

Benzodiazepines – drugs of first choice for treating anxiety and insomnia

Buspirone – an anxiolytic drug that differs significantly from the benzodiazepines

Generalized anxiety disorder – difficult-to-control, excessive anxiety that lasts six months or more

Hypnotics – drugs given to promote sleep

Insomnia – the inability to fall asleep or stay asleep

Melatonin – an important hormone secreted from the pineal gland that is believed to induce sleep

Obsession – a recurrent, persistent thought, impulse, or mental image that is unwanted and distressing, and comes involuntarily to mind despite attempts to ignore or suppress it

Obsessive-compulsive disorder – anxiety characterized by recurrent, repetitive behaviors that interfere with normal activities or relationships

Panic attacks – sudden-onset, intense episodes that may include trembling, shortness of breath, heart palpitations, chest pain (or chest tightness), sweating, nausea, dizziness (or slight vertigo), light-headedness, hyperventilation, paresthesias (tingling sensations), and sensations of choking or smothering

Panic disorder – anxiety characterized by recurrent, intensely uncomfortable episodes known as panic attacks

Post-traumatic stress disorder – anxiety that develops following a traumatic event that elicited an immediate reaction of fear, helplessness, and horror

Sedative-hypnotics – drugs that when given in lower doses, produce a calming effect, and when given in higher doses, produce sleep

Social anxiety disorder – an intense, irrational fear of situations in which one might be scrutinized by others, or might do something that is embarrassing or humiliating; also known as *social phobia*

Social phobia – an intense, irrational fear of situations in which one might be scrutinized by others, or might do something that is embarrassing or humiliating; also known as *social anxiety disorder*

OVERVIEW

Medical Terminology Review

preanesthetic
pre- = before
an- = without, not
-esthesi/o = feeling, sensation
-tic = pertaining to
a drug administered before an anesthetic

Anxiety disorders are common occurrences in society today. These disorders can prove stressful and disruptive to those suffering from them. There are a variety of anxiety disorders for which drug therapy may be therapeutic. Antianxiety drugs or hypnotics are the most common classifications of medications that may be used to treat these disorders.

Sleep disturbances are also extremely common. If chronic, they have the potential to seriously disrupt normal day-to-day living. Many people suffering from a sleep disorder want to turn to drugs to solve their problem. The use of drugs in many of these situations is usually undesirable.

Many of the medications discussed in this chapter are also administered as muscle relaxants, preanesthetic medications, anticonvulsants, and therapeutic aids in psychiatry.

ANXIETY

According to the Anxiety Disorders Association of America, anxiety disorders are the most common psychiatric illnesses in the United States, affecting 40 million people, with a higher incidence in women than in men. **Anxiety** is an uncomfortable state that has both psychological and physical components. The psychological component can be characterized by fear, apprehension, dread, and uneasiness. The physical component may cause tachycardia, palpitations, trembling, dry mouth, sweating, weakness, fatigue, and shortness of breath. Fortunately, anxiety disorders respond well to treatment with behavior therapy, psychotherapy, or drug therapy.

Anxiety disorders may be classified as generalized anxiety disorder, panic disorder, obsessive-compulsive disorder, social anxiety disorder, or post-traumatic stress disorder. Brief explanations of the different types of anxiety follow.

Medical Terminology Review

tachycardia
tachy- = fast, rapid
cardia = the heart
rapid heart beat

Generalized Anxiety Disorder

Generalized anxiety disorder is a chronic condition characterized by uncontrollable worrying. Most patients with generalized anxiety disorder also have another psychiatric disorder, usually depression. The hallmark of this disorder is unrealistic or excessive anxiety about several events or activities (e.g., work or school performance). Generalized anxiety disorder may last for six months or longer.

Panic Disorder

Panic disorder is characterized by recurrent, intensely uncomfortable episodes known as **panic attacks. Panic attacks** have a sudden onset, reaching peak intensity within ten minutes. Symptoms may include trembling, shortness of breath, heart palpitations, chest pain (or chest tightness), sweating, nausea, dizziness (or slight vertigo), light-headedness, hyperventilation, paresthesias (tingling sensations), and sensations of choking or smothering. These symptoms typically disappear within 30 minutes. Many patients go to an emergency department because they think they are having a heart attack. Some patients experience panic attacks daily; others have only one or two per month. According to the *American Journal of Psychiatry,* the incidence of panic disorders in women is two to three times than seen in men. Onset of panic disorder usually occurs in the late teens or early twenties.

Obsessive-Compulsive Disorder

Obsessive-compulsive disorder is a potentially disabling condition characterized by persistent obsessions and compulsions that cause marked distress, consume at least one hour per day, and significantly interfere with daily living. An **obsession** is defined as a recurrent, persistent thought, impulse, or mental image that is unwanted and distressing, and comes involuntarily to mind despite attempts to ignore or suppress it. A **compulsion** is a ritualized behavior or mental act that a person is driven to perform in response to his or her obsessions.

Social Anxiety Disorder

Social anxiety disorder, formerly known as **social phobia**, is characterized by an intense, irrational fear of situations in which one might be scrutinized by others, or might do something that is embarrassing or humiliating. Exposure to the feared situation almost always elicits anxiety. As a result, the person avoids the situation, or, if it cannot be avoided, endures it with intense anxiety. Manifestations include blushing, stuttering, sweating, palpitations, dry throat, and muscle tension.

Social anxiety disorder is one of the most common psychiatric disorders and the most common anxiety disorder. This disorder typically begins during the teenage years and, if left untreated, is likely to be lifelong.

Post-Traumatic Stress Disorder

Post-traumatic stress disorder develops following a traumatic event that elicited an immediate reaction of fear, helplessness, or horror. It is more common in women than in men and is the fourth most common psychiatric disorder. Traumatic events that involve interpersonal violence (e.g., assault, rape, or torture) are more likely to cause post-traumatic stress disorder than are traumatic events that do not (e.g., car accidents or natural disasters).

SLEEP DISORDERS

Medical
Terminology
Review

insomnia
in- = lack of
-somnia = ability to sleep
lacking the ability to sleep

Insomnia is the inability to fall asleep or stay asleep. Difficulty in falling asleep or disturbed sleep patterns both result in insufficient sleep. Sleep disorders are common and may be short in duration or longstanding. They may have little or no apparent relationship to other immediate disorders. Sleep disorders can be secondary to emotional problems, pain, physical disorders, and the use or withdrawal of drugs. Excess alcohol consumed in the evening can shorten sleep and lead to withdrawal effects in the early morning.

SEDATIVES AND HYPNOTICS

The **sedative-hypnotics** are agents that depress central nervous system (CNS) function. These drugs are widely used primarily to treat anxiety and insomnia. Agents given to relieve anxiety are known as **antianxiety agents** or **anxiolytics**. They were previously known as tranquilizers. Drugs given to promote sleep are known as **hypnotics**. The distinction between antianxiety and hypnotic effects is often a matter of dosage. Sedative-hypnotics relieve anxiety in low doses and induce sleep in higher doses. Therefore, a single drug may be considered both an antianxiety agent and a hypnotic agent, depending upon the reason for its use and the dosage employed.

Sedative-hypnotic drugs include barbiturates, benzodiazepines, and benzodiazepine-like drugs. Anxiety and insomnia are treated primarily with the benzodiazepines. Benzodiazepines are used primarily for one condition (generalized anxiety disorder). In contrast, the selective serotonin reuptake inhibitors (SSRIs) are now used for all anxiety disorders. It should be noted that, although SSRIs were developed as antidepressants, they are highly effective against anxiety (with or without depression). SSRIs are discussed in Chapter 5. Table 6-1 shows the first-line drugs that are used for specific anxiety disorders. Table 6-2 shows sedative-hypnotics, including barbiturates, benzodiazepines, and miscellaneous agents used to treat anxiety and insomnia.

TABLE 6-1	First-Line Drugs for Anxiety Disorders		
Type of Anxiety Disorder	**Benzodiazepines (all are Schedule C-IV)**	**SSRIs**	**Others**
Generalized Anxiety Disorder	alprazolam (C-IV) **(al-PRAY-zoh-lam)**	escitalopram (Rx) **(ee-sih-TAH-loh-pram)**	buspirone (Rx) **(byoo-SPY-rohn)**
	chlordiazepoxide (C-IV) **(klor-dy-ah-zeh-POK-syd)**	paroxetine (Rx) **(pah-ROK-seh-teen)**	venlafaxine (Rx) **(ven-lah-FAK-seen)**
	clorazepate (C-IV) **(klo-RAH-zeh-payt)**		

Table 6-1 continued

	diazepam (C-IV) **(dy-AH-zeh-pam)**		
	lorazepam (C-IV) **(loh-RAH-zeh-pam)**		
	oxazepam (C-IV) **(ok-ZAH-zeh-pam)**		
Panic Disorder	alprazolam (C-IV) **(al-PRAY-zoh-lam)**	paroxetine (Rx) **(pah-ROK-seh-teen)**	
	clonazepam (C-IV) **(klo-NAH-zeh-pam)**	sertraline (Rx) **(SER-trah-leen)**	
	lorazepam (C-IV) **(loh-RAH-zeh-pam)**		
Obsessive-Compulsive Disorder		citalopram (Rx) **(sy-TAH-loh-pram)**	
		escitalopram (Rx) **(ee-sih-TAH-loh-pram)**	
		fluoxetine (Rx) **(floo-OK-seh-teen)**	
		fluvoxamine (Rx) **(floo-VOK-sah-meen)**	
		paroxetine (Rx) **(pah-ROK-seh-teen)**	
		sertraline (Rx) **(SER-trah-leen)**	
Post-Traumatic Stress Disorder		paroxetine (Rx) **(pah-ROK-seh-teen)**	
		sertraline (Rx) **(SER-trah-leen)**	

TABLE 6-2	**Drugs for Anxiety and Insomnia**		
Generic Name	**Trade Name**	**Route of Administration**	**Average Adult Dosage**
Barbiturates (Short-Acting) (both are Schedule C-II)			
pentobarbital **(pen-toh-BAR-bih-tal)**	Nembutal®	PO	Sedative: 20–30 mg bid
			Hypnotic: 120–200 mg/day
secobarbital **(say-koh-BAR-bih-tal)**	Seconal®	PO	Sedative: 100–300 mg/day in 3 divided doses
			Hypnotic: 100–200 mg/day

continued on next page

Table 6-2 continued

(Intermediate-Acting) (either Schedule C-II or C-III)			
amobarbital (C-II) **(ah-moh-BAR-bih-tal)**	Amytal®	PO	Sedative: 30–50 mg bid–tid
			Hypnotic: 65–200 mg (max: 500 mg/day)
			Hypnotic: 40–160 mg/day
butabarbital (C-III) **(byoo-tah-BAR-bih-tal)**	Butisol®	PO	Sedative: 15–30 mg tid–qid
			Hypnotic: 50–100 mg hs
(Long-Acting) (both are Schedule C-IV)			
mephobarbital **(meh-foh-BAR-bih-tal)**	Mebaral®	PO	Sedative: 32–100 mg tid
phenobarbital **(fee-noh-BAR-bih-tal)**	Luminal®	PO	Sedative: 30–120 mg/day
Benzodiazepines (all are Schedule C-IV)			
alprazolam **(al-PRAY-zoh-lam)**	Xanax®	PO	0.25–2 mg tid
chlordiazepoxide **(klor-dy-ah-zeh-POK-syd)**	Librium®	PO	5–25 mg tid–qid
clonazepam **(kloh-NAH-zeh-pam)**	Klonopin®	PO	1–2 mg/day in divided doses (max: 4 mg/day)
clorazepate **(kloh-RAH-zeh-payt)**	Tranxene®	PO	7.5–30 mg/day in divided doses (max: 60 mg/day)
diazepam **(dy-AH-zeh-pam)**	Valium®	PO	2–10 mg bid–qid
estazolam **(eh-STAH-zoh-lam)**	ProSom®	PO	1 mg hs (max: 2 mg prn)
flurazepam **(floo-RAH-zeh-pam)**	Dalmane®	PO	15–30 mg hs
lorazepam **(loh-RAH-zeh-pam)**	Ativan®	PO	1–3 mg bid–tid
midazolam **(mih-DAH-zoh-lam)**	Midazolam Injection®	IM, IV	IM: 0.07–0.08 mg/kg; IV: 1–2.5 mg over 2 min – *Black Box Warning 1*
oxazepam **(ok-ZAH-zeh-pam)**	Serax®	PO	10–30 mg tid–qid
quazepam **(KWAY-zeh-pam)**	Doral®	PO	7.5–15 mg hs
temazepam **(teh-MAH-zeh-pam)**	Restoril®	PO	15 mg hs
triazolam **(try-AH-zoh-lam)**	Halcion®	PO	0.125–0.25 mg hs (max: 0.5 mg/day)

Table 6-2 continued

Benzodiazepine-Like Drugs			
eszopiclone (Rx) **(eh-soh-PIH-klohn)**	Lunesta®	PO	2–3 mg hs
ramelteon (Rx) **(rah-MEL-tee-on)**	Rozerem®	PO	8 mg within 30 min of hs
zaleplon (C-IV) **(ZAH-leh-plon)**	Sonata®	PO	5–10 mg hs
zolpidem (C-IV) **(ZOL-pih-dem)**	Ambien®	PO	10 mg hs
Miscellaneous Drugs: Antiseizure Medication			
valproic acid (Rx), (divalproex sodium, sodium valproate) **(val-PROH-ik AH-sid)** **(dy-val-PROH-eks SOH-** **dee-um) (SOH-dee-um** **val-PROH-ayt)**	Depakote®, Depakene®, Depacon®	PO PO PO	250 mg tid (max: 60 mg/kg/day)
Special Anxiolytic (Azaspirodecanedione)*			
buspirone (Rx) **(byoo-SPY-rohn)**	BuSpar®	PO	7.5–15 mg in divided doses (max: 60 mg/day)
Beta-Blockers (rarely indicated for treatment of anxiety)			
atenolol (Rx) **(ah-TEH-noh-lol)**	Tenormin®	PO	25–100 mg once daily
propranolol (Rx) **(proh-PRAH-noh-lol)**	Inderal®	PO	40 mg bid (max: 320 mg/day)

*NOTE: Buspirone has an extremely complex mechanism of action in comparison to the other drugs in this table, and therefore, this separate classification.

Black Box Warning 1 – Associated with respiratory depression and respiratory arrest, especially when used for sedation in noncritical care settings.

Benzodiazepines

Benzodiazepines are the drugs of first choice for treating anxiety and insomnia. The popularity of the benzodiazepines as sedatives and hypnotics stems from their clear superiority over the alternatives, such as barbiturates and other general CNS depressants. The benzodiazepines are safer than the general CNS depressants and have a lower potential for abuse. Note that all benzodiazepines are Schedule IV controlled substances.

Mechanism of Action

The mechanism of action of benzodiazepines on the CNS appears to be closely related to their ability to potentiate GABA (gamma-aminobutyric acid)-mediated neural inhibition. Recent research has identified specific

Key Concept

Elderly patients need smaller doses of hypnotics because, in some instances, a sedative dose may produce sleep.

binding sites for benzodiazepines in the CNS, and has established the close relationship between the sites of action of the benzodiazepines and GABA.

Indications

Benzodiazepines are useful for the short-term treatment of panic disorder, generalized anxiety, phobias, and insomnia. Chlordiazepoxide (Librium) and diazepam (Valium) are among the most widely prescribed benzodiazepines. The benzodiazepines are categorized as Schedule IV drugs. Benzodiazepines are also used in absence seizures and myoclonic seizures. Parenteral diazepam is used to terminate status epilepticus.

Adverse Effects

Adverse effects of benzodiazepines include drowsiness, ataxia, impaired judgment, dry mouth, fatigue, visual disturbances, rebound insomnia, and development of tolerance. The use of any of the benzodiazepines during pregnancy is likely to cause fetal abnormalities. Although benzodiazepines produce considerably less physical dependence and result in less tolerance than barbiturates, overdosage may result in CNS and respiratory depression as well as hypotension and coma. Gradual withdrawal of these drugs is recommended.

Contraindications and Precautions

Benzodiazepines are contraindicated in patients with known hypersensitivity to the drugs. They are also contraindicated in patients with acute narrow-angle glaucoma, psychosis, liver or kidney disease, and neurological disorders.

Benzodiazepines should be used cautiously during pregnancy (category D), and in elderly or debilitated patients. The use of flurazepam is entirely contraindicated during pregnancy.

Drug Interactions

Benzodiazepines increase CNS depression with alcohol and omeprazole. They also increase pharmacological effects if combined with cimetidine, disulfiram, or hormonal contraceptives. The effects of benzodiazepines decrease when given with theophyllines and ranitidine.

Benzodiazepine-Like Drugs

Nonbenzodiazepines have become quite popular as sleep aids. They are not indicated for anxiety (see Table 6-2).

Mechanism of Action

Benzodiazepine-like drugs are structurally different from the benzodiazepines, but nonetheless share the same mechanism of action. They all act as agonists at the benzodiazepine receptor site on the GABA receptor-chloride channel complex. These drugs are highly effective hypnotics and have a low potential for tolerance, dependence, or abuse. Ramelteon has a unique mechanism of action that activates the **melatonin receptors**.

Medical Terminology
Review

ataxia
a- = without, not
tax/o = order
-ia = condition
without muscular coordination

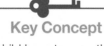
Key Concept
A child born to a mother taking benzodiazepines can develop withdrawal symptoms after birth.

Indications

Benzodiazepine-like drugs, especially zolpidem (Ambien), and the *special anxiolytic* called buspirone (BuSpar), are widely used for sleep disorders and anxiety. Buspirone is discussed in detail later in this chapter. Benzodiazepine-like drugs are approved only for short-term management of insomnia, except eszopiclone, which was approved by the FDA in 2005 with no limitation on how long it can be used. Ramelteon is approved for treating chronic insomnia, and long-term use is permitted.

Adverse Effects

Zolpidem has adverse effects similar to those of benzodiazepines. Daytime drowsiness and dizziness are the most common, and these occur in only 1% to 2% of patients. At therapeutic doses, benzodiazepine-like drugs cause little or no respiratory depression. Safety during pregnancy has not been established.

Zaleplon and eszopiclone are well tolerated. The most common side effects are headache, nausea, drowsiness, dizziness, myalgia, and abdominal pain.

Ramelteon can increase levels of prolactin and reduce levels of testosterone. As a result, the drug has the potential to cause galactorrhea, amenorrhea, reduced libido, and fertility problems.

Contraindications and Precautions

Benzodiazepine-like drugs are contraindicated in patients with a known hypersensitivity, acute narrow-angle glaucoma, shock, and psychoses. These drugs are also contraindicated in patients with acute alcoholic intoxication or depressed vital signs, and in comatose patients.

Benzodiazepine-like agents are contraindicated in patients during pregnancy (category B), and the drug metabolite freely crosses the placenta. These drugs are used with caution in patients who have impaired liver or kidney function, and in the elderly.

Drug Interactions

Benzodiazepine-like drugs cause less additive CNS depression than other antianxiety drugs but should still be avoided with concurrent use of a CNS depressant. Buspirone may increase serum digoxin levels, increasing the risk of digitalis toxicity.

Barbiturates

The **barbiturates** depress multiple aspects of CNS function and can be used for sleep, seizures, and general anesthesia. Barbiturates cause tolerance and dependence, have high abuse potential, and are subject to multiple drug interactions. Moreover, barbiturates are powerful respiratory depressants that can be fatal in overdose. Because of these undesirable properties, barbiturates are used much less often today than in the past, having been replaced by newer and safer drugs—primarily the benzodiazepines and benzodiazepine-like

---

Key Concept

Ramelteon is the only sedative-hypnotic not regulated as a controlled substance.

Medical Terminology Review

myalgia
my/o- = muscle
-algia = pain
muscle pain

Medical Terminology Review

metabolite
metabol- = metabolism
-ite = produced substance
substance produced through metabolism

drugs. However, although their use has declined greatly, barbiturates still have important applications in seizure control and anesthesia.

Mechanism of Action

All barbiturates exert a depressant effect on the CNS. These drugs act by changing the action of GABA, the primary inhibitory neurotransmitter in the brain. Barbiturates mimic the effects of GABA by stimulating an influx of chloride ions that interact with the GABA receptor through chloride channel molecules. When the receptors of barbiturate are stimulated, chloride ions move into the cells, therefore suppressing the ability of neurons to fire.

Indications

Barbiturates are used as sedatives and as hypnotics (short term, up to two weeks) for insomnia. Long-term treatment with certain barbiturates is prescribed for generalized tonic-clonic and cortical focal seizures. They are also indicated for emergency control of some acute convulsive episodes such as occur in status epilepticus, eclampsia, meningitis, tetanus, and toxic reactions to local anesthetics. Thiopental and other highly lipid-soluble barbiturates are given to induce general anesthesia. Unconsciousness develops within seconds of intravenous injections. After prolonged use of barbiturates, withdrawal symptoms may occur.

Phenobarbital and mephobarbital are used for seizure disorders, congenital hyperbilirubinemia, and neonatal jaundice. Indications for intermediate-acting barbiturates are regional anesthesia, sedation, and hypnosis. Ultra-short-acting barbiturates are used for intravenous general anesthesia.

Adverse Effects

Barbiturates may cause numerous adverse effects on several different body systems. The manifestations of adverse effects include ataxia, drowsiness, dizziness, and hangover effect. Some patients may have nausea and vomiting, insomnia, constipation, headache, night terrors, and faintness. Long-term use of barbiturates may cause bone pain, anorexia, muscle pain, and weight loss.

Contraindications and Precautions

Barbiturates are contraindicated in patients with known hypersensitivity to these agents, pregnancy (category D), or lactation. Barbiturates are also contraindicated in parturition, fetal immaturity, and uncontrolled pain.

Barbiturates should be used cautiously in patients with liver or kidney impairments and in those with neurological disorders. These drugs are used with caution in patients with pulmonary disorders and in hyperactive children.

Drug Interactions

Barbiturates increase serum levels and therapeutic and toxic effects when given with valproic acid. They also increase CNS depression with alcohol, narcotic analgesics, and antidepressants. Barbiturates decrease effects of the following drugs: theophyllines, oral anticoagulants, beta-blockers, doxycycline, griseofulvin, corticosteroids, hormonal contraceptives, and metronidazole.

Miscellaneous Drugs

Several CNS drugs used for anxiety and insomnia are categorized as miscellaneous drugs. These agents are chemically unrelated to the benzodiazepines, benzodiazepine-like drugs, or barbiturates.

The antiseizure drug valproic acid (see Chapter 9), the beta-blockers atenolol and propranolol (see Chapter 12), and the CNS depressant buspirone are also used for anxiety or sleep disorders (see Table 6-2). Buspirone is unique and is commonly prescribed for its antianxiety effects.

Buspirone

Buspirone (BuSpar) is an anxiolytic drug that differs significantly from the benzodiazepines. Buspirone is as effective as the benzodiazepines and has three distinct advantages:

- It does not cause sedation
- It has no abuse potential
- It does not intensify the effects of CNS depressants

Mechanism of Action The anxiolytic effect of buspirone is mainly on the brain's D_2-dopamine receptors. It has agonist effects on presynaptic dopamine receptors. It also has a high affinity for serotonin receptors.

Indications Buspirone is prescribed for management of anxiety disorders and for short-term treatment of generalized anxiety.

Adverse Effects Buspirone is generally well tolerated. The most common reactions are dizziness, nausea, headache, nervousness, lightheadedness, and excitement. The drug is nonsedating and does not interfere with daytime activities.

Contraindications and Precautions Buspirone is contraindicated in patients with known hypersensitivity to this medication. It is also contraindicated with concomitant use of alcohol because of rare fatalities that have occurred, though the exact reason for this is not fully understood. Safety during pregnancy (category B), labor, delivery, lactation, and in children younger than 18 years is not established. Buspirone should be used with caution in patients with moderate to severe renal or hepatic impairment.

Drug Interactions Blood levels of buspirone can be greatly increased by erythromycin and ketoconazole. Levels of buspirone can also be increased by grapefruit juice. Buspirone does not enhance the depressant effects of alcohol, barbiturates, and other general CNS depressants. However, since rare fatalities have occurred when buspirone was combined with alcohol, concurrent use is contraindicated.

SUMMARY

Sedatives affect the CNS, which can relieve anxiety; hence they are often called anxiolytics. Hypnotic is the term used to describe a substance that induces sleep. Both anxiety and insomnia are extremely common in the United States.

There are three major groups of anxiolytics and hypnotics: barbiturates, benzodiazepines, and benzodiazepine-like drugs. Benzodiazepines act on the GABA receptor complex. These drugs are relatively nontoxic, but can have several undesirable adverse effects. With most anxiolytics, the antianxiety effect is related to their sedative effect. The use of barbiturates as hypnotics is no longer advised, and they are gradually being phased out from use. Their major use today is in the treatment of epilepsy, and as anesthetics. Hypnotic drugs should be used for short-term therapy only.

Nonbenzodiazepine drugs have become very popular as sleep aids. They are not indicated for anxiety use. Benzodiazepine-like drugs are structurally different from the benzodiazepines, but their mechanism of action is the same. Nonbenzodiazepine drugs, especially zolpidem and buspirone, are widely used for anxiety and sleep disorders.

Miscellaneous drugs that are used for anxiety and insomnia are chemically unrelated to either benzodiazepines or barbiturates. These agents include antiseizure drugs (valproic acid) and beta-blockers (atenolol and propranolol).

EXPLORING THE WEB

Visit **www.medicinenet.com**

- Search using the term *post-traumatic stress disorder*. Review relevant articles related to the treatment of this disorder.

Visit **www.nlm.nih.gov**

- Choose one of the disorders discussed in this chapter and research the treatments used to address the disorder.

Visit **www.justice.gov**

- Search using the term *benzodiazepines*. Look for information published by the Drug Enforcement Administration on this drug. What are the concerns with use of this drug? What is the potential for abuse?

REVIEW QUESTIONS

Multiple Choice

1. Which of the following are the first-line drugs used in the treatment of anxiety and insomnia?

   A. benzodiazepines and barbiturates

   B. benzodiazepines and SSRIs

   C. benzodiazepines and MAOIs

   D. benzodiazepines and chloral hydrate

2. Which of the following is the main concern for a patient who stops taking barbiturates suddenly?

   A. shock

   B. hypotension

   C. severe withdrawal

   D. respiratory depression

3. Which of the following may increase the effects of sedatives?

   A. chocolate

   B. cheese

   C. nicotine

   D. alcohol

4. Benzodiazepines act by binding to the GABA receptor of which of the following channel molecules?

   A. chloride

   B. sodium

   C. potassium

   D. calcium

5. Generalized anxiety disorder may last for:

   A. 3 weeks or less

   B. 6 weeks

   C. 3 months

   D. 6 months or more

6. Symptoms of panic disorder typically disappear within:

   A. 30 seconds

   B. 30 minutes

   C. 30 days

   D. 90 days

7. Benzodiazepine-like drugs are the preferred agents for treating:

   A. insomnia

   B. depression

   C. panic disorder

   D. obsessive-compulsive disorder

8. Which of the following benzodiazepine-like drugs may increase levels of prolactin and reduce levels of testosterone?

   A. ramelteon

   B. zolpidem

   C. zaleplon

   D. all of the above

9. The newest drugs used for anxiety and sleep disorders include which of the following?

   A. Nembutal® and Depakote®

   B. Seconal® and Inderal®

   C. Amytal® and Mebaral®

   D. ProSom® and Ambien®

10. Adverse effects of zolpidem (Ambien®) are similar to which of the following?

   A. antihypertensives

   B. barbiturates

   C. benzodiazepines

   D. beta-blockers

11. The indications for barbiturates have declined greatly, but they still have important applications in which of the following disorders or conditions?

   A. insomnia

   B. major depression

   C. anxiety

   D. anesthesia

12. Which of the following hormones is believed to induce sleep?

   A. prolactin

   B. thyroxin

   C. melanin

   D. melatonin

13. The trade name of diazepam is:

   A. Librium®

   B. Valium®

   C. Xanax®

   D. Serax®

14. The generic name of Luminal® is:

   A. butabarbital

   B. pentobarbital

   C. phenobarbital

   D. secobarbital

15. Long-term treatment with certain barbiturates is prescribed for which of the following disorders?

    A. insomnia

    B. anxiety attacks

    C. general anesthesia

    D. generalized tonic-clonic seizures

Fill in the Blank

1. Benzodiazepines are the drugs of first choice for treating _____ and _____.

2. Barbiturates cause tolerance and _____.

3. All barbiturates act by changing the action of _____.

4. Panic disorder is characterized by episodes known as _____.

5. The sedative-hypnotics are used primarily to treat _____ and _____.

6. Antianxiety agents were previously known as _____.

7. Barbiturates are contraindicated in pregnancy because they are in category _____.

Critical Thinking

Kaleen is a nurse who was assaulted by an unknown man on her way home from the hospital where she works. She was hospitalized for three weeks and developed post-traumatic stress disorder after approximately six months.

1. What would be the first-line drug for this condition?

2. If she also developed a panic disorder, does her physician have to change her medication or add other drugs to her regimen?

3. If her physician is prescribing the correct first-line drug, what would be the most severe adverse effect?

Drug Therapy for the Autonomic Nervous System

OBJECTIVES

After completing this chapter, the reader should be able to:

1. Describe the subdivisions of the autonomic nervous system (ANS).
2. Explain the various types of receptors.
3. Differentiate sympathomimetics from sympatholytic agents and give two examples for each.
4. Outline five beta$_2$-adrenergic drugs.
5. Explain the action of adrenergic blockers.
6. Describe the use of cholinergic agonist drugs.
7. Differentiate between cholinergics and cholinergic blockers.
8. Explain the major adverse effects of anticholinergic drugs.
9. Explain the contraindications of cholinergic blockers.
10. List three neurotransmitters that employ the ANS.

GLOSSARY

Adrenergic blocker agents – drugs that antagonize the secretion of epinephrine and norepinephrine from sympathetic terminal neurons; also known as *sympatholytics*

Adrenergic receptors – receptors that mediate responses to epinephrine (adrenaline) and norepinephrine

Alpha-receptor – an adrenergic receptor; there are two types: alpha$_1$ and alpha$_2$

Beta-receptor – an adrenergic receptor; there are two types: beta$_1$ and beta$_2$

Catecholamines – a group of chemically related compounds having a sympathomimetic action

Cholinergic receptors – receptors that mediate responses to acetylcholine

Congenital megacolon – congenital dilation and hypertrophy of the colon due to reduction in motor neurons of the parasympathetic nervous system, resulting in extreme constipation, and if untreated, growth retardation; also known as *Hirschsprung's disease*

Cycloplegia – paralysis of the ciliary muscles of the eye, resulting in loss of visual accommodation

Dopamine receptor – an adrenergic receptor

Epinephrine – produced by the medulla of the adrenal glands, and often called the "fight or flight" hormone because it is released when danger threatens

Iritis – inflammation of the iris

Miosis – contraction of the pupil of the eye

Mydriasis – dilation of the pupil

Necrosis – death of a group of cells or tissues

Parasympathomimetic – producing effects similar to those produced when a parasympathetic nerve is stimulated

Pheochromocytoma – a vascular tumor of chromaffin tissue of the adrenal medulla or sympathetic preganglia, characterized by hypersecretion of epinephrine and norepinephrine, causing persistent hypertension. Only a small percentage of the lesions are malignant.

Somnolence – prolonged drowsiness that may last hours to days

Sympatholytic – inhibiting or opposing adrenergic nerve function; sympatholytic agents are also known as *adrenergic blocker agents*

Sympathomimetic – adrenergic, or producing an effect similar to that obtained by stimulation of the sympathetic nervous system

Uveitis – inflammation of the uvea (the vascular middle layer of the eye, including the iris, ciliary body, and choroid)

OVERVIEW

The peripheral nervous system regulates both voluntary and involuntary functions in the human body. This chapter focuses on drugs that are used to regulate and control disorders of the involuntary functions. The therapeutic agents discussed here are used to treat many disorders and conditions such as hypertension, hypotension, asthma, dysrhythmia, glaucoma, and even runny nose.

ANATOMY REVIEW

- The peripheral nervous system has two divisions: the somatic nervous system (SNS) and the autonomic nervous system (ANS) (Figure 7-1).

- The SNS regulates voluntary or conscious functions such as motor movement.

- The ANS regulates all involuntary functions such as secretion of hormones; contraction of the heart muscle, blood vessels, and bronchioles; and the ability to move substances through the digestive tract.

- The ANS can be further divided into the sympathetic and parasympathetic nervous systems (PNS) (Figures 7-2 and 7-3).

- These divisions work antagonistically; for example, activation of the sympathetic division will increase heart rate while activation of the parasympathetic division will decrease it.

- The sympathetic division responds in emergencies or during stressful situations and is called the fight-or-flight response.

- The parasympathetic division responds as a restorative function and is called the rest-and-digest response.

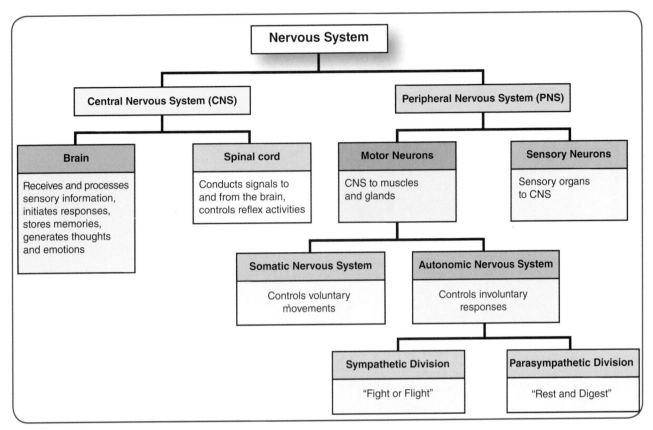

Figure 7-1 Divisions of the nervous system.

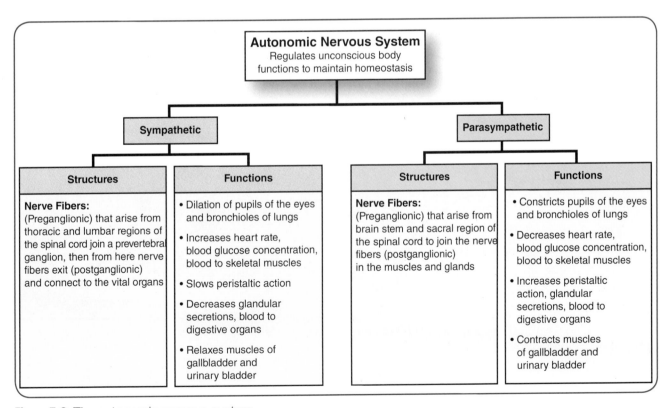

Figure 7-2 The autonomic nervous system.

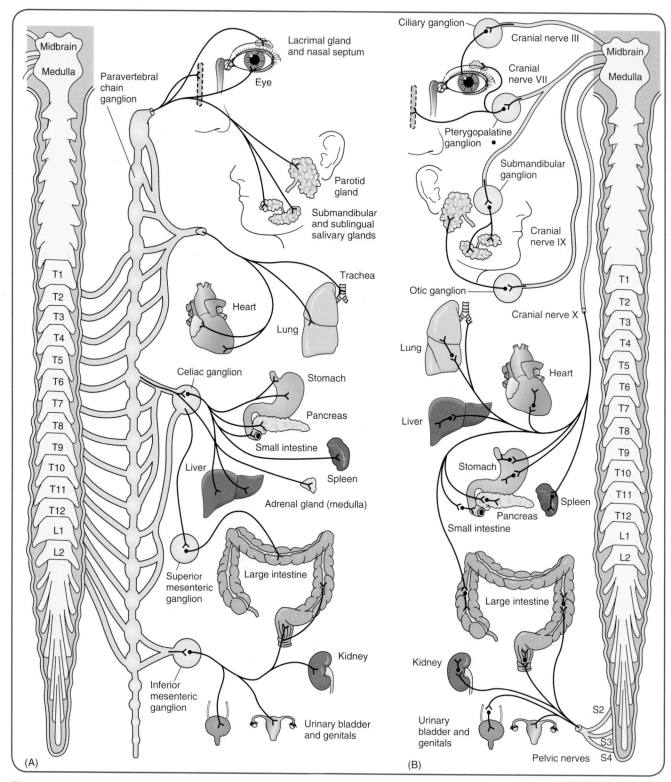

Figure 7-3 (A) The sympathetic division of the autonomic nervous system. (B) The parasympathetic division of the autonomic nervous system.

NEUROTRANSMITTERS ASSOCIATED WITH THE AUTONOMIC NERVOUS SYSTEM

Previous chapters discussed the role of altered neurotransmitter production and function in psychiatric illnesses and the treatments of these illnesses. This chapter focuses on the role of these important biochemicals in the involuntary body functions regulated by the ANS. The three main neurotransmitters discussed are acetylcholine, norepinephrine, and epinephrine. Any given junction in the ANS uses only one of these transmitter substances. A fourth compound, dopamine, may also serve as a transmitter, but this role has not been demonstrated conclusively.

In order to understand the mechanism of action of drugs that act upon these neurotransmitters, it is necessary to know the identity of the transmitter employed at each of the junctions of the ANS (Figure 7-4).

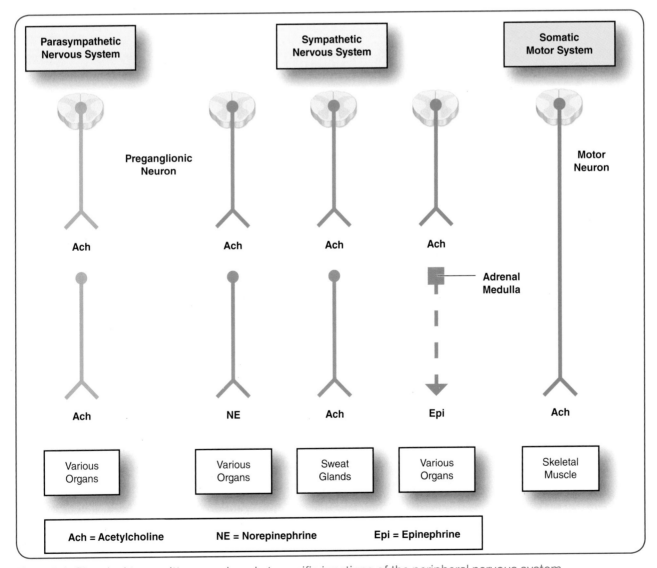

Figure 7-4 Chemical transmitters employed at specific junctions of the peripheral nervous system.

Acetylcholine is the chemical transmitter employed at most junctions of the ANS as well as at the skeletal muscles. Acetylcholine is the transmitter released by:

1. All preganglionic neurons of the PNS
2. All preganglionic neurons of the SNS
3. All postganglionic neurons of the PNS
4. Most postganglionic neurons of the SNS that go to sweat glands
5. All motor neurons to skeletal muscles

Norepinephrine is the chemical transmitter released by all postganglionic neurons of the SNS. It is also referred to as "noradrenaline." The only exceptions are the postganglionic sympathetic neurons that go to sweat glands, which employ acetylcholine as their transmitter. **Epinephrine** is a major transmitter released by the adrenal medulla, and is also referred to as "adrenaline."

RECEPTORS

The PNS and ANS work through various types of receptors. Understanding these receptors is essential to understanding nervous system pharmacology.

There are two basic types of receptors associated with the PNS: cholinergic and adrenergic receptors. Each of these receptors is divided into different subtypes. Activation of each subtype of these receptors causes a characteristic set of physiological responses. Some drugs affect all receptor subtypes while others only affect one type of receptor. Different doses of a drug may activate one type of receptor, while increased doses may activate other receptor subtypes. It is important to memorize the various receptor types and their responses.

Cholinergic Receptors

Cholinergic receptors are defined as receptors that mediate responses to acetylcholine. These receptors mediate responses at all junctions where acetylcholine is the transmitter. There are three major subtypes of cholinergic receptors, which are referred to as nicotinic$_N$, nicotinic$_M$, and muscarinic.

Adrenergic Receptors

Adrenergic receptors are defined as receptors that mediate responses to epinephrine and norepinephrine. These receptors mediate responses at all junctions where norepinephrine or epinephrine is the transmitter. Adrenergic receptors are divided into two types: **alpha-receptors** (α-receptors) and **beta-receptors** (β-receptors). Alpha-receptors are divided into alpha$_1$ and alpha$_2$ receptors, and beta-receptors are divided into beta$_1$ and beta$_2$ receptors.

In addition to the four major subtypes of adrenergic receptors, there is another adrenergic receptor type, referred to as the **dopamine receptor**. Dopamine receptors respond only to dopamine, a neurotransmitter found

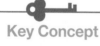

Key Concept

Although dopamine receptors are classified as adrenergic, these receptors do not respond to epinephrine or norepinephrine.

primarily in the CNS. Tables 7-1 and 7-2 summarize functions of cholinergic and adrenergic receptor subtypes.

TABLE 7-1	Cholinergic Receptor Subtype Functions	
Receptor Subtype	**Location**	**Response to Receptor Stimulation**
nicotinic$_N$	all autonomic nervous system ganglia and the adrenal medulla	stimulation of both parasympathetic and sympathetic postganglionic nerves and release of epinephrine from the adrenal medulla
nicotinic$_M$	neuromuscular junction	contraction of skeletal muscle
muscarinic	all parasympathetic target organs:	
	eyes	contraction of the ciliary muscle focuses the lens for near vision, and contraction of the iris sphincter muscle causes **miosis** (contraction of the pupil)
	heart	decreased rate
	lungs	constriction of bronchi and increased secretions
	GI tract	salivation, increased gastric secretions, increased intestinal tone and motility, defecation
	sweat glands	generalized sweating
	urinary bladder	increased bladder pressure, relaxation of smooth muscles and sphincter, allowing urine to leave the bladder
	sex organs	erection
	blood vessels	vasodilation

TABLE 7-2	Adrenergic Receptor Subtype Functions	
Receptor Subtype	**Location**	**Response to Receptor Stimulation**
alpha$_1$	pancreas	inhibition of insulin secretion
	blood vessels	constriction
	intestine, bladder	relaxation
alpha$_2$	presynaptic sympathetic nerve terminals	inhibition of norepinephrine release
beta$_1$	heart	increased rate and force of contraction
	kidneys	renin release
beta$_2$	arterioles of the heart	dilation
	bronchioles	dilation
	uterus	relaxation
	skeletal muscle	increased contraction
	liver	glycogenesis, gluconeogenesis
	pancreas	insulin secretion
dopamine	kidneys	dilation of kidney vasculature

DRUGS AFFECTING THE AUTONOMIC NERVOUS SYSTEM

Drugs that affect the ANS may be classified into four categories:

- Sympathomimetics (adrenergics)
- Sympatholytics (adrenergic blockers)
- Parasympathomimetics (cholinergics)
- Parasympatholytics (anticholinergics)

Sympathomimetics (Adrenergic Agonists)

Sympathomimetic agents are also called adrenergic agonists. These agents produce their effects by activating adrenergic receptors. Since the SNS acts through these same receptors, responses to adrenergic agonists and responses to stimulation of the SNS are very similar.

Adrenergic agonist drugs may affect both alpha- and beta-receptors. The classification seems confusing; therefore, the effects of adrenergic drugs on each receptor will be discussed separately. Selected adrenergic agonist drugs are listed in Table 7-3.

Mechanism of Action

Adrenergic drugs stimulate $alpha_1$, $beta_1$, and $beta_2$ receptor sites. The alpha-adrenergic receptor sites are located in the smooth muscle of blood vessels, the gastrointestinal tract, and the genitourinary tract. They produce vasoconstriction when stimulated by adrenergic drugs. The $beta_1$-adrenergic receptors are located in the heart muscle. When stimulated by adrenergic drugs, they produce increased contractility (resulting in increased heart rate).

Beta$_2$-adrenergic receptors in the respiratory system, located in the bronchial muscle, produce bronchodilation when stimulated by adrenergic agents.

Indications

Adrenergic agonist drugs that affect alpha-adrenergic receptors are used in patients with hypotension, hemostasis, to relieve nasal congestion, as adjuncts to local anesthesia (to reduce bleeding), and for dilation of the pupils (which facilitates eye examinations and ocular surgery). The beta-adrenergic drugs are used in the treatment of asthma and bronchitis.

Adverse Effects

All the adverse effects caused by $alpha_1$ activation result directly or indirectly from vasoconstriction. The most common adverse effects include hypertension, **necrosis** (death of a group of cells or tissues) if an intravenous line is employed to administer an $alpha_1$ agonist, and slowness of the heart rate.

TABLE 7-3   Sympathomimetics (Adrenergic Agonists)

Generic Name and Classification	Trade Name	Route of Administration	Average Adult Dosage
albuterol **(al-BYOO-teh-rol)** (beta$_2$)	Proventil®, Ventolin®	PO, Inhalation	PO: 2.4 mg 3–4 times daily; Inhalation: 1–2 inhalations q4–6h
dobutamine **(doh-BYOO-tah-meen)** (beta$_1$)	Dobutrex®	IV	2.5–10 mcg/kg/min
dopamine hydrochloride **(DOH-pah-meen hy-droh-KLOR -ryd)** (dopaminic$_1$, dopaminic$_2$, dopaminic$_3$, dopaminic$_4$, dopaminic$_5$)	Intropin®, Dopamine®	IV	2–5 mcg/kg/min
epinephrine **(eh-pih-NEH-frin)** (primarily beta$_2$, also beta$_1$)	EpiPen®, Primatene Mist Suspension ®	SC, Inhalation	SC: 0.1–0.5 mL of 1:1000 q10–15 min prn; Inhalation: 1 inhalation q4h prn
isoproterenol hydrochloride **(eye-soh-proh-TEH-reh-nol hy-droh-KLOR-ryd)** (beta$_1$)	Isuprel®	IV, Metered dose inhaler (MDI)	IV: 0.01–0.02 mg prn; MDI: 1–2 inhalations 4–6 times daily
metaproterenol sulfate **(meh-tah-proh-TEH-reh-nol SUL-fayt)** (beta$_2$)	Alupent®, Metaprel®	PO, MDI, Nebulizer	PO: 20 mg q6–8h; MDI: 2–3 inhalations q3–4h; Nebulizer: 5–10 inhalations
methyldopa **(meh-thil-DOH-pah)** (alpha$_2$)	Aldomet®	PO, IV	PO/IV: 250–500 mg bid or tid
norepinephrine bitartrate **(nor-eh-pih-NEH-frin by-TAR-trayt)** (alpha$_1$, alpha$_2$, beta$_1$)	Levarterenol®, Levophed®	IV	Initial: 8–12 mcg/min; Maint: 2–4 mcg/min
oxymetazoline **(ok-see-meh-TAH-zoh-lin)** (selective alpha$_1$ and partial alpha$_2$)	Afrin®	Intranasal	2–3 drops or 2–3 sprays of 0.05% solution bid
phenylephrine hydrochloride **(feh-nil-EH-freen hy-droh-K-LOR-ryd)** (alpha$_1$)	Neo-Synephrine®	IM, IV, SC	IM/SC: 1–10 mg q10–15 min prn; IV: 0.1–0.18 mg/min
pseudoephedrine hydrochloride **(soo-doh-eh-FEH-drin hy-droh-KLOR-ryd)** (all alpha, and also beta$_2$)	Sudafed®, Cenafed®	PO	60 mg q4–6h
salmeterol xinafoate **(sal-MEH-the-rol zih-NAH-foh-ayt)** (beta$_2$)	Serevent®	Inhalation	2 inhalations of aerosol (42 mcg) bid
terbutaline sulfate **(ter-BYOO-tah-leen SUL-fayt)** (beta$_2$)	Brethine®, Brethaire®	PO, Inhalation, SC	PO: 2.5–5 mg tid; Inhalation: 2 inhalations q4–6h; SC: 0.25 mg q15–30 min up to 0.5 mg in 4h

Common adverse effects of beta-adrenergic drugs include headache, tremors, mild leg cramps, nervousness, fatigue, hypertension, palpitation, nausea, vomiting, and shortness of breath.

Contraindications and Precautions

Adrenergic drugs are contraindicated in patients with known hypersensitivity to these agents. These drugs are also contraindicated in the elderly, who are more sensitive to the effects of adrenergic drugs. These drugs should not be given to patients with symptoms such as blurred vision, seizures, chest pain, and palpitations.

Alpha-adrenergic drugs are contraindicated in children younger than 2 years. Safe use during pregnancy (category C) or lactation is not established.

Beta-adrenergic drugs are contraindicated in patients with cardiac arrhythmias associated with tachycardia, hyperthyroidism, pregnancy (category C), and lactation.

Adrenergic drugs should be used with caution in older adults and in patients with hypertension, cardiovascular disorders (including coronary artery disease), hyperthyroidism, and diabetes.

Drug Interactions

No clinically significant drug interactions have been established for alpha-adrenergic agents. Beta-adrenergic drugs may interact with general anesthetics (especially cyclopropane and halothane).

Sympatholytics (Adrenergic Blockers)

Sympatholytic agents (or **adrenergic blocker agents**) produce many of the same responses as the parasympathomimetics. These drugs are the most commonly prescribed class of autonomic drugs. Adrenergic blocker agents are also effective on all adrenergic alpha- and beta-receptors. Selected adrenergic antagonists or adrenergic blockers are listed in Table 7-4.

Mechanism of Action

Adrenergic blockers reduce delivery of **catecholamines** to the adrenergic receptors by disrupting catecholamine synthesis, storage, or release.

Indications

Adrenergic blockers are used in the treatment of hypertension, dysrhythmias, angina, heart failure, glaucoma, and migraines.

Adverse Effects

Adverse effects of adrenergic blockers include orthostatic hypotension, edema, headache, dizziness, vertigo, **somnolence** (prolonged drowsiness),

---

Medical Terminology Review

sympatholytic
sympatho- = related to the sympathetic nervous system
-lytic = opposing effects
a drug that acts to oppose the actions of the sympathetic nervous system

TABLE 7-4   Sympatholytics (Adrenergic Blockers)

Generic Name and Classification	Trade Name	Route of Administration	Average Adult Dosage
acebutolol **(ah-seh-BYOO-toh-lol)** (beta$_1$)	Sectral®	PO	400–800 mg/day
atenolol **(ah-TEH-noh-lol)** (beta$_1$)	Tenormin®	PO	25–50 mg/day
carteolol **(kar-TAY-oh-lol)** (nonselective, beta$_1$ or beta$_2$)	Cartrol®	PO	2.5 mg once daily
carvedilol **(kar-VEH-dih-lol)** (nonselective beta$_1$, beta$_2$, and alpha$_1$)	Coreg®	PO	3.125 mg bid
doxazosin mesylate **(dok-SAY-zoh-sin MEH-sih-layt)** (alpha$_1$)	Cardura®	PO	116 mg hs
esmolol hydrochloride **(EZ-moh-lol hy-droh-KLOR-ryd)** (beta$_1$)	Brevibloc®	IV	500 mcg/kg loading dose followed by 50 mcg/kg/min
metoprolol tartrate **(meh-toh-PROH-lol TAR-trayt)** (beta$_1$)	Lopressor®	PO	50–100 mg/day
nadolol **(nay-DOH-lol)** (nonselective, beta$_1$ and beta$_2$)	Corgard®	PO	40 mg once daily
phentolamine **(fen-TAW-lah-meen)** (primarily alpha$_1$, also alpha$_2$)	Regitine®	IM, IV	IM/IV: 5 mg 1–2h before surgery
prazosin hydrochloride **(PRAY-zoh-sin hy-droh-KLOR-ryd)** (alpha$_1$)	Minipress®	PO	Start with 1 mg hs, then 1 mg bid or tid
propranolol hydrochloride **(pro-PRAH-noh-lol hy-droh-KLOR-ryd)** (nonselective, beta$_1$ and beta$_2$)	Inderal®	PO, IV	PO: 10–40 mg bid; IV: 0.5–3 mg q4h prn
sotalol hydrochloride **(SOH-tah-lol hy-droh-KLOR-ryd)** (nonselective, beta$_1$ and beta$_2$)	Betapace®	PO	40-160 mg bid
tamsulosin hydrochloride **(tam-soo-LOH-sin hy-droh-KLOR-ryd)** (alpha$_1$)	Flomax®	PO	0.4 mg qd 30 min after a meal
terazosin **(teh-RAY-zoh-sin)** (alpha$_1$)	Hytrin®	PO	1–5 mg/day
timolol maleate **(TY-moh-lol MAH-lee-ayt)** (nonselective, beta$_1$ and beta$_2$)	Blocadren®, Timoptic®	PO	10–60 mg bid

fatigue, nervousness, and anxiety. These agents may also cause abdominal pain, nausea, vomiting, diarrhea, and exacerbation of peptic ulcer.

Adverse effects of beta-adrenergic blockers include respiratory disturbances, bradycardia, peripheral vascular insufficiency, palpitations, postural hypotension, behavioral changes, blurred vision, and dry eyes.

Contraindications and Precautions

Alpha-adrenergic blockers are contraindicated in patients with known hypersensitivity to these agents, and in patients with hypotension or syncope. Safe use during pregnancy (category D) or in children is not established.

Beta-adrenergic blockers are contraindicated in patients with sinus bradycardia, heart failure, peripheral vascular disease, hypotension, or pulmonary edema. Safety during pregnancy (category D) or lactation is not established.

Alpha-adrenergic blockers must be used cautiously in patients with hepatic impairment, renal disease, or lactation.

Beta-adrenergics are used with caution in hypertensive patients with congestive heart failure controlled by digitalis, and with diuretics; in vasospastic angina, asthma, bronchitis, emphysema, major depression, diabetes mellitus, impaired renal function, myasthenia gravis, hyperthyroidism, and **pheochromocytoma**; as well as in older adults.

Drug Interactions

Atropine and other anticholinergics may increase absorption of adrenergic blockers from the gastrointestinal (GI) tract.

Parasympathomimetics (Cholinergic Agonists)

Parasympathomimetic or cholinergic agonist drugs are able to mimic actions of the PNS. Table 7-5 shows selected parasympathomimetic drugs.

Mechanism of Action

Some cholinergic drugs increase the concentration of acetylcholine at cholinergic transmission sites, which prolongs and exaggerates their action. Others produce reversible cholinesterase inhibition and have direct stimulant action on voluntary muscle fibers.

Indications

Cholinergic agonist drugs are used most commonly in glaucoma to induce miosis. Specific muscarinic agonist drugs may be used in the treatment of atonic constipation, **congenital megacolon**, and in postoperative or postpartum adynamic intestinal ileus. Bethanechol has been used to increase the tone of the lower esophageal sphincter in the diagnosis or treatment of reflux esophagitis. Muscarinic agonists are useful in the treatment of non-obstructive urinary retention and neurogenic atony of the urinary bladder

> **Medical Terminology Review**
>
> **pheochromocytoma**
> pheo- = dusky or gray
> chromo = related to chromaffin cells
> -cytoma = cell tumor
> a pigmented tumor of the chromaffin cells (adrenal gland)

TABLE 7-5 Parasympathomimetics (Cholinergic Agonists)

Generic Name and Classification	Trade Name	Route of Administration	Average Adult Dosage
bethanechol chloride **(beh-THAY-neh-kol KLOR-ryd)** (nonselective, muscarinic)	Urecholine®	PO	10–50 mg bid–qid
cevimeline hydrochloride **(seh-VIH-meh-leen hy-droh-KLOR-ryd)** (muscarinic$_1$, muscarinic$_3$)	Evoxac®	PO	30 mg tid
neostigmine **(nee-oh-STIG-meen)** (nonselective, muscarinic)	Prostigmin®	PO, IM, IV	PO: 15–375 mg/day; IM: 0.022 mg/kg; IV: 0.5–2.5 mg slowly
physostigmine salicylate **(fy-soh-STIG-meen sah-LIH-sih-layt)** (nonselective, nicotinic and muscarinic)	Antilirium®	IM, IV	IM/IV: 0.5–3 mg
pilocarpine hydrochloride **(py-loh-KAR-peen hy-droh-KLOR-ryd)** (muscarinic$_3$)	Isopto Carpine®, Salagen®	PO, Ophthalmic	PO: 5–10 mg tid; Ophthalmic: 1 drop of 1–2% solution in affected eye q5–10 min for 3–6 doses
pyridostigmine **(py-rih-doh-STIG-meen)** (nonselective, nicotinic and muscarinic)	Mestinon®	PO	60 mg–1.5 g/day
rivastigmine tartrate **(rih-vah-STIG-meen TAR-trayt)** (undetermined)	Exelon®	PO	1.5–6 mg bid

with retention. Cholinergic agonist drugs are also used for dysrhythmias, Alzheimer's disease, and for myasthenia gravis.

Adverse Effects

Undesirable effects of cholinergic agonist drugs include flushing, sweating, abdominal cramps, difficulty in visual accommodation, headache, and convulsions (at high doses). Specific GI adverse effects include epigastric distress, diarrhea, involuntary defecation, nausea and vomiting, and colic. Other adverse effects are asthma and excessive salivary, nasopharyngeal, and bronchial secretions.

Contraindications and Precautions

Cholinergic agonist drugs are contraindicated in patients with known hypersensitivity to these agents, hypertension, coronary insufficiency, pheochromocytoma (benign tumor of adrenal medulla that increases production of epinephrine and norepinephrine), hyperthyroidism, asthma, and peptic ulcer.

Muscarinic drugs should be used cautiously in patients with hypertension, coronary disease, asthma, and hyperthyroidism.

Drug Interactions

Procainamide, quinidine, atropine, and epinephrine antagonize the effects of bethanechol. Beta-adrenergic agonists may cause conduction disturbances that may have additive effects with cholinergic drugs.

Neostigmine antagonizes effects of tubocurarine, atracurium, procainamide, quinidine, and atropine. Physostigmine may antagonize effects of echothiophate and isoflurophate.

Parasympatholytics (Anticholinergics or Cholinergic Blockers)

All parasympathetic effectors, some sympathetic effectors, all autonomic ganglia, and voluntary muscles bear cholinergic receptors. As a consequence, cholinergic drugs may affect the function of both divisions of the ANS. Anticholinergic drugs are shown in Table 7-6.

Mechanism of Action

Cholinergic blockers act by selectively blocking all muscarine responses to acetylcholine, whether excitatory or inhibitory. Cholinergic blockers depress the CNS. Antisecretory action of cholinergic blockers includes suppression of sweating, lacrimation, salivation, and secretions from the nose, mouth, and bronchi.

Indications

Cholinergic blockers relieve rigidity and tremor of Parkinson's syndrome. They are used as adjuncts in the symptomatic treatment of GI disorders (e.g., peptic ulcer, pylorospasm, GI hypermotility, irritable bowel syndrome, and spastic disorders of the biliary tract). Cholinergic blockers are prescribed to produce **mydriasis**, **cycloplegia** (paralysis of the ciliary muscles of the eye) before refraction, and for the treatment of anterior **uveitis** (inflammation of the middle layer of the eye) and **iritis** (inflammation of the iris). These agents are also used in general anesthesia, bradycardia, or asystole during cardiopulmonary resuscitation.

Adverse Effects

The main adverse effects of cholinergic blockers include headache, ataxia, dizziness, excitement, irritability, convulsions, drowsiness, fatigue, weakness, mental depression, confusion, disorientation, hallucinations, hypertension or hypotension, ventricular fibrillation, inability to swallow, difficulty passing urine, skin eruption, and loss of power in the ciliary muscles of the eye.

TABLE 7-6   Parasympatholytics (Anticholinergics or Cholinergic Blockers)

Generic Name and Classification	Trade Name	Route of Administration	Average Adult Dosage
atropine sulfate **(AH-troh-peen SUL-fayt)** (muscarinic₁, muscarinic₂, muscarinic₃, muscarinic₄, muscarinic₅)	Atropisol®, Isopto Atropine®	IV, IM, SC, Ophthalmic	IV/IM/SC: 0.4–0.6 mg 30–60 min before surgery; Ophthalmic: 1–2 drops tid
benztropine mesylate **(BENZ-troh-peen MEH-si-h-layt)** (muscarinic₁)	Cogentin®	PO	0.5–6 mg/day
cyclopentolate **(sy-kloh-PEN-toh-late)** (nonselective, muscarinic)	Cyclogyl®	Topical	1 drop of 1% solution in eye 40–50 min before procedure, followed by 1 drop in 5 min
dicyclomine hydrochloride **(dy-SY-klo-meen hy-droh-KLOR-ryd)** (primarily muscarinic₁, also muscarinic₂)	Bentyl®	PO, IM	PO: 20–40 mg qid; IM: 20 mg qid
glycopyrrolate **(gly-ko-PY-roh-layt)** (nonselective, muscarinic₁, muscarinic₂, muscarinic₃)	Robinul®	PO, IM, IV	PO: 1–2 mg tid; IM/IV: 0.1–0.2 mg as single dose tid or qid
ipratropium bromide **(ih-pro-TROH-pee-um BROH-myd)** (nonselective, muscarinic)	Atrovent®	Inhalation	2 inhalations of MDI qid at no less than 4h intervals
oxybutynin **(ok-see-BYOO-tih-nin)** (muscarinic₁, muscarinic₂, muscarinic₃)	Ditropan®	PO	5 mg bid or tid
propantheline **(proh-PAN-theh-leen)** (nonselective, muscarinic)	Pro-Banthine®	PO	15 mg 30 min ac and 30 mg hs
scopolamine **(skoh-PAW-lah-meen)** (muscarinic₁)	Hyoscine®, Transderm-Scop®	PO, IM, IV, SC	PO: 0.5–1 mg; IM/IV/SC: 0.3–0.6 mg
tiotropium bromide **(ty-oh-TROH-pee-um BROH-myd)** (nonselective, but primarily muscarinic₃)	Spiriva®	Inhalation	Inhale contents of 1 capsule daily using hand inhaler device provided

Contraindications and Precautions

Cholinergic blockers are contraindicated in patients with hypersensitivity to belladonna alkaloids, synechiae, angle-closure glaucoma, parotitis, obstructive uropathy, intestinal atony, paralytic ileus, obstructive GI tract diseases, severe ulcerative colitis, toxic megacolon, tachycardia, acute hemorrhage, or myasthenia gravis. Safety during pregnancy (category C) or lactation is not established.

Cholinergic blockers are used with caution in patients with myocardial infarction, hypertension or hypotension, coronary artery disease, congestive heart failure, and irregular heart rhythms. Other conditions in which cholinergic blockers should be used cautiously include gastric ulcer, GI infections, hiatal hernia with reflux esophagitis, hyperthyroidism, chronic lung disease, and hepatic or renal disease. These blockers should be used cautiously in the following types of patients: older adults, debilitated patients, children younger than 6 years, Down syndrome patients, those with autonomic neuropathy or spastic paralysis, children with brain damage, those exposed to high environmental temperatures, and in patients with fever.

Drug Interactions

Cholinergic blockers may interact with amantadine, antihistamines, tricyclic antidepressants, quinidine, and procainamide, which may add to the anticholinergic effects. The effects of levodopa are decreased with cholinergic blockers. Methotrimeprazine may precipitate extrapyramidal effects. The antipsychotic effects of phenothiazines are decreased due to decreased absorption.

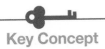

Key Concept

Because the thermal regulatory system in elderly patients declines, hyperthermia is possible with anticholinergics. This happens because these drugs decrease sweating.

SUMMARY

The portion of the PNS serving involuntary effectors is called the autonomic nervous system or ANS. The sympathetic and parasympathetic nervous systems are subdivisions of the ANS.

Three neurotransmitters play a role in the functions regulated by the autonomic nervous system: acetylcholine, norepinephrine, and epinephrine. Dopamine may also serve as a nervous system transmitter.

There are two basic types of receptors associated with the ANS: cholinergic receptors and adrenergic receptors. There are three major subtypes of cholinergic receptors, which are referred to as $nicotinic_N$, $nicotinic_M$, and muscarinic. There are four major subtypes of adrenergic receptors: $alpha_1$, $alpha_2$, $beta_1$, and $beta_2$.

Drugs that affect the ANS may be classified into four categories: sympathomimetics (adrenergic agonists), sympatholytics (adrenergic blockers), parasympathomimetics (cholinergic agonists), and parasympatholytics (anticholinergics).

EXPLORING THE WEB

Visit **http://cvpharmacology.com**

- Click on the link "Vasodilator." Research additional information on this drug class and the variations of drugs within this class. Record your findings to help further your understanding of the topics discussed in this chapter.

Visit **www.anaesthetist.com**

- Click on the link "Autonomic physiology." Read additional information about the autonomic nervous system to enhance your understanding of its functions.

Visit **www.pharmacology2000.com**

- Scroll down, read the printed disclaimer, then click on the link "I have read the disclaimer below and am ready to go to the Table of Contents (*Click Here to Continue*). Scroll down, then click on the link "Chapter 4: Pharmacology of the Autonomic Nervous System: Introduction." Explore the discussions related to the autonomic nervous system and the drug classes that affect this system.

REVIEW QUESTIONS

Multiple Choice

1. Dopamine, epinephrine, and isoproterenol are classified as which of the following types of drug?
   A. sympatholytics
   B. anticholinergics
   C. adrenergics
   D. cholinergic blockers

2. Which of the following agents are used to treat patients with myasthenia gravis?
   A. sympathomimetics (adrenergics)
   B. sympatholytics (adrenergic blockers)
   C. parasympatholytics (anticholinergics)
   D. parasympathomimetics (cholinergics)

3. Propranolol, metoprolol, and atenolol are:

   A. parasympathomimetics

   B. adrenergic drugs

   C. anticholinergic drugs

   D. beta-adrenergic blocking drugs

4. Elderly patients receiving anticholinergic drugs should be monitored closely for which of the following adverse effects?

   A. hyperthermia

   B. diuresis

   C. bradycardia

   D. hypothermia

5. The ANS employs all of the following neurotransmitters, *except*:

   A. epinephrine

   B. serotonin

   C. norepinephrine

   D. acetylcholine

6. Sympathomimetic drugs are also known as:

   A. cholinergics

   B. anticholinergics

   C. adrenergics

   D. adrenergic blockers

7. Which of the following adrenergic receptor subtypes may cause mydriasis?

   A. $alpha_1$

   B. $alpha_2$

   C. $beta_1$

   D. $beta_2$

8. Dobutamine is used to treat cardiac decompensation because of its action as a(n):

   A. adrenergic agonist

   B. adrenergic blocking agent

   C. anticholinergic

   D. cholinergic

9. Atenolol may best be described as a(n):

   A. $beta_2$-adrenergic blocker

   B. $alpha_1$-adrenergic blocker

   C. $beta_1$-and $beta_2$-adrenergic blocker

   D. $beta_1$-adrenergic blocker

10. Which of the following agents is indicated for the treatment of anterior uveitis and iritis?

    A. timolol

    B. atropine

    C. nadolol

    D. bethanechol

11. Which of the following drugs are contraindicated in patients with hypertension, asthma, hyperthyroidism, or peptic ulcer?

    A. cholinergic agonists

    B. anticholinergics

    C. adrenergic blockers

    D. adrenergic agonists

12. Which of the following describes pilocarpine?

    A. $nicotinic_1$ cholinergic agonist

    B. $muscarinic_3$ cholinergic agonist

    C. reduces the delivery of catecholamine

    D. stimulates alpha receptor sites

13. Which of the following agents is classified as a sympatholytic?

    A. neostigmine (Prostigmin®)

    B. cevimeline (Evoxac®)

    C. pilocarpine (Isopto Carpine®)

    D. prazosin (Minipress®)

14. Which of the following statements is true of scopolamine?

    A. it is an anticholinergic

    B. it is an anticoagulant

    C. it is a thrombolytic agent

    D. it is an adrenergic blocker

15. Which of the following agents is used prior to anesthesia?

    A. scopolamine

    B. cyclopentolate

    C. atropine

    D. oxybutynin

True or False

_____ 1. All the adverse effects caused by alpha$_1$ activation result in vasoconstriction.

_____ 2. Sympathomimetics are also called adrenergic blockers.

_____ 3. Adrenergic blockers are used in the treatment of hypotension.

_____ 4. The sympathetic nervous system's responses are also called rest-and-digest responses.

_____ 5. Norepinephrine is released by all postganglionic neurons of the sympathetic nervous system.

_____ 6. Muscarinic cholinergics may cause miosis.

_____ 7. Adrenergic agonist drugs may affect both alpha- and beta-receptors.

_____ 8. Prostigmin is the trade name of neostigmine.

_____ 9. All preganglionic neurons of the parasympathetic nervous system release acetylcholine.

_____ 10. Acetylcholine is a major transmitter released by the adrenal medulla.

Critical Thinking

A 61-year-old man has been diagnosed with glaucoma. He has recently had abdominal surgery. He has developed postoperative adynamic intestinal ileus.

1. Which class of autonomic nervous system drugs is the best for use in a patient with glaucoma and postoperative adynamic intestinal ileus?

2. If the patient is taking the drug of choice for these two conditions, what would be the most common adverse effects?

3. If the patient has asthma and hyperthyroidism, can the drug of choice still be used?

Drug Therapy for Parkinson's and Alzheimer's Diseases

OBJECTIVES

After completing this chapter, the reader should be able to:

1. Identify the most common degenerative diseases of the central nervous system.
2. Explain the cause of Parkinson's disease.
3. Classify the drugs that are used for the treatment of Parkinson's disease.
4. Describe the roles of dopamine and acetylcholine in Parkinson's disease.
5. Identify the characteristics of dopamine and levodopa.
6. Discuss the actions and adverse effects of dopaminergic drugs when used in the treatment of Parkinson's disease.
7. Discuss the actions and contraindications of cholinergic blocker drugs when used in the treatment of Parkinson's disease.
8. Identify the characteristics of Alzheimer's disease.
9. Explain the role of acetylcholinesterase inhibitors in the treatment of Alzheimer's disease.
10. Explain possible preventive therapies for Alzheimer's disease.

GLOSSARY

Alzheimer's disease – a disorder causing severe cognitive dysfunction in older persons in which the brain experiences atrophy (shrinkage) and exhibits senile plaques

Atrophy – meaning "without development"; wasting away

Basal nuclei – clusters of nerve cells at the base of the brain; responsible for body movement and coordination

Bradykinesia – extremely slow movement, as seen in Parkinson's disease or because of certain drug toxicities.

Corpus striatum – layers of nervous tissue within the brain

Encephalitis – inflammation of the brain

Parkinson's disease – a neurological syndrome usually resulting from deficiency of dopamine and characterized by degenerative, vascular, or inflammatory changes in the basal ganglia

Substantia nigra – pigmented cells in the midbrain responsible for the production of dopamine

Tremor – repetitive, often regular, oscillatory movements caused by alternate, or synchronous, but irregular contraction of opposing muscle groups

OVERVIEW

Degenerative diseases of the central nervous system include Alzheimer's disease, multiple sclerosis, Huntington's chorea, and Parkinson's disease. The focus in this chapter will be on Parkinson's and Alzheimer's diseases, which are more common than other related diseases and affect millions of people (mostly elderly) in the United States.

PARKINSON'S DISEASE

Parkinson's disease is a progressive degenerative disorder that affects motor function as a consequence of the loss of extrapyramidal activity. This disease is characterized by muscle **tremor at rest**, muscle rigidity, and **bradykinesia**, and disturbances of posture and equilibrium are often present (Figure 8-1).

According to the National Parkinson's Alliance, it is estimated that as many as 1.5 million Americans have Parkinson's disease. This disorder causes dysfunction and changes in the **basal nuclei** (clusters of nerve cells at the base of the brain), principally in the **substantia nigra** (pigmented cells in the midbrain responsible for the production of dopamine). In this condition, a decreased number of neurons in the brain secrete dopamine, an inhibitory neurotransmitter, leading to an imbalance between excitation and

> **Medical Terminology Review**
>
> **bradykinesia**
> brady- = slow
> -kinesia = ability of movement
> slowing in the ability to move

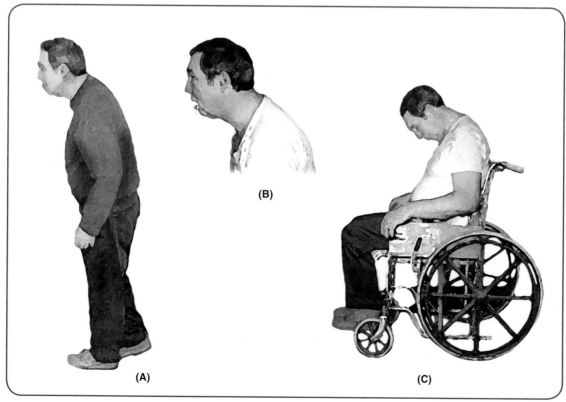

(B)

(A)   (C)

Figure 8-1 Parkinson's disease is characterized by a shuffling gait and early postural changes.

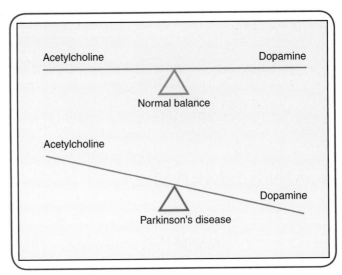

Figure 8-2 Dopamine imbalance exhibited in Parkinson's disease.

inhibition in the basal nuclei. The cause of the disease is not fully understood, but it is believed to be associated with an imbalance of the neurotransmitters acetylcholine and dopamine in the brain (Figure 8-2).

The excess stimulation affects movement and posture by increasing muscle tone and activity, leading to resting tremors, muscular rigidity, difficulty in initiating movement, and postural instability. Parkinson's disease usually develops after age 60 and occurs in both men and women. It may occur following **encephalitis**, trauma, or vascular disease. Drug-induced Parkinson's disease is particularly linked to use of phenothiazines (e.g., chlorpromazine). Pharmacotherapy is often successful in reducing some of the distressing symptoms of this disease.

> **Medical Terminology Review**
>
> **encephalitis**
> encephal- = brain
> -itis = inflammation
> inflammation of the brain

PHARMACOTHERAPY FOR PARKINSON'S DISEASE

Several drugs can be used for Parkinson's disease; the goal of drug therapy for this condition is to increase the ability of the patient to perform daily activities. Pharmacotherapy does not cure Parkinson's disease, but it can dramatically reduce symptoms in some patients.

Antiparkinsonism drugs are administered to restore the balance of dopamine and acetylcholine in the **corpus striatum** (layers of nervous tissue in the brain). Dopaminergic drugs and anticholinergics (cholinergic blockers) are the mainstays of antiparkinsonism (see Tables 8-1 and 8-2).

> **Medical Terminology Review**
>
> **dopaminergic**
> dopamin- = dopamine
> -ergic = related to drugs affecting dopamine

Dopaminergic Drugs

The group of drugs classified as dopaminergic drugs are used to increase dopamine levels in the brain. Levodopa (L-Dopa) is the drug of choice for

TABLE 8-1   Dopaminergic Drugs for Parkinsonism

Generic Name	Trade Name	Route of Administration	Average Adult Dosage
amantadine hydrochloride **(ah-MAN-tah-deen hy-droh-KLOR-ryd)**	Symmetrel®	PO	200 mg/day or 100 bid
bromocriptine mesylate **(broh-moh-KRIP-teen MEH-sih-layt)**	Parlodel®	PO	1.25–2.5 mg/day (max: 7.5 mg/day in divided doses)
carbidopa-levodopa **(kar-bih-DOH-pah LEE-voh-doh-pah)**	Sinemet®	PO	1 tablet of 10 mg carbidopa/100 mg levodopa, or 25 mg carbidopa/100 mg levodopa tid (max: 6 tablets/day)
carbidopa-levodopa-entacapone **(kar-bih-DOH-pah LEE voh-doh-pah en-TAK-ah-pohn)**	Stalevo® (in formulations ranging from 50 to 200).	PO	Optimum daily dosage is determined by careful, individualized titration; max daily dose depends on strength used; a patient taking 1 tablet of carbidopa-levodopa 25 mg/100 mg and 1 tablet of entacapone 200 mg at each administration (up to 8 per day) can switch to 1 Stalevo 100 tablet per administration, which contains the same mixture; max dose is 1600 mg/day
entacapone **(en-TAK-ah-pohn)**	Comtan®	PO	One 200-mg tablet administered at same time with each carbidopa-levodopa dose (up to 8 per day); max dose is 1600 mg/day
levodopa **(LEE-voh-doh-pah)**	Larodopa®	PO	500 mg–1 g/day, may be increased by 750 mg q3–7 days
pergolide mesylate **(PER-goh-lyd MEH-sih-layt)**	Permax®	PO	Start with 0.05 mg/day for 2 days, increase by 0.1–0.15 mg/day q3 days for 12 days, then increase by 0.25 mg every third day (max: 5 mg/day)
pramipexole **(prah-mih-PEK-sohl)**	Mirapex®	PO	Start with 0.125 mg tid for 1 week; double dose for the next week, increasing by 0.25 mg/dose tid q week to a max dose of 1.5 mg tid
ropinirole hydrochloride **(roh-PIH-nih-rohl hy-droh-KLOR-ryd)**	Requip®	PO	Start with 0.25 mg tid, increasing by 0.25 mg/dose tid q week to a max dose of 1 mg tid
selegiline hydrochloride **(seh-LEH-jih-leen hy-droh-KLOR-ryd)**	Carbex®, Eldepryl®	PO	5 mg/dose bid; *Note:* doses greater than 10 mg/day are potentially toxic
tolcapone **(TOL-cah-pohn)**	Tasmar®	PO	100 mg tid (max: 600 mg/day)

TABLE 8-2	Anticholinergic Drugs for Parkinsonism		
Generic Name	Trade Name	Route of Administration	Average Adult Dosage
benztropine mesylate **(BENZ-troh-peen MEH-sih-layt)**	Cogentin®	PO	0.5–1 mg/day, increasing prn (max: 6 mg/day)
biperiden hydrochloride **(by-PAIR-ih-den hy-droh-KLOR-ryd)**	Akineton®	PO	2 mg/day to qid
diphenhydramine hydrochloride **(dy-fen-HY-drah-meen hy-droh-KLOR-ryd)**	Benadryl®	PO	25–50 mg tid–qid (max: 300/day)
procyclidine hydrochloride **(pro-SY-klih-deen hy-droh-KLOR-ryd)**	Kemadrin®	PO	2.5 mg tid pc; may increase to 5 mg tid if tolerated, with an additional 5 mg at bedtime (max: 45–60 mg/day)
trihexyphenidyl **(try-hek-see-FEH-nih-dihl)**	Artane®, Trihexy®	PO	1 mg for day 1; doubled for day 2; increased by 2 mg q3–5 days up to 6–10 mg/day (max: 15 mg/day)

Parkinson's disease. Levodopa is a precursor of dopamine formation and stimulates this process.

Mechanism of Action

Dopaminergic agents restore the neurotransmitter dopamine in the extrapyramidal region of the brain. Levodopa can cross the blood-brain barrier, but dopamine cannot. Therefore, dopamine by itself is not used for the treatment of Parkinson's disease. The mechanism of action of amantadine and selegiline in the treatment of parkinsonism is not fully understood. L-Dopa should be taken on an empty stomach because large neutral amino acids will compete with it for absorption from the gut and the drug will be transported across the blood-brain barrier.

Indications

Levodopa is considered the drug of choice for Parkinson's disease. Either carbidopa is combined with levodopa, or they are prescribed as two separate drugs. Amantadine is less effective than levodopa as a drug therapy for Parkinson's disease, but more effective than the cholinergic blockers. Amantadine is given alone or in combination with another antiparkinsonism drug with cholinergic activity. Amantadine is also indicated for drug therapy for viral disorders.

Key Concept

Hallucinations occur commonly in older adults when taking dopamine receptor agonists.

Key Concept

Patients taking levodopa should be monitored for orthostatic hypotension and cardiac arrhythmias, and also watched for psychiatric disturbances.

Key Concept

Patients taking levodopa should avoid foods and medications containing substantial amounts of pyridoxine (vitamin B$_6$).

Adverse Effects

Adverse effects of levodopa include increased, uncontrollable rhythmic hand shaking or trembling, grinding of teeth (bruxism), muscle incoordination, numbness, fatigue, and headache. Levodopa may also cause upright position hypotension, tachycardia, hypertension, nausea, vomiting, dry mouth, bitter taste, and hepatotoxicity.

Adverse effects of bromocriptine include headache, dizziness, vertigo, fainting, sedation, nightmares, and insomnia. It may also produce blurred vision, hypertension, palpitation, arrhythmias, nausea, vomiting, and diarrhea. The most serious adverse effects of amantadine are orthostatic hypotension, congestive heart failure, depression, psychosis, convulsions, leukopenia, and urinary retention.

Contraindications and Precautions

The dopaminergic drugs are contraindicated in patients with known hypersensitivity to these agents. Levodopa should be avoided in patients with narrow-angle glaucoma, those receiving a monoamine oxidase inhibitor (MAOI), and during lactation.

Dopaminergic drugs are used with caution in patients with renal or hepatic disease, bronchial asthma, cardiovascular disease, and peptic ulcer. These agents should be used cautiously during pregnancy (category C) and lactation.

Drug Interactions

Levodopa increases therapeutic effects and the possibility of a hypertensive crisis with MAOIs. Withdrawal of MAOIs is necessary at least 14 days before levodopa therapy is started. Levodopa exhibits decreased efficacy with pyridoxine (vitamin B$_6$) and phenytoin.

Cholinergic Blockers

Cholinergic blockers, or anticholinergic drugs, are able to change the balance between dopamine and acetylcholine in the brain.

Mechanism of Action

Cholinergic blockers act by inhibiting excess cholinergic stimulation of neurons in the brain. Anticholinergic drugs inhibit acetylcholine in the central nervous system.

Indications

Cholinergic blockers are used as adjunctive therapy to relieve symptoms of parkinsonism and in the control of drug-induced disorders such as postural tremor and chorea.

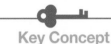

Medical Terminology
Review

dysuria
dys- = difficult
-uria = characteristic
of urine
difficult urination

Key Concept

Elderly people are very sensitive to anticholinergics, and these drugs must be used only when the patient can be carefully observed, because confusion and disorientation are often reported.

Adverse Effects

Cholinergic blockers produce dry mouth, blurred vision, sedation, dizziness, tachycardia, and constipation. Other adverse effects include urinary retention, dysuria, muscle weakness, confusion, disorientation, and skin rash.

Contraindications and Precautions

Anticholinergic drugs are contraindicated in patients with known hypersensitivity to these agents. These drugs are also contraindicated in those with peptic ulcers, duodenal obstruction, angle-closure glaucoma, prostatic hypertrophy, myasthenia gravis, and an extreme dilation of the large intestine.

Anticholinergic drugs should be used cautiously in patients with cardiac arrhythmias, hypertension, hypotension, and liver or kidney dysfunction.

Drug Interactions

Cholinergic blockers interact with many drugs. These agents should not be taken with alcohol, MAOIs, procainamide, phenothiazines, quinidine, or the nutraceutical supplement Tricycline® because of combined sedative effects.

ALZHEIMER'S DISEASE

Alzheimer's disease (senile disease complex) has been demonstrated to be one of the most common causes of severe cognitive dysfunction in older persons. Pathologically, the brain experiences **atrophy** (shrinkage) and exhibits senile plaques. The exact cause of Alzheimer's disease is unknown, but current theories include loss of neurotransmitter stimulation by choline acetyltransferase.

Alzheimer's disease is a devastating illness characterized by progressive memory failure, impaired thinking, confusion, disorientation, personality changes, restlessness, speech disturbances, hallucinations, and the inability to perform routine tasks. The patient may become hypomanic, refuse food, and lose sphincter control even though there is no impairment of the autonomic nervous system. Although it occurs with equal frequency in men and women, the familial risk is four times that of the general population. Typical pathologic features are spreading amyloid plaques in the cortex and fibrillary degeneration in the layers containing pyramidal ganglion cells.

Unfortunately, the disease is incurable and, according to the American Health Assistance Foundation, affects about 350,000 new individuals per year in the United States. The current pharmacotherapy is focused on improving cognitive functioning or limiting the disease progression and controlling symptoms. In Alzheimer's disease, acetylcholine is decreased (this chemical substance is necessary for neurotransmission and for forming memories). There is no specific test for this disease, but other tests are performed to rule out any other cause of dementia. However, a definitive diagnosis is possible only upon autopsy. Diagnostic criteria consist of a failure in at least three cognitive functions, including memory, use of language, visuo-spatial skills, personality, and calculating skills.

PHARMACOTHERAPY FOR ALZHEIMER'S DISEASE

The FDA has approved a few medications for Alzheimer's disease, although there is no cure. Table 8-3 lists drugs currently used in the treatment of this disease. These agents are classified as acetylcholinesterase inhibitors. Recent studies focusing on the prevention of Alzheimer's disease have indicated that nondrugs such as Axona® and Cerefolin® may prevent or slow the onset of the disease. Axona contains fractionated coconut oil as caprylic triglyceride. Cerefolin contains the vitamins folate (as L-methylfolate), vitamin B_{12} (as cyanocobalamin), vitamin B_2 (as riboflavin), and vitamin B_6 (as pyridoxine).

Mechanism of Action

Acetylcholinesterase inhibitors are centrally acting agents, leading to elevated acetylcholine levels in the brain. Therefore, their action slows the

TABLE 8-3	Drugs Used to Treat Alzheimer's Disease		
Generic Name	Trade Name	Route of Administration	Average Adult Dosage
donepezil hydrochloride **(doh-NEH-peh-zihl hy-droh-KLOR-ryd)**	Aricept®	PO	5–10 mg hs
galantamine hydrobromide **(gah-LAN-tah-meen hy-droh-BROH-myd)**	Razadyne®	PO	Start with 4 mg bid (at least 4 weeks); increase by 4 mg bid q4wk to 12 mg bid (max: 8–16 mg bid)
memantine **(meh-MAN-teen)**	Namenda®	PO	Start with 5 mg once daily, increasing in 5 mg increments to 10 mg/day (5 mg twice daily), 15 mg/day (5 mg and 10 mg as separate doses), and 20 mg/day (10 mg twice daily); minimum interval between dose increases is 1 week
memantine and donepezil hydrochloride **(meh-MAN-teen and doh-NEH-peh-zihl hy-droh-KLOR-ryd)**	Namzaric®	PO	Patients stabilized on memantine hydrochloride (10 mg bid or 28 mg extended-released once daily) and donepezil hydrochloride (10 mg) can be switched to this medication, taken once a day in the evening. Begin the following day after last dose of the separate medications. No divided doses or doubled-up doses permitted.
rivastigmine tartrate **(rih-vah-STIG-meen TAR-trayt)**	Exelon®	PO	Start with 1.5 mg bid with food; increase by 1.5 mg bid q2wk if tolerated to 3–6 mg bid (max: 12 mg bid)

neuronal degradation that occurs in Alzheimer's disease, and improves memory in cases of mild to moderate Alzheimer's dementia. Patients should receive pharmacotherapy for at least six months prior to assessing the maximum benefits of drug therapy.

Indications

Acetylcholinesterase inhibitors are used in the treatment of mild to moderate dementia of the Alzheimer's type.

Adverse Effects

Adverse effects of acetylcholinesterase inhibitors generally include nausea and vomiting, diarrhea, heartburn, muscle pain, and headache. Donepezil may cause darkened urine. Other adverse effects of acetylcholinesterase inhibitors include an inability to sleep, a sudden drop in blood pressure, depression, and irritability.

Contraindications and Precautions

Acetylcholinesterase inhibitors are contraindicated in patients with known hypersensitivity to these agents. These agents are also contraindicated in patients with liver or kidney impairment, in pregnancy (category B), and lactation.

Acetylcholinesterase inhibitors should be used cautiously in patients with cardiac disorders, asthma, enlargement of the prostate, a history of seizures or gastrointestinal (GI) bleeding, and renal or hepatic disease.

Drug Interactions

Donepezil, which is a cholinesterase inhibitor, increases effects and risk of toxicity with theophylline. This is because theophylline concentrations and toxicity increase via cholinesterase inhibition of the CYP1A2 enzyme, which is responsible for theophylline metabolism. When this occurs, toxicity is severe because of the narrow therapeutic index of theophylline.

Though cholinesterase inhibitors are not usually prescribed with other drugs in the same class, when this occurs in rare instances, the drug interactions involve an increase in cholinergic adverse effects. Drugs such as donepezil decrease effects of anticholinergics and increase risk of GI bleeding with nonsteroidal anti-inflammatory drugs. Phenobarbital, phenytoin, dexamethasone, and rifampin may speed elimination of donepezil.

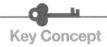

Key Concept

Ginkgo is a natural remedy and one of the oldest known herbs in the world. Gingko extract is most commonly used in treating dementia. Adverse effects include gastrointestinal upset, muscle cramps, bleeding, and headache.

Key Concept

As part of the prevention of Alzheimer's disease, adequate sleep helps in the production of melatonin, which eliminates beta-amyloids from the brain. These abnormal proteins are known to accumulate in the brains of Alzheimer's patients. Also, by sleeping at least 7 hours every night, the cerebrospinal fluid is able to remove waste materials from the brain, including beta-amyloids. Therefore, adequate sleep is very important in preventing Alzheimer's disease.

SUMMARY

Parkinson's and Alzheimer's diseases are among the most common degenerative diseases of the central nervous system. Multiple sclerosis and Huntington's chorea are other degenerative diseases. Parkinson's disease results in the death of neurons that produce dopamine. It affects over 1.5 million Americans, is primarily seen in patients older than the age 60, and occurs in both men and women.

The goal of drug therapy for Parkinson's disease is to increase the ability of the patient to perform daily activities. Antiparkinsonism agents are given to restore the balance of dopamine and acetylcholine in the brain. Dopaminergic drugs and anticholinergics are the mainstays of antiparkinsonism.

Alzheimer's disease is characterized by progressive memory failure, impaired thinking, confusion, disorientation, and speech disturbances. It is very common, affecting about 350,000 new individuals per year in the United States. In Alzheimer's disease, acetylcholine (which is necessary for forming memories) is decreased. Unfortunately, the disease is incurable. The FDA has approved only a few medications for Alzheimer's disease to reduce its symptoms. These drugs are known as acetylcholinesterase inhibitors.

EXPLORING THE WEB

Visit **http://jaapa.com**

- Search for the article "Pharmacotherapy for Parkinson's Disease: Current Options, Promising Future Therapies."

Visit **www.alz.org**

- Learn more about Alzheimer's disease and review information on treatments and research related to pharmacological therapies.

Visit **www.nlm.nih.gov**

- Click on the link "Medline Plus." Search for additional information on Parkinson's disease and Alzheimer's disease.

REVIEW QUESTIONS

Multiple Choice

1. Which of the following drugs may induce Parkinson's disease?

    A. pyridoxine (vitamin B_6)

    B. chlorpromazine

    C. dopamine

    D. levodopa

2. The mechanism of action of amantadine in the treatment of parkinsonism is:

    A. to inhibit the effect of GABA

    B. to prevent the production of dopamine

    C. to inhibit the effect of acetylcholine

    D. unknown

3. Which of the following agents is the drug of choice for Parkinson's disease?

    A. levodopa

    B. aspirin

    C. amantadine

    D. pyridoxine

4. Anticholinergic drugs are contraindicated in patients who have which of the following conditions?

   A. parkinsonism

   B. glaucoma

   C. hypocalcemia

   D. cataracts

5. Dopaminergic drugs should be used cautiously during pregnancy because they are included in which of the following pregnancy categories?

   A. D

   B. C

   C. B

   D. A

6. Which of the following brain chemicals, necessary for forming memories, is decreased in Alzheimer's disease?

   A. dopamine

   B. epinephrine

   C. melatonin

   D. acetylcholine

7. Which of the following agents is used in Alzheimer's disease?

   A. bromocriptine (Parlodel®)

   B. amantadine (Symmetrel®)

   C. memantine (Namenda®)

   D. ropinirole (Requip®)

8. A patient with Alzheimer's disease is given donepezil. Which of the following adverse effects is unique to this drug?

   A. constipation

   B. darkened urine

   C. increased drowsiness

   D. muscle weakness

9. Cholinesterase inhibitors are used to treat which of the following conditions associated with Alzheimer's disease?

   A. depression

   B. dementia

   C. urinary incontinence

   D. peripheral paralysis

10. Which of the following is an adverse effect of gingko (an herbal substance used for Alzheimer's disease)?

    A. insomnia and dizziness

    B. tremors

    C. gastrointestinal upset and headache

    D. an inability to speak normally

Fill in the Blank

1. Parkinson's disease causes dysfunction and changes in the_____ of the brain.

2. Parkinson's disease usually develops after age _____.

3. Antiparkinsonism drugs are given to restore the balance of dopamine and _____.

4. Acetylcholinesterase inhibitors are used in the treatment of mild dementia for _____.

5. Agents used for Alzheimer's disease are classified as _____ inhibitors.

6. The commonly prescribed medications for Alzheimer's disease, such as Aricept®, are contraindicated if these patients also have _____ or _____ impairment.

7. Levodopa should be avoided in patients with _____, those receiving a monoamine oxydase inhibitor (MAOI), and during lactation.

8. Cholinergic blockers are used as adjunctive therapy to relieve _____ symptoms.

9. Dopamine is a precursor of norepinephrine and _____.

10. Patients taking levodopa should avoid foods and medications containing substantial amounts of vitamin _____.

11. Aside from ruling out other forms of dementia, there is no specific test for _____, and a definitive diagnosis is possible only upon autopsy.

12. Levodopa is considered the drug of choice for _____.

Critical Thinking

A 72-year-old woman is diagnosed with Parkinson's disease. In her past medical history, she has had chronic hepatitis C and hypertension.

1. What are the chances that levodopa will be able to cure Parkinson's disease in this patient?

2. With the history of hepatitis C, what precautions should be taken if the physician ordered this drug of choice?

3. If levodopa is not effective for this patient, can dopamine be substituted?

Drug Therapy for Seizures

OBJECTIVES

After completing this chapter, the reader should be able to:

1. Distinguish between partial and generalized seizures.
2. Classify generalized seizures.
3. Explain tonic-clonic (grand mal) seizures.
4. Discuss the most commonly used anti-seizure drugs.
5. Discuss indications and major adverse effects of phenytoin.
6. Explain the mechanism of action of succinimides and their indications.
7. Recognize major phenytoin-like drugs.
8. Discuss treatment of status epilepticus.
9. Explain the type of seizures that are common in children.
10. List the drugs that may increase the toxicity of valproic acid.

GLOSSARY

Absence seizures – generalized seizures that do not involve motor convulsions; also referred to as *petit mal*

Anticonvulsants – drugs that prevent or stop convulsive seizures

Convulsions – abnormal motor movements

Electrical threshold – an individual's balance between excitatory and inhibitory forces in the brain; also known as the *seizure threshold*

Epilepsy – an older term that describes a condition characterized by periodic or recurrent seizures or convulsions

Generalized seizures – seizures originating in and involving both cerebral hemispheres

Grand mal – a generalized seizure characterized by full-body tonic and clonic motor convulsions

Partial seizures – seizures originating in one area of the brain that may spread to other areas

Seizure – abnormal discharge of brain neurons that causes alteration of behavior or motor activity, or both

Status epilepticus – an emergency situation characterized by continual seizure activity with no interruptions

Tonic-clonic seizures – generalized seizures characterized by alternating contraction (tonic phase) and relaxation (clonic phase) of muscles, loss of consciousness, and abnormal behaviors

OVERVIEW

According to the National Institute of Neurological Disorders and Stroke (NINDS), nearly 2.3 million people in the United States today have been diagnosed with **epilepsy** (a condition characterized by seizures) in one of its many forms. The terms *epilepsy*, *convulsions*, and *seizures* are commonly used interchangeably, although each has a slightly different medical meaning. The term *epilepsy* is used less often today because of the stigma once attached to patients suffering from this disorder. Instead, the term *recurrent seizures* is preferred. **Seizure** is a term used to refer to all epileptic events, whereas **convulsion** relates to abnormal motor movements. NINDS statistics indicate that 75% to 90% of seizure patients have their first seizure before age 20. Fortunately, scientific discoveries about how the brain works have enabled about 80% of those diagnosed with a seizure disorder to benefit from modern medicines, and implantable devices regulated by the FDA can help many patients to live productive lives. Anti-seizure drugs prevent or stop a convulsive seizure.

CLASSIFICATIONS OF SEIZURES

Seizures are characterized by hyperexcitability of neurons in the brain. The abnormal stimuli can produce many symptoms, from short periods of unconsciousness to violent convulsions. Seizures are usually brief, with a beginning and an end. The activity may be localized or generalized. Seizures may result acutely from any of a number of neurological disorders, as well as from metabolic disturbances, trauma, and exposure to certain toxins. Each seizure lasts for a few seconds or minutes, and the excessive activity of the neurons then ceases spontaneously. The altered pattern of electrical activity, or brain waves, during a seizure can be demonstrated on the electroencephalogram (EEG), indicating the type of seizure. Patients may experience post-seizure impairment.

Seizure disorders are classified by their location in the brain and their clinical features, including characteristic EEG patterns during and between seizures. The international classification of seizures is summarized in Table 9-1. This is a commonly accepted classification that incorporates current terminology and divides seizures into two basic categories: generalized and partial.

Generalized seizures have multiple foci that may cause loss of consciousness, whereas **partial seizures** have a single or focal origin, often in the cerebral cortex (Figure 9-1). Partial seizures may or may not involve altered consciousness. However, partial seizures may progress to generalized seizures.

Complications may arise from generalized **tonic-clonic (grand mal)** seizures that are severe and frequent. Injuries may occur during a seizure. Recurrent or continuous seizures that occur without recovery of

Medical Terminology Review

electroencephalogram
electro- = electronic
encephalo = brain
-gram = x-ray
electronic x-ray of the brain

TABLE 9-1	Classifications of Seizures
Partial Seizures (focal)	**Generalized Seizures**
A. Simple	A. Tonic-clonic (grand mal)
1. Motor (includes Jacksonian)	B. Absence (petit mal)
2. Sensory (e.g., visual, auditory)	C. Myoclonic
3. Autonomic	D. Infantile spasms
4. Psychic	E. Atonic (akinetic)
B. Complex (impaired consciousness)	
1. Psychomotor	

Key Concept

Absence seizures (generalized seizures that do not involve motor convulsions; also referred to as *petit mal*), which are common in children, may decrease or be replaced by tonic-clonic or psychomotor seizures.

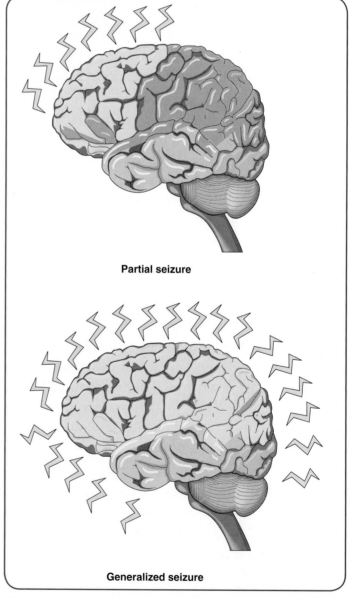

Partial seizure

Generalized seizure

Figure 9-1 A partial seizure is characterized by chaotic firing occurring in one portion of the brain, while a generalized seizure is characterized by chaotic firing all over the brain.

consciousness are termed status epilepticus. This condition may lead to serious consequences if not treated promptly, and it is always an emergency condition.

ANTI-SEIZURE DRUGS

Several major groups of medications are used to treat seizure disorders. The choice of medication varies according to individual patient conditions and physician preference. In treatment of recurrent seizures, it takes weeks to establish drug plasma levels and to determine the adequacy of therapeutic improvement. Usually the most effective drug with the least adverse effects is used initially. Drug treatment is not always necessary for the lifetime of the patient. Medications for seizures include barbiturates and benzodiazepines, which are the most useful anticonvulsants (drugs that stop or prevent a convulsant seizure). Other medications include hydantoins, phenytoin-like agents, and succinimides, which are detailed below. Valproic acid, carbamazepine, and phenytoin are the drugs of choice for generalized tonic-clonic (grand mal) seizures.

Phenobarbital is now considered to be an alternative drug for adults, but continues to be the primary drug for infants. Ethosuximide and valproic acid are the drugs of choice for absence seizures. Clonazepam is also effective as an alternative drug. The drugs of first choice for partial seizures are carbamazepine, phenytoin, and lamotrigine.

Myoclonic seizures are usually treated with valproic acid. Drugs that may also be used include clonazepam, levetiracetam, topiramate, and zonisamide. For short-term control of status epilepticus, intravenous diazepam or lorazepam can be used. However, for prolonged therapy, intravenous phenytoin is used. This must be done carefully since phenytoin may cause cardiotoxicity.

Barbiturates

Barbiturates are chemical derivatives of barbituric acid. They are classified into four groups: ultra-short-acting, short-acting, intermediate-acting, and long-acting. They are also classified as either Schedule II or III medications. More than 2500 barbiturates have been synthesized, but only about 50 have been approved for clinical use in the United States, and fewer than a dozen are commonly used. Barbiturates were discussed in detail in Chapter 6. Specific barbiturates used solely in the treatment of seizures are summarized in Table 9-2.

Benzodiazepines

Benzodiazepines are one of the most widely prescribed classes of drugs. They are used not only to control seizures but also for the treatment of anxiety,

TABLE 9-2	Summary of Barbiturates Used in Seizure Disorders		
Generic Name	Trade Name	Route of Administration	Average Adult Dosage
phenobarbital (C-IV) **(fee-noh-BAR-bih-tahl)**	Barbital®, Solfoton®	PO	50–100 mg bid–tid
phenobarbital sodium (C-IV) **(fee-noh-BAR-bih-tahl SOH-dee-um)**	Luminal®	IM, IV	30–320 mg; may repeat in 6 h

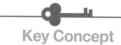

Key Concept

Phenytoin is administered orally, and fosphenytoin is administered intravenously.

skeletal muscle spasms, and alcohol withdrawal symptoms. Benzodiazepines are drugs of choice to treat anxiety and are used for hypnosis because of their great margin of safety. Benzodiazepines were discussed in detail in Chapter 6. Specific benzodiazepines used in the treatment of seizures are listed in Table 9-3.

Hydantoins

The most recognizable and used drug in the hydantoin class is phenytoin, and fosphenytoin is the newest. Phenytoin is a potent broad-spectrum anti-seizure medication. Fosphenytoin is used parenterally when substitution for oral anti-seizure medications is necessary, such as after surgery (Table 9-4).

Mechanism of Action

Hydantoins act by desensitizing sodium channels in the central nervous system responsible for neuronal responsiveness. This desensitization prevents the spread of disruptive electrical charges in the brain that cause seizures.

TABLE 9-3	Benzodiazepines Used in Seizure Disorders		
Generic Name	Trade Name	Indications	Average Adult Dosage
clonazepam (C-IV) **(kloh-NAH-zeh-pam)**	Klonopin®	Seizure disorders	0.5–1.5 mg/day in divided doses
clorazepate dipotassium (C-IV) **(kloh-RAH-zeh-payt dy-poh-TAH-see-um)**	Tranxene®	Partial seizures	15–60 mg/day in divided doses
diazepam (C-IV) **(dy-AH-zeh-pam)**	Valium®	Status epilepticus	2–10 mg bid–qid

TABLE 9-4   Hydantoins, Phenytoin-Like Drugs, and Succinimides

Generic Name	Trade Name	Route of Administration	Average Adult Dosage
Hydantoins			
fosphenytoin sodium (Rx) **(fos-feh-nih-TOH-in SOH-dee-um)**	Cerebyx®	IV	Initial: 15–20 mg/kg at 100–150 mg/min; then 4–6 mg/kg/day
phenytoin sodium (Rx) **(feh-nih-TOH-in SOH-dee-um)**	Dilantin®	PO	15–18 mg/kg or 1 g initial dose, then 300 mg/day in 1–3 divided doses; may be gradually increased by 100 mg/week
Phenytoin-Like Drugs			
carbamazepine (Rx) **(kar-bah-MAH-zeh-peen)**	Tegretol®	PO	200 mg bid, gradually increased to 800–1200 mg/day in 3–4 divided doses
felbamate (Rx) **(FEL-bah-mayt)**	Felbatol®	PO	Initial: 1200 mg/day in 3–4 divided doses; may increase by 600 mg/day q2 weeks (max: 3600 mg/day)
lamotrigine (Rx) **(lah-MOH-trih-jeen)**	Lamictal®	PO	50 mg/day for 2 weeks, then 50 mg bid for 2 weeks; may increase gradually to 300–500 mg/day in 2 divided doses (max: 700 mg/day)
pregabalin (C-V) **(pray-GAH-bah-lihn)**	Lyrica®	PO	100 mg/day in 3 divided doses
primidone (Rx) **(PRY-mih-dohn)**	Mysoline®	PO	Up to 500 mg qid
tiagabine hydrochloride (Rx) **(ty-AH-goh-been hy-droh-KLOR-ryd)**	Gabitril®		4–56 mg/day
topiramate (Rx) **(toh-PEER-ah-mayt)**	Topamax®		200–400 mg/day in divided doses
valproic acid (Rx) **(val-PROH-ik AH-sid)**	Depakene®	PO, IV	15 mg/kg/day in divided doses when total is > 250 mg/day; increase by 5–10 mg q week (max: 60 mg/kg/day)
zonisamide (Rx) **(zoh-NIH-sah-myd)**	Zonegran®	PO	100–600 mg/day
Succinimides			
ethosuximide (Rx) **(ee-thoh-SUK-sih-myd)**	Zarontin®	PO	250 mg bid, increased q4–7 days (max: 1.5 g/day)
methsuximide (Rx) **(meth-SUK-sih-myd)**	Celontin®	PO	300 mg/day, may increase q4–7 days (max: 1.2 g/day in divided doses)

Key Concept

Gingival hyperplasia is one of the major adverse effects of long-term use of phenytoin (Dilantin®). Patients who use this agent should be periodically examined for an excessive growth of gum tissue.

Indications

Phenytoin is used for **tonic-clonic seizures**, psychomotor seizures, and seizures after head trauma. Fosphenytoin is converted to phenytoin in the body and is used parenterally for control of status epilepticus; it is a short-term substitute for oral phenytoin.

Adverse Effects

Adverse effects of phenytoin are related to plasma concentrations and include inability to coordinate muscle activity, mental confusion, dizziness, inability to sleep, headache, uncontrollable rhythmic movement of the eyes, gingival hyperplasia, toxic hepatitis, and reduction of the blood cells. Phenytoin may also cause dysrhythmias such as slow heart rate or ventricular fibrillation, abnormally low blood pressure, and hyperglycemia (excess blood glucose).

Contraindications and Precautions

Hydantoin products are contraindicated in patients with known hypersensitivity to these drugs. Hydantoin products are also contraindicated in patients with rash, seizures due to low blood glucose, pregnancy (category D), and lactation.

Hydantoin products should be used cautiously in older adults and in patients with impaired liver or kidney function, alcoholism, blood dyscrasias, hypotension, bradycardia, severe myocardial insufficiency, pancreatic adenoma, and diabetes mellitus.

Drug Interactions

Phenytoin has increased pharmacological effects with chloramphenicol, cimetidine, isoniazid, and sulfonamides. Complex drug interactions and effects occur when phenytoin and valproic acid are given together. Severe hypotension may occur when phenytoin is given intravenously with dopamine. Alcohol decreases fosphenytoin effects. This drug may decrease absorption and increase metabolism of oral anticoagulants.

Phenytoin-Like Agents

Several commonly used drugs are classified as phenytoin-like drugs, including carbamazepine and valproic acid. Newer anti-seizure drugs, which have more limited uses, include zonisamide, felbamate, and lamotrigine, which are categorized as phenytoin-like drugs (see Table 9-4).

Mechanism of Action

In general, the mechanisms of action of phenytoin-like agents are not known, but resemble the mechanism of action of phenytoin.

Indications

Phenytoin-like drugs are useful for a wide range of seizure types, including **absence seizures** and mixed types of seizures. Valproic acid is used for prevention of migraine headaches and treatment of bipolar disorder.

Adverse Effects

Phenytoin-like drugs may result in adverse effects such as drowsiness, sedation, gastrointestinal upsets, and prolonged bleeding time. Other adverse effects are visual disturbances, muscle weakness, bone marrow suppression, rash, fatal liver toxicity, weight gain, loss of hair, and abdominal pain.

Contraindications and Precautions

Phenytoin-like drugs are contraindicated in patients with known hypersensitivity to these agents, and in cardiac, hepatic, or renal disease. These drugs are also contraindicated in pregnancy (category D) and lactation. Carbamazepine should be used with caution in older adults and those with a history of cardiac disease. Valproic acid is used cautiously in patients with a history of kidney disease or renal impairment. This drug should be used with caution in patients with severe recurrent seizures and hypoalbuminemia.

Drug Interactions

Valproic acid interacts with many drugs. For example, chlorpromazine, felbamate, erythomycin, cimetidine, and aspirin may increase valproic acid toxicity. Lamotrigine, phenytoin, and rifampin lower valproic acid levels.

Succinimides

Succinimide drugs are another class of anticonvulsant drugs. Ethosuximide is generally considered to be the safest of the succinimide drugs, and is the most commonly prescribed drug in this class. The succinimide drugs are also listed in Table 9-4.

Mechanism of Action

Succinimides delay the entry of calcium into neurons by blocking calcium channels. Put simply, anti-seizure drugs of this group increase the **electrical threshold**. Succinimides suppress the EEG pattern associated with lapses of consciousness in absence (petit mal) seizures. Their mechanism of action is not understood, but these drugs may act to inhibit neuronal systems.

Indications

Succinimide drugs are used to control absence seizures and myoclonic seizures. They may be given in combination with other anticonvulsants.

Medical Terminology Review

hypoalbuminemia
hypo- = low; under; beneath
albumin = plasma protein
-emia = blood condition
low albumin in the blood plasma

Medical Terminology Review

myoclonic
myo- = muscle
-clonic = contraction and relaxation
contraction and relaxation of the muscles

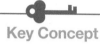

Adverse Effects

Adverse effects of succinimides include ataxia, dizziness, nervousness, headache, and blurred vision. Behavioral changes are more prominent in patients with a history of psychiatric illness. Ethosuximide can also cause abnormal reduction of all circulating blood cells, depression, vaginal bleeding, gingival hyperplasia, muscle weakness, and abnormal liver and kidney function tests.

Contraindications and Precautions

Succinimide drugs are contraindicated in patients with known hypersensitivity to these agents. Succinimides are also contraindicated in patients with bone marrow depression, or with hepatic or renal dysfunction. Ethosuximide should be used cautiously in pregnancy (category C) and lactation.

Drug Interactions

Levels of ethosuximide can be decreased or increased if used with valproates. Even so, combinations of ethosuximide with valproates have a greater protective index than either drug alone. Ethosuximide may elevate serum phenytoin levels. Methsuximide should not be used with barbiturates or hydantoins, since these drugs can increase its adverse effects. Also, methsuximide may decrease the effectiveness of lamotrigine.

SUMMARY

Seizures are a group of disorders that are characterized by hyperexcitability of neurons in the brain. Nearly 2.3 million people in the United States have seizure disorders. *Seizure* is a term for all epileptic events, whereas *convulsion* relates to abnormal motor movements.

Seizure disorders are classified into two basic categories: generalized and partial. Generalized seizures include tonic-clonic (grand mal), absence (petit mal), myoclonic, infantile spasms, and atonic (akinetic). Partial seizures (focal) may be divided into two categories: simple or complex (psychomotor).

Anti-seizure drugs are classified into five groups: barbiturates, benzodiazepines, hydantoins, phenytoin-like agents, and succinimides. Phenytoin is the most recognizable and most used drug in the class of hydantoins. The newest drug in this class is fosphenytoin. Phenytoin is used for tonic-clonic and psychomotor seizures. Fosphenytoin is used for control of status epilepticus. Phenytoin-like drugs are useful for a wide range of seizure types, including absence seizures and mixed types of seizures.

EXPLORING THE WEB

Visit **http://professionals.epilepsy.com**

- Under the heading "Diagnosis & Treatment," look for additional information on drug therapies used to treat epilepsy.

Visit **www.brainexplorer.org**

- Click on the link to "Focus on brain disorders," then click on the link to epilepsy. Read more about this disorder and how the brain is affected.

Visit **www.livestrong.com**

- Search for "benzodiazepines" or "seizures" and review for additional information on these topics.

Visit **www.webmd.com**

- Search for "seizures and epilepsy." Choose articles related to this topic to read for a greater understanding of the disorder and methods used to treat it.

Visit **www.mayoclinic.com**

- Click on "Patient Care & Health Info," then under "Diseases & Conditions A-Z," click on the letter "E," and then "Epilepsy." Review the additional information available on this topic.

Visit **www.nlm.nih.gov**

- Click on "Medline Plus" and search for information related to seizures and epilepsy.

REVIEW QUESTIONS

Multiple Choice

1. Which of the following adverse effects can be caused by ethosuximide (Zarontin®)?

   A. tremors

   B. depression

   C. gingival hyperplasia

   D. hyperplasia of the prostate

2. Which of the following seizures is characterized by alternating contractions and relaxation of the muscles?

   A. febrile

   B. absence

   C. psychomotor

   D. tonic-clonic

3. Which of the following anti-seizure drugs increases phenytoin serum levels?

   A. carbamazepine (Tegretol®)

   B. valproic acid (Depakene®)

   C. ethosuximide (Zarontin®)

   D. felbamate (Felbatol®)

4. Which of the following seizures is classified as a simple seizure?

   A. infantile spasms

   B. absence (petit mal)

   C. psychic

   D. tonic-clonic (grand mal)

5. Which of the following seizures is the most dangerous, and requires prompt treatment?

   A. status epilepticus

   B. Jacksonian

   C. psychomotor

   D. absence

6. The newest drugs in the group of hydantoins is:

   A. phenytoin (Dilantin®)

   B. fosphenytoin (Cerebyx®)

   C. felbamate (Felbatol®)

   D. valproic acid (Depakene®)

7. Most anti-seizure drugs should be used cautiously in pregnancy because they are in which of the following categories?

   A. A

   B. B

   C. C

   D. D

8. Which of the following is the trade name for ethosuximide?

   A. Milontin®

   B. Celontin®

   C. Zarontin®

   D. Zonegran®

9. A specific barbiturate used solely in the treatment of seizures is:

   A. clonazepam

   B. clorazepate

   C. phenobarbital

   D. diazepam

10. Which of the following hydantoins is used for tonic-clonic, psychomotor, and head trauma–related seizures?

    A. carbamazepine

    B. phenytoin

    C. valproic acid

    D. fosphenytoin

11. Diazepam (Valium®) is indicated for which type of seizure disorder?

    A. partial

    B. tonic-clonic

    C. absence

    D. status epilepticus

12. The most recognizable and most used drug in the category of hydantoins is:

    A. ethosuximide

    B. valproic acid

    C. phenytoin

    D. carbamazepine

13. Ethosuximide delays the entry of which of the following minerals into neurons by blocking its channels?

    A. calcium

    B. sodium

    C. potassium

    D. chloride

14. Which of the following agents is the drug of choice for absence seizures?

    A. clonazepam (Klonopin®)

    B. ethosuximide (Zarontin®)

    C. felbamate (Felbatol®)

    D. phenytoin (Dilantin®)

15. Which of the following agents is the trade name of primidone?

    A. Gabitril®

    B. Mysoline®

    C. Lyrica®

    D. Topamax®

Fill in the Blank

1. The trade name of valproic acid is_____.

2. The choice of drugs to treat seizure disorders depends on patient conditions and _____ preference.

3. Tonic-clonic seizures are classified as_____ seizures.

4. A complex seizure that impairs consciousness is also known as a _____ seizure.

5. Fosphenytoin is the newest drug of the hydantoin group and is converted to_____ in the body.

6. Absence seizures are also known as_____.

7. Examples of phenytoin-like drugs include carbamazepine, felbamate, lamotrigine, pregabalin, primidone, tiagabine hydrochloride, topiramate, _____, and _____.

Critical Thinking

A 36-year-old woman has been suffering from migraine headaches for almost two years. Her physician orders an anti-seizure, phenytoin-like medication for prevention of migraines.

1. Which of the phenytoin-like drugs is used for the prevention of migraines?

2. If this patient were suffering from absence seizures, what phenytoin-like drugs might be prescribed?

3. Name the most dangerous adverse effects for a patient who is taking phenytoin-like drugs.

Anesthetic Drugs

OBJECTIVES

After completing this chapter, the reader should be able to:

1. List the stages of anesthesia.
2. Define the importance of preanesthesia.
3. Outline the effects of general anesthetics.
4. Explain the mechanism of action of local anesthetics.
5. List the problems associated with the use of local anesthetics.
6. Describe the common local anesthetics and their uses.
7. Compare and contrast the five major routes for administering local anesthetics.
8. Define malignant hyperthermia.
9. Explain a malignant hyperthermia kit.
10. Define balanced anesthesia.

GLOSSARY

Anesthesia – a loss of feeling or sensation

Anesthetics – agents that partially or completely numb or eliminate sensitivity with or without loss of consciousness

Epidural anesthesia – injection of an anesthetic into the space immediately outside of the dura mater that contains a supporting cushion of fat and other connective tissues

General anesthetics – agents that provide a pain-free state for the entire body

Hypermetabolic – burning energy and nutrients at a higher rate than normal

Infiltration anesthesia – anesthesia produced by injecting a local anesthetic drug into tissues

Lipophilic – able to dissolve much more easily in lipids than in water

Local anesthetics – agents that provide a pain-free state in a specific area of the body

Malignant hyperthermia – a rare, genetic hypermetabolic condition that is characterized by severe overproduction of body heat with rigidity of skeletal muscles

Nystagmus – rhythmical oscillation of the eyeballs

Preanesthetic medications – drugs given before the administration of anesthesia

Spinal anesthesia – a type of regional anesthesia produced by injecting a local anesthetic drug into the subarachnoid space of the spinal cord

Volatile liquids – liquids that evaporate upon exposure to the air

OVERVIEW

For several centuries, opiates and alcohol were the mainstays of **anesthetics** (substances used to reduce sensation of pain) in the control of pain. These substances had limited success, but were probably better than nothing. It was not until the 1840s that surgical **anesthesia** (reduction or elimination of pain) became possible, with the introduction of three agents: chloroform, ether, and nitrous oxide. These three substances, upon inhalation, quickly lead to a state of unconsciousness in which pain is not felt. Nitrous oxide is still one of the most widely used gaseous anesthetics, and diethyl ether is still occasionally used. Chloroform is rarely used today because of its toxicity, but other, newer halogenated hydrocarbons, such as halothane, are extremely common.

Gaseous anesthetics are the principal agents used in the maintenance of anesthesia, but agents given by other routes are still used in the induction of anesthesia. Anesthesia is basically characterized by four reversible action consciousness, analgesia, immobility, and amnesia. The critical factor is that there should be no significant impairment of cardiovascular or respiratory functions, especially those supplying the brain and other vital organs with adequate blood, nutrients, and gases.

General anesthetics are used to produce loss of consciousness before and during surgery. **Local anesthetics** numb small areas of the body tissue where a minor procedure is to be done, and are commonly used in dentistry for minor surgery. Regional anesthesia affects a larger (but still limited) part of the body, but does not make the person unconscious. Spinal and epidural anesthesia are examples of regional anesthesia.

> **Medical Terminology Review**
>
> **epidural**
> epi- = on; upon; at; near; among
> -dural = dura mater; the outermost layer of the meninges
> near the outermost layer of the meninges

PREANESTHETIC MEDICATIONS

Preanesthetic medications are used prior to the administration of an anesthetic to facilitate induction of anesthesia and to relieve anxiety and pain. They may also be used to minimize some of the undesirable effects of anesthetics, such as excessive salivation, bradycardia, and vomiting. To accomplish these objectives, several drugs are often used at the same time. The following medications are commonly used as preoperative drugs:

- Sedative-hypnotics such as hydroxyzine and promethazine (see Chapter 6 for discussion of this classification)

- Antianxiety agents such as droperidol and diazepam (see Chapter 6)

- Opioid analgesics such as morphine, meperidine, and fentanyl (see Chapter 22)

- Anticholinergics such as atropine and scopolamine (see Chapter 7)

> **Key Concept**
>
> Preanesthetic drugs may not be used in patients older than 60 years of age because many of the medical conditions or disorders for which these drugs are contraindicated occur in this age group.

STAGES AND PLANES OF ANESTHESIA

Before patients reach surgical anesthesia, they go through several stages. The use of these stages and planes of anesthesia helps to describe the levels and progression of anesthesia produced by anesthetics. There are four stages of general anesthesia:

Stage I

This stage begins when the agent is administered and lasts until loss of consciousness. Stage I is characterized by:

- Analgesia
- Euphoria
- Perceptual distortions
- Amnesia

Stage II

Delirium begins with loss of consciousness and extends to the beginning of surgical anesthesia. There may be excitement and involuntary muscular activity. The skeletal muscle tone increases and breathing is irregular. At this stage, hypertension and tachycardia may occur. It is important that the passage from stage I to stage III be attained as quickly as possible. Sudden death can occur during stage II.

Stage III

Surgical anesthesia lasts until spontaneous respiration ceases. It is further divided into four planes based on:

- Respiration
- The size of the pupils
- Reflex characteristics
- Eyeball movements

This stage is characterized by progressive muscular relaxation. Muscle relaxation is important during many surgical procedures as reflex movements can occur when a scalpel slices through the tissues.

Stage IV

Medullary paralysis begins with respiratory failure and can lead to circulatory collapse. Through careful monitoring, this stage is avoided.

Key Concept

In the induction of anesthesia with intravenous anesthetic agents, stages I and III merge so quickly into one another that they are not apparent.

GENERAL ANESTHETICS

General anesthetics are drugs that immediately produce unconsciousness and complete analgesia. These agents are generally administered by intravenous or inhalation routes. Preanesthetic and adjunct drugs are given before, during, and after surgery.

Inhalation Anesthetics

Certain drugs that are gases or **volatile liquids** at room temperature are administered by inhalation in combination with air or oxygen. The only gas used routinely for anesthesia is nitrous oxide, commonly called laughing gas. It is usually administered in combination with oxygen. Nitrous oxide provides analgesia equivalent to 10 mg of morphine sulfate but may cause occasional episodes of nausea and vomiting. Volatile liquids are converted into a vapor and inhaled to produce their anesthetic effects. Commonly administered volatile agents are halothane, enflurane, and isoflurane. The most potent of these is halothane (Table 10-1).

Mechanism of Action

Inhaled general anesthetics are all very **lipophilic** (able to dissolve much more easily in lipids than in water). When the lipophilic anesthetic enters the lipid membrane, the whole membrane is slightly distorted and closes the sodium channels, causing a marginal blockage, which prevents neural conduction.

Indications

Volatile anesthetics are rarely used as the sole agents for both induction and maintenance of anesthesia. Most commonly, they are combined with

Medical Terminology
Review
lipophilic
lipo- = lipids (fats)
-philic = having an affinity for
having an affinity for fats

TABLE 10-1	Inhaled General Anesthetics	
Generic Name	**Trade Name**	**Uses**
Gas		
nitrous oxide **(NY-truhs OK-syd)**	(generic only)	Used alone in dentistry, obstetrics, and short medical procedures; used in combination with more potent inhaled anesthetics
Volatile Liquids		
desflurane **(des-FLOO-rayn)**	Suprane®	Induction and maintenance of general anesthesia
enflurane **(en-FLOO-rayn)**	Ethrane®	Induction and maintenance of general anesthesia
halothane **(HAL-loh-thayn)**	Fluothane®	Induction and maintenance of general anesthesia; since safer agents have become available, its use has declined
isoflurane **(eye-soh-FLOO-rayn)**	Forane®	Induction and maintenance of general anesthesia; it is the most widely used inhalation anesthetic
methoxyflurane **(meh-thok-see-FLOO-rayn)**	Penthrane®	Used during labor; it does not suppress uterine contractions as greatly as other agents
sevoflurane **(see-voh-FLOO-rayn)**	Ultane®	Induction and maintenance of general anesthesia

intravenous agents in regimens of the so-called balanced anesthesia. Of the inhaled anesthetics, nitrous oxide, desflurane, and sevoflurane are the most commonly used in the United States.

Adverse Effects

Nitrous oxide at higher doses causes anxiety, excitement, and aggressiveness. It also produces nausea, vomiting, and difficulty in breathing. Volatile anesthetics may cause headache, shivering, muscle pain, mental or mood changes, sore throat, and nightmares.

Contraindications and Precautions

Inhaled general anesthetics are contraindicated in patients with known hypersensitivity to these agents. They are also contraindicated in patients who have received monoamine oxidase inhibitors (MAOIs) within the previous 14 days (refer to Chapter 5). They should not be used by those who are intolerant to benzodiazepines, or have myasthenia gravis, acute narrow-angle glaucoma, acute alcohol intoxication, status asthmaticus, and acute intermittent porphyria.

Inhaled general anesthetics should be used cautiously during pregnancy, and in children younger than 12.

Drug Interactions

Inhaled general anesthetic drugs may interact with levodopa and increase the level of dopamine in the central nervous system. Skeletal muscle weakness, respiratory depression, or apnea may occur if halothane is administered with polymyxins, lincomycin, or aminoglycosides.

Injectable General Anesthetics

Intravenous anesthetics are often administered with inhaled general anesthetics. Administration of intravenous and inhaled anesthetics together allows the dose of the inhaled drug to be reduced, resulting in a decreased probability of serious side effects. Intravenous anesthetics also provide more analgesia and muscle relaxation than is provided by an inhaled anesthetic alone. Drugs used as intravenous anesthetics include opioids, barbiturates, and benzodiazepines (Table 10–2).

LOCAL ANESTHETICS

Local anesthetics are drugs that block the transmission of nerve impulses between the peripheral nervous system and the central nervous system. Their main purpose is to prevent pain impulses from pain receptors reaching the higher centers. They are mainly used in minor surgical procedures

TABLE 10-2 **Intravenous Anesthetics**

Generic Name	Trade Name	Comments
Barbiturates and Barbiturate-Like Agents		
etomidate (eh-TAW-mih-dayt)	Amidate®	For induction of anesthesia and for short medical procedures
methohexital sodium (meh-thoh-HEK-sih-tahl SOH-dee-um)	Brevital®	Ultra–short-acting; for induction of anesthesia and as a supplement to other anesthetics
propofol (PROH-poh-fahl)	Diprivan®	For induction and maintenance of general anesthesia, and for short medical procedures
thiopental sodium (thy-oh-PEN-tahl SOH-dee-um)	Pentothal®	Ultra–short-acting; for induction of anesthesia and as a supplement to other anesthetics
Benzodiazepines		
diazepam (dy-AH-zeh-pam)	Valium®	For induction of anesthesia; the prototype benzodiazepine
lorazepam (loh-RAH-zeh-pam)	Ativan®	For induction of anesthesia, to produce conscious benzodiazepine sedation, and for short medical procedures or surgery
midazolam hydrochloride (mih-DAH-zoh-lam hy-droh-KLOR-ryd)	Versed®	For induction of anesthesia; to produce conscious sedation, and for short diagnostic procedures
Opioids		
alfentanil hydrochloride (al-FEN-tah-nihl hy-droh-KLOR-ryd)	Alfenta®	Rapid onset and short onset of action; for induction of anesthesia; used as a supplement to other anesthetics
fentanyl citrate (FEN-tah-nihl SY-trayt)	Sublimaze®	Short-acting; used during operative and perioperative periods; to supplement both general and regional anesthesia
remifentanil hydrochloride (reh-mih-FEN-tah-nihl hy-droh-KLOR-ryd)	Ultiva®	Short-acting; for induction and maintenance of general anesthesia
sufentanil citrate (soo-FEN-tah-nihl SY-trayt)	Sufenta®	For induction and maintenance of anesthesia; approximately 7 times as potent as fentanyl with more rapid onset and duration of action
Others		
ketamine hydrochloride (KEE-tah-meen hy-droh-KLOR-ryd)	Ketalar®	For sedation, amnesia, analgesia in short diagnostic, therapeutic, or surgical procedures; most often used in children

and are especially common in dentistry. Many minor surgical procedures such as suturing, excision of superficial growths, and removal of cataracts are commonly performed using a local anesthetic injected intradermally or subcutaneously. Even deeper-excision operations such as hernias are performed occasionally using local anesthetics. Local anesthesia is more accurately called surface anesthesia or regional anesthesia. Neuromuscular blocking agents, which interfere locally with impulses from motor nerves to skeletal muscles, are discussed in Chapter 11.

Classification of Local Anesthetics

The two major groups of local anesthetics are esters and amides (Table 10–3). The ester-type anesthetics, represented by procaine, contain an ester linkage in their chemical structure. The esters are classified as long-acting (tetracaine), short-acting (procaine), and surface-acting (benzocaine, cocaine). In contrast, the amide-type drugs, represented by lidocaine, contain an amide linkage. They are of two groups: long-acting (bupivacaine, ropivacaine) and medium-acting (lidocaine).

The amides have several advantages over the esters. Hypersensitivity to amide local anesthetics is rare. Most of the local anesthetics in common use today belong to the amide class.

Ester-type local anesthetics have been in use longer than amides. They tend to have a rapid onset and short duration of activity (except tetracaine). Esters are associated with a higher incidence of allergic reactions due to one of their metabolites, para-amino benzoic acid (PABA). PABA is structurally similar to methylparaben.

Mechanism of Action

Local anesthetics stop nerve conduction by inhibiting movement of sodium through channels in the membrane of a neuron. Therefore, neurons cannot fire because these agents block sodium channels.

Indications

Local anesthetics are used for minor surgery, dental procedures, suturing small wounds, or making an incision into a small area for removing a superficial tissue sample for biopsy. Local anesthetics may also be used for obstetrics during labor and delivery, for diagnostic procedures such as gastrointestinal endoscopy, wart treatment, vasectomy, and neonatal circumcision.

Adverse Effects

True allergic reactions to local anesthetics are rare and usually involve ester agents. Toxic effects are usually dose-related. Adverse effects include restlessness, dizziness, disorientation, light-headedness, **nystagmus** (rhythmical oscillation of the eyeballs), and psychosis. Slurred speech and tremors

TABLE 10-3 | **Common Local Anesthetics**

Generic Name	Trade Name	Use	Comments
Esters			
benzocaine (**BEN-zoh-kayn**)	Americaine®, Solarcaine®	Topical	For earache, hemorrhoids, sore throat, sunburn, and minor skin conditions
chloroprocaine (**klor-oh-PROH-kayn**)	Nesacaine®	Epidural, infiltration, and nerve block	Short duration
cocaine (**ko-KAYN**)	(generic only)	Topical	For ear, nose, and throat procedures
procaine hydrochloride (**PROH-kayn hy-droh-KLOR-ryd**)	Novocain®	Epidural, infiltration, nerve block, and spinal	Short duration
tetracaine (**TEH-trah-kayn**)	Pontocaine®	Spinal and topical	Long duration
Amides			
bupivacaine hydrochloride (**byoo-PIH-vah-kayn**)	Marcaine®	Epidural and infiltration	Long duration
dibucaine (**DY-byoo-kayn**)	Nupercainal®	Spinal and topical	Long duration
lidocaine hydrochloride (**LY-doh-kayn hy-droh-KLOR-ryd**)	Xylocaine®	Epidural, infiltration, nerve block, spinal, and topical	May be combined with prilocaine (EMLA cream) for topical application
mepivacaine (**meh-PIH-vah-kayn**)	Carbocaine®	Epidural, infiltration, and nerve block	Intermediate duration
prilocaine (**PRY-loh-kayn**)	Citanest®	Epidural, infiltration, and nerve block	Intermediate duration
ropivacaine (**roh-PIH-vah-kayn**)	Naropin®	Epidural, infiltration, and nerve block	Long duration
Miscellaneous Agents			
dyclonine (**DY-kloh-neen**)	Dyclone®	Topical	For ear, nose, and throat procedures
pramoxine (**prah-MOK-seen**)	Tronolane®	Topical	For minor medical procedures

often precede seizures. Severe convulsions may be followed by coma, with respiratory depression, cardiovascular depression, and cardiac arrest.

Contraindications and Precautions

Local anesthetics are contraindicated in patients with known hypersensitivity, in the elderly, and in severe hemorrhage, hypotension, and shock. These agents are also contraindicated in patients with cerebrospinal deformities, blood dyscrasias, and hypertension.

Drug Interactions

Barbiturates may decrease the activity of lidocaine. Increased effects of lidocaine may occur if taken with beta-blockers, cimetidine, and quinidine. If lidocaine is used on a regular basis, its effectiveness may diminish when used with other medications.

Routes of Administration of Local Anesthetics

There are five major routes for applying local anesthetics (Figure 10-1). These routes are summarized as follows:

1. Topical
2. Nerve block
3. Infiltration
4. Spinal
5. Epidural

Topical Anesthesia

Topical anesthesia acts as a nerve conduction–blocking agent on the skin or mucous membranes. This procedure can provide anesthesia on skin and

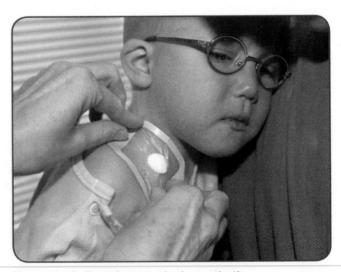

Figure 10-1A Tegaderm topical anesthetic.

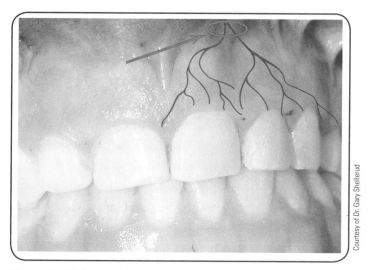

Figure 10-1B Nerve block anesthesia.

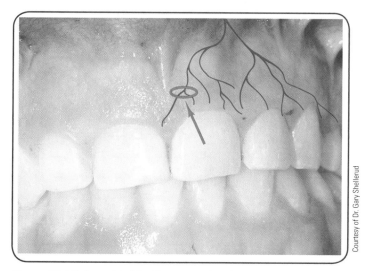

Figure 10-1C Local infiltration anesthesia.

the mucous membranes of the rectum, urethra, and vagina. Lidocaine is an example of a topical anesthetic agent.

Nerve Block Anesthesia

Nerve block anesthesia affects the bundle of nerves serving the area to be operated upon. This method is used to block sensation in a limb or large area such as the face.

Local Infiltration Anesthesia

Local **infiltration anesthesia** blocks a specific group of nerves in a small area very close to the area to be operated on. Local infiltration is probably the most common route used to administer local anesthetics and is the simplest form of regional anesthesia. Lidocaine is a popular choice for infiltration anesthesia, but bupivacaine is used for longer procedures.

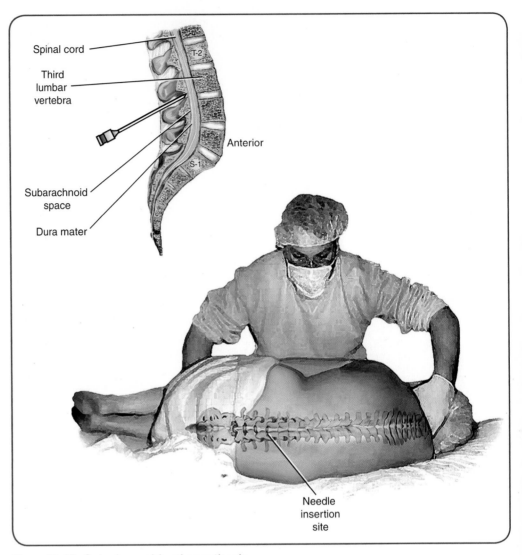

Figure 10-1D Spinal or epidural anesthesia.

Spinal Anesthesia

During **spinal anesthesia**, an anesthetic agent is injected into the subarachnoid space (beneath the arachnoid membrane or between the arachnoid and pia mater, and filled with cerebrospinal fluid) through a spinal needle. Drugs injected in this manner affect large regional areas such as the lower abdomen and legs.

Epidural Anesthesia

Epidural anesthesia involves injection of the local anesthetic into the epidural (lumbar or caudal) space by means of a catheter that allows repeated infusions. After injection, the anesthetic agent is very slowly absorbed into the cerebrospinal fluid. This method is most commonly used in obstetrics during labor and delivery.

Medical Terminology Review

arachnoid
arach- = spider
-noid = like
spider-like

MALIGNANT HYPERTHERMIA

Malignant hyperthermia is a rare, genetic **hypermetabolic** condition that is characterized by severe overproduction of body heat with rigidity of skeletal muscles. It is a serious adverse effect of anesthesia (relating to inhalation anesthetics) that must be treated immediately. Drugs that are known triggers of malignant hyperthermia include desflurane, enflurane, ether, halothane, isoflurane, methoxyflurane, sevoflurane, and succinylcholine. Treatment includes administration of large doses of dantrolene sodium and 100% oxygen, followed by immediate cooling, cessation of surgery, and correction of hyperkalemia.

Dantrolene has a very short shelf life and must be restocked regularly so that, when needed, its action will be potent. The drug is stored in a freeze-dried form that is reconstituted with sterile water that does not contain a bacteriostatic agent. This sterile water should be stored in 100-mL vials, not bags, to avoid accidental intravenous administration of this hypotonic solution. Reconstitution involves injecting 60 mL of sterile water per bottle of dantrolene. The bottle must be shaken vigorously to dissolve the dantrolene, and to help warm the mixture. The mixture is then injected rapidly through intravenous lines. (**NOTE: A source for this procedure is http://www .mhaus.org/faqs/dantrolene**)

Malignant hyperthermia may cause the death of the patient due to brain damage, cardiac arrest, internal bleeding, or damage to other body systems. A malignant hyperthermia kit must include:

- Dantrolene
- Furosemide
- Glucose
- Procainamide
- Sodium bicarbonate (7.5%)
- Sterile water

Medical Terminology Review

hyperkalemia
hyper- = over; above; beyond
-kalemia = condition of potassium ions in the blood
increased number of potassium ions in the blood

Key Concept

Patients susceptible to malignant hyperthermia must be informed of the condition and potentially susceptible relatives of the patient should also be screened.

SUMMARY

Preanesthetic drugs are used to facilitate induction of anesthesia and to relieve anxiety and pain. There are four stages of anesthesia. Stage I is characterized by analgesia, euphoria, and amnesia. Stage II increases the skeletal muscle tone and breathing is irregular. It is important that the passage from stage I to stage III be attained as quickly as possible. Stage III is called surgical anesthesia, which produces muscular relaxation. Stage IV causes medullary paralysis, and this stage should be avoided.

General anesthesia is a reversible stage of unconsciousness as a result of medication. It can be induced by inhalation or by injection of drugs. The combination of injectable anesthetics together with inhaled general anesthetics allows a decreased probability of serious side effects.

The two major groups of local anesthetics are esters and amides. The amides have several advantages over the esters. Local anesthetics are used for minor surgery, dental procedures, suturing small wounds, or removing a superficial tissue sample for biopsy.

EXPLORING THE WEB

Visit **www.webmd.com**

• Search for "toxicology" and look for information related to the drugs covered in this chapter.

Visit **www.healthline.com**

• Search for "anesthesia," and review information that related to this topic.

Visit **www.mayoclinic.com**

• Search for "anesthesia," and review information that related to this topic.

REVIEW QUESTIONS

Multiple Choice

1. The main purpose of local anesthetics is to prevent which of the following?
   A. falling asleep and muscle contraction
   B. allergic reaction and anaphylactic shock
   C. pain impulses from pain receptors reaching the lower limbs
   D. pain impulses from pain receptors reaching the higher centers

2. The ester-type anesthetics are represented by which of the following substances?
   A. procaine
   B. prolactin
   C. pro-hormone
   D. pro-vitamin

3. Which of the following is the most common route used to administer local anesthetics?
   A. epidural
   B. topical
   C. local infiltration
   D. nerve block

4. Which of the following stages of anesthesia must be avoided?

    A. Stage I

    B. Stage II

    C. Stage III

    D. Stage IV

5. Which of the following preanesthetic medications relieve anxiety?

    A. scopolamine

    B. promethazine

    C. diazepam

    D. atropine

6. Which of the following stages of anesthesia is characterized by euphoria and perceptual distortions?

    A. Stage I

    B. Stage II

    C. Stage III

    D. Stage IV

7. Which of the following is the only gas that is routinely used for anesthesia?

    A. chloroform

    B. ether

    C. nitrous oxide

    D. halothane

8. Which of the following volatile agents is the most potent?

    A. isoflurane

    B. halothane

    C. sevoflurane

    D. enflurane

9. All of the following agents are used as inhaled anesthetics, *except*:

    A. desflurane

    B. nitrous oxide

    C. propofol

    D. sevoflurane

10. Local anesthesia is more accurately called:

    A. surface anesthesia

    B. preanesthetic medication

    C. maintenance of anesthesia

    D. surgical anesthesia

11. Which of the following agents is in the local anesthetic amide group?

    A. procaine (Novocain®)

    B. lidocaine (Xylocaine®)

    C. tetracaine (Pontocaine®)

    D. benzocaine (Americaine®)

12. Which of the following is the stage of surgical anesthesia?

    A. Stage I

    B. Stage IV

    C. Stage II

    D. Stage III

Matching

Generic Names

_____ 1. sevoflurane

_____ 2. isoflurane

_____ 3. halothane

_____ 4. enflurane

_____ 5. desflurane

_____ 6. methoxyflurane

Trade Names

A. Penthrane®

B. Suprane®

C. Fluothane®

D. Ethrane®

E. Forane®

F. Ultane®

Fill in the Blank

1. A woman in labor will most likely receive _____ anesthesia.

2. Anticholinergics used to minimize some of the undesirable after effects of anesthetics, such as excessive salvation, vomiting, and bradycardia, include_____ and _____.

3. Nitrous oxide is also called _____.

4. Hypersensitivity to amide local anesthetics is _____.

Critical Thinking

A 65-year-old man is going under local anesthesia for two dental implants. His medical history is satisfactory, but he is taking three different medications: Zocor® 10 mg and niacin 1000 mg (for hypercholesterolemia), and Allegra® 180 mg (for allergies).

1. What would be the best type of local anesthesia for this patient?

2. If his dentist is using the preferred local anesthesia for this procedure, would there be any drug interactions with the medications that the patient is taking?

3. What may be the adverse effects for local anesthesia used in this procedure?

Drug Therapy for the Musculoskeletal System

OBJECTIVES

After completing this chapter, the reader should be able to:

1. Compare and define the terms *rheumatoid arthritis*, *gout*, and *osteoarthritis*.

2. Discuss skeletal muscle relaxants.

3. Discuss neuromuscular blocking agents.

4. Explain the goals of pharmacotherapy with skeletal muscle relaxants.

5. Define centrally acting skeletal muscle relaxants.

6. Explain the major side effect of dantrolene (direct-acting skeletal muscle relaxant).

7. Discuss drugs used to treat gout.

8. Explain the mechanism of action of corticosteroids.

9. Explain gold compounds and their indications.

10. Define the newer drugs (DMARDs and biologics) used in the treatment of rheumatoid arthritis.

GLOSSARY

Articular – related to the joints of the body

Contusions – injuries to body parts or tissues without a break in the skin

Exfoliative dermatitis – a skin disorder characterized by reddening and scaling of 100% of the skin; erythroderma

Gout – a disease caused by a congenital disorder of uric acid metabolism; metabolic arthritis

Hematomas – collections of blood that has seeped from a blood vessel and entered tissues, organs, or body spaces

Lacerations – cuts or breaks in the skin

Periosteum – a thick, fibrous membrane covering the entire surface of a bone except its articular cartilage and where it attaches to tendons and ligaments

Psoriatic arthritis – a form of arthritis associated with psoriatic lesions of the skin and nails, particularly at the distal interphalangeal joints of the fingers and toes

Osteoarthritis (OA) – arthritis characterized by erosion of articular cartilage that mainly affects weight-bearing joints in older adults

Rheumatoid arthritis (RA) – a chronic and progressive condition that affects more women than men, producing inflammation mainly of the joints of the hands and feet, and leading to deformity and disability

Spasticity – a type of increase in muscle tone at rest, characterized by increased resistance of the muscles to stretching

Sprain – an injury to supporting ligaments of joints

Strain – an injury caused by overstretching a muscle, resulting in a tear of the muscle or muscle and tendon

Synapse – acting as the point of contact between two neurons, or between a neuron and an effector organ, across which nerve impulses are transmitted through the action of a neurotransmitter

OVERVIEW

Muscle spasms, spasticity, and joint disorders are some of the most common disorders in humans of any age. Medications used to treat these conditions may be classified in two broad categories: skeletal muscle relaxants and nonsteroidal anti-inflammatory drugs (NSAIDs). In this chapter, we will focus on drugs such as skeletal muscle relaxants (for disorders such as muscular spasticity due to neurological disorders), gold salts (for arthritis), disease-modifying anti-rheumatic drugs (DMARDs), biologics, and agents used to treat gout. NSAIDs will be discussed with more depth in Chapter 22.

ANATOMY REVIEW

- The musculoskeletal system consists of several separate body systems: the skeletal system, the muscular system, and the **articular** system (Figure 11-1).

- The skeletal system consists of 206 bones as well as the cartilages, ligaments, and tendons associated with the bones (Figure 11-2).

- Functions of the skeletal system include support and stabilization, protection of organs, assistance with movement, manufacture of blood cells, and storage of minerals.

- The muscular system consists of three types of muscle: skeletal, smooth, and cardiac (Figure 11-3).

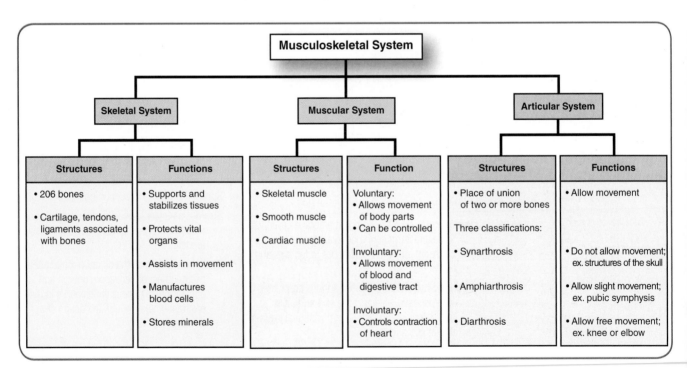

Figure 11-1 The musculoskeletal system.

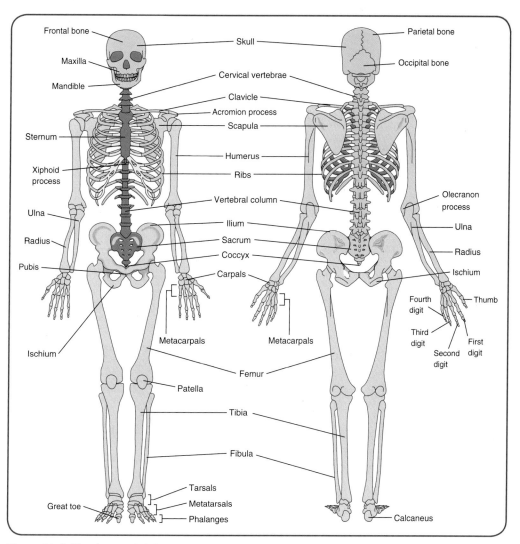

Figure 11-2 The bones of the human body.

- Skeletal muscle allows voluntary movement such as flexion and extension of the legs. Smooth muscle allows involuntary movement in particular body organs such as movement of the nutrients through the digestive tract. Cardiac muscle is found only in the heart and controls the involuntary contractions of the heart.

- The articular system consists of three types of joints: synarthrosis, amphiarthrosis, and diarthrosis (Figure 11-4).

- Synarthrosis joints, such as the sutures in the skull, do not allow movement.

- Amphiarthrosis joints, such as the pubic symphysis, allow slight movement.

- Diarthrosis joints allow free range of motion such as the movements around the shoulder girdle.

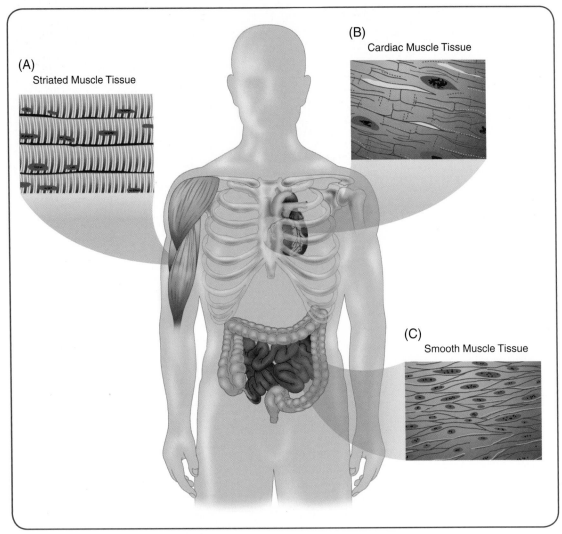

Figure 11-3 Types of muscle: (A) skeletal (striated) muscle, (B) cardiac muscle, (C) smooth muscle.

MUSCULOSKELETAL DISORDERS

The musculoskeletal system is subject to a large number of disorders. These disorders affect persons of all age groups and occupations. They are a major cause of pain and disability.

Injury and Trauma of the Musculoskeletal System

A broad spectrum of musculoskeletal injuries results from numerous physical forces, including blunt tissue trauma, disruption of tendons and ligaments, and fractures of bony structures. Many of the forces that cause injury to the musculoskeletal system are typical for a particular environmental setting, activity, or age group. Trauma resulting from high-speed motor accidents is a common cause of injury in adults younger than 45. The most common causes of childhood injuries are falls, bicycle-related injuries, and sports injuries. Falls are the most common causes of injury in people of

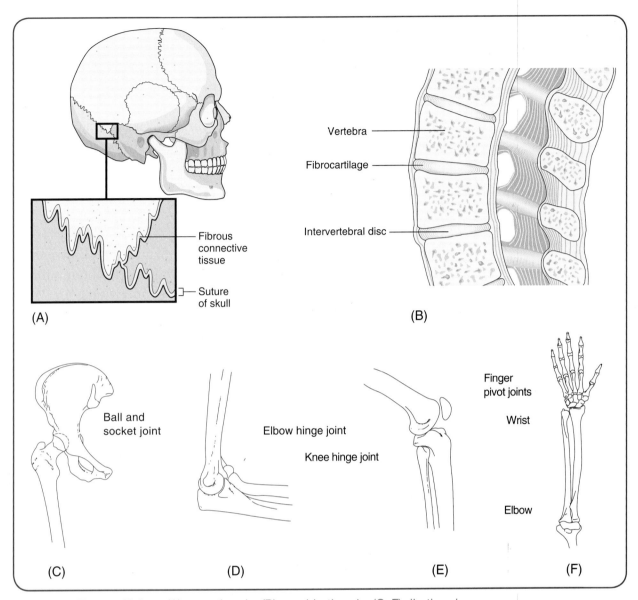

Figure 11-4 Types of joints: (A) synarthrosis, (B) amphiarthrosis, (C–F) diarthrosis.

65 years of age and older, with fractures of the hip and proximal humerus particularly common in this age group.

Most skeletal injuries are accompanied by soft tissue (muscle, tendon, or ligament) injuries. These injuries include **contusions** (injuries of body parts without a break in the skin), **hematomas** (collections of blood that has seeped from the blood vessels to become trapped in organs, spaces, or tissues), and **lacerations** (cuts or breaks in the skin).

Joints are sites where two or more bones meet. Joints are supported by tough bundles of collagenous fibers called ligaments that attach to the joint capsule and bind the articular ends of bones together. They are also supported by tendons that join muscles to the **periosteum** of an articulating bone. Joint injuries involve mechanical overloading or forcible twisting or stretching.

Sprains and strains are both musculoskeletal injuries, but they differ in terms of the tissue that is affected. A **sprain** involves the supporting ligaments of a joint. A complete tear in a muscle or tendon is described as a rupture. A **strain** is a stretching or a partial tear in a muscle or a muscle-tendon unit. Strains commonly result from the sudden stretching of a muscle that is actively contracting. Strains can occur at any age, but are more common in middle-aged and older adults. Muscle strains are usually characterized by pain, stiffness, swelling, and local tenderness. Pain is increased with stretching of the muscle group.

Rheumatoid Arthritis

Rheumatoid arthritis (RA) is a systemic inflammatory disease that attacks joints by producing inflammation of the synovial membranes that leads to the destruction of the articular cartilage and underlying bone. Women are affected by this condition two to three times more frequently than men. Although the disease occurs in all age groups, its prevalence increases with age. The peak incidence among women is between the ages of 40 and 60 years, with the onset at 30 to 50 years of age.

The cause of RA has not been established. However, evidence points to a genetic predisposition and the development of joint inflammation that is immunologically mediated. Unknown environmental factors such as viral infections are believed to play a role in RA.

Onset of RA is insidious. Joint involvement usually is systemic and involves more than one joint. The patient may complain of joint pain, swelling, redness, warmth, and stiffness, beginning in the early morning, which lasts for 30 minutes or longer, and frequently for several hours. The most commonly affected joints initially are the fingers, hands, wrists, knees, and feet. Later, other joints may become involved, including those of the shoulders, elbows, and hips. Spinal involvement usually is limited to the cervical region. There is generalized afternoon fatigue and malaise, generalized weakness, anorexia, and sometimes, a low-grade fever. This disease progresses most quickly during the first six years, particularly in the first year. Within 10 years, 80% of patients develop permanent joint abnormalities. It progresses unpredictably, but are usually symmetric.

Extra-articular manifestations include subcutaneous rheumatoid nodules in one-third of patients, and visceral nodules that are usually asymptomatic. In some patients, vasculitis, pericarditis, myocarditis, pulmonary nodules, or lymphadenopathy develop.

Gout

Gout is actually a group of diseases known as the gout syndrome. It includes acute gouty arthritis with recurrent attacks of severe joint inflammation, and the accumulation of crystalline deposits in joint surfaces, bones, soft tissue, and cartilage. Gout also may cause gouty nephropathy or renal impairment, and uric acid kidney stones.

Uric acid is a waste product of purine metabolism, normally excreted through the kidneys. A sudden increase in serum uric acid levels usually precipitates an attack of gout. Gout often affects a single joint, such as in the big toe. When acute inflammation develops from uric acid deposits, the joint cartilage is damaged. The inflammation causes redness and swelling of the joint, accompanied by severe pain.

Osteoarthritis

Osteoarthritis (OA) is by far the most common form of arthritis among the elderly. It is the greatest cause of disability and limitation of activity in older adults. It has been suggested that osteoarthritis begins at a very young age, expressing itself in the elderly only after a long period of latency. Osteoarthritis presents a major management problem, but there is much that can be done to help lessen its effects. Self-control, by maintaining a positive attitude and a sense of self-esteem, is a frequent coping strategy. Treatment of osteoarthritis in the elderly focuses on relief of pain and improvement of functional status.

Psoriatic Arthritis

Psoriatic arthritis is a chronic, inflammatory condition that occurs in 5% to 40% of patients who have psoriasis of the skin or nails. It is often asymmetric, and may affect the distal interphalangeal joints of the fingers and toes. The condition is more common in patients who also have AIDS.   It is of unknown etiology and pathophysiology.

Signs and symptoms include skin lesions in the scalp, gluteal folds, or umbilicus, and back or spinal pain, since the other joints that may be affected include those of the sacroiliacs and spine. Joint and skin symptoms may lessen or worsen at the same time. Joint deformities are often "sausage" shaped. Remissions of the condition are usually faster, more complete, and occur more frequently than those of rheumatoid arthritis. However, psoriatic arthritis may progress to chronic arthritis and crippling deformities. Patients suspected of having this condition should be tested for *rheumatoid factor*. Treatments are similar to those used for rheumatoid arthritis, and may also include phototherapy with a substance called *psoralen* plus ultraviolet A exposure.

SKELETAL MUSCLE RELAXANTS

Most muscle strains and spasms are self-limited and respond to rest, physical therapy, and short-term use of aspirin and other analgesics. However, spasticity (a form of muscular contraction), as the result of closed head injuries, stroke, cerebral palsy, multiple sclerosis, spinal cord injury, and other neurological conditions, requires long-term use of muscle relaxants. The skeletal muscles are voluntary muscles. They are under control of the central nervous system (CNS). Skeletal muscle relaxants work by blocking somatic motor nerve impulses through depression of the neurons within the CNS. Transmission of an impulse from the motor nerve to each muscle cell occurs across a space known as the neuromuscular junction (Figure 11-5). This space is sensitive to chemical changes in its immediate environment. Therefore, the somatic motor nerve impulses cannot be generated. This mechanism may also decrease the availability of calcium ions to the myofibrillar contractile system. Discontinuity of certain afferent reflex pathways by local anesthesia may also effect relaxation of limited muscle groups; local anesthetic block of efferent somatic motor outflow also is used occasionally to relieve localized skeletal muscle spasms.

Neuromuscular Blocking Agents

Neuromuscular blocking agents are chemical substances that interfere locally with the transmission or reception of impulses from motor nerves to skeletal muscles. Table 11-1 shows some popular neuromuscular blocking agents.

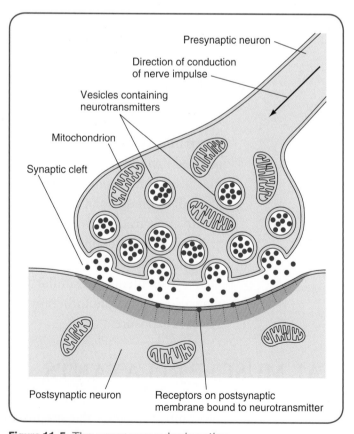

Figure 11-5 The neuromuscular junction.

TABLE 11-1	Neuromuscular Blocking Agents		
Generic Name	Trade Name	Route of Administration	Average Adult Dosage
Short Duration			
succinylcholine chloride **(suk-sih-nihl-KOH-leen KLOR-ryd)**	Anectine®, Quelicin®	IM, IV	IV: 0.3–1.1 mg/kg; IM: 2.5–4 mg/kg
Intermediate Duration			
atracurium besylate **(ah-trah-KYOO-ree-um BEH-sih-layt)**	Tracrium®	IV	Initial: 0.4–0.5 mg/kg; then 0.08–0.1 mg/kg
cisatracurium besylate **(sih-sah-trah-KYOO-ree-um BEH-sih-layt)**	Nimbex®	IV	0.15–0.20 mg/kg
rocuronium bromide **(raw-kyoo-ROH-nee-um BROH-myd)**	Zemuron®	IV	0.6 mg/kg
Extended Duration			
doxacurium chloride **(dok-sah-KYOO-ree-um KLOR-ryd)**	Nuromax®	IV	Initial: 0.025–0.05 mg/kg; then 0.005–0.01 mg/kg
mivacurium chloride **(my-vah-KYOO-ree-um KLOR-ryd)**	Mivacron®	IV	0.15–0.25 mg/kg
pancuronium bromide **(pan-kyoo-ROH-nee-um BROH-myd)**	Pavulon®	IV	0.06–0.1 mg/kg
pipecuronium bromide **(pih-peh-kyoo-ROH-nee-um BROH-myd)**	Arduan®	IV	0.07–0.85 mg/kg
tubocurarine chloride **(too-boh-kyoo-RAH-reen KLOR-ryd)**	(tubocurarine systemic, generic only)	IV	0.1–0.3 mg/kg, administered slowly

Mechanism of Action

Neuromuscular blocking agents prevent somatic motor nerve impulses, which affect the skeletal muscles. Some agents occupy receptor sites on the motor end plate and are able to block the action of acetylcholine. These agents are called competitive neuromuscular blocking agents. The action of other neuromuscular blocking agents resembles that of acetylcholine by depolarizing the muscle fiber. These agents are not immediately destroyed by cholinesterase. Therefore, their action is more prolonged than that of acetylcholine. Examples of these agents include succinylcholine, atracurium, and doxacurium.

Indications

The principal use of neuromuscular blocking drugs is to provide adequate skeletal muscular relaxation during surgery, controlled respiration, and orthopedic manipulations. The short-acting drugs are used to relax the laryngeal muscles during endotracheal intubation and bronchoscopy. They may also be used to decrease the severity of muscle contractions during electroconvulsive treatment. Neuromuscular blocking agents have been used in the management of tetanus and for various spastic disorders, but the results usually have been dissatisfying. Neuromuscular blocking agents are not effective for rigidity and spasticity of muscles caused by neurological disease or trauma.

Adverse Effects

The most commonly reported adverse effects of neuromuscular blocking agents include drowsiness, increased occurrence of seizures in patients with epilepsy, dry mouth, loss of strength, hypotension, muscle weakness, occasional hepatitis, and cardiac arrhythmias.

Contraindications and Precautions

Neuromuscular blocking agents are contraindicated in patients with hypersensitivity to these drugs or a family history of malignant hyperthermia. Atracurium is contraindicated in patients with myasthenia gravis. Neuromuscular blocking drugs are not safe during pregnancy (category C), lactation, or in children younger than two years of age.

These agents should be used cautiously in patients with asthma, significant cardiovascular disease, impaired pulmonary function, dehydration, and acid-base imbalance. These drugs must be stored away from other types of medications due to the potential for harm.

Drug Interactions

Neuromuscular blocking agents play an important role in severe adverse reactions occurring during anesthesia. Most reactions to these agents are of immunological origin, and tests for possible hypersensitivity to these drugs must be conducted before administration of anesthesia. Neuromuscular blocking agents should not be used with muscle relaxants such as succinylcholine, volatile, intravenous, or local anesthetics, antibiotics, anticonvulsants, magnesium, diuretics, corticosteroids, or acetylcholine esterase inhibitors (reversal drugs).

Centrally Acting Skeletal Muscle Relaxants

Skeletal muscles are voluntarily controlled by impulses originating in the CNS. Impulses are conducted through the spinal cord in somatic neurons

TABLE 11-2	Centrally Acting Skeletal Muscle Relaxants		
Generic Name	**Trade Name**	**Route of Administration**	**Average Adult Dosage**
baclofen **(BAK-loh-fen)**	Lioresal®	PO	5 mg tid
carisoprodol **(kah-rih-SAW-proh-dahl)**	Soma®	PO	350 mg tid
chlorphenesin carbamate **(klor-FEN-eh-sihn KAR-bah-mayt)**	Maolate®	PO	800 mg tid until effective; reduce to 400 mg qid or less
chlorzoxazone **(klor-ZOK-sah-zohn)**	Paraflex®, Parafon Forte®	PO	250–500 mg tid
cyclobenzaprine hydrochloride **(sy-kloh-BEN-zah-preen hy-droh-KLOR-ryd)**	Flexeril®	PO	10–15 mg tid
diazepam **(dy-AH-zeh-pam)**	Valium®, Valrelease®	PO, IM, IV	PO: 2–10 mg bid–qid; IM/IV: 5–10 mg up to 30 mg
methocarbamol **(meh-thoh-KAR-bah-mahl)**	Robaxin®	PO	1.5 g qid for 2–3 days, then reduce to 1 g qid
orphenadrine citrate **(or-FEN-ah-dreen SIH-trayt)**	Norflex®, Banflex®, Myolin®	PO, IM, IV	PO: 100 mg bid; IM/IV: 60 mg

that eventually **synapse** with the muscle in a neuromuscular junction. Table 11-2 shows some examples of the centrally acting skeletal muscle relaxants.

Mechanism of Action

The exact mechanism of centrally acting muscle relaxants is unknown. The neurotransmitter acetylcholine (ACh) is released to combine with ACh receptors on the muscle cell membrane. When an adequate number of ACh receptors are bound, the cell then experiences sodium ion influx, causing an impulse to travel over the cell, which causes a contraction. Relaxation occurs when ACh is broken down by acetylcholinesterase. Centrally acting muscle relaxants may act in the CNS at various levels to depress polysynaptic reflexes; sedative effects may be responsible for relaxation of muscle spasms.

Indications

Use of the centrally acting muscle relaxants is uncertain, owing to their limited selectivity. Involuntary movement of skeletal muscles, such as occurs in palsies, chorea, or parkinsonism, is mostly the result of impairment of feedback control within the brain. These agents may be used to reduce muscle spasms in patients with cerebral palsy, multiple sclerosis, and spinal cord injury.

Adverse Effects

Common adverse effects of centrally acting agents include weakness, fatigue, drowsiness, and dizziness. Baclofen is often the drug of first choice because of its wide safety margin.

Contraindications and Precautions

Centrally acting skeletal muscle relaxants are contraindicated in patients with hypersensitivity to these agents. Cyclobenzaprine should be avoided in the acute recovery phase of myocardial infarction, cardiac arrhythmias, and hyperthyroidism. Centrally acting skeletal muscle relaxants are contraindicated during pregnancy (category B or C), lactation, and in children younger than five years of age.

These agents should be used cautiously in patients with liver or kidney impairment, bipolar disorder, seizure disorders, stroke, cerebral palsy, depression, head trauma, and diabetes mellitus.

Drug Interactions

Alcohol, phenothiazines, or CNS depressants may cause additive sedation if they are used with centrally acting skeletal muscle relaxants. Cyclobenzaprine should not be used within two weeks of a monoamine oxidase inhibitor (MAOI) because hyperpyretic crisis and convulsions may occur.

Direct-Acting Skeletal Muscle Relaxants

These agents directly relax the spastic muscle. Direct-acting skeletal muscle relaxants produce about a 50% decrease in contractility of skeletal muscles, but they have no effect on smooth or cardiac muscles. Examples of direct-acting antispasmodic drugs are botulinum toxin type A and B, dantrolene, and quinine sulfate (Table 11-3).

Medical Terminology Review

hyperpyretic
hyper- = over, excessive
pyr/e = fire, heat
-tic = pertaining to
pertaining to overheating

Medical Terminology Review

spastic
spas- = spasms
-tic = condition of
the presence of spasms

TABLE 11-3	Direct-Acting Antispasmodic Agents		
Generic Name	Trade Name	Route of Administration	Average Adult Dosage
botulinum toxin type A **(baw-choo-LYE-num TOK-sin)**	Botox®, Dysport®	IM	20–50 units injected directly into target muscle
botulinum toxin type B **(baw-choo-LYE-num TOK-sin)**	Myobloc®	IM	2500–5000 units/dose injected directly into target muscle
dantrolene sodium **(DAN-troh-leen SOH-dee-um)**	Dantrium®	PO	25 mg/day; increased to 25 mg bid–qid; may increase q4–7 days up to 100 mg bid–tid
quinine sulfate **(KWY-nyn SUL-fayt)**	Quinamm®, Quiphile®	PO	260–300 mg at bedtime

Mechanism of Action

Direct-acting skeletal muscle relaxants do not interfere with neuromuscular transmission or the electrical excitability of muscles. They inhibit the release of calcium ions from storage areas inside skeletal muscle cells. This action makes the muscle less responsive to nerve impulses. Dantrolene is an example of a direct-acting skeletal muscle relaxant that will be discussed in detail.

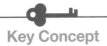

Key Concept

Quinine sulfate is an antimalarial drug that is used for nocturnal leg cramps or congenital tonic spasms.

Indications

Dantrolene is used to treat spasticity resulting from upper motor neuron lesions such as those in spinal cord injury, stroke, multiple sclerosis, and cerebral palsy, but not spasticity resulting from musculoskeletal injury, lumbago, or rheumatoid disorders. The drug is also used to treat malignant hyperthermia.

Adverse Effects

The major adverse effects of dantrolene include muscle weakness, drowsiness, dizziness, nausea, diarrhea, seizures, tachycardia, erratic blood pressure, and pericarditis.

Contraindications and Precautions

Dantrolene is contraindicated in patients with liver disease and respiratory muscle weakness. It may color the urine orange to red. Safe use during pregnancy (category C), lactation, or in children younger than five years of age is not established.

Dantrolene should be used cautiously in patients with impaired cardiac or pulmonary function, and in patients younger than 35 years of age (especially women).

Drug Interactions

The use of dantrolene with alcohol and other CNS depressants causes increased CNS depression. Estrogen increases the risk of hepatotoxicity in women younger than 35 years of age. The use of intravenous dantrolene with verapamil and other calcium channel blockers increases the risk of ventricular fibrillation and cardiovascular collapse.

ANTI-RHEUMATIC DRUGS

Drugs used to treat rheumatoid arthritis are of several types, based upon their actions. They include disease-modifying anti-rheumatic drugs (DMARDs), biologics, and slow-acting anti-rheumatic drugs. Altering the disease course is attempted initially with **the DMARDs**, often along with biologics. The slow-acting anti-rheumatic drugs are then used if required.

Disease-Modifying Anti-Rheumatic Drugs (DMARDs)

These agents slow the progression of joint damage from rheumatoid arthritis and similar conditions, by affecting the immune system. The most commonly used DMARD is *methotrexate*, but it must be used with caution because of its many adverse effects (see later discussion). Hydroxychloroquine and sulfasalazine are less potent DMARDs, but also produce fewer adverse effects. Minocycline is an antibiotic DMARD that acts by stopping inflammation, but up to one year of treatment is needed for its full effects to be seen. Leflunomide is a DMARD that works nearly as well as methotrexate and is more effective when combined with it. Table 11-4 shows examples of DMARDs.

Mechanism of Action

Methotrexate may exert its immunosuppressive effects by inhibiting replication and function of T lymphocytes, and possibly B lymphocytes. It also slows quickly growing cells, possibly because of its inhibition of the enzyme dihydrofolate reductase. The mechanism of action of hydrochloroquine is not fully understood, but it is believed to inhibit enzymes, resulting in cytotoxicity to cells, causing their death. Leflunomide also acts by inhibiting enzyme actions. Minocycline acts by inhibiting bacterial protein synthesis through RNA binding. The mechanism of action of sulfasalazine is not fully understood, but the drug is believed to act primarily inside the intestine.

TABLE 11-4	Disease-Modifying Anti-Rheumatic Drugs (DMARDs)		
Generic Name	Trade Name	Route of Administration	Average Adult Dosage
hydroxychloroquine **(hy-drok-see-KLOR -oh-kween)**	Plaquenil®	PO	400–600 mg daily, taken with food or a glass of milk; dosage may need to be temporarily reduced due to adverse effects, then gradually increased to optimum response level
leflunomide **(leh-FLOO-no-myd)**	Arava®	PO	Loading: one 100 mg tablet/day for 3 days; Maint: 20 mg/day
methotrexate **(meh-thoh-TREK-sayt)**	Rheumatrex Dose Pack®, Trexall®	PO	Single: 7.5 mg once/week; Divided: 2.5 mg q12h for 3 doses once/week (max weekly dose: 20 mg)
minocycline **(my-no-SY-kleen)**	Minocin®	PO, IV	Initial: 200 mg, followed by 100 mg q12h (max: 400 mg/day)
sulfasalazine **(sul-fah-SAH-lah-zeen)**	Azulfidine®	PO	Initial: 3–4 g/day in divided doses with dosage intervals not exceeding 8 h; Maint: 2 g/day

Indications

Methotrexate is indicated for severe rheumatoid arthritis and active polyarticular juvenile idiopathic arthritis. Hydrochloroquine is used to treat rheumatoid arthritis and other rheumatic disorders, such as Sjögren's syndrome and porphyria cutanea tarda. Leflunomide relieves symptoms of active rheumatoid arthritis, improving physical function and slowing disease progression. Minocycline may improve the signs and symptoms of rheumatoid arthritis. Sulfasalazine is used for rheumatoid arthritis as well as other types of inflammatory arthritis, such as psoriatic arthritis.

Adverse Effects

The common, severe adverse effects of methotrexate include azotemia, bacterial infections, visceral bleeding, canker sores, decreased blood platelets or white blood cells, intestinal ulcers, gum or mouth inflammation, stomach or intestinal inflammation, and sensitivity to ultraviolet radiation. Less serious, yet still common, adverse effects include dizziness, nausea and vomiting, anorexia, reduced energy, and malaise. The most common adverse effects of hydrochloroquine are mild nausea, occasional stomach cramps, and mild diarrhea. Its most serious adverse effects involve toxicity to the cornea and macula of the eye. The most common adverse effects of leflunomide include bloody or cloudy urine, coughing, breathing problems, urination problems, dizziness, fever, headache, anorexia, nausea, vomiting, sneezing, sore throat, chest tightness, and jaundice.

The most significant adverse effects of minocycline include black, tarry stools, skin changes, blood in urine or stools, vision changes, radiating chest pain, confusion, diarrhea, dizziness, eye pain, tachycardia, general malaise, tiredness, skin rash, joint or muscle pain, swelling (of face, throat, or extremities), anorexia, nausea, vomiting, severe headache or stomach pain, breathing difficulty, mouth lesions, unusual bleeding, and jaundice. The most common adverse effects of sulfasalazine include joint aches, fever, continuing headache, increased sensitivity of the skin to sunlight, skin rash, itching, and vomiting.

Contraindications and Precautions

Methotrexate is contraindicated in hypersensitivity to the drug or its components, pregnancy (category X), and lactation. Hydrochloroquine is contraindicated in corneal or macular eye diseases, visual field defects, liver disease, psoriasis, hypoglycemia, certain anemias, porphyria, alcoholism, and in patients with abnormally low neutrophil counts. Contraindications to leflunomide include hypersensitivity and pregnancy (category X). Contraindications to minocycline include hypersensitivity to this drug or any tetracyclines or their components. Contraindications to sulfasalazine include hypersensitivity to this drug, salicylates, sulfonamides, chemically related drugs, and their components. Sulfasalazine is also contraindicated in patients with intestinal or urinary obstruction, and porphyria.

Drug Interactions

DMARDs are associated with many potentially serious drug interactions. Administration of methotrexate concurrently with alcohol, azathioprine, or sulfasalazine increases the risk of hepatotoxicity. Chloramphenicol, salicylates, NSAIDs, sulfonamides, phenylbutazone, phenytoin, tetracyclines, penicillin, and probenecid may increase methotrexate levels, resulting in increased toxicity. Folic acid may reduce adverse effects caused by methotrexate. Major drug interactions with hydrochloroquine include auranofin, aurothioglucose, deferiprone, gold sodium thiomalate, leflunomide, teriflunomide, thioridazine, and vigabatrin. Iron and antibiotics may alter sulfasalazine absorption. Drugs and substances that interact with leflunomide include activated charcoal, cholestyramine, live-virus vaccines, methotrexate, NSAIDs, rifampin, and tolbutamide.

Drugs and substances that interact with minocycline include antacids, calcium supplements, salicylates, preparations containing iron, laxatives containing magnesium, sodium bicarbonate, cholestyramine, colestipol, cimetidine, digoxin, insulin, iron salts, lithium, methoxyflurane, oral anticoagulants, oral contraceptives containing estrogen, penicillin, and vitamin A. Interactions with sulfasalazine include bone marrow depressants, digoxin, folic acid, hepatotoxic drugs, hydantoins, oral anticoagulants, oral antidiabetic drugs, methotrexate, phenylbutazone, and sulfinpyrazone.

Biologics

Biologic agents are the newest drugs used for rheumatoid arthritis and similar conditions. These drugs are injected either under the skin or directly into a vein and work by neutralizing the immune system signals that result in joint damage. Biologics are very effective when used in combination with methotrexate. Examples of biologics include abatacept, adalimumab, anakinra, certolizumab, etanercept, golimumab, infliximab, rituximab, and tocilizumab (Table 11-5).

Mechanism of Action

Abatacept inhibits T-cell activation by binding to proteins involved in this activation, which is a key component in the development of rheumatoid arthritis. Adalimumab binds to tumor necrosis factor (TNF) to block interaction with its receptors. TNF is a major component of inflammation and joint destruction in rheumatoid arthritis. Anakinra inhibits binding of interleukin-1 to its type 1 receptor (1R), blocking its activity, which is linked to rheumatoid symptoms. Certolizumab acts by binding and inhibiting TNF-alpha. Etanercept acts similarly to adalimumab. Golimumab and infliximab act similarly to certolizumab. Rituximab binds specifically to a B-cell antigen believed to

TABLE 11-5	Biologics		
Generic Name	Trade Name	Route of Administration	Average Adult Dosage
abatacept (ah-BAY-tah-sept)	Orencia®	IV infusion, SC	IV: based on weight, 500–1000 mg over 30 min, repeated in 2–4 weeks; SC: following a single IV loading dose and based on body weight, 125 mg given within 1 day, followed by 125 mg once/week
adalimumab (ad-ah-LIM-yoo-mab)	Humira®	SC	40 mg every other week
anakinra (an-ah-KIN-rah)	Kineret®	SC	100 mg daily
certolizumab (ser-toh-LIZ-oo-mab)	Cimzia®	SC	Initial: 400 mg (as two 200 mg injections), repeated at weeks 2 and 4. Maint: 200 mg every other week or 400 mg (as two 200 mg injections) q 4 weeks if clinical response occurs
etanercept (ih-TAN-er-sept)	Enbrel®	SC	50 mg once/week on same day each week
golimumab (go-LIM-yoo-mab)	Simponi®	SC, IV infusion	SC: 50 mg monthly. IV: 2 mg/kg infused over 30 min at weeks 0 and 4, then q 8 weeks thereafter
infliximab (in-FLIK-zih-mab)	Remicade®	IV infusion	3 mg/kg, with methotrexate, repeated 2 and 6 weeks after first infusion, then q 8 weeks thereafter
rituximab (rih-TUK-zih-mab)	Rituxan®	IV infusion	Two 1000 mg infusions separated by 2 weeks
tocilizumab (toh-sih-LIZ-oo-mab)	Actemra®	IV infusion, SC	IV: 4 mg/kg over 60 min q 4 weeks, increased prn to 8 mg/kg over 60 min q 4 weeks (maximum: 800 mg per infusion). SC: based on body weight, 162 mg every other week, followed by increased dosage frequency to every week prn, up to 162 mg every week

play a role in rheumatoid arthritis, interrupting the antigen's functions. Tocilizumab binds to interleukin-6 receptors to interrupt their signaling.

Indications

Abatacept is indicated for patients with moderate to severe active rheumatoid arthritis who have inadequately responded to methotrexate or other drugs. Adalimumab, certolizumab, and infliximab are prescribed for patients with moderate to severe rheumatoid arthritis, psoriatic arthritis, and ankylosing spondylitis. Anakinra is indicated for patients with moderate to severe rheumatoid arthritis who have not responded to DMARDs. Etanercept is indicated for rheumatoid arthritis and psoriatic arthritis, alone or in combination with methotrexate. Golimumab is indicated for psoriatic arthritis or ankylosing spondylitis with or without methotrexate or other DMARDs.

Rituximab is indicated for moderate to severe rheumatoid arthritis, in combination with methotrexate, when the patient has not responded to one or more TNF-antagonist therapies. Tocilizumab is indicated for moderate to severe active rheumatoid arthritis as monotherapy in patients who have had an inadequate response to one or more DMARDS, or as adjunct with methotrexate or other DMARDs.

Adverse Effects

The most severe adverse effects of abatacept include hypertension or hypotension, diarrhea, diverticulitis, acute pyelonephritis, pneumonia, cellulitis, anaphylaxis, malignancies, and systemic infections. Adverse effects of adalimumab include stroke, hypertensive encephalopathy, subdural hematoma, arrhythmias, cardiac arrest, deep vein thrombosis, hypertension, myocardial infarction, diverticulitis, hemorrhage, liver damage or failure, large bowel perforation, nausea and vomiting, hematuria, kidney dysfunction, pneumonia, pulmonary embolism, and anaphylaxis. Anakinra has adverse effects that include diarrhea, neutropenia, serious bone and joint infections, pneumonia, cellulitis, hypersensitivity reaction, and malignancies.

The most severe adverse effects of certolizumab include bipolar disorder, fainting, suicidal ideation, angina, arrhythmias, heart failure, myocardial infarction, retinal hemorrhage, hepatitis, kidney disorders, pneumonia, Stevens-Johnson syndrome, toxic epidermal necrolysis, severe infections, and malignancies. Adverse effects of etanercept include multiple sclerosis, seizures, congestive heart failure, hypertension or hypotension, hepatitis, diarrhea, nausea and vomiting, pneumonia, cellulitis, malignancies, Stevens-Johnson syndrome, toxic epidermal necrolysis, and serious infections. Golimumab's adverse effects include hypertension, oral herpes, pneumonia, tuberculosis, cellulitis, malignancies, anaphylaxis, serious infections, influenza, and sepsis.

The most severe adverse effects of infliximab include Guillain-Barré syndrome, meningitis, seizures, stroke, arrhythmias, hypertension or hypotension, myocardial infarction, thrombophlebitis, acute hepatic failure, diarrhea, gastrointestinal hemorrhage, hepatitis, nausea and vomiting, renal failure, pneumonia, tuberculosis, severe bronchospasm, malignancies, anaphylaxis, serious infections, and sepsis. Adverse effects of rituximab include hepatitis, progressive multifocal leukoencephalopathy, tumor lysis syndrome, infections, arrhythmias, renal toxicity, and bowel obstruction or perforation. Tocilizumab has adverse effects that include hypertension, diverticulitis, gastrointestinal perforation, pneumonia, cellulitis, anaphylaxis, herpes zoster, malignancies, opportunistic infections, sepsis, and tuberculosis.

Contraindications and Precautions

Abatacept is contraindicated in hypersensitivity to any of its components. Adalimumab is contraindicated in active infections, lactation, and hypersensitivity to its components. Anakinra is contraindicated in active infections, hypersensitivity to its components, or hypersensitivity to *Escherichia coli*-derived proteins. Certolizumab is contraindicated in active infections, use of DMARDs or TNF blockers, hypersensitivity to this drug or its components, and intravenous drug administration. Etanercept is contraindicated in hypersensitivity to its components or to hamster protein, an in patients with or at risk of sepsis. Golimumab is contraindicated in hypersensitivity to any of its components. Infliximab is contraindicated in lactation, hypersensitivity to its components or murine proteins, and class III or IV heart failure.

There are no contraindications for rituximab, but this drug can cause severe or even fatal infusion reactions such as hypotension, hypoxia, bronchospasm, acute respiratory distress syndrome, myocardial infarction, ventricular fibrillation, cardiogenic shock, and anaphylaxis. Tocilizumab is contraindicated in hypersensitivity to its components, an absolute neutrophil count below $2000/mm^3$, a platelet count below $100,000/mm^3$, or a serum alanine aminotransferase or aspartate aminotransferase level more than 1.5 times the upper limit of normal.

Drug Interactions

Abatacept may interact with immunosuppressants, live-virus vaccines, and TNF antagonists. Adalimumab may interact with abatacept, anakinra, rituximab, azathioprine, 6-mercaptopurine, and live-virus vaccines. Anakinra may interact with etancercept, infliximab, and other drugs that block TNF, as well as live-virus vaccines. Certolizumab may interact with anakinra, immunosuppressants, and live-virus vaccines. Etancercept may interact with cyclophosphamide or sulfasalazine. Golimumab may interact with abatacept, anakinra, rituximab, cytochrome P-450 substrates (e.g., cyclosporine, theophylline, and warfarin), live-virus vaccines, and therapeutic infectious agents such as bacillus Calmette-Guerin (BCG), used in bladder installation for treatment of cancer.

Infliximab may interact with abatacept, anakinra, etanercept, tocilizumab, live-virus vaccines, and therapeutic infectious agents such as BCG. Formal drug interaction studies have not been performed with rituximab, but there have been reported interactions with amphotericin, belatacept, cisplatin, denosumab, fingolimod, ioversol, and sipuleucel. Tocilizumab may interact with anti-CD20 monoclonal antibodies, interleukin-1R antagonists, selective co-stimulation modulators, TNF antagonists, atorvastatin, cytochrome P-450 substrates with a narrow therapeutic index (e.g., cyclosporine, theophylline, and warfarin), CYP3A4 substrates such as lovastatin, oral contraceptives, simvastatin, omeprazole, and live-virus vaccines.

TABLE 11-6	Second-Line Agents for Rheumatoid Arthritis		
Generic Name	Trade Name	Route of Administration	Average Adult Dosage
auranofin (or-AN-oh-fin)	Ridaura®	PO	3 mg bid
gold sodium thiomalate (GOLD SOH-dee-um thy-oh-MAH-layt)	Aurolate®	IM	10 mg week 1; 1.25 mg week 2; then 25–50 mg/week
penicillamine (peh-nih-SIL-lah-meen)	Depen®	PO	125–250 mg/day, may increase after several months

Slow-Acting Anti-Rheumatic Drugs

Slow-acting anti-rheumatic drugs may be prescribed for patients with rheumatoid arthritis that is unresponsive to first-line therapy with DMARDs or biologics, or progresses to deformity. Table 11-6 shows these second-line agents for rheumatoid arthritis.

Mechanism of Action

The exact mechanisms of action of slow-acting anti-rheumatic drugs are not known. Gold compounds (auranofin and gold sodium thiomalate) suppress or prevent inflammation in the acute forms of arthritis, but do not cure the disease. Penicillamine is a chelating drug that is a metabolite of penicillin. It is also classified as an anti-inflammatory drug. The mechanism of action of penicillamine is unknown.

Indications

Slow-acting anti-rheumatic drugs may be prescribed for advanced states of some rheumatoid disorders. The oral gold compound is available as auranofin, whereas gold sodium thiomalate is a parenteral preparation, administered intramuscularly. Gold compounds that retard destruction of bone and joints by an unknown mechanism are long-latency drugs used in more advanced stages of some rheumatoid diseases.

Corticosteroids are used in severe, progressive rheumatoid arthritis. Prednisone may afford some degree of control, but corticosteroids are usually recognized as agents of last resort. Corticosteroids do not alter the course of rheumatoid arthritis. They may be occasionally used for elderly patients as alternatives to avoid the risks of second-line agents, for patients who cannot tolerate NSAIDs, and for patients with significant systemic manifestations of rheumatoid arthritis.

Medical Terminology Review

corticosteroids
cortico- = (adrenal) cortex
-steroids = hormones
hormones produced in the adrenal cortex

Adverse Effects

Common adverse effects of gold compounds and penicillamine include GI disturbances, dermatitis, and lesions of mucous membranes. Less common side effects include aplastic anemia and nephritic syndrome. It is important to note that, except for diarrhea, serious toxicity occurs most commonly when parenteral therapy is used. If toxicity occurs gold therapy should be stopped immediately.

Long-term administration of corticosteroids may cause gastrointestinal (GI) bleeding, poor wound healing, hyperglycemia, hypertension, and osteoporosis.

Contraindications and Precautions

These preparations are contraindicated in patients with a history of gold-induced necrotizing enterocolitis, renal disease, **exfoliative dermatitis**, or bone marrow aplasia, in patients who have recently received radiation therapy, and in those with a history of severe toxicity from previous exposure to gold or other heavy metals. Safety during pregnancy (various categories) or lactation and in children is not established.

These agents must be used with caution in patients who have inflammatory bowel disease, rash, liver disease, a history of bone marrow depression, diabetes mellitus, congestive heart failure, and in older adults.

Drug Interactions

Gold compounds may have drug interactions with antimalarials and immunosuppressants. Penicillamine increases the risk of blood dyscrasias. The combination of penicillamine with antimalarials and gold therapy may potentiate hematological and renal adverse effects. Iron may decrease penicillamine absorption.

DRUGS FOR GOUTY ARTHRITIS

There are two types of clinical gouty arthritis: acute and chronic. The initial attack for acute gout is abrupt, usually occurring at night or in the early morning as synovial fluid is reabsorbed. The most common site of the initial attack is the big toe. Other sites that may be affected include the ankle, heel, knee, wrist, elbow, and fingers. There are two choices for therapy: general therapeutic drugs and specific drugs. In acute gout, immobilization of the affected joint is essential. Anti-inflammatory drug therapy should begin immediately, and urate-lowering drugs should not be given until the acute attack is controlled. Specific drugs include colchicines, NSAIDs (see Chapter 22), and corticosteroids. Colchicine and allopurinol are detailed below selectively.

Colchicine

Colchicine is a gout suppressant with antimitotic and indirect anti-inflammatory properties.

Mechanism of Action

Colchicine is not an analgesic, and its precise mechanism of action is not known. The drug is well absorbed after oral administration. It is often combined with probenecid to improve prophylactic therapy of chronic gouty arthritis. Both urinary and fecal routes eliminate colchicine.

Indications

Colchicine is the traditional drug of choice for relieving pain and inflammation and ending the acute gout attack. It is most effective when initiated 12 to 36 hours after symptoms begin. It is also used in combination with either phenylbutazone or allopurinol in the management of acute gout.

Adverse Effects

The drug is very toxic, and it should be stopped at the first symptom of toxicity, such as nausea, vomiting, diarrhea, and abdominal pain. Adverse effects of oral colchicine include nausea, abdominal cramps, and diarrhea.

Contraindications and Precautions

Colchicine is contraindicated in patients with peptic ulcers. Local pain and necrosis can occur with administration of intravenous colchicines.

Drug Interactions

Colchicine may decrease intestinal absorption of vitamin B_{12}.

> **Medical Terminology Review**
>
> **uricosuric**
> urico- = related to uric acid
> -suric = increasing excretion
> increased excretion of uric acid

Allopurinol

Allopurinol is a xanthine oxidase inhibitor uricosuric agent.

Mechanism of Action

This drug is not analgesic, but it relieves gouty pain because it blocks the formation of or enhances the excretion of uric acid.

Indications

Allopurinol is used in the treatment of gout, primary or secondary uric acid nephropathy, uric acid stone formation, and renal calculi.

Adverse Effects

Adverse effects of allopurinol include drowsiness, headache, vertigo, nausea, vomiting, diarrhea, abdominal discomfort, indigestion, malaise, thrombocytopenia, urticaria or pruritus, pruritic maculopapular rash, toxic epidermal necrolysis, hepatotoxicity, and renal insufficiency. In rare cases, allopurinol may cause agranulocytosis, aplastic anemia, and bone marrow depression.

Contraindications and Precautions

Allopurinol is contraindicated in children, except those with hyperuricemia secondary to cancer. It should not be used by nursing mothers, or by patients who develop a severe reaction to the drug.

Drug Interactions

Alcohol may inhibit renal excretion of uric acid. Ampicillin and amoxicillin increase the risk of skin rash. Allopurinol enhances anticoagulant effects of warfarin. Toxicity from azathioprine, mercaptopurine, cyclophosphamide, and cyclosporin increase with allopurinol.

Medical Terminology
Review

hyperuricemia
hyper- = over; above; beyond
uric = uric acid
-emia = blood condition
excessive uric acid in the blood

SUMMARY

Skeletal muscle relaxants and non-narcotic analgesics may be classified in two broad categories: skeletal muscle relaxants and NSAIDs (discussed in Chapter 22). Most muscle strains and spasms are self-limited and respond to rest, physical therapy, and aspirin. Spasticity resulting from closed head injuries, stroke, cerebral palsy, and others require long-term use of muscle relaxants. Neuromuscular blocking agents prevent somatic motor nerve impulses, which affect the skeletal muscles. Rheumatoid arthritis is treated with DMARDs and biologics, followed by slower acting agents such as gold compounds. The drug of choice for acute gouty arthritis is colchicine.

EXPLORING THE WEB

Visit **www.drugs.com**

- Search for "skeletal muscle relaxants." Review the material presented to gain a better understanding of the drugs that fall within this category.

Visit **www.medicinenet.com** or **www.nlm.nih.gov**

- Search by the disorders or drugs discussed in this chapter to enhance your understanding of the reading.

REVIEW QUESTIONS

Multiple Choice

1. The type of muscle that attaches to bones and joints by connective tissue is which of the following?

   A. smooth

   B. skeletal

   C. myocardium

   D. tendon

2. Which of the following refers to disease of the joints?

   A. bursa

   B. osteoporosis

   C. arthritis

   D. connective

3. Skeletal muscles are voluntary muscles that are under the control of the:

   A. central nervous system

   B. peripheral nervous system

   C. environment

   D. calcium ions

4. One of the principal uses of neuromuscular blocking agents is to provide adequate skeletal muscular relaxation during:

   A. surgery

   B. rest

   C. epileptic seizures

   D. exercise

5. The abbreviation ACh stands for:

   A. ache

   B. aluminum chloride

   C. acetylcholine

   D. acetaminophen

6. A centrally acting skeletal muscle relaxant commonly used to alleviate signs and symptoms of spasticity from multiple sclerosis is:

   A. carisoprodol

   B. baclofen

   C. barbiturate

   D. codeine

7. Which of the following drugs may cause urine discoloration from orange to purple-red?

   A. dantrolene

   B. diazepam

   C. chlorzoxazone

   D. cortisol

8. Which of the following is the generic name for Norflex®?

   A. cyclobenzaprine

   B. orphenadrine citrate

   C. dantrolene sodium

   D. baclofen

9. Pain-relieving drugs are also known as:

   A. anaphylactics

   B. antiemetics

   C. analgesics

   D. antitoxins

10. Which of the following is a xanthine oxidase inhibitor agent?

    A. auranofin

    B. allopurinol

    C. acetaminophen

    D. colchicine

11. Gold compounds are indicated in which of the following?

    A. exfoliative dermatitis

    B. rheumatoid arthritis

    C. bone marrow aplasia

    D. exposure to heavy metals

12. The trade name of botulinum toxin type B is:

    A. Botox

    B. Dantrium

    C. Dysport

    D. Myobloc

13. Allopurinol is used in the treatment of all of the following disorders, *except*:

    A. temporary relief of mild to moderate pain

    B. secondary uric acid nephropathy

    C. uric acid stone formation

    D. gout

14. Which of the following is an example of a direct-acting antispasmodic drug?

    A. Soma

    B. Robaxin

    C. Dantrium

    D. Flexeril

15. An example of a disease-modifying anti-rheumatic drug (DMARD) is:

    A. dantrolene

    B. auranofin

    C. baclofen

    D. methotrexate

Fill in the Blank

1. Skeletal muscle relaxants work by blocking _____ nerve impulses.

2. Neuromuscular blocking drugs are not safe during pregnancy because they are in category _____.

3. Baclofen is often the drug of first choice as a centrally acting skeletal muscle relaxant because of its wide _____.

4. Name three anti-inflammatory drugs that are classified as slow-acting anti-rheumatic drugs:

   A. _____

   B. _____

   C. _____

5. Name five adverse effects of long-term administration of corticosteroids:

   A. _____

   B. _____

   C. _____

   D. _____

   E. _____

6. The precise mechanism of action of colchicine is _____.

7. The most common site of the initial attack of gout is the metatarsophalangeal _____.

Critical Thinking

A 48-year-old woman has been diagnosed with gouty arthritis. She also has a history of hypertension and a chronic peptic ulcer.

1. Though it should be used cautiously, which of the medications for gouty arthritis discussed in this chapter should be prescribed?

2. What would be the treatment choices for acute gouty arthritis?

3. If she received the drug of choice for acute gouty arthritis, what would be the most common adverse effects?

12 Drug Therapy for Cardiovascular Disorders

OUTLINE

OBJECTIVES

After completing this chapter, the reader should be able to:

1. Describe normal cardiac function related to contractility and blood flow.
2. Explain the pathophysiology of angina pectoris.
3. Explain the different types of coronary vasodilators.
4. Explain the common adverse effects associated with each antianginal drug class.
5. Identify the various types of antiarrhythmics and their adverse effects.
6. Describe myocardial infarction and three steps that should be taken to limit myocardial necrosis.
7. List medications that are used in congestive heart failure.
8. Describe vasoconstrictors and their purpose.
9. Discuss the action of digitalis and its side effects.
10. Explain the consequences of congestive heart failure for the cardiovascular system.

GLOSSARY

Angina pectoris – an episodic, reversible oxygen insufficiency of the heart

Arrhythmias – deviations from the normal pattern of the heartbeat; also called *dysrhythmias*

Arteriosclerosis – degenerative changes in small arteries, commonly occurring in older individuals and diabetic patients, in which the walls of arteries lose elasticity and become thickened and hard

Atherosclerosis – disease of the arteries characterized by the presence of atheromas (plaques) inside the walls of large arteries

Atheromas – plaques consisting of lipids, cells, and cell debris, often with attached thrombi, which form inside the walls of large arteries

Beta-adrenergic blockers – drugs used to reverse sympathetic heart action caused by exercise, stress, or physical exertion

Calcium channel blockers – drugs used to treat stable angina

Congestive heart failure (CHF) – a condition in which the heart is not able to pump enough blood to meet the body's metabolic demands

Coronary arterial bypass graft (CABG) – a procedure in which a vein graft is surgically implanted to bypass the area of occlusion in a coronary artery

Coronary artery disease (CAD) – a condition in which there is an insufficient supply of oxygen to the myocardium (cardiac muscle); also referred to as *coronary heart disease* and *ischemic heart disease*

Coronary heart disease (CHD) – a condition in which there is an insufficient supply of oxygen to the myocardium (cardiac muscle); also referred to as *coronary artery disease* and *ischemic heart disease*

Ischemic heart disease (IHD) – a condition in which there is an insufficient supply of oxygen to the myocardium (cardiac muscle); also referred to as *coronary artery disease* and *coronary heart disease*

Myocardial infarction (MI) – destruction of an area of cardiac muscle tissue, with or without hemorrhage, as a result of obstruction of a coronary artery

Nitrates – drugs used for the treatment of angina

Percutaneous transluminal coronary angioplasty (PTCA) –use of invasive procedures requiring cardiac catheterization to reduce obstruction in a coronary artery; the catheter contains an inflatable balloon that flattens the obstruction

Silent angina – a condition that occurs in the absence of angina pain

Vasospastic angina – decubitus angina; characterized by periodic attacks of cardiac pain that occur when a person is lying down

OVERVIEW

Cardiovascular disorders are among the most common causes of death in the United States. There are many factors that contribute to heart disease, such as age, genetics, and lifestyle. Proper diet, exercise, avoiding cigarette smoking, and getting enough rest can do a lot to keep the heart functioning for a long time. Heart disease may also be caused by other conditions or disorders such as high blood pressure, high blood cholesterol levels, obesity, and diabetes mellitus. A pharmacy technician should be familiar with the most common disorders of the cardiovascular system and the most effective agents used in the treatment of each of them.

ANATOMY REVIEW

- The cardiovascular system consists of the heart, blood vessels, and blood (Figure 12-1).

- The heart is a hollow muscular organ consisting of the myocardium, pericardium, and endocardium. Four valves control blood flow into and out of the heart (Figure 12-2).

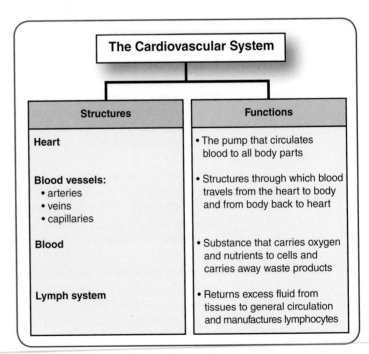

Figure 12-1 The cardiovascular system.

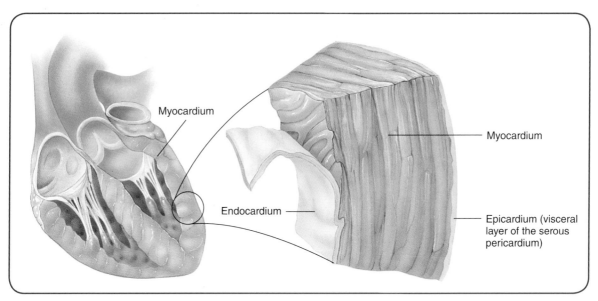

Figure 12-2 The walls and valves of the heart.

- Coronary arteries provide blood flow and nutrients to the heart muscle itself (Figure 12-3).

- The largest of the blood vessels are the arteries, which carry oxygenated blood away from the heart to the capillaries. The pulmonary arteries are the exceptions; they carry deoxygenated blood from the heart to the lungs.

- The capillaries are the smallest of the blood vessels. They are the sites of oxygen and nutrient exchange between the blood and the organs of the body.

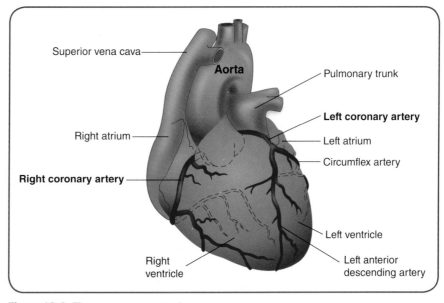

Figure 12-3 The coronary arteries.

- The veins carry deoxygenated blood away from the capillaries to the heart.

- There are two circuits for blood flow: the left side of the heart pumps blood to the systemic circuit, while the right side of the heart pumps blood through the pulmonary circuit (Figure 12-4).

- The myocardium conducts its own electrical impulse, which serves to regulate the heartbeat (Figure 12-5).

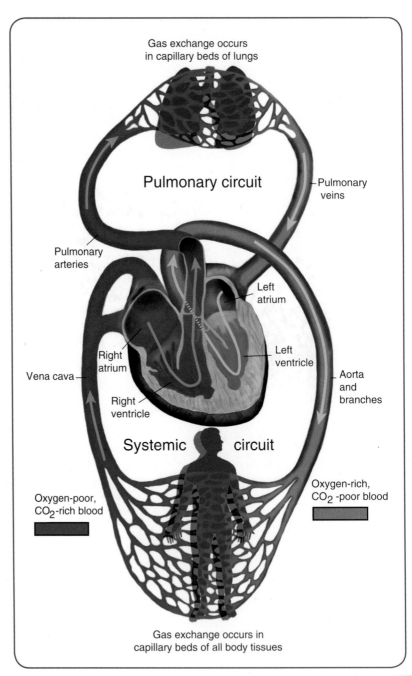

Figure 12-4 The left side of the heart pumps blood to the entire systemic circuit, while the right side pumps blood to the pulmonary circuit.

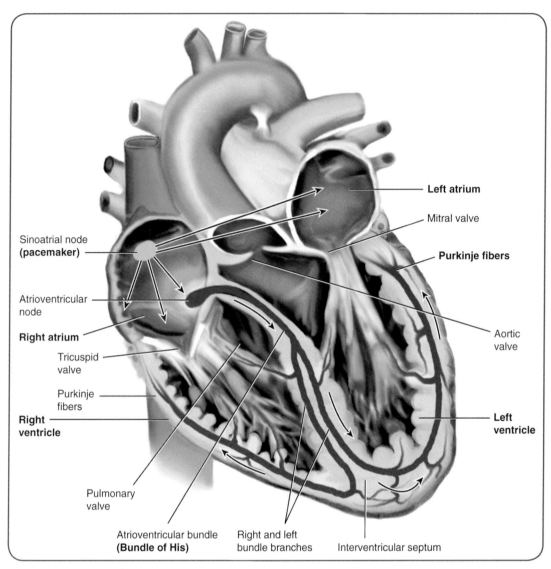

Figure 12-5 The heart's conduction system.

- The autonomic nervous system (ANS) and the drugs that stimulate or inhibit it influence heart contractions. The sympathetic nervous system and the drugs that stimulate it increase heart rate, whereas the parasympathetic nervous system and the drugs that stimulate it decrease heart rate.

ISCHEMIC HEART DISEASE

In **ischemic heart disease (IHD)** (most commonly called **coronary artery disease [CAD],** and also referred to as **coronary heart disease [CHD]**) or in a myocardial infarction (heart attack), part of the heart muscle is damaged because of obstruction in an artery. The basic problem is insufficient oxygen for the needs of the heart muscle.

TABLE 12-1	Factors Affecting Cardiac Parameters that Control Myocardial Oxygen Demand	
Factors	Heart Rate	Blood Pressure
Beta-Blockers	Decrease	Decrease
Cold	Increase	Increase
Exercise	Increase	Increase
Nitroglycerin	Increase	Decrease
Smoking	Increase	Increase

A common cause of disability and death, coronary artery disease may ultimately lead to heart failure, serious arrhythmias, or sudden death. It is the leading cause of death in men and women in the United States. There are several factors that may affect functions that control myocardial oxygen demand (Table 12-1).

Arteriosclerosis and Atherosclerosis

Arteriosclerosis is the term used to describe degenerative changes in small arteries, commonly occurring in older individuals and diabetic patients. Elasticity is lost, and the walls of the arteries become thickened and hard. The lumen gradually narrows and may become obscured. This leads to diffuse ischemia and death in various tissues, such as those of the heart, kidneys, or brain.

Atherosclerosis is differentiated by the presence of **atheromas** (plaques consisting of lipids, cells, and cell debris, often with attached thrombi, which form inside the walls of large arteries). Atheromas form primarily in large arteries such as the aorta and the coronary arteries. Figure 12-6 illustrates accumulation of lipids in blood vessels, causing occlusion.

Angina Pectoris

Angina pectoris is an episodic, reversible oxygen insufficiency of the heart. This condition is the most common form of IHD. Angina pectoris is applied to varying forms of transient chest pain that are attributable to insufficient myocardial oxygen. Atherosclerotic lesions that produce a narrowing of the coronary arteries are the major cause of angina. However, tachycardia (increased heart rate), anemia, hyperthyroidism, and hypotension can cause an oxygen imbalance. According to the American Heart Association, angina occurs more commonly in women than in men. There are several types of angina: stable (classic), unstable, decubitus (nocturnal), and silent angina. The most common form is classic angina, which may occur, with predictable frequency, from exertion (often from exercising), emotional stress, or a heavy meal. Classic angina is relieved by rest, nitroglycerin, or both.

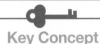

Medical Terminology Review

myocardial
my/o- = muscle
cardi/a = heart
-al = pertaining to
the heart muscle

Key Concept

Every health care professional should be certified in cardiopulmonary resuscitation (CPR) because heart disease is the number one cause of death in the United States. It is vital that CPR be applied correctly to patients with suspected heart attacks in order to save their lives.

Key Concept

The drugs that are commonly found on a hospital crash cart include acetaminophen, adenosine, amiodarone, atropine, dexamethasone, diphenhydramine, dobutamine, dopamine, epinephrine, furosemide, heparin, ipecac, lidocaine, naloxone, nitroglycerin, norepinephrine, oxygen, phenytoin, procainamide, sodium bicarbonate, and verapamil.

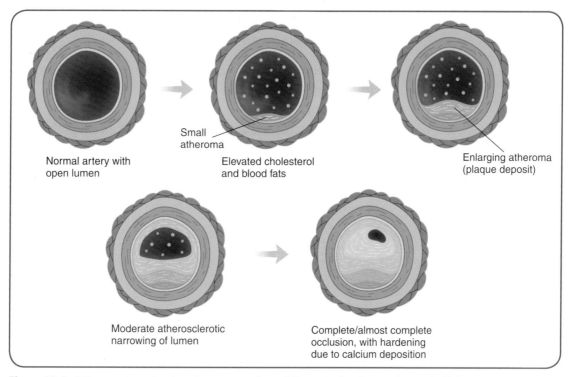

Figure 12-6 Atherosclerosis showing narrowing of the arteries from plaque buildup.

Normal artery with open lumen

Small atheroma

Elevated cholesterol and blood fats

Enlarging atheroma (plaque deposit)

Moderate atherosclerotic narrowing of lumen

Complete/almost complete occlusion, with hardening due to calcium deposition

Medical Terminology Review

arteriosclerosis
arteri/o- = artery
sclera/o = hard
-sis = condition
hardening of the arteries

Key Concept

According to recent research, the buildup of calcium plaque in the arteries carries an increased risk of heart attacks and death in multiple ethnic groups.

Unstable angina is a medical emergency, and the patient must be treated in a hospital. It typically has a sudden onset, sudden worsening, and stuttering reoccurrence over days and weeks, and carries a more severe short-term prognosis than stable chronic angina. Unstable angina occurs during periods of rest. Signs of unstable angina include changes in blood pressure, transient heart murmur, and arrhythmias. Note: unstable angina is the only form of angina that may also be treated with angiotensin-converting enzyme (ACE) inhibitors. Examples of these agents include benazepril (Lotensin®), captopril (Capoten®), and enalapril (Vasotec®).

Decubitus angina is a condition characterized by periodic attacks of cardiac pain that occur when a person is lying down, but not necessarily while sleeping. It is also known as **vasospastic angina**. Decubitus angina occurs when the decreased myocardial blood flow is caused by spasms of the coronary arteries.

Silent angina is a condition that occurs in the absence of angina pain. One or more coronary arteries are occluded, but the individual remains asymptomatic.

Nocturnal angina is caused by coronary artery spasms and can be treated by calcium channel blockers and nitrates. It occurs during the REM period of sleep.

Treatment goals for angina include:

- Reducing the risk of sudden death
- Preventing myocardial infarction

- Increasing myocardial oxygen supply
- Reducing pain and anxiety associated with an angina attack

Treatment for angina includes surgery and drug therapy. If the coronary arteries are significantly occluded or blocked, **coronary arterial bypass graft (CABG)** or **percutaneous transluminal coronary angioplasty (PTCA)** is performed. CABG is a procedure in which a vein graft is surgically implanted to bypass the area of occlusion in a coronary artery. PTCA reduces obstruction by means of invasive procedures requiring cardiac catheterization. The catheter contains an inflatable balloon that flattens the obstruction. Newer techniques use laser angioplasty.

>
> **Medical Terminology**
> ### Review
> **angioplasty**
> angio- = blood and lymph vessel
> -plasty = molding or forming surgically
> a procedure involving the molding or forming of a blood vessel surgically

ANTIANGINAL DRUG THERAPY

> **Key Concept**
> According to a recent study, aggressive drug therapy now appears to be just as effective as angioplasty for patients with stable heart disease.

There are three groups of medications that may meet the treatment goals for angina pectoris:

1. Nitrates
2. Beta-adrenergic blockers
3. Calcium channel blockers

For chronic angina, the drug ranolazine (Ranexa®) also may be used. This is a newer sodium channel blocker that is used as a first-line treatment for chronic angina.

Nitrates

Nitrates were the first agents used to relieve angina. This group of drugs reduces myocardial ischemia, but may cause hypotension. Nitrates are still an important part of antianginal therapy. Table 12-2 shows nitrates and other agents commonly used in the treatment of angina.

Mechanism of Action

Nitrates primarily are effective in the venous circulation by relaxing vascular smooth muscle and reducing the work of the left ventricle. These agents are administered to dilate the blood vessels and stop attacks of angina (Figure 12-7).

Indications

Nitrates are used in the treatment of angina as coronary vasodilators. Nitrate preparations should be based on onset of action, duration of action, and patient compliance. Nitrate preparations are available in sublingual tablets, nitroglycerin spray bottles, topical nitroglycerin ointments, and transdermal patches.

The sublingual route is the most common route of administration for nitroglycerin. This agent begins to work rapidly and lasts for about an hour.

TABLE 12-2   Commonly Used Combination Drugs for Angina and Myocardial Infarction

Generic Name	Trade Name	Route of Administration	Average Adult Dosage
Beta-Adrenergic Blockers			
atenolol **(ah-TEH-noh-lol)**	Tenormin®	PO	25–50 mg/day (max: 100 mg/day)
metoprolol tartrate **(meh-TOH-proh-lol TAR-trayt)**	Lopressor®	PO	100 mg bid (max: 400 mg/day)
propranolol hydrochloride **(proh-PRAH-noh-lol hy-droh-KLOR-ryd)**	Inderal®, Inderal LA®	PO	10–20 mg bid–tid (max: 320 mg/day)
timolol maleate **(TIH-moh-lol MAH-lee-ayt)**	Betimol®, Blocadren®	PO	15–45 mg tid (max: 60 mg/day)
Calcium Channel Blockers			
amlodipine **(am-LOH-dih-peen)**	Norvasc®	PO	5–10 mg/day (max: 10 mg/day)
bepridil **(BEE-prih-dihl)**	Vascor®	PO	200 mg/day (max: 360 mg/day)
diltiazem hydrochloride **(dihl-TY-ah-zem hy-droh-KLOR-ryd)**	Cardizem®, Dilacor XR®	PO	30 mg qid (max: 360 mg/day)
nicardipine hydrochloride **(ny-KAR-dih-peen hy-droh-KLOR-ryd)**	Cardene®	PO	20–40 mg tid or 30–60 mg sustained release (SR) bid (max: 120 mg/day)
nifedipine **(ny-FEH-dih-peen)**	Adalat®, Procardia®	PO	10–20 mg tid (max: 180 mg/day)
verapamil hydrochloride **(veer-AH-pah-mihl hy-droh-KLOR-ryd)**	Calan®, Covera-HS®	PO	80 mg tid–qid (max: 480 mg/day) taken at bedtime
Organic Nitrates			
amyl nitrate **(AY-mihl NY-trayt)**	(generic only)	Inhalation	1 ampule (0.18–0.3 mL) prn
isosorbide dinitrate **(eye-soh-SOR-byd dy-NYE-trayt)**	Isordil®	PO	2.5–30 mg qid
isosorbide mononitrate **(eye-soh-SOR-byd maw-noh-NYE-trayt)**	Imdur®, ISMO®	PO	20 mg bid
nitroglycerin **(ny-troh-GLIH-sir-rihn)**	Nitrostat®, Nitro-Dur®	SL, Topical	1 tablet (0.3–0.6 mg) or 1 spray (0.4–0.8 mg) q3–5 min (max: 3 doses in 15 min) applied transdermally daily

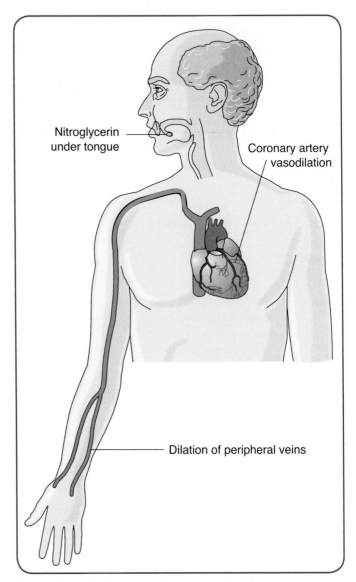

Figure 12-7 Mechanism of action of nitroglycerin.

This is an ideal preparation for use in patients with acute anginal pain. Administration should begin as soon as the pain begins, and should not be delayed until the pain is severe. If one tablet is not sufficient, one or two additional tablets should be taken at five-minute intervals. For persistent pain, the patient should see a physician, because he or she may have signs of a myocardial infarction. The shelf life of nitroglycerin is greater when the medication is kept in a dark, tightly closed container. After the container is opened, the drug is effective for approximately 30 days, and the date on which it was opened should be written on the container. Thirty days after the container is opened, the medication should be discarded and replaced with a new bottle.

Transdermal patches contain a reservoir of nitroglycerin. This agent is slowly released for absorption through the skin (Figure 12-8). The patches

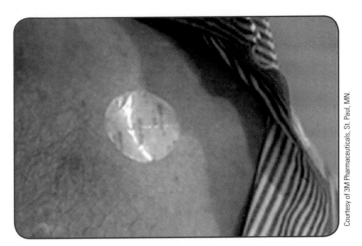

Courtesy of 3M Pharmaceuticals, St. Paul, MN.

Figure 12-8 Transdermal nitroglycerin patch.

have a slow onset and are not effective for an ongoing anginal attack. The application site of the patch should be rotated daily to prevent irritation.

Topical ointment can also be used on the skin; the ointment should be applied using an applicator, and then covered with plastic wrap that is held in place with adhesive tape. The sites should be rotated to prevent local irritation.

Adverse Effects

Abrupt discontinuation of long-acting nitroglycerin preparations may cause angina. Vasodilation can lead to orthostatic hypotension, tachycardia, headache, dizziness, weakness, syncope, and blushing. Nitrate-induced headache occurs as a result of the dilation of cerebral blood vessels. Nitrates may also increase intraocular and intracranial pressure. Continuous exposure to nitrates may lead to tolerance. Large doses of nitrate drugs can produce methemoglobinemia (the presence of methemoglobin in the blood).

Contraindications and Precautions

These agents are contraindicated in patients with hypersensitivity to nitrates, severe anemia, head trauma, and increased intracranial pressure. Nitrates are also contraindicated in patients with glaucoma, hypotension, hyperthyroidism, and alcoholism. Safety during pregnancy (category C) and lactation is not established. Nitrate drugs should also be used cautiously in patients with severe liver or kidney disease.

Drug Interactions

A combination of nitrates and sildenafil (Viagra®) can cause prolonged and *potentially life-threatening hypotension*. Sildenafil therapy is therefore contraindicated in patients who use nitrates. This is important to remember because sildenafil and similar drugs used for erectile dysfunction are also

Medical Terminology Review

hyperthyroidism
hyper- = over; above; beyond
thyroid = the thyroid gland
-ism = action; process; practice
overactive thyroid gland

sometimes used for hypertension. Beta-blockers, calcium channel blockers, vasodilators, and alcohol can enhance the hypotensive effect of nitrates. Intravenous nitroglycerin may antagonize the effects of heparin.

Beta-Adrenergic Blockers

Beta-adrenergic blockers (beta-blockers) block the beta$_1$ receptor site. Beta-blockers decrease the effects of the sympathetic nervous system by blocking the release of the catecholamines epinephrine and norepinephrine, thereby decreasing the heart rate and blood pressure. (They are listed in both Tables 12-2 and 12-4.)

Mechanism of Action

Beta-blockers reduce oxygen demand both at rest and during exertion in the myocardium, and prevent myocardial infarction.

Indications

The beta-blockers reduce the frequency and severity of exertional angina that is not controlled by nitrates. Therefore, these agents are an important part of therapy for angina pectoris. Combined therapy with nitrates is often preferred in the treatment of angina pectoris, because of a decrease in the side effects of both agents.

Adverse Effects

Beta-blockers have few adverse effects on the respiratory and cardiovascular systems. Common adverse effects of these drugs include dyspnea, bronchospasm, hypotension, bradycardia, and hypoglycemia. These agents may also cause insomnia and depression.

Contraindications and Precautions

Beta-blockers are contraindicated in patients with a known hypersensitivity to these agents. Beta-blockers are also contraindicated in patients with asthma, congestive heart failure, heart block, bradycardia, and diabetes mellitus. These drugs should be avoided in patients with cardiogenic shock, pulmonary edema, and peripheral vascular disease.

Beta-adrenergic blockers should be used with caution in patients prone to non-allergenic bronchospasm (e.g., chronic bronchitis, emphysema), major surgery, stroke, renal disease, or hepatic disease. Beta-blockers are used cautiously in elderly patients, patients with diabetes mellitus, and in patients prone to hypoglycemia.

Drug Interactions

These agents may interact with atropine and other anticholinergics, nonsteroidal anti-inflammatory drugs, insulin, sulfonylureas, lidocaine, verapamil, prazosin, and terazosin.

Medical Terminology Review

hypoglycemia
hypo- = under; beneath; down
glyc = carbohydrate and especially sugar
-emia = condition of having low blood sugar levels

Medical Terminology Review

bronchospasm
broncho = windpipe; bronchial (tube)
spasm = an involuntary and abnormal muscular contraction
abnormal muscular contractions of the windpipe

Calcium Channel Blockers

Calcium channel blockers are considered third-choice agents in the treatment of stable angina, certain dysrhythmias, and hypertension. Calcium channel blockers are also listed in Tables 12-2 and 12-4.

Mechanism of Action

Calcium channel blockers are a type of drug that blocks the entry of calcium into smooth muscle cells as well as myocytes. They produce arterial vasodilation and thereby reduce arterial blood pressure. They also reduce myocardial contractility, resulting in reduction of myocardial oxygen consumption.

Indications

Calcium channel blockers are used to treat exertional angina that is not controlled by nitrates, and in combination with beta-blockers. This combination provides the most effective therapy. They are considered the drug of choice in the treatment of angina at rest. Diltiazem and verapamil will reduce the heart rate. Nifedipine, amlodipine, and felodipine are among the most potent calcium-blocking agents. Beta-blockers are recommended as the first-line treatment of angina pectoris, but if they are not tolerated, calcium channel blockers can be administered. Diltiazem and verapamil can be used, but they have the disadvantage of depressing contractility more than dihydropyridines do. The therapeutic goal in medication use is to reduce the frequency and intensity of anginal attacks without suppressing the cardiac action too much.

Adverse Effects

Common adverse effects related to the use of calcium channel blockers include flushing, headaches, dizziness, hypotension, ankle edema, constipation, and palpitations. Combinations of nitrates, beta-blockers, and calcium channel blockers are often preferred for treatment of angina pectoris, because these agents have fewer adverse effects.

Contraindications and Precautions

Calcium channel blockers are contraindicated in patients with a history of hypersensitivity to these drugs, hypotension, or cardiogenic shock. The major contraindications to combination therapy are associated with the use of beta-blockers and calcium channel blockers, which may cause excessive cardiac depression. Calcium channel blockers should be used with caution during pregnancy (category C) and lactation, and in patients with congestive heart failure, hepatic or renal dysfunction, and hypotension.

Drug Interactions

Calcium channel blockers increase the risk of orthostatic hypotension with prazosin. Increased blood pressure may occur with aspirin, bismuth subsalicylate, or magnesium salicylate. Some calcium channel blockers increase serum levels and toxicity of cyclosporine.

MYOCARDIAL INFARCTION

A **myocardial infarction (MI)** is an area of dead cardiac muscle tissue, with or without hemorrhage, resulting from an obstruction of a coronary artery. Coronary heart disease is the primary cause of death in American men and women, as well as a major cause of disability. Those who survive an MI have a notably greater risk of a second MI, congestive heart failure, or a stroke occurring within a short time.

An MI (heart attack) occurs when obstruction of a coronary artery causes prolonged ischemia (reduction of blood supply to the heart). The resulting lack of oxygen to the tissue leads to cell death, or infarction, of the heart wall (Figure 12-9).

After an MI, three goals should be achieved expeditiously and simultaneously to limit myocardial necrosis and mortality:

- Relief of pain
- Confirmation of diagnosis by electrocardiogram (ECG) and measurements of serum markers
- Assessment and treatment of hemodynamic abnormalities

Pain relief is best achieved with oxygen (2 L/min by nasal cannula), nitroglycerin, and morphine sulfate. The rationale for reperfusion therapy (thrombolytic therapy) is based on the high prevalence of occlusive thrombi in early treatment. The greatest benefit is seen when this therapy is performed within the first four hours of the onset of pain. Antithrombotic agents should be considered for all patients with an acute MI. Antithrombotic medications

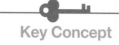

Key Concept

During an acute MI, women are less likely to experience chest pain than men. Common acute symptoms in women include dyspnea, weakness, fatigue, nausea or vomiting, palpitations, and indigestion.

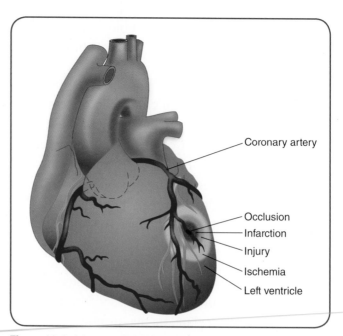

Coronary artery

Occlusion
Infarction
Injury
Ischemia
Left ventricle

Figure 12-9 Myocardial infarction.

TABLE 12-3	Arrhythmias
Type of Arrhythmia	**Beats per Minute**
Bradycardia	Less than 60
Tachycardia	150 to 250
Atrial flutter	200 to 350
Atrial fibrillation	More than 350
Ventricular fibrillation	Variable
Premature atrial contraction	Variable
Premature ventricular contraction	Variable

include unfractionated heparin, low-molecular-weight heparin, warfarin, aspirin, and antiplatelet drugs (see Chapter 15).

CARDIAC ARRHYTHMIAS

Medical Terminology
Review

dysrhythmia
dys- = abnormal
rhythm = regular recurrence of action
-ia = pathological condition
abnormal heart rhythm

Arrhythmias (dysrhythmias) are deviations from the normal cardiac rate or rhythm (Table 12-3). They may result from damage to the heart's conduction system or from systemic causes such as electrolyte abnormalities, fever, hypoxia, stress, and drug toxicity.

Arrhythmias reduce the efficiency of the heart's pumping cycle. A slight increase in heart rate increases cardiac output, but a very rapid heart rate prevents adequate filling during diastole, reducing cardiac output. A very slow heart rate also reduces output to the tissues, including the brain and the heart itself. Irregular contractions are inefficient because they interfere with the normal filling and emptying cycle. Table 12-3 summarizes various cardiac arrhythmias.

Key Concept

According to a recent study, patients who are diagnosed for the first time with atrial fibrillation have a significantly greater early risk of dying compared with those who do not have this condition. Factors that are strongly associated with death in atrial fibrillation patients include a faster heart rate at diagnosis, being thin, a history of chronic kidney disease, and malignancy.

ANTIARRHYTHMIC DRUGS

Antiarrhythmic agents do not cure the dysrhythmia, but the goal of treatment is to restore normal cardiac function. These agents are classified into four distinct groups, according to their effects (Table 12-4):

- Class I (sodium channel blockers), which are further subclassified into three groups—IA, IB, and IC
- Class II (beta-adrenergic blockers)
- Class III (potassium channel blockers, which interfere with potassium outflow)
- Class IV (calcium channel blockers)

There are also other agents that may be used for the treatment of arrhythmias, such as digoxin, atropine, and magnesium.

TABLE 12-4 **Classifications of Antiarrhythmic Drugs**

Generic Name	Trade Name	Route of Administration	Average Adult Dosage
Class IA (sodium channel blockers)			
disopyramide phosphate **(dy-soh-PEER-ah-myd FOS-fayt)**	Norpace®	PO	100–200 mg q6h or 300 mg SR capsule q12h
procainamide hydrochloride **(pro-KAY-nah-myd hy-droh-KLOR-ryd)**	Procan SR®, Procanbid®, Pronestyl®	PO, IM, IV	PO: 50 mg/kg/day in divided doses; IM: 0.5–1g q4–8h; IV: 100 mg q5 min at a rate of 25–50 mg/min until arrhythmia is controlled
quinidine gluconate **(KWIH-nih-deen GLOO-koh-nayt)**	Quinaglute®	PO	200–300 mg q3–4h for 4 or more doses until arrhythmia terminates
Class IB			
lidocaine hydrochloride **(LY-doh-kayn hy-droh-KLOR-ryd)**	Xylocaine®	IV	immediately after 1st bolus
mexiletine **(mek-SIH-lih-teen)**	Mexitil®	PO	200–300 mg q8h (max: 1200 mg/day)
phenytoin **(feh-nih-TOH-in)**	Dilantin®	IV	50–100 mg q10–15 min until dysrhythmia is terminated
Class IC			
flecainide acetate **(fleh-KAY-nyd AH-seh-tayt)**	Tambocor®	PO	100 mg q12h, may increase 50 mg bid q4d (max: 400 mg/day)
moricizine hydrochloride **(mor-RIH-sih-zeen hy-droh-KLOR-ryd)**	Ethmozine®	PO	600–900 mg/day
propafenone **(pro-PAH-feh-nohn)**	Rythmol®	PO	150–300 mg/tid; increase dosage slowly, prn (max: 900 mg/day)
Class II (beta-adrenergic blockers)			
acebutolol **(ah-seh-BYOO-toh-lol)**	Sectral®	PO	200–600 mg bid increased to 1200 mg/day
atenolol **(ah-TEH-noh-lol)**	Tenormin®	PO	25–50 mg/day, may increase to 100 mg/day
esmolol hydrochloride **(EZ-moh-lol hy-droh-KLOR-ryd)**	Brevibloc®	IV	50 mcg/kg/min (max: 200 mcg/kg/min)
nadolol **(nay-DOH-lol)**	Corgard®	PO	40 mg once daily, increase to 240–320 mg/day in 1–2 divided doses
propranolol hydrochloride **(pro-PRAH-noh-lol hy-droh-KLOR-ryd)**	Inderal®	PO	10–30 mg tid or qid

Table 12-4 continued

Class III (potassium channel blockers)			
amiodarone hydrochloride (ah-mee-OH-dah-rohn hy-droh-KLOR-ryd)	Cordarone®	PO	400–1600 mg/day in 1–3 divided doses
bretylium tosylate (breh-TIH-lee-um TOH-sih-layt)	Bretylol®	IV	Rapid injection (5–10 mg/kg), or 1–2 mg/min as continuous infusion
dofetilide (doh-FEH-tih-lyd)	Tikosyn®	PO	125–500 mcg bid
ibutilide fumarate (eye-BYOO-tih-lyd FYOO-mah-rayt)	Corvert®	IV	1 mg infused over 10 min
Class IV (calcium channel blockers)			
diltiazem (dihl-TY-ah-zem)	Cardizem®	IV	0.25–15 mg/kg bolus over 2 min, may repeat in 15 min with 0.35 mg/kg
verapamil hydrochloride (veer-AH-pah-mihl hy-droh-KLOR-ryd)	Calan®	IV	2.5–5 mg initial dose, then 5–10 mg after 15–30 min
Others			
atropine (AH-troh-peen)	Atropisol®	IM, IV	0.5–1 mg q1–2h prn (max: 2 mg)
digoxin (dih-JOK-sihn)	Lanoxin®	PO, IV	PO: 0.75–1.5 mg/kg; IV: 0.5–1 mg/kg

Mechanism of Action

Class I Fast (sodium) channel blockers decrease the fast sodium influx to the cardiac cells. These drugs decrease conduction velocity in the cardiac tissue, suppress automaticity, and increase recovery time (repolarization). There are three subgroups of fast channel blockers: IA slows conduction and prolongs repolarization (e.g., disopyramide, quinidine, procainamide); IB slows conduction and shortens repolarization (e.g., lidocaine, mexiletine); and IC prolongs conduction with little to no effect on repolarization (e.g., flecainide).

Class II Beta-adrenergic blockers inhibit adrenergic stimulation of the heart, and depress myocardial excitability and contractility. Therefore, they decrease conduction velocity in cardiac tissue. Major beta-adrenergic blockers are listed in Tables 12-2 and 12-4.

Class III Antiarrhythmics interfere with potassium outflow during repolarization. They prolong the action potential duration and effective refractory period. The prolonged period decreases the frequency of the heart rate. Amiodarone decreases automaticity, prolongs atrioventricular (AV) conduction, and may even block the exchange of sodium and potassium.

Class IV

Antiarrhythmics selectively block slow calcium channels. Therefore, these agents can prolong nodal conduction and effective refractory period. These calcium antagonists may also decrease the ability of the heart to produce forceful contractions, leading to congestive heart failure. Antiarrhythmic drugs also relax smooth muscle and cause vasodilation. Verapamil works on the sinoatrial node to decrease its activity, thus decreasing the heart rate. It also decreases AV node conduction and is used for AV node dysrhythmias.

Indications

Quinidine is used to treat supraventricular arrhythmias, such as atrial flutter and atrial fibrillation, acute ventricular dysrhythmias, and life-threatening ventricular dysrhythmias. This agent also exhibits antimalarial, antipyretic, and oxytocic actions. Procainamide is safer to use intravenously and has fewer gastrointestinal adverse effects. Disopyramide has been approved for the treatment of ventricular arrhythmias. Generally, it is reserved for patients who are intolerant of quinidine or procainamide. Lidocaine doses must be adjusted in patients with congestive heart failure or hepatic disease. Mexiletine is used primarily for chronic treatment of ventricular arrhythmias associated with previous myocardial infarction. Phenytoin is an antiepileptic drug (see Chapter 9) that has proved to be useful in treating digitalis-induced tachyarrhythmias.

Beta-adrenergic blockers are useful in treating tachyarrhythmias resulting from increased sympathetic activity, and also are used for a variety of other arrhythmias, atrial flutter, and atrial fibrillation. These agents are sometimes used for patients experiencing digitalis toxicity. Propranolol is the most common beta-blocker that is used as an antiarrhythmic. Amiodarone is useful for severe refractory supraventricular and ventricular tachyarrhythmias. Amiodarone also possesses antianginal effects.

Calcium channel blockers are useful for angina and for hypertension. Verapamil is useful for reentrant supraventricular tachycardia.

Digitalis drugs are the principal medications used in the treatment of congestive heart failure (discussed later in this chapter) and certain arrhythmias. Digoxin is most often prescribed because it can be administered orally and parenterally. It has an intermediate duration of action.

Adverse Effects

Quinidine can lead to skeletal muscle weakness, especially in patients with myasthenia gravis. Rapid infusion of quinidine may cause severe hypotension and shock. It can produce ringing of the ears, dizziness, diarrhea, thrombocytopenia, and ventricular arrhythmias.

Key Concept

The process of establishing the correct therapeutic dose of digitalis that maintains optimal functioning of the heart without inducing toxic effects is referred to as *digitalization*. The margin between effective therapy and dangerous toxicity is very narrow. Careful monitoring of the cardiac rate and rhythm (with an ECG), cardiac function, adverse effects, and the blood digitalis level is required to determine the therapeutic maintenance dose.

A high incidence of adverse reactions to procainamide is seen with chronic use. Severe or irreversible heart failure has been produced more frequently by procainamide than by quinidine. Procainamide also often causes drug-induced lupus syndrome.

Disopyramide may cause dry mouth, blurred vision, constipation, and urinary retention.

High doses of lidocaine can cause cardiovascular depression, confusion, and light-headedness. Otherwise, there is a low level of cardiotoxicity with the use of lidocaine. The most common side effects are neurological, in contrast to quinidine and procainamide. Lidocaine has little effect on the autonomic nervous system. The common adverse effects of phenytoin use are nystagmus, blurred vision, vertigo, and hyperplasia of the gums.

Adverse effects of the use of beta-adrenergic blockers include bronchospasm. Bradycardia and myocardial depression may occur. Atropine or isoproterenol may be used to alleviate bradycardia. The most frequent cardiovascular adverse effects with use of propranolol are hypertension and bradycardia. It may also cause mental confusion and skin rashes.

Contraindications and Precautions

Class I antiarrhythmics agents are contraindicated in patients with hypersensitivity to these drugs, pregnancy (category B or C), and lactation. They should be avoided in patients with complete AV block, thyrotoxicosis, acute rheumatic fever, extensive myocardial damage, hypotensive states, myasthenia gravis, and digitalis intoxication. Quinidine should be used cautiously in patients with incomplete heart block, impaired kidney or liver function, bronchial asthma, myasthenia gravis, and potassium imbalance. Procainamide is used with caution in patients with hypotension, cardiac enlargement, congestive heart failure, heart attack, coronary occlusion, and hepatic or renal insufficiency.

Class II antiarrhythmics drugs (e.g., propranolol and others) are contraindicated in patients with congestive heart failure, right ventricular failure secondary to pulmonary hypertension, ventricular dysfunction, sinus bradycardia, bronchial asthma or bronchospasm, pulmonary edema, and allergic rhinitis during pollen season. Beta-adrenergic blockers are used cautiously in elderly patients and patients prone to nonallergic bronchospasm (e.g., chronic bronchitis, emphysema), stroke, major surgery, renal or hepatic disease, and diabetes mellitus.

Class III antiarrhythmic drugs (e.g., bretylium) have no contraindications for use in life-threatening ventricular arrhythmias. Safety during pregnancy (category C), lactation, or in children is not established. Amiodarone is contraindicated in patients with hypersensitivity to this agent. Amiodarone should be avoided in cardiogenic shock, severe sinus bradycardia, severe liver disease, and children. Safety during pregnancy (category D) or

Medical Terminology Review

bradycardia
brady- = slow
-cardia = heart action
slow heart rate

lactation is not established. Amiodarone is given to patients cautiously if they have cirrhosis of the liver, goiter, hypersensitivity to iodine, electrolyte imbalance, hypokalemia, hypovolemia, and open-heart surgery. It also must be used with caution in elderly patients. Bretylium is used with caution in patients with severe aortic stenosis or severe pulmonary hypertension, and angina pectoris.

Class IV antiarrythmic drugs (calcium channel blockers) are contraindicated in patients with severe hypotension, cardiogenic shock, cardiomegaly, digitalis toxicity, atrial flutter and fibrillation, and severe congestive heart failure. Safe use of these agents during pregnancy (category C) or lactation, and in children, is not established. Calcium channel blockers are used cautiously in patients with hepatic or renal impairment, patients who have had an MI (heart attack) caused by coronary occlusion, and in those with aortic stenosis.

Drug Interactions

Two antiarrhythmic agents used concurrently may cause additive effects and may increase the risk for drug toxicity. If quinidine and procainamide are given with digitalis, the risk of digitalis toxicity may be increased. Quinidine may interact with cimetidine or barbiturates, causing quinidine blood levels to be increased. Quinidine that is given concurrently with verapamil increases the risk of hypotension. Lidocaine and procainamide may interact and cause additive cardiodepressant effects. Inderal may also increase the risk of lidocaine toxicity.

CONGESTIVE HEART FAILURE

Congestive heart failure (CHF) is one of the most common cardiovascular disorders. This condition occurs when the heart is not able to pump enough blood to meet the body's metabolic demands. Signs and symptoms of CHF differ depending on which side of the heart is affected but generally include distended neck veins, lower leg edema, splenomegaly, hepatomegaly, ascites, and pulmonary edema (Figure 12-10). Heart failure may be caused by any disorder that affects the heart's ability to receive or eject blood. The symptoms of left-sided heart failure include cough, decreased urine production, difficulty lying down, fatigue, weakness, faintness, irregular or rapid pulse, palpitations, shortness of breath (often causing the patient to awaken from sleep), and weight gain. The symptoms of right-sided heart failure include shortness of breath, swelling of feet and ankles, urinating more frequently at night, distended neck veins, palpitations, irregular and fast heartbeat, fatigue, weakness, and fainting.

Because there is no cure for heart failure, the treatment goals are to prevent, treat, or remove the underlying causes when possible. Drugs can

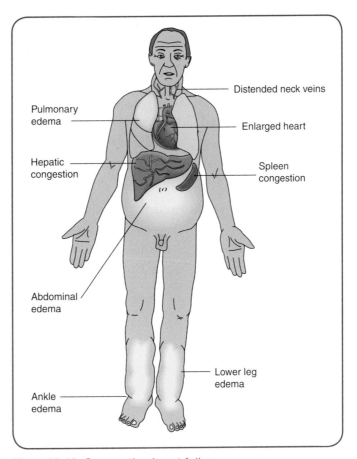

Figure 12-10 Congestive heart failure.

relieve the symptoms of heart failure by a number of different mechanisms, including slowing the heart rate, increasing contractility, and reducing its workload. Drugs used for heart failure include ACE inhibitors, diuretics, vasodilators, and cardiac glycosides. In this section, cardiac glycosides will be discussed in detail. The other drugs also used for heart failure are discussed in Chapter 13and 14.

CARDIAC GLYCOSIDES

Cardiac glycosides are among the oldest drugs used in the treatment of heart diseases (having been in use in some form for over 2000 years). A number of plants contain cardiac glycosides. Digoxin is extracted from the leaves of the purple foxglove (*Digitalis purpura*). In fact, the generic term *digitalis* is often used to represent all cardiac glycosides used in the clinical setting.

Cardiac glycosides increase the speed of myocardial contractions in both normal and failing hearts. Under normal cardiac conditions, treatment with these drugs results in an increase in systemic vascular resistance and the constriction of smooth muscles in veins (cardiac output may decrease).

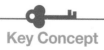

Key Concept

Patients should never stop taking digoxin without first consulting a physician. A sudden absence of this drug can cause a serious change in heart function. Digoxin usually must be taken for long periods of time, and sometimes lifelong.

In heart failure, cardiac glycosides increase the force of myocardial contractions, slow the heart rate, and slow the conduction of electrical impulses. The increased force of contractions improves the efficiency of the heart without increasing oxygen consumption. As a result, more blood is pumped from the heart, decreasing congestion. Normal blood circulation is restored, and kidney function is increased. Cardiac glycosides are able to strengthen the myocardium within a short period of time. The most common cardiac glycosides are digoxin and digitoxin.

Digitalis drugs are principal medications for the treatment of CHF and certain arrhythmias (atrial fibrillation, flutter, and paroxysmal atrial tachycardias) discussed earlier in this chapter (see also Table 12–4). Digoxin is prescribed most often but requires careful dosage calculation and adjustment (digitalization), as well as monitoring, to ensure that the correct therapeutic dosage is maintained.

Mechanism of Action

Cardiac glycosides act by increasing the force and velocity of myocardial systolic contraction (positive inotropic effect). They also decrease conduction velocity through the AV node.

Indications

Cardiac glycosides are used principally in the prophylactic management and treatment of heart failure, and to control the ventricular rate in patients with atrial fibrillation or flutter. These drugs are also used to treat and prevent recurrent atrial tachycardia, cardiogenic shock, and angina pectoris.

Because individual cardiac glycosides have similar pharmacological and therapeutic properties, the choice of a preparation depends on the onset of action required, desired route of administration, and duration of action. Digoxin is the most commonly used cardiac glycoside, primarily because it may be administered by various routes, and it has an intermediate duration of action.

Adverse Effects

The most dangerous adverse effect of digoxin is its ability to cause dysrhythmias, particularly in patients who have hypokalemia. Common adverse effects of digoxin therapy include nausea, vomiting, anorexia, and abnormalities of the nervous system such as headache, blurred vision (yellow-green halos), diplopia, photophobia, drowsiness, fatigue, and confusion.

Contraindications and Precautions

Cardiac glycosides are contraindicated in patients with known hypersensitivity to these agents, ventricular tachycardia, or ventricular failure, and in the presence of digitalis toxicity.

Cardiac glycosides are used cautiously in patients with renal insufficiency, hypokalemia, advanced heart disease, acute MI, severe lung disease, hypothyroidism, pregnancy (category A), and lactation. Fetal toxicity and neonatal death have been reported from maternal digoxin overdosage.

Drug Interactions

Cardiac glycosides react with many different drugs, including antacids, cholestyramine, and diuretics. Colestipol decreases digoxin absorption.

SUMMARY

Diseases of the cardiovascular system are among the leading causes of death in the United States. Numerous medications are available for the treatment of cardiovascular disease, some of which effect the myocardium itself, while others affect the blood vessels of the vascular system. Vasodilators, such as nitrates, increase the size of blood vessels to improve circulation of the blood in the management of angina pectoris. Cardiac glycosides, derived from digitalis, are used to increase the force of myocardial contractions in congestive heart failure. Antiarrhythmics are used to treat disorders of cardiac rhythm. These disorders may occur as a result of coronary artery disease, electrolyte imbalances, cardiac conduction abnormalities, or even from endocrine disease (thyroid disorders).

EXPLORING THE WEB

Visit **www.livestrong.com**

- Search for "cardiac drugs." Read some of the related articles on disorders of the heart and cardiovascular system and the drug therapies used to treat them.

Visit **www.heart.org**

- Research the diseases and conditions discussed within this chapter for further understanding of them.

REVIEW QUESTIONS

Multiple Choice

1. Which of the following antianginal drugs are also used as antihypertensives and antiarrhythmics?

   A. nitrates

   B. vasoconstrictors

   C. diuretics

   D. beta-adrenergic blockers

2. Which of the following drugs is in the class of calcium channel blockers?

   A. propranolol

   B. isosorbid

   C. verapamil

   D. atenolol

3. Early signs of toxicity of digitalis include:

   A. mental disorders

   B. nausea and vomiting

   C. tachycardia

   D. seizures

4. Which of the following medications is not used for dysrhythmia?

   A. beta-adrenergic blockers

   B. digoxin

   C. heparin

   D. atropine

5. A combination of nitrates and sildenafil (Viagra) can cause:

   A. stroke

   B. hypotension

   C. heart murmur

   D. hypertension

6. An example of a class II antiarrhythmic drug is:

    A. propranolol

    B. digoxin

    C. bretylium

    D. quinidine

7. Which of the following are common adverse effects of antiarrhythmic drugs?

    A. fatigue, diarrhea, hypertension

    B. dizziness, hypotension, and weakness

    C. anorexia, fatigue, and constipation

    D. fatigue, hypertension, and headache

8. An antiarrhythmic drug may cause:

    A. increased hepatic insufficiency

    B. decreased cardiac output

    C. increased cardiac output

    D. increased renal insufficiency

9. Which of the following administration routes for nitroglycerin is the most common?

    A. sublingual

    B. transdermal patch

    C. topical ointment

    D. parenteral

10. Combined therapy with nitrates is often preferred in treatment of angina pectoris because it results in which of the following?

    A. better toleration

    B. fewer adverse effects

    C. less expense

    D. increased blood volume

11. The generic name of Lopressor® is:

    A. metoprolol

    B. atenolol

    C. propranolol

    D. timolol

12. Blocadren® is the trade name of:

    A. propranolol

    B. metoprolol

    C. atenolol

    D. timolol

13. Calan® (verapamil) is classified as a(n):

    A. beta-adrenergic blocker

    B. calcium channel blocker

    C. organic nitrate

    D. potassium channel blocker

14. Cordarone® (amiodarone) is an example of a(n):

    A. beta-adrenergic blocker

    B. calcium channel blocker

    C. potassium channel blocker

    D. sodium channel blocker

15. Norpace® (disopyramide) is an example of a:

    A. sodium channel blocker

    B. potassium channel blocker

    C. beta-adrenergic blocker

    D. calcium channel blocker

Fill in the Blank

1. Beta-blockers reduce the frequency and severity of exertional angina that is not controlled by _____.

2. Class I antiarrhythmic drugs are also called _____.

3. Calcium channel blockers are in class _____ of the antiarrhythmic drugs.

4. Common side effects of phenytoin use are _____, _____, _____, and _____.

5. Cardiac glycosides act by increasing the force and velocity of _____.

Matching

_____ 1. Subclass IA

_____ 2. Subclass IB

_____ 3. Subclass IC

_____ 4. Class III (potassium channel blockers)

_____ 5. Class IV (calcium channel blockers)

A. diltiazem (Cardizem®)

B. lidocaine (Xylocaine®)

C. bretylium (Bretylol®)

D. procainamide (Pronestyl®)

E. flecainide (Tambocor®)

Critical Thinking

A 67-year-old man has been diagnosed with congestive heart failure. His physician orders digitalis for him.

1. For what other cardiovascular conditions is digitalis used?

2. What is the mechanism of action of digitalis?

3. What are the contraindications and precautions for digitalis?

CHAPTER 13

Antihypertensive Agents and Hyperlipidemia

OBJECTIVES

After completing this chapter, the reader should be able to:

1. Describe the effects of cardiac output, peripheral resistance, and blood volume on blood pressure.

2. Identify the major risk factor associated with hypertension.

3. Explain the role of the kidneys and renin-angiotensin-aldosterone system in blood pressure regulation.

4. Describe the classification of antihypertensives.

5. Describe the mechanisms of action of all drug groups used in the treatment of hypertension.

6. State common adverse effects of the antihypertensive drug groups.

7. Discuss the angiotensin-converting enzyme (ACE).

8. Identify three types of antihyperlipidemic drugs.

9. Describe combination drug therapy for hyperlipidemia.

GLOSSARY

Angiotensin-converting enzyme inhibitors – drugs that competitively inhibit conversion of angiotensin I to angiotensin II, a potent vasoconstrictor, through the activity of angiotensin-converting enzyme, with resultant lower levels of angiotensin II

Angiotensin II receptor antagonists – drugs that block the binding of angiotensin II to the angiotensin II type 1 receptor

Cardiac output – the amount of blood the heart pumps to the body in one minute

Diastolic blood pressure – the pressure measured at the moment the ventricles relax

Essential hypertension – idiopathic (occurring spontaneously from an unknown cause); also known as *primary hypertension*

Hyperlipidemia – an increase in triglycerides and cholesterol

Hypertension – an abnormal increase in arterial blood pressure

Lipoprotein – a class of blood chemicals whose molecules are composed of a lipid portion and a protein portion

Malignant hypertension – an uncontrollable, severe, and rapidly progressive form of hypertension with many complications

Niacin – vitamin B_3, nicotinic acid

Primary hypertension – idiopathic (occurring spontaneously from an unknown cause); also known as essential hypertension

Rhabdomyolysis – a potentially fatal destruction of skeletal muscle, characterized by the presence of myoglobin in the urine; it is also associated with acute renal failure in heatstroke

Sclerotic – hardening, toughening

Secondary hypertension – a type of hypertension that results from renal (e.g., nephrosclerosis) or endocrine (e.g., hyperaldosteronism) disease, or pheochromocytoma, a benign tumor of the adrenal medulla; in this type of hypertension, the underlying problem must be resolved

Statins –a class of drugs (HMG-CoA reductase inhibitors) that inhibits the activity of an enzyme that forms cholesterol in the body;

so named because all of their generic names end with "-statin" (e.g., lovastatin)

Steatorrhea – elimination of large amounts of fat in the stool

Stroke volume – the volume of blood pumped with each heartbeat

Systolic blood pressure – the pressure measured at the moment the heart contracts

Vasodilators – drugs used to relax or dilate vessels throughout the body

OVERVIEW

Hypertension (high blood pressure) is the most common cardiovascular disease. The prevalence varies with age, race, education, and many other variables. Sustained arterial hypertension damages blood vessels in the kidneys, heart, and brain, leading to an increased incidence of cardiac failure, coronary diseases, stroke, and renal failure. Effective pharmacological lowering of blood pressure has been shown to prevent damage to blood vessels and to substantially reduce morbidity and mortality rates.

Metabolic disorders that involve elevation in levels of any of the **lipoproteins** (a class of blood chemicals whose molecules are comprised of a lipid portion and a protein portion) are termed **hyperlipidemias**. The term *hyperlipidemia* denotes increased levels of triglycerides and cholesterol in the plasma. Analysis of serum lipids includes assessment of all of the subgroups (total cholesterol, triglycerides, low-density lipoproteins, and high-density lipoproteins), because the proportions in which these groups are found in the blood indicate the risk factors for the individual. The danger associated with elevated cholesterol levels occurs when cholesterol collects on blood vessel walls and calcifies. This hardening of the arteries causes the vessels to narrow, lose resiliency, and become rough enough to damage passing blood cells. Damaged blood cells trigger clotting, which can result in stroke or myocardial infarction.

Medical Terminology Review

hyperlipidemia
hyper- = over; above; beyond
lipid = fat
-emia = blood condition
condition in which there are increased levels of fat in the blood

BLOOD PRESSURE

Key Concept

The main factors determining blood pressure are cardiac output and systemic vascular resistance (the total amount of resistance the blood has to overcome to travel throughout the body). Blood pressure is regulated by an interaction between the nervous, humoral, and renal systems.

Blood pressure is a measurement of the pressure exerted on the walls of arteries as the heart pumps. The pressure measured at the moment the heart contracts is called **systolic blood pressure**. The pressure measured at the moment the ventricles relax is called **diastolic blood pressure**. The arteries closest to the heart maintain the highest pressures. Pressure decreases in the arteries the farther the arteries are from the heart.

Blood pressure is determined by **cardiac output** and **stroke volume**. The amount of blood the heart pumps to the body in one minute is the cardiac output. The stroke volume is the volume of the blood pumped with each heartbeat. Cardiac output is dependent upon stroke volume and the rate at which the heart beats. Therefore, cardiac output can be increased by increasing the heart rate, increasing the stroke volume, or increasing both factors.

HYPERTENSION

Hypertension is defined as an abnormal increase in arterial blood pressure, the incidence of which increases with age. According to the American Heart Association, in approximately 90% of cases, the cause is unknown, and more than a third of those affected have no idea that they have hypertension. Risk factors for hypertension include family history, stress, obesity, smoking, lifestyle, diabetes mellitus, and excessive lipid blood levels. Hypertension must be diagnosed in early stages (Table 13-1). When it is not properly treated, the risk of stroke, coronary artery disease, congestive heart failure, and renal failure increases.

There are three classifications of hypertension:

1. **Primary** or **essential hypertension** is idiopathic (occurring spontaneously from an unknown cause) and is the form discussed in this section.

2. **Secondary hypertension** results from renal (e.g., nephrosclerosis) or endocrine (e.g., hyperaldosteronism) disease, or pheochromocytoma, a mostly benign tumor of the adrenal medulla. In this type of hypertension, the underlying problem must be resolved.

3. **Malignant hypertension**, the third type, is an uncontrollable, severe, and rapidly progressive form of hypertension with many complications.

Hypertension is sometimes classified as systolic or diastolic depending on the measurement that is elevated. For example, elderly people with loss of elasticity in the arteries frequently have high systolic pressure and a low diastolic value.

Essential hypertension develops when the blood pressure is consistently above 140/90 mm Hg. This figure may be adjusted for the individual's age. The diastolic pressure is important because it indicates the degree of peripheral resistance and the increased workload of the left ventricle. The condition may be mild, moderate, or severe.

TABLE 13-1	Blood Pressure and Hypertension	
Classification	**Systolic (mm Hg)**	**Diastolic (mm Hg)**
Normal	Less than 120	Less than 80
Prehypertension	120–139	80–89
Stage I hypertension	140–159	90–99
Stage II hypertension	160 or higher	100 or higher

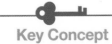

In essential hypertension, there is an increase in arteriolar vasoconstriction, which is attributed variously to increased susceptibility to stimuli or increased stimulation, or perhaps a combination of factors. A very slight decrease in the diameter of the arterioles causes a major increase in peripheral resistance, reduces the capacity of the system, and increases the diastolic pressure. Frequently, vasoconstriction leads to decreased blood flow through the kidneys, leading to increased renin, angiotensin, and aldosterone secretion. These substances increase vasoconstriction and blood volume, further increasing blood pressure. Figure 13-1 illustrates the development of hypertension. If this cycle is not broken, blood pressure can continue to increase. Renal failure is increased during hypertension because the flow of the blood through the kidneys is reduced. Kidneys are very important in maintaining electrolyte balances, especially those of sodium and water.

The increased blood pressure causes damage to the arterial walls, which become hardened and thick (**sclerotic**), narrowing the lumen. Blood supply to the involved area is reduced, leading to ischemia and necrosis with loss of function. The areas most commonly damaged are the kidneys, brain, and retinas.

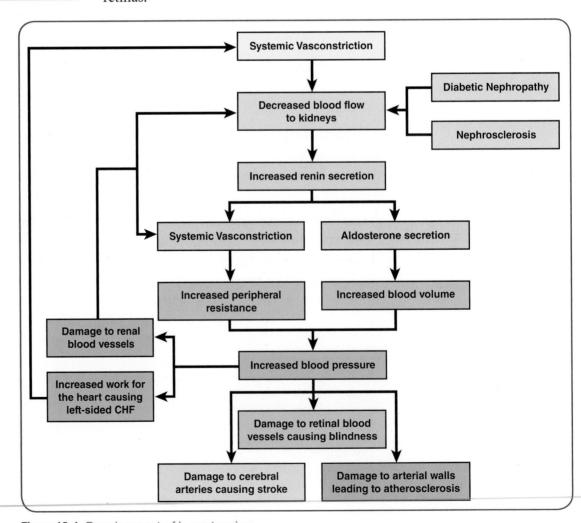

Figure 13-1 Development of hypertension.

ANTIHYPERTENSIVE THERAPY

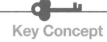

Key Concept

Blood pressure reduction is done in a step-wise approach, often beginning with nonpharmacological methods that include weight loss, dietary, and lifestyle modifications.

Key Concept

Drugs that primarily lower systemic vascular resistance include ACE inhibitors, alpha-antagonists, and peripheral vasodilators.

In primary hypertension, long-term therapy is necessary to prevent the morbidity and mortality associated with uncontrolled hypertension. Treatment primarily aims to lower the blood pressure toward "normal" with minimal side effects, and to prevent or reverse organ damage. Antihypertensive drugs do not cure hypertension. They only control it. After withdrawal of the drug, the blood pressure will return to levels similar to those before treatment with medication, if all other factors remain the same. Numerous antihypertensive drugs are used in the treatment and management of all degrees of hypertension. In mild cases of hypertension, the initial treatment regimen usually includes diet modification (reducing salt), weight reduction, mild exercise programs, smoking cessation, and stress reduction. Drugs prescribed to lower blood pressure act in various ways. The drug of choice varies according to the degree of hypertension (mild, moderate, or severe). Antihypertensives are sometimes combined for greater effectiveness and to reduce side effects. There are five groups of drugs that act to lower blood pressure in the following manner: (1) angiotensin-converting enzyme (ACE) inhibitors, (2) angiotensin II receptor antagonists, (3) adrenergic blockers, centrally and peripherally acting blockers (sympatholytics), (4) peripheral **vasodilators**, and (5) diuretics. They are explained below in more detail.

Angiotensin-Converting Enzyme Inhibitors

Angiotensin-converting enzyme inhibitors (ACE inhibitors) competitively inhibit conversion of angiotensin I to angiotensin II, a potent vasoconstrictor, through the activity of angiotensin-converting enzyme (ACE), with resultant lower levels of angiotensin II. Lower angiotensin II levels increase plasma renin activity and reduce aldosterone secretion.

Mechanism of Action

Angiotensin-converting enzyme inhibitors slow the formation of angiotensin II, which reduces vascular resistance, blood volume, and blood pressure. Renin is an enzyme that is released by the kidneys in response to reduced renal blood circulation or hyponatremia. It acts in the plasma, splitting the protein angiotensinogen to produce angiotensin I, which is then converted to angiotensin II, mostly in the lungs. Angiotensin II is a vasoconstricting agent. It causes sodium retention through the release of aldosterone. In the adrenal gland, angiotensin II is converted to angiotensin III. Both angiotensin II and angiotensin III stimulate the release of aldosterone. Angiotensin I is inactive in the cardiovascular system. Angiotensin II has several cardiovascular-renal actions. The most important site of ACE activity is in the lungs, but ACE also is found in the kidneys, central nervous system, and elsewhere. ACE inhibitors may affect the renin-angiotensin system to increase urine

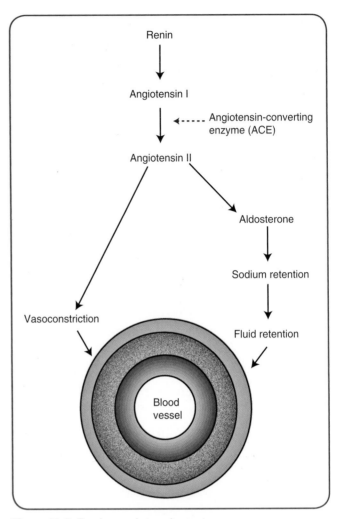

Figure 13-2 Renin-angiotensin system.

output. Figure 13-2 shows the renin-angiotensin system. Examples of ACE inhibitors are shown in Table 13-2.

Indications

Angiotensin-converting enzyme inhibitors are becoming the drugs of choice in the first-line treatment of essential hypertension.

Adverse Effects

Although ACE inhibitors as a group are relatively free of side effects or toxicities in most patients, they do occur, and some can be life-threatening. The adverse effects of ACE inhibitors may include dizziness, angioedema, loss of taste, photosensitivity, severe hypotension, dry cough, hyperkalemia, blood dyscrasias, and renal impairment.

Contraindications and Precautions

Angiotensin-converting enzyme inhibitors are contraindicated in patients with hypersensitivity to these agents, kidney damage, heart failure, hepatic

TABLE 13-2	Examples of ACE Inhibitors		
Generic Name	Trade Name	Route of Administration	Average Adult Dosage
benazepril hydrochloride **(beh-NAY-zeh-prihl hy-droh-KLOR-ryd)**	Lotensin®	PO	10–40 mg/day in 1–2 divided doses
captopril **(KAP-toh-prihl)**	Capoten®	PO	6.25–25 mg tid; may increase to 50 mg tid
enalapril maleate **(eh-NAH-lah-prihl MAH-lee-ayt)**	Vasotec®	PO	5–40 mg/day
fosinopril **(foh-SIH-noh-prihl)**	Monopril®	PO	5–40 mg/day (max: 80 mg/day)
lisinopril **(ly-SIH-noh-prihl)**	Prinivil®, Zestril®	PO	10–40 mg/day (max: 80 mg/day)
moexipril hydrochloride **(moh-EK-sih-prihl hy-droh-KLOR-ryd)**	Univasc®	PO	7.5–30 mg/day
perindopril erbumine **(pair-IN-doh-prihl ER-byoo-meen)**	Aceon®	PO	4 mg once daily; may increase to 8 mg/day
quinapril hydrochloride **(KWIH-nah-prihl hy-droh-KLOR-ryd)**	Accupril®	PO	10–20 mg once daily, may increase to 80 mg/day in 1–2 divided doses
ramipril **(RAH-mih-prihl)**	Altace®	PO	2.5–5 mg/day
trandolapril **(tran-DOH-lah-prihl)**	Mavik®	PO	1–4 mg/day

impairment, and diabetes mellitus. These drugs should be avoided during pregnancy (category D). Safety during lactation or in children is not established.

The ACE inhibitors should be used cautiously in patients with renal impairment or hypovolemia, as well as those who are receiving diuretics or undergoing dialysis. These drugs are used with caution in patients with congestive heart failure, hepatic impairment, and diabetes mellitus.

Drug Interactions

Angiotensin-converting enzyme inhibitors increase the risk of hypersensitivity reactions with allopurinol. They decrease antihypertensive effects with indomethacin. The ACE inhibitors also increase captopril effects with probenecid. Some ACE inhibitors may increase coughing if combined with capsaicin. Fosinopril increases the risk of high potassium levels if taken with potassium-sparing diuretics. Quinapril may increase digoxin levels and decrease tetracycline absorption.

Angiotensin II Receptor Antagonists

Angiotensin II receptor antagonists block the binding of angiotensin II to the angiotensin I receptor. Angiotensin II receptor antagonists have beneficial effects on the symptoms and hemodynamics of patients with congestive heart failure.

Mechanism of Action

Angiotensin II receptor antagonist drugs work by blocking the binding of angiotensin II to the angiotensin I receptors. By blocking the receptor site, these agents inhibit the vasoconstrictor effects of angiotensin II as well as preventing the release of aldosterone due to angiotensin II from the adrenal glands.

Indications

This class of drugs has been one of the most rapidly growing groups of drugs for the treatment of hypertension. Currently, seven agents are available: candesartan cilexetil, eprosartan, irbesartan, losartan, telmisartan, and valsartan (Table 13-3).

Adverse Effects

Angiotensin II receptor antagonists may cause dizziness, headache, hypotension, drowsiness, and depression. These drugs can also cause hepatitis, and

TABLE 13-3	Angiotensin II Receptor Antagonists		
Generic Name	Trade Name	Route of Administration	Average Adult Dosage
candesartan cilexetil **(KAN-deh-sar-tan sih-LEK-sih-tihl)**	Atacand®	PO	8–32 mg/day
eprosartan mesylate **(eh-proh-SAR-tan MEH-sih-layt)**	Teveten®	PO	400–800 mg/day
irbesartan **(ear-beh-SAR-tan)**	Avapro®	PO	150–300 mg/day
losartan potassium **(loh-SAR-tan poh-TAH-see-um)**	Cozaar®	PO	25–50 mg/day
olmesartan medoxomil **(ohl-meh-SAR-tan meh-DOK-soh-mihl)**	Benicar®	PO	20–40 mg/day
telmisartan **(tel-mih-SAR-tan)**	Micardis®	PO	40–80 mg/day
valsartan **(val-SAR-tan)**	Diovan®	PO	80–160 mg/day

elevated blood urea nitrogen (BUN) and serum creatinine. Using these medications may result in arrhythmias, abdominal pain, oliguria, and urinary tract infections, as well as hyperkalemia and hyponatremia.

Contraindications and Precautions

Angiotensin II receptor antagonists are contraindicated in patients with a known hypersensitivity to these agents, and should not be used in special hypertensive populations, such as diabetic patients with nephropathy or congestive heart failure, unless the patient cannot tolerate an ACE inhibitor. These drugs are also contraindicated in pregnancy (category C, first trimester; category D, second and third trimesters) and lactation.

Angiotensin II receptor antagonists are used cautiously in patients with concurrent administration of high-dose diuretics, potassium-sparing diuretics, or potassium salt substitutes; in those with diabetes mellitus, and during lactation. They should be used with caution in patients with hepatic or renal impairment, or in elderly patients.

Drug Interactions

Some of these drugs, such as losartan, decrease serum levels and effectiveness if taken concurrently with phenobarbital. Losartan is converted to an active metabolite by cytochrome P450, which may decrease the antihypertensive effects of losartan. Telmisartan increases serum levels and risk of toxicity of digoxin if combined.

Adrenergic Blockers, Centrally and Peripherally Acting Blockers (Sympatholytics)

The **sympatholytic** drugs include four main groups of medications: alpha-/beta-blockers, beta-blockers, centrally acting blockers, and peripherally acting blockers. These drugs are summarized in Table 13-4.

Mechanism of Action

Beta-blockers reduce peripheral resistance and inhibit cardiac function. They also block renin secretion. Centrally acting antiadrenergic blockers act primarily within the central nervous system on alpha$_2$ receptors to decrease sympathetic outflow to the cardiovascular system. Methyldopa decreases total peripheral resistance while having little effect on cardiac output or heart rate (except in older patients). Clonidine stimulates alpha$_2$ receptors centrally, and decreases vasomotor tone and heart rate. Guanabenz and guanfacine are centrally acting alpha$_2$-adrenergic agonists that have actions similar to clonidine.

Peripherally acting blockers may interfere with the release of norepinephrine from nerve endings or may block receptors in the vascular smooth muscle. This class of antihypertensive drug is best avoided unless it is

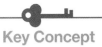

Key Concept

Beta-blockers, calcium channel antagonists, angiotensin II antagonists, combined alpha- and beta-antagonists, and centrally acting sympathetic depressants all act to lower both cardiac output and systemic vascular resistance.

TABLE 13-4 **Sympatholytic Drugs**

Generic Name	Trade Name	Route of Administration	Average Adult Dosage
Alpha-/Beta-Blocker			
labetalol hydrochloride **(lah-BEH-tah-lol hy-droh-KLOR-ryd)**	Trandate®	PO, IV	PO: Initial: 100 mg bid; Maint: 200–400 mg bid; IV: 20 mg slowly over 2 min with 40–80 mg over 10 min if needed
Beta-Blockers			
acebutolol hydrochloride **(ah-seh-BYOO-toh-lol hy-droh-KLOR-ryd)**	Sectral®	PO	200–800 mg/day in 2 divided doses
atenolol **(ah-TEH-noh-lol)**	Tenormin®	PO	25–100 mg once daily
betaxolol hydrochloride **(beh-TAK-soh-lol hy-droh-KLOR-ryd)**	Kerlone®	PO	5–10 mg/day (max: 20 mg/day)
bisoprolol fumarate **(by-soh-PROH-lol FYOO-mah-rayt)**	Zebeta®	PO	2.5–20 mg/day
carteolol hydrochloride **(kar-TEE-oh-lol hy-droh-KLOR-ryd)**	Cartrol®	PO	2.5–10 mg/day
metoprolol tartrate **(meh-TOH-proh-lol TAR-trayt)**	Lopressor®	PO, IV	PO: 50–450 mg/day; IV: 40–320 mg/day
nadolol **(nay-DOH-lol)**	Corgard®	PO	40 mg once daily; may increase to 240–320 mg/day
penbutolol **(pen-BYOO-toh-lol)**	Levatol®	PO	10–20 mg/day; may increase to 40–80 mg/day
propranolol hydrochloride **(pro-PRAH-noh-lol hy-droh-KLOR-ryd)**	Inderal®	PO	40–60 mg bid; usually requires 160–480 mg/day
timolol maleate **(TIH-moh-lol MAH-lee-ayt)**	Blocadren®	PO	10 mg bid; may increase to 60 mg/day
Centrally Acting Blockers			
clonidine hydrochloride **(KLAW-nih-deen hy-droh-KLOR-ryd)**	Catapres®	PO, Transdermal system	Initial: 0.1 mg bid; Maint: 0.1–0.2 mg/day
guanabenz acetate **(GWAH-nah-benz AH-seh-tayt)**	Wytensin®	PO	Initial: 4 mg bid (max: 32 mg bid)
guanfacine hydrochloride **(GWAN-fah-seen hy-droh-KLOR-ryd)**	Tenex®	PO	1–3 mg/day

Table 13-4 continued

methyldopa (meh-thil-DOH-pah)	Aldomet®	PO, IV	Initial: 250 mg bid; Maint: 500 mg to 3 g/day in 2–4 doses
Peripherally Acting Blockers			
doxazosin mesylate (dok-ZAH-zoh-sihn MEH-sih-layt)	Cardura®	PO	Initial: 1 mg/day; Maint: 2–16 mg once daily
guanadrel (GWAH-nah-drehl)	Hylorel®	PO	Initial: 10 mg/day; most patients require 20–75 mg/day
guanethidine (gwah-NEH-thih-deen)	Ismelin®	PO	Initial: 10 mg/day; average 25–50 mg/day
prazosin hydrochloride (PRAH-zoh-sin hy-droh-KLOR-ryd)	Minipress®	PO	First dose limited to 1 mg hs; then 1 mg bid–tid; may increase to 20 mg/day
reserpine (REH-ser-peen)	Serpalan®	PO	0.1–0.25 mg/day
terazosin (teh-RAH-zoh-sihn)	Hytrin®	PO	Initial: 1 mg hs, then 1–5 mg/day

necessary to treat severe hypertension that is unresponsive to all other medications, because agents in this class are poorly tolerated by most patients. Guanethidine is one of the most potent antihypertensive drugs currently in clinical use. It acts in peripheral neurons, where it first produces a sympathetic blockade. Guanadrel is chemically and pharmacologically similar to guanethidine.

Indications

Beta-blockers are used for the initial treatment of hypertension. These medications can be used for angina, acute myocardial infarction, and hypertension. Propranolol was the first beta-blocking agent shown to block both beta$_1$ and beta$_2$ receptors. It is available as both a fast-acting product and a long-acting product. Nadolol was the first beta-blocker that allowed once-daily dosing. It also blocks both beta$_1$ and beta$_2$ receptors. Timolol was the first beta-blocker shown to be effective after an acute myocardial infarction to prevent sudden death.

Alpha-/beta-blockers are drugs available for hypertensive patients who have not responded to initial antihypertensive therapy. These agents are similar to beta-blockers.

Centrally acting antiadrenergic drugs have been used in the past as alternatives to initial antihypertensives, but their use in mild to moderate hypertension has decreased primarily because of the availability of other drugs.

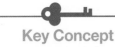

Key Concept

The control of malignant hypertension is usually achieved using direct-acting peripheral vasodilators, in particular, sodium nitroprusside.

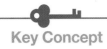

Key Concept

Postural hypotension is a common adverse effect of antihypertensive drugs. Abrupt withdrawal of treatment may lead to rebound hypertension.

Clonidine is effective in patients with renal impairment, although a reduced dose or a longer dosing interval may be required. Clonidine is also available as a transdermal patch (Catapres-TTS®), which releases the drug slowly over seven days. Guanabenz and guanfacine are recommended as adjunctive therapy with other antihypertensives for additive effects when initial therapy has failed.

Adverse Effects

Beta-blockers are not totally safe in patients with bronchospastic diseases such as asthma and chronic obstructive pulmonary disease (COPD). Suddenly stopping beta-blocker therapy puts the patient at risk for a withdrawal syndrome.

The adverse effects of alpha-/beta-blockers include postural hypotension, nausea, dizziness, headache, and bronchospasm.

The use of methyldopa is limited because it may produce sedation and must be administered two to four times daily. Other less common adverse effects include hemolytic anemia, hypotension and drowsiness, nausea, vomiting, sore tongue, sexual dysfunction, nasal congestion, and hepatic dysfunction. Sedation and dry mouth are common with use of clonidine but usually disappear with continued therapy. Clonidine has a tendency to cause or worsen depression. Its action is apparent within 30 to 60 minutes after administration of an oral dose. Adverse effects of guanabenz and guanfacine include sedation, dry mouth, dizziness, and reduced heart rate.

Reserpine is derived from the *Rauwolfia serpentina* plant. Because of the high incidence of adverse effects, other drugs are usually chosen first. When used, reserpine is given in low doses and in conjunction with other antihypertensive agents. Common adverse effects include drowsiness, dizziness, weakness, lethargy, memory impairment, sleep disturbances, and weight gain. Postural and exercise hypotension, fluid retention, and sexual dysfunction are common side effects when using guanethidine. Guanadrel should be avoided in patients with congestive heart failure, angina, and stroke. Adverse effects include fainting, orthostatic hypotension, and diarrhea.

Contraindications and Precautions

Beta-blockers are contraindicated in patients with a known hypersensitivity to the individual agents. Use of beta-blockers should be avoided in patients with uncompensated heart failure, cardiogenic shock, hypotension, and pulmonary edema. Safety of these drugs during pregnancy (category B) or lactation is not established.

Alpha-/beta-blockers are contraindicated in bronchial asthma, uncontrolled cardiac failure, cardiogenic shock, and severe bradycardia. Safe use during pregnancy (category C), lactation, or in children is not established. Centrally acting blockers (e.g., clonidine patch) are contraindicated in patients with collagen diseases (such as systemic lupus erythematosus) and during pregnancy (category C).

Beta-blockers should be used with caution in patients with hepatic or renal impairment, diabetes mellitus, and bronchospastic disease (asthma, emphysema), and in patients undergoing major surgery involving general anesthesia. Abrupt withdrawal of beta-blockers should be avoided, since sudden withdrawal may result in rebound hypertension, angina, and heart attack. This drug dose should be tapered over several weeks.

Drug Interactions

Patients taking guanethidine should avoid over-the-counter preparations that contain adrenergic substances such as cold medicines, because the combination may potentiate an acute hypertensive effect.

Peripheral Vasodilators

Vasodilators are used to relax or dilate vessels throughout the body. Some work on either veins or arteries; others work on both. Vasodilators are prescribed as second-line agents to initial therapy in patients taking diuretics, beta-blockers, ACE inhibitors, calcium channel blockers, alpha-adrenergic blockers, or alpha-/beta-adrenergic blockers.

Mechanism of Action

Vasodilators block the movement of calcium into the smooth muscle of the blood vessels to cause relaxation of the smooth muscle and dilation of the resistance vessels.

Indications

Vasodilator agents are reducers of hypertension. A peripheral vasodilator is frequently used in the treatment of moderate to severe hypertension.

Hydralazine and minoxidil may be used in the treatment of moderate essential or early malignant hypertension and hypertensive emergencies, virtually always in conjunction with other antihypertensive drugs. However, mainly because of side effects, they are generally not used until other, safer therapy has failed. Because they increase renal blood flow, they are often used to treat toxemia of pregnancy. They are sometimes used in acute congestive heart failure or after myocardial infarction. These drugs are shown in Table 13-5.

Adverse Effects

Toxic effects of hydralazine are syndromes resembling rheumatoid arthritis or lupus erythematosus, the appearance of which necessitates the withdrawal

TABLE 13-5	Vasodilators		
Generic Name	Trade Name	Route of Administration	Average Adult Dosage
diazoxide **(dy-ah-ZOK-syd)**	Hyperstat®, Proglycem®	IV	1–3 mg/kg up to 150 mg, repeat at 5–15 min intervals prn
fenoldopam mesylate **(feh-NOHL-doh-pam MEH-sih-layt)**	Corlopam®	IV	0.025–0.3 mcg/kg/min by continuous infusion for up to 48 h
hydralazine hydrochloride **(hy-DRAH-lah-zeen hy-droh-KLOR-ryd)**	Apresoline®	PO, IM, IV	PO: 10–50 mg qid; IM: 10–50 mg q4–6h; IV: 10–20 mg q4–6h, may increase to 40 mg
minoxidil **(mih-NOK-sih-dihl)**	Rogaine®	PO	5 mg/day, increased q3–5 days up to 40 mg/day in single or divided doses prn (max: 100 mg/day)
nitroprusside sodium **(ny-troh-PRUS-syd SOH-dee-um)**	Nitropress®	IV	0.3–0.5 mcg/kg/min (max: 10 mcg/kg/min)
prazosin hydrochloride **(PRAH-zoh-sihn hy-droh-KLOR-ryd)**	Minipress®	PO	1 mg bid–tid up to 20 mg/day

Medical Terminology Review

hyponatremia
hypo- = below; beneath; under
natr = sodium
-emia = blood condition
low sodium levels in the blood

Key Concept

Nitroprusside sodium, diazoxide, and fenoldopam can be administered only parenterally. Minoxidil and hydralazine are used orally for long-term outpatient therapy. Hydralazine can also be administered IM or IV.

of the drug. Common adverse effects of vasodilator drugs include headache, dizziness, tachycardia, palpitations, anxiety, nausea, vomiting, disorientation, depression, edema, impotence, and allergic reactions.

Contraindications and Precautions

Vasodilators are contraindicated in patients with coronary artery disease, mitral valvular rheumatic heart disease, atriovenous shunt, and myocardial infarction. Safe use of vasodilators during pregnancy (category C) or lactation is not established.

Vasodilators are used cautiously in patients with stroke, hepatic insufficiency, advanced renal impairment, hyponatremia, and in the elderly.

Drug Interactions

Hydralazine should be used with caution in patients receiving monoamine oxidase inhibitors (MAOIs). Profound hypotensive episodes may occur when hydralazine is used along with diazoxide injections.

Diuretics

Diuretics increase sodium excretion and lower blood volume. Diuretics are divided into five categories according to their action: thiazide diuretics, loop diuretics, potassium-sparing diuretics, osmotic diuretics, and carbonic anhydrase inhibitors. The type of diuretic used is determined by the condition being treated. For example, carbonic anhydrase inhibitors, such as acetazolamide (Diamox®) are used to lower intraocular pressure. The most common diuretics are discussed in Chapter 14.

HYPERLIPIDEMIA

Lipids or fats, which are usually transported in various combinations with proteins (lipoproteins), play a key role in cardiovascular disorders. Lipids, including cholesterol and triglycerides, are essential elements in the body. They are synthesized in the liver; therefore, they can never be eliminated from the body. Excessive lipid content in the blood is called hyperlipidemia.

Dietary or drug therapy of elevated plasma cholesterol levels can reduce the risk of atherosclerosis, and subsequent cardiovascular disease. A patient with high serum cholesterol and increased low-density lipoprotein (LDL) is at risk of atherosclerotic coronary disease and myocardial infarction. Atherosclerosis is a disorder in which lipid subgroups (total cholesterol, triglycerides, LDL, and high-density lipoproteins [HDL]) in various proportions indicate risk factors for the individual. Comparison of HDL ("good cholesterol") and LDL ("bad cholesterol") is shown in Figure 13-3. Table 13-6 shows an analysis of cholesterol and triglycerides.

Analysis of serum lipids includes assessment of all the deposits that accumulate on the lining of the blood vessels, resulting in degenerative changes

Medical Terminology
Review

atherosclerosis
athero- = deposit
sclero = hard or hardened
-sis = state or condition
a condition of hardened deposits in the arteries

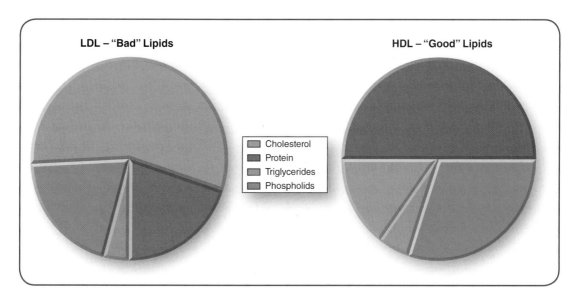

Figure 13-3 Comparison of HDL to LDL.

TABLE 13-6	Normal Values of Cholesterol and Triglyceride Levels
Cholesterol Level	**Cholesterol Category**
Less than 200 mg/dL	Desirable
200–239 mg/dL	Borderline
240 mg/dL or higher	High
HDL Cholesterol Level	**HDL Cholesterol Category**
Less than 40 mg/dL (for men) and less than 50 mg/dL (for women)	Low HDL cholesterol. A major risk factor for heart disease.
60 mg/dL or higher	High HDL cholesterol. An HDL of 60 mg/dL and above is considered protective against heart disease.
LDL Cholesterol Level	**LDL Cholesterol Category**
Less than 100 mg/dL	Optimal
100–129 mg/dL	Above optimal
130–159 mg/dL	Borderline high
160–189 mg/dL	High
190 mg/dL or higher	Very high
Triglyceride Level	**Triglyceride Category**
Less than 150 mg/dL	Normal
150–199 mg/dL	Borderline high
200–499 mg/dL	High
500 mg/dL or higher	Very high

and obstruction of blood flow (Figure 13-4). Obstructions may be partial or complete, and emboli are common. Factors such as genetic conditions, high-cholesterol diet, elevated serum LDL levels, and elevated blood pressure predispose patients to development of this condition.

Diseases of plasma lipids can be manifested as an elevation in triglycerides, or as an elevation in cholesterol. Elevated triglycerides can produce life-threatening pancreatitis.

ANTIHYPERLIPIDEMIC DRUGS

Medications are not the first line of treatment for hyperlipidemia. Antihyperlipidemic drugs are used only if diet modification and exercise programs fail to lower LDL to normal levels. When medications are started, diet therapy must continue. Antihyperlipidemics are the group of drugs prescribed in adjuvant therapy to reduce elevated cholesterol levels in patients with high cholesterol and LDL levels in the blood. These medications are used to

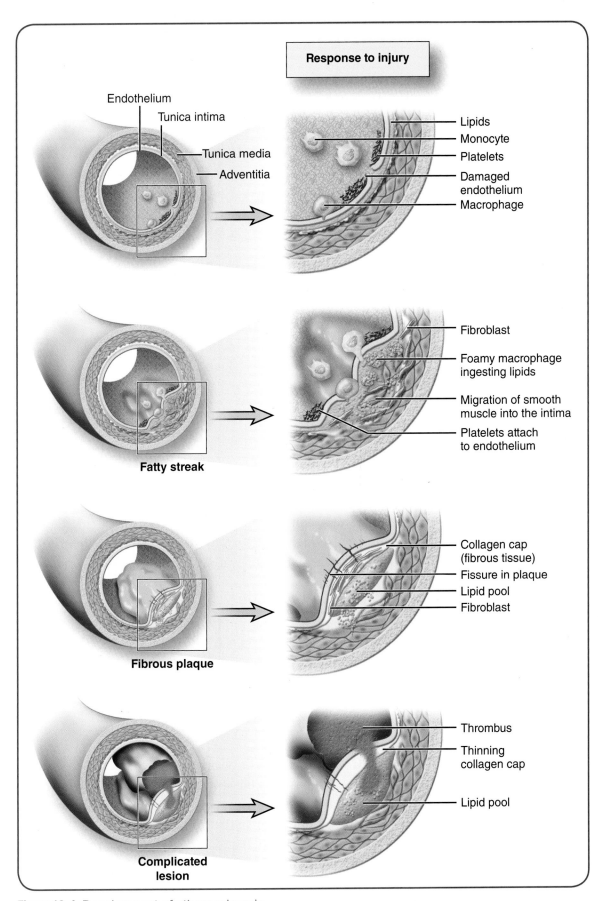

Figure 13-4 Development of atherosclerosis.

decrease the risk of arteriosclerosis. The major drugs for reduction of LDL cholesterol levels are bile acid sequestrants and nicotinic acid. The fibric acid derivatives and clofibrate (Atromid-S®) are less effective in reducing LDL cholesterol. The most effective agents for reducing plasma LDL levels are the statins. Table 13-7 lists the drugs commonly used to lower lipid levels.

HMG-CoA Reductase Inhibitors (Statins)

Statins have become the mainstay of LDL-reducing therapy, and they are the most effective agents for reducing plasma LDL levels. The statins include atorvastatin, fluvastatin, lovastatin, pravastatin, and simvastatin. These statins are extremely effective and well tolerated.

Mechanism of Action

Statins inhibit HMG co-enzyme A, the enzyme that catalyzes the first step in the cholesterol synthesis pathway, resulting in a decrease in serum cholesterol and serum LDLs.

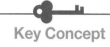

Key Concept

HMG-CoA reductase inhibitors are usually well-tolerated. A rare but serious adverse effect is rhabdomyolysis (destruction of skeletal muscle).

Indications

The statin drugs are used as adjuncts to diet in treatment of elevated total cholesterol, serum triglycerides, and LDL cholesterol in patients with primary hypercholesterolemia.

Adverse Effects

HMG-CoA reductase inhibitors may cause headache, flatulence, abdominal pain, cramps, constipation, nausea, and heartburn. They have an impressively low frequency of serious adverse effects. The most important side effects are transaminase elevation and acute myositis.

Contraindications and Precautions

HMG-CoA reductase inhibitors are contraindicated in patients with hypersensitivity to these agents, serious liver disorders, and during pregnancy (category X) and lactation. HMG-CoA reductase inhibitors should be used with caution in patients with acute infection, visual disturbances, hypotension, endocrine disorders, and a history of alcoholism.

Drug Interactions

HMG-CoA reductase inhibitors may have decreased effects if taken with rifamycin. There is possible severe myopathy (disorders of the striated muscles) or **rhabdomyolysis** if taken with cyclosporine, erythromycin, gemfibrozil, niacin, and other statins. When the HMG-CoA reductase inhibitors are given with oral anticoagulants, the effect of the anticoagulants will be increased. These drugs have a Black Box Warning since they can interact with grapefruit and grapefruit juice, leading to potentially dangerous and increased drug effects.

TABLE 13-7   Lipid-Lowering Drugs

Generic Name	Trade Name	Route of Administration	Average Adult Dosage
HMG-CoA Reductase Inhibitors (Statins)			
atorvastatin calcium **(ah-TOR-vah-stah-tihn KAL-see-um)**	Lipitor®	PO	10–20 mg hs; may increase to 80 mg/day in 1–2 divided doses
fluvastatin sodium **(FLOO-vah-stah-tihn SOH-dee-um)**	Lescol®, Lescol XL®	PO	20–40 mg once or twice daily
lovastatin **(loh-vah-STAH-tihn)**	Mevacor®, Altoprev®	PO	20–40 mg once or twice daily
pravastatin sodium **(prah-vah-STAH-tihn SOH-dee-um)**	Pravachol®	PO	10–80 mg/day
rosuvastatin calcium **(roh-SOO-vah-stah-tihn KAL-see-um)**	Crestor®	PO	5–40 mg/day
simvastatin **(SIM-vah-stah-tihn)**	Zocor®	PO	10–80 mg/day
Bile Acid Sequestrant (binding) Agents			
cholestyramine resin **(koh-leh-STEER-ah-meen REH-zin)**	Questran®, LoCHOLEST®, Prevalite®	PO	4–24 g bid–qid
colesevelam hydrochloride **(koh-leh-SEH-veh-lam hy-droh-KLOR-ryd)**	Welchol®	PO	3 tablets bid with meals or 6 tablets qd
colestipol hydrochloride **(koh-LES-tih-pahl hy-droh-KLOR-ryd)**	Colestid®	PO	15–30 g bid
Fibric Acid Derivatives			
clofibrate **(kloh-FY-brayt)**	Atromid-S®	PO	2 g/day in divided doses
dextrothyroxine sodium **(deks-troh-thy-ROK-seen SOH-dee-um)**	Choloxin®	PO	4–8 mg/day
fenofibrate **(feh-noh-FY-brayt)**	Tricor®	PO	54–160 mg/day
gemfibrozil **(jem-FY-broh-zihl)**	Lopid®	PO	600 mg bid
Miscellaneous Preparations			
niacin (nicotinic acid) **(NY-ah-sin) (nih-koh-TEE-nik AH-sid)**	Niaspan®	PO	1–3 g in divided doses; or extended release: 500–2000 mg/day

BILE ACID SEQUESTRANTS

Bile acid sequestrants are a group of drugs that chemically combine with bile acids in the intestine, causing these bile acids to be eliminated from the body. Bile acid sequestrants are prescribed to lower blood cholesterol and other blood lipid levels. Cholestyramine (Questran®) and colestipol (Colestid®) are examples of bile acid sequestrants.

Mechanism of Action

Bile acid sequestrant drugs bind to bile acids to form an insoluble substance that cannot be absorbed by the intestine. Therefore, it is excreted in the feces. This action increases loss of bile acids, and the liver uses cholesterol to manufacture more bile. This leads to lowered serum cholesterol levels.

Indications

Bile acid sequestrants are used as adjuncts to diet therapy in management of patients with primary hypercholesterolemia with a significant risk of atherosclerotic heart disease and myocardial infarction. These agents may also be prescribed to relieve pruritus associated with partial biliary obstruction.

Adverse Effects

Constipation is a common problem associated with bile acid sequestrants. Other adverse effects are fecal impaction, hemorrhoids, nausea, and abdominal pain. Additional adverse effects include weight loss or gain; vitamin A, D, and K deficiencies (from poor absorption); and bleeding tendencies caused by depletion of vitamin K.

Contraindications and Precautions

Bile acid sequestrants are contraindicated in patients with a known hypersensitivity to the medications. Bile acid sequestrants are avoided in those with complete biliary obstruction, pregnancy (category C), and lactation. Safe use of these drugs in children younger than 16 years is not established.

Bile acid sequestrants should be used cautiously in patients with bleeding disorders, hemorrhoids, peptic ulcer, and malabsorption states (e.g., **steatorrhea**). These agents are used with caution in patients with liver or kidney impairment, and during pregnancy or lactation.

Drug Interactions

Bile acid sequestrants decrease the absorption of oral anticoagulants, digoxin, tetracyclines, penicillins, and phenobarbital. Therefore, bile acid sequestrants should be given alone and other drugs administered at least one hour before or four hours later.

FIBRIC ACID DERIVATIVES

These agents reduce hepatic synthesis of cholesterol and result in a reduction in the plasma concentration of very-low-density lipoprotein (VLDL) and triglycerides. Because more successful medications are on the market, clofibrate is no longer the hypolipidemic drug of choice, although it is still used for patients who may not respond to other medications.

Mechanism of Action

Fibric acid derivatives stimulate the liver to increase breakdown of VLDL to LDL, and decrease liver synthesis of VLDL by inhibiting cholesterol formation.

Indications

Primary indication of clofibrate is for hyperlipidemia that does not respond to diet. Clofibrate is also prescribed for patients with very high serum triglycerides with abdominal pain and pancreatitis that does not respond to diet.

Adverse Effects

Adverse effects of fibric acid derivatives include angina, arrhythmias, swelling, phlebitis, and pulmonary emboli. These agents also cause nausea, vomiting, diarrhea, flatulence, gastritis, and gallstones (with long-term therapy). Clofibrate may produce impotence, dysuria, hematuria, leukopenia, and anemia.

Contraindications and Precautions

Fibric acid derivatives are contraindicated in patients with hypersensitivity to these agents, impaired renal or hepatic function, primary biliary cirrhosis, pregnancy (category C), and lactation. Safe use of fibric acid derivatives in children younger than 14 years is not established.

Fibric acid derivatives are used cautiously in patients with a history of jaundice or hepatic disease, gallstones, peptic ulcer, hypothyroidism, and cardiovascular disease.

Drug Interactions

Fibric acid derivatives may increase anticoagulant effects by lowering plasma protein binding. They increase the effect of antidiabetic agents, and exaggerate diuretic response to furosemide. Clofibrate increases the effects of insulin. With probenecid, the therapeutic and toxic effects of clofibrate are increased. With ursodiol, there is increased risk of gallstone formation.

Niacin

Niacin (vitamin B_3, nicotinic acid) can exert cholesterol- and triglyceride-lowering effects at high concentrations, resulting in a decrease of LDL and VLDL levels, and an increase in HDL levels, but its use is limited by its side effects.

Mechanism of Action

Nicotinic acid may partially inhibit the release of free fatty acids from adipose tissue and increase lipoprotein activity, which could increase the rate of triglyceride removal from plasma. These actions reduce the total LDL and triglycerides, resulting in increased HDL.

Indications

Niacin may be prescribed as an adjunct to diet for treatment of adults with very high serum triglyceride levels who present a risk of pancreatitis, and who do not respond adequately to dietary control.

Adverse Effects

Nicotinic acid may cause headache, anxiety, hypotension, flushing or burning feelings in the skin, dry skin, peptic ulcer, or abnormal liver function tests. Other adverse effects of this agent include hyperuricemia, glucose intolerance, nausea, vomiting, diarrhea, hyperglycemia, and elevated plasma uric acid.

Contraindications and Precautions

Niacin is contraindicated in patients with hypersensitivity to this agent, hepatic impairment, severe hypotension, or arterial bleeding. Niacin also is contraindicated in patients with active peptic ulcer, pregnancy (category C), lactation, and in children younger than 16 years of age.

Niacin is used cautiously in individuals with a history of gallbladder disease, liver impairment, and peptic ulcer. This agent should be used with caution in glaucoma, angina, coronary artery disease, and diabetes mellitus.

Drug Interactions

Niacin can increase the effectiveness of antihypertensive or vasoactive drugs. It also increases the risk of bleeding with anticoagulants. Niacin *decreases absorption with bile acid sequestrants and separate doses must be at least four to six hours apart.*

Combination Drug Therapy

Certain combinations of medications can be useful in treating markedly elevated LDL cholesterol levels. Combination therapy can maximize the reduction in LDL levels. It can also allow for decreased dosages of individual LDL-reducing drugs, thus limiting side effects. For patients with elevations

> **Medical Terminology Review**
>
> **hyperuricemia**
> hyper- = over; above; beyond
> uric = relating to uric acid or urine
> -emia = blood condition
> excess blood in the urine

in both triglycerides and LDL, the addition of nicotinic acid or a fibric acid derivative to control triglyceride levels can allow the use of a bile acid sequestrant to help reduce LDL levels. The following are the most effective combinations for lowering LDL:

- A statin plus a bile acid sequestrant
- A statin plus nicotinic acid
- Nicotinic acid plus a bile acid sequestrant
- A statin plus a bile acid sequestrant plus nicotinic acid

The combination of a fibric acid derivative with a statin should usually be avoided because of an increased risk of myopathy.

SUMMARY

Antihypertensive drugs include diuretics (to lower blood volume), ACE inhibitors, beta-blockers, and vasodilators. In some cases, calcium channel blockers must be used, but care must be taken when patients are elderly. Medications are used only when lifestyle changes have not adequately lowered elevated blood pressure.

To reduce the circulating hyperlipidemia, medications may be required. Statins reduce the enzyme necessary for cholesterol production. Nicotinic acid reduces LDL and VLDL levels. The fibric acid derivatives decrease triglyceride and VLDL levels while raising HDL levels. These medications for hyperlipidemia are long-term therapy.

EXPLORING THE WEB

Visit **www.heart.org**

- Search for information on management of hypertension and hyperlipidemia.

Visit **www.womenheart.org**

- What are some of the challenges related to managing cardiovascular health for women that are different than for men?

Visit **www.cvphysiology.com**

- Click on "Hypertension" and review additional information to further your understanding of this condition.

Visit **www.hypertension-facts.org**

- For additional resources and information on hypertension.

Visit **www.medicinenet.com** or **www.nlm.nih.gov/ medlineplus**

- Search for the disorders or drugs discussed in this chapter. What additional information can you find?

REVIEW QUESTIONS

Multiple Choice

1. Which of the following antianginal drugs are also used as antihypertensives?

   A. nitrates

   B. vasoconstrictors

   C. diuretics

   D. beta-adrenergic blockers

2. Which of the following body organs is very important in maintaining sodium and water balance?

   A. brain

   B. kidney

   C. heart

   D. liver

3. Hydralazine (Apresoline®) is a(n):

   A. vasodilator

   B. vasoconstrictor

   C. anticoagulant

   D. antiarrhythmic

4. An example of a angiotensin-converting enzyme (ACE) inhibitor is:

   A. captopril (Capoten®)

   B. acebutolol (Sectral®)

   C. lidocaine (Xylocaine®)

   D. procainamide (Pronestyl®)

5. Hypertension with an unknown etiology is referred to as:

   A. secondary hypertension

   B. malignant hypertension

   C. familial hypertension

   D. primary hypertension

6. The trade names of clonidine include which of the following?

   A. Corgard®

   B. Catapres®

   C. Aldomet®

   D. Lopressor®

7. Which of the following agents have become the mainstay of LDL-reducing therapy?

   A. calcium channel blockers

   B. cardiac glycosides

   C. angiotensin II receptor antagonists

   D. HMG-CoA reductase inhibitors

8. Which of the following is the initial treatment of hypertension?

   A. beta-blockers

   B. antiarrhythmic drugs

   C. antihyperlipidemic drugs

   D. cardiac glycosides

9. Which of the following is the generic name of Kerlone®?

   A. carteolol

   B. betaxolol

   C. metoprolol

   D. atenolol

10. Which of the following may be caused as a result of ACE inhibitor therapy?

    A. hyperglycemia

    B. hypercalcemia

    C. hyperkalemia

    D. hypernatremia

11. Which of the following type of antihypertensive drugs may affect the renin-angiotensin system to increase urine output?

    A. vasodilators

    B. ACE inhibitors

    C. direct-acting vasodilators

    D. adrenergic blockers

12. The generic name of Minipress® is:

    A. prazosin

    B. guanethidine

    C. doxazosin

    D. reserpine

13. Which of the following is a common adverse effect of a bile acid sequestrant?

    A. double vision

    B. constipation

    C. insomnia

    D. hypotension

14. Which of the following is the first drug of choice to lower hyperlipidemia?

    A. statins

    B. fibric acids

    C. bile acids

    D. nicotinic acids

15. Which of the following is a potent vasoconstrictor?

    A. renin

    B. angiotensin I

    C. angiotensin II

    D. aldosterone

Matching

Generic Name	Trade Name

_____ 1. simvastatin

_____ 2. gemfibrozil

_____ 3. fenofibrate

_____ 4. pravastatin

_____ 5. cholestyramine

_____ 6. atorvastatin

_____ 7. colesevelam

A. Welchol®

B. Lipitor®

C. Pravachol®

D. Tricor®

E. Questran®

F. Lopid®

G. Zocor®

Critical Thinking

A 48-year-old woman who was diagnosed with essential hypertension five years ago has avoided taking her medication for the last four months because she claims that she feels fine without it. She has decreased her regular exercise due to taking care of her new home business, and has noticed occasional nosebleeds, blurred vision, dizziness, and overall tiredness. Her physician examines her and finds her blood pressure to be 185/115 mm Hg. He also hears crackling noises (rales) when he listens to her lungs, and notices that she has ruptures in the capillaries of the retinas in her eyes. He prescribes blood pressure medication, urinary tests to check her kidneys, rest and relaxation, and instructs her to see a nutritionist.

1. What is the pathophysiology of essential hypertension?

2. Since the patient has high diastolic pressure, what possible problems may be associated with her condition?

3. The physician suspects mild congestive heart failure. Explain how this can develop as a result of hypertension.

Diuretics

OBJECTIVES

After completing this chapter, the reader should be able to:

1. Explain the main function of the urinary system.
2. Identify different sections of the nephron.
3. Describe and compare the five types of diuretics.
4. Explain the mechanisms of drug action and important adverse effects of loop diuretics.
5. Explain the contraindications of thiazide diuretics.
6. Describe the use of osmotic diuretics.
7. Identify the major diuretic groups used in the treatment of different disorders or conditions.
8. Explain the mechanisms of action of the carbonic anhydrase inhibitors.
9. Describe the most important indications for the use of loop diuretics.
10. Explain potassium-sparing diuretics.

GLOSSARY

Anuria – inability to produce urine

Diuretics – drugs that increase the secretion of urine from the kidneys

Gynecomastia – enlargement of breast tissue in males

Hyperkalemia – high blood level of potassium

Hypokalemia – low blood level of potassium

Hyponatremia – low blood level of sodium

Hypotonic – having a lesser osmotic pressure than a reference solution

Impotence – inability to achieve or maintain penile erection

OVERVIEW

The kidneys are the major organs of the body involved with water balance. They have the ability to regulate their output according to the amount of fluid ingested, and the amounts lost from the body by other routes. In conditions such as hypertension, heart failure, liver disorders, or kidney disorders, fluid may accumulate in the body's tissues and diuretics should be used.

Diuretics are mainly used to remove the excess extracellular fluid from the body that can result in edema (abnormal fluid accumulation) of the tissues, and in hypertension. These conditions occur in diseases of the heart, liver, and kidneys. In order to understand the action of diuretics, it is important to have some knowledge of the basic processes that take place in the nephron.

ANATOMY REVIEW

- The structures of the urinary system include two kidneys, two ureters, a bladder, and a urethra (Figures 14-1 and 14-2).
- The urinary system functions to remove waste materials from the body tissues and fluids, to maintain the acid-base balance, and to discharge the waste products from the body.
- The kidneys are the most important of the excretory organs (Figure 14-3). Kidney failure can result in the buildup of toxic wastes in the body and may lead to death.
- The nephron is the basic structural and functional unit of the kidney.
- The renal corpuscle is a capillary network also the glomerulus, where the process of filtration occurs. In this process, blood pressure forces water and dissolved solutes out of the glomerular capillaries and into a chamber known as the capsular space (Figure 14-4).
- The formation of urine follows this path: blood enters the afferent arteriole → passes through the glomerulus → to Bowman's capsule → now it becomes filtrate (blood minus the red blood cells and plasma proteins) → continues through the proximal convoluted tubule → to the loop of Henle → to the distal convoluted tubule → to the collecting duct (at this time about 99% of the filtrate has been reabsorbed) → approximately 1 mL of urine is formed per minute → the 1 mL of urine goes to the renal pelvis → to the ureter → to the bladder → to the urethra → to the urinary meatus.

DIURETICS

Diuretics are a group of drugs that promote water loss from the body into the urine. As urine formation takes place in the kidneys, it is not surprising that diuretics have their principal action at the level of the nephron.

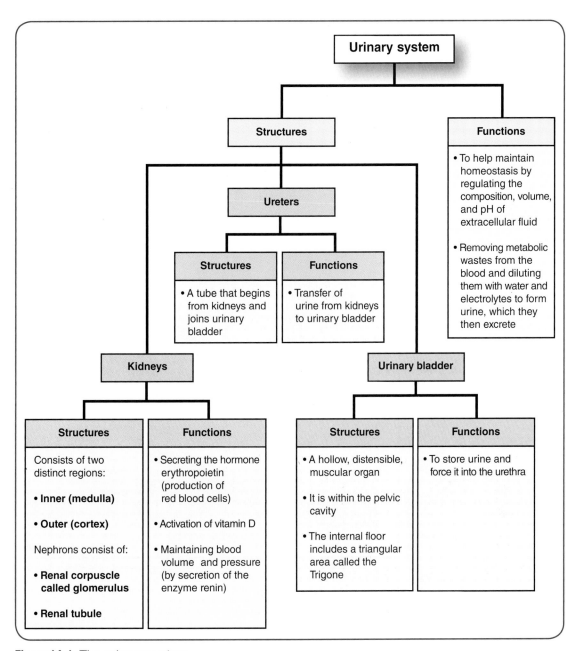

Figure 14-1 The urinary system.

However, the action of some diuretics is not confined to their action on the kidneys: they also act elsewhere in the body.

Diuretic drugs are an important part of heart failure management. In heart failure, diuretics are primarily used to clear fluid overload and to sustain normal blood volume. Diuretics are divided into five categories according to their action: loop, thiazide and thiazide-like, potassium-sparing, osmotic, and carbonic anhydrase inhibitors. The type of diuretic used is determined by the condition being treated. For example, carbonic anhydrase inhibitors, such as acetazolamide (Diamox®), which is recognized as a diuretic compound, are used to lower intraocular pressure.

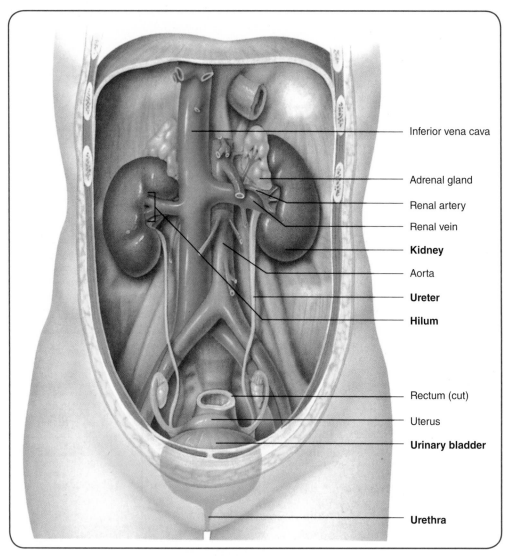

Figure 14-2 The structures of the urinary system.

Loop Diuretics

Good control of water balance is achieved by alterations in the permeability of the collecting duct system of the kidney to water by the presence of antidiuretic hormone from the posterior pituitary gland. This is one of the major control systems for water balance, and slight interference here will completely upset the normal function of the kidney and result in a variation in urine output. Loop diuretics are the most effective diuretics available (Table 14-1). They act similarly to thiazide diuretics, but their effects are more rapid and effective, resulting in a greater diuresis.

Mechanism of Action

Loop diuretics act on the medullary part of the ascending limb of the loop of the nephron (loop of Henle). These drugs inhibit the reabsorption of chloride and sodium ions from the loop into the interstitial fluid. The result

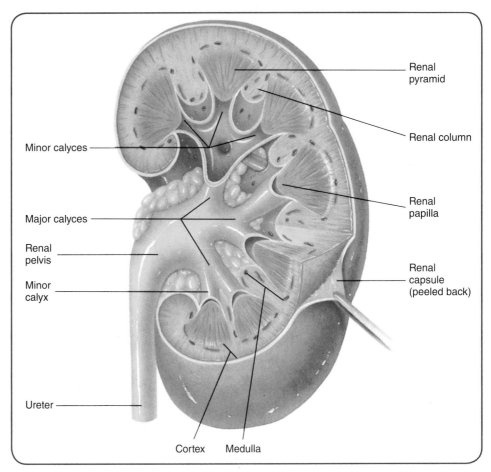

The labels on the figure read:

Renal pyramid

Renal column

Minor calyces

Renal papilla

Major calyces

Renal pelvis

Renal capsule (peeled back)

Minor calyx

Ureter

Cortex   Medulla

Figure 14-3 The structures of the kidney.

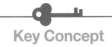

Key Concept

Loop diuretics are the most efficacious diuretic agents available and are rapidly absorbed.

is that the interstitial fluid becomes relatively **hypotonic** (having a lower osmotic pressure than a reference solution, such as water).

Indications

Loop diuretics are used in patients with edematous states associated with impaired renal function or liver disease, and can be given intravenously for immediate action. The most important indications for the use of loop diuretics include acute pulmonary edema, other edematous conditions, and acute hypercalcemia. These agents can also be used in patients with hypertension, but other types of diuretics are probably better choices in most of these patients. Loop diuretics are sometimes used in combination with other antihypertensives when thiazide diuretics are ineffective in the treatment of hypertension. In renal failure, they can also be effective in helping to normalize urine output. Loop diuretics, such as furosemide, are potent but relatively short-acting diuretics used in the management of severe chronic heart failure. They are also useful in the treatment of acute heart failure, and are commonly prescribed for the treatment of congestive heart failure, and ascites caused by malignancy or cirrhosis.

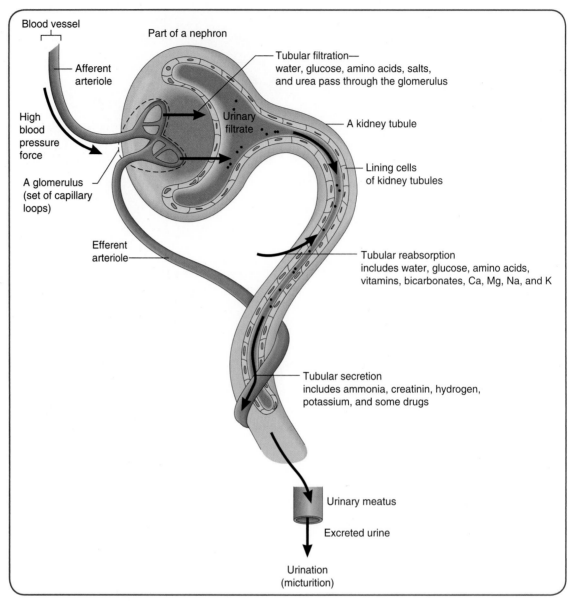

Figure 14-4 Processes and structures of the nephron.

TABLE 14-1	**Loop Diuretics**		
Generic Name	Trade Name	Route of Administration	Average Adult Dosage
bumetanide **(byoo-MEH-tah-nyd)**	Bumex®	PO	0.5–2 mg/day
ethacrynic acid **(eh-thah-KRY-nik AH-sid)**	Edecrin®	PO, IV	50–100 mg once or twice daily; adjust in 25–50 mg increments; Maint: 50–200 mg/day
furosemide **(fyoo-ROH-seh-myd)**	Lasix®	PO	20–80 bid (max: 600 mg/day)
torsemide **(TOR-seh-myd)**	Demadex®	PO, IV	10–20 mg once daily, up to 200 mg/day

Key Concept

Routine administration of loop diuretics, and probably all diuretics, should be done before late afternoon to avoid severe nocturnal enuresis (bedwetting).

Medical Terminology Review

hypokalemia
hypo- = low
-kalemia = blood levels of potassium
low levels of potassium in the blood

Adverse Effects

A major problem of loop diuretics is the loss of electrolytes from the body. Potassium and sodium are the main ions affected. Potassium loss often leads to **hypokalemia**, which can result in abnormal cardiac rhythms and even death. Other electrolyte changes can occur, especially with high doses of loop diuretics, and the periodic assessment of blood calcium and magnesium levels is required. Uric acid levels may rise during loop diuretic therapy, which can be problematic for people with gout. Additional adverse effects may include dehydration, hypotension, collapse, nausea, vomiting, anorexia, diarrhea, hyperglycemia, blurred vision, and hearing impairment.

Contraindications and Precautions

Loop diuretics are contraindicated in patients with known hypersensitivity to these drugs. Loop diuretics should be avoided in patients with **anuria** (inability to produce urine), hepatic coma, severe electrolyte deficiency, and during lactation or pregnancy (category C).

Loop diuretics should be used with caution in older adults, cardiac patients, and patients with hepatic cirrhosis, diabetes mellitus, history of gout, and pulmonary edema associated with acute myocardial infarction.

Drug Interactions

Loop diuretics may increase the effectiveness of anticoagulants or thrombolytics. Loop diuretics may increase the risk of glycoside toxicity and ototoxicity if taken with an aminoglycoside. Plasma levels of propranolol can increase when the drug is given with furosemide.

Thiazide and Thiazide-Like Diuretics

Thiazide diuretics are a group of drugs that are chemically similar and the most commonly prescribed class of diuretics. They are the most commonly used type of diuretic. All of the thiazide diuretics have equivalent effectiveness (Table 14-2).

Mechanism of Action

Key Concept

The optimum therapeutic effects of thiazide diuretics are seen in 15 to 30 minutes when given intravenously. When given orally, these drugs may take as long as four weeks to be effective.

Thiazide drugs act on the cortical segment of the ascending loop and the distal convoluted tubules of the nephron, and decrease sodium reabsorption. This results in a more concentrated fluid entering the collecting ducts, and therefore decreases water reabsorption and results in a diuresis. These agents increase excretion of water, sodium, chloride, and potassium. Thiazide diuretics have an effect on the peripheral arterioles, which results in vasodilation. This, combined with their diuretic effects, makes them particularly suitable in hypertensive patients (see Chapter 13). This action of these drugs is not completely understood.

TABLE 14-2	Thiazide and Thiazide-Like Diuretics		
Generic Name	Trade Name	Route of Administration	Average Adult Dosage
Thiazide Diuretics			
bendroflumethiazide (ben-droh-floo-meh-THY-ah-zyd)	Naturetin®	PO	2.5–20 mg, once or twice daily
chlorothiazide sodium (klor-oh-THY-ah-zyd SOH-dee-um)	Diuril®	PO	250 mg–1 g, in 1–2 divided doses
hydrochlorothiazide (hy-droh-klor-oh-THY-ah-zyd)	HydroDIURIL®, HCTZ®	PO	12.5–100 mg, 1–3 times/day
hydroflumethiazide (hy-droh-floo-meh-THY-ah-zyd)	Diucardin®, Saluron®	PO	25–100 mg, once or twice daily
methyclothiazide (meh-thih-kloh-THY-ah-zyd)	Aquatensin®, Enduron®	PO	2.5–10 mg/day
metolazone (meh-TOL-lah-zohn)	Mykrox®	PO	5–20 mg/day
polythiazide (pol-lee-THY-ah-zyd)	Renese®	PO	1–4 mg/day
trichlormethiazide (try-klor-meh-THY-ah-zyd)	Diurese®, Metahydrin®	PO	1–4 mg, once or twice daily
Thiazide-Like Diuretics			
chlorthalidone (klor-THAL-lih-dohn)	Thalitone®, Hygroton®	PO	12.5-25 mg/day (max: 100 mg/day)
indapamide (in-DAH-pah-myd)	Lozol®	PO	2.5 mg once daily; may increase to 5 mg/day

Indications

Thiazide diuretics are still considered to be in the front line for the treatment of mild to moderate hypertension either on their own or combined, usually with a beta-blocker. These drugs are also used to treat edema due to heart failure, liver disease, hypertension, and corticosteroid or estrogen therapy.

Adverse Effects

Adverse effects of thiazide diuretics, as with loop diuretics, include potassium and sodium loss. Thiazide diuretics may also cause hypokalemia, hypochloremia, and muscle weakness. Thiazides occasionally cause a rise in blood uric acid levels, which can be problematic in those predisposed to gout. These drugs can also cause hyperglycemia, which is potentially dangerous in diabetic patients. Lactation can be suppressed, and thiazide drugs have been used for this purpose. **Impotence** in men can also occur.

Other adverse effects of thiazide diuretics are dehydration, electrolyte imbalances, loss of appetite, dizziness, vertigo, postural hypotension, headache, fatigue, lethargy, hyperuricemia, increased sensitivity to sun exposure, and pruritus.

Contraindications and Precautions

Thiazide diuretics are contraindicated in patients with known hypersensitivity to these agents. These drugs are also contraindicated in patients with electrolyte imbalances, anuria, hepatic coma, and renal impairment. Thiazide diuretics should be given with caution during pregnancy (category C) and lactation, in children, and in those with liver or kidney impairment.

Drug Interactions

If thiazide diuretics are used with alcohol, nitrates, or other antihypertensive drugs, they may cause additive hypotensive effects. Anesthetic agents may increase the effects of thiazides. The effects of anticoagulants may be decreased when given with thiazide diuretics.

Potassium-Sparing Diuretics

There are two types of potassium-sparing diuretics: the aldosterone antagonists and those independent of aldosterone. The best-known aldosterone antagonist is spironolactone. These agents are not very powerful as diuretics (Table 14-3), but their most important feature is that they promote potassium retention.

Mechanism of Action

Potassium-sparing diuretics (such as spironolactone) inhibit the action of aldosterone on the distal convoluted tubule of the nephron. Spironolactone is effective only when aldosterone is present, but triamterene and amiloride

TABLE 14-3	Potassium-Sparing Diuretics		
Generic Name	Trade Name	Route of Administration	Average Adult Dosage
amiloride hydrochloride **(ah-MIL-lor-ryd hy-droh-KLOR-ryd)**	Midamor®	PO	5 mg/day; may increase to 20 mg/day in 1–2 divided doses
spironolactone **(spy-ron-oh-LAK-tohn)**	Aldactone®	PO	25–200 mg, once or twice daily
triamterene **(try-AM-teh-reen)**	Dyrenium®	PO	100 mg bid (max: 300 mg/day)

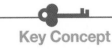

exert their effects independent of the presence or absence of aldosterone. Aldosterone is the sodium-retaining hormone secreted from the adrenal cortex. If it acts on the distal tubule, the body retains more sodium ions, and water is passively conserved at the same time. When sodium is retained by the nephron at this site, potassium is lost. Therefore, if aldosterone is blocked, potassium is retained and sodium is lost along with a slight increase in diuresis.

Indications

Potassium-sparing diuretics are not usually required for patients who are taking loop or thiazide diuretics. Spironolactone has proved to be of tremendous value in the treatment of congestive heart failure. Potassium-sparing diuretics are sometimes administered under conditions in which potassium depletion can be dangerous. They are used in the management of edema associated with congestive heart failure, hepatic cirrhosis with ascites, nephrotic syndrome, and idiopathic edema. Since their effects are less pronounced than other types of diuretics, they are used mainly in combination with other drugs in the management of hypertension, and to correct hypokalemia often caused by other diuretic agents. Spironolactone is also used in primary hyperaldosteronism.

Adverse Effects

Adverse effects that occur with this type of diuretic are related to their mode of action, and include **hyperkalemia** (which may lead to cardiac arrhythmias), dehydration, weakness, fatigue, lethargy, weight loss, nausea, vomiting, diarrhea, hypotension, acute renal failure, kidney stones, and **hyponatremia**. In men, spironolactone can produce **gynecomastia** due to its estrogenic effect, as well as carcinoma of the breast.

Contraindications and Precautions

Potassium-sparing diuretics are contraindicated in patients with hypersensitivity to these drugs, anuria, acute renal insufficiency, and hyperkalemia, and during pregnancy (category D) or lactation. These drugs should be used cautiously in patients with impaired kidney or liver function, history of gouty arthritis, diabetes mellitus, or a history of kidney stones.

Drug Interactions

Alcohol, nitrate, and other antihypertensive agents may have increased hypotensive effects when a potassium-sparing diuretic is given. Potassium-sparing diuretics may cause severe hyperkalemia when potassium preparations are also given.

Osmotic Diuretics

Osmotic diuretic drugs are capable of being filtered by the glomerulus, but have a limited capability of being reabsorbed into the bloodstream (Table 14-4).

TABLE 14-4	Osmotic Diuretics		
Generic Name	Trade Name	Route of Administration	Average Adult Dosage
glycerin (GLIH-ser-rihn)	Glycerol®, Osmoglyn®	PO	1–1.8 g/kg given 1–1.5 h before ocular surgery
mannitol (MAN-nih-tahl)	Osmitrol®	IV	100 g as a 10%–20% solution over 2–6 h
urea (yoo-REE-ah)	Ureaphil®	IV	1–1.5 g/kg of 30% solution infused slowly over 1–2.5 h

Mechanism of Action

Osmotic diuretics work by directly interfering with osmosis. They elevate plasma osmolality, causing water to flow from tissues such as the brain and eyes, and also from the cerebrospinal fluid (CSF), into the extracellular fluid. This decreases the intracranial and intraocular pressure. Mannitol is an osmotic diuretic that increases the osmolarity of the glomerular filtrate, which decreases water reabsorption. This leads to increased excretion of water, sodium, chloride, and toxic substances.

Indications

Osmotic diuretics can be used to reduce increased intracranial pressure and to promote prompt removal of renal toxins. These agents can be used to maintain urine volume and to prevent anuria. Mannitol, an osmotic diuretic, has been shown to increase renal plasma flow and glomerular hydrostatic pressure. Mannitol and urea are most commonly used to reduce intracranial or intraocular pressure. Mannitol has also been used to prevent and treat acute renal failure or during certain cardiovascular surgical procedures. It is also used alone or with other diuretics to promote excretion of toxins in cases of drug poisoning.

Adverse Effects

Adverse effects of osmotic diuretics are related to the amount of solute administered. They include fluid and electrolyte imbalance and the potential for dehydration. This potential for dehydration is similar to that which would occur from the drinking of seawater. Additional adverse effects may include headache, mental confusion, nausea, vomiting, tachycardia, hypertension, hypotension, allergic reactions, and severe pulmonary edema.

Contraindications and Precautions

Osmotic diuretics are contraindicated in patients with known hypersensitivity to these drugs. They should be avoided in patients with severe dehydration, anuria, and electrolyte imbalances. Mannitol is contraindicated in patients with intracranial bleeding.

Osmotic diuretics should be used with caution in patients with electrolyte imbalances or renal impairment. These drugs must be given cautiously to pregnant women (category C) and during lactation.

Drug Interactions

Osmotic diuretics increase urinary excretion of lithium, salicylates, barbiturates, potassium, and imipramine.

Carbonic Anhydrase Inhibitors

When patients are taking carbonic anhydrase inhibitors, it is important that their fluid input, fluid output, glucose levels, and electrolyte levels be monitored. See Table 14-5 for these agents.

Mechanism of Action

Carbonic anhydrase is an enzyme that speeds up the conversion of carbon dioxide into bicarbonate ions and vice versa, according to the following equation:

$$CO_2 + H_2O \leftrightarrow H_2CO_3 \leftrightarrow H^+ + HCO_3^-$$

This reaction occurs in the kidney as well as in other parts of the body. In the kidney, the reaction occurs mainly in the proximal tubule and, as it involves bicarbonate loss, is concerned with acid-base balance. The tubular cells are not very permeable to bicarbonate ions or carbonic acid, but are

TABLE 14-5	Carbonic Anhydrase Inhibitors		
Generic Name	Trade Name	Route of Administration	Average Adult Dosage
acetazolamide **(ah-see-tah-ZOH-lah-myd)**	Diamox®	PO, IM, IV	For glaucoma: PO: 250 mg 1–4 times/day, 500 mg sustained release bid; IM/IV: 500 mg, may repeat in 2–4 h; for edema: PO: 250–375 mg every AM (5 mg/kg)
dichlorphenamide **(dy-klor-FEN-ah-myd)**	Daranide®, Oratrol®	PO	100–200 mg, 1–2 times/day
methazolamide **(meh-thah-ZOH-lah-myd)**	Neptazane®	PO	50–100 mg bid–tid

very permeable to carbon dioxide. Under normal circumstances, carbonic anhydrase in the tubular cell converts the carbonic acid into carbon dioxide and water, which are promptly reabsorbed. If the enzyme is inhibited, there will be a net loss of bicarbonate from the body with a consequent loss of water. The drug acetazolamide is a noncompetitive inhibitor of this enzyme and has been used as a diuretic.

Indications

The carbonic anhydrase inhibitors are used in the treatment of open-angle glaucoma, secondary glaucoma, and preoperative treatment of acute closed-angle glaucoma. These agents are also prescribed in the treatment of edema resulting from congestive heart failure, and drug-induced edema. Another use of carbonic anhydrase inhibitors is the treatment of altitude sickness.

Adverse Effects

Carbonic anhydrase inhibitors may cause acidosis (a clinical state where the pH of the blood drops significantly, below 7.35), renal stones, hypokalemia, drowsiness (following large doses), and hypersensitivity reactions.

Contraindications and Precautions

Carbonic anhydrase inhibitors are contraindicated in patients with known hypersensitivity, anuria, severe renal or liver impairment, and imbalance of electrolytes.

Carbonic anhydrase inhibitors should be used cautiously in patients with kidney impairment, and during lactation and pregnancy (category C).

These drugs need to be given with caution in patients with respiratory acidosis, emphysema, or chronic respiratory disease as diuresis can be diminished in the presence of acidotic conditions.

Drug Interactions

Carbonic anhydrase inhibitors interact with renal excretion of amphetamines, ephedrine, quinidine, and procainamide. Carbonic anhydrase inhibitors may decrease the effects of tricyclic antidepressants, thereby enhancing or prolonging their effects. These diuretics also decrease the renal excretion of lithium.

SUMMARY

Diuretics have their principal action at the level of the kidneys' nephrons. These drugs are mainly used to remove the excess extracellular fluid from the body that can result in edema of the tissues and in hypertension. The urinary system has three major functions: excretion, elimination, and homeostatic regulation of the volume of blood plasma.

Diuretic drugs are an important part of heart failure, hypertension, and edema management. These agents are divided into five categories according to their action: loops, thiazide and thiazide-like, potassium-sparing, osmotic, and carbonic anhydrase inhibitors.

Loop diuretics are major controllers for water balance and result in a variation in urine output. Thiazide and thiazide-like diuretics are the most commonly prescribed types of diuretics. The best-known potassium-sparing diuretic is spironolactone, which is an aldosterone antagonist. Osmotic diuretics work by directly interfering with osmosis, which causes the kidneys to keep water in the renal tubules, resulting in water loss. Carbonic anhydrase is an enzyme that speeds up the conversion of carbon dioxide into bicarbonate ions and vice versa. If the enzyme is inhibited, there will be a net loss of bicarbonate from the body with a consequent loss of water.

EXPLORING THE WEB

Visit **http://nephron.com**

- Explore articles related to the types of diuretics discussed in this chapter.

Visit **www.mayoclinic.com** and **www.medicinenet.com**

- Look for information related to diuretics.

REVIEW QUESTIONS

Multiple Choice

1. Thiazide diuretics are contraindicated in patients with all of the following conditions, *except:*

   A. impaired liver function

   B. edema caused by heart failure

   C. diabetes mellitus

   D. a history of gout

2. Which of the following substances may alter the permeability of the collecting duct of the nephron to water?

   A. antidiuretic hormone

   B. insulin

   C. vitamin C

   D. calcitonin

3. Which of the following is the major problem with the loop diuretics?

   A. decrease of uric acid

   B. hyperkalemia

   C. loss of glucose from the kidneys

   D. loss of electrolytes from the body

4. Thiazide drugs act on which of the following segments of the nephron?

   A. descending loop

   B. ascending loop

   C. proximal convoluted tubule

   D. collecting duct

5. Which of the following is an aldosterone antagonist?

   A. mannitol

   B. furosemide

   C. spironolactone

   D. acetazolamide

6. Which of the following is a trade name of acetazolamide?

   A. Osmitrol®

   B. Diamox®

   C. Ureaphil®

   D. Aldactone®

7. Diuretics are mainly used in which of the following?

   A. diabetes

   B. encephalitis

   C. hepatitis B

   D. hypertension

8. Which of the following diuretics are used in the treatment of open-angle glaucoma?

   A. carbonic anhydrase inhibitors

   B. potassium-sparing diuretics

   C. thiazide and thiazide-like diuretics

   D. loop diuretics

9. Which of the following time periods are required for optimum therapeutic effects of orally administered thiazides?

   A. 15 to 30 minutes

   B. 2 to 4 days

   C. 1 to 2 weeks

   D. 3 to 4 weeks

10. The most commonly used osmotic drug is:

    A. ethacrynic acid

    B. furosemide

    C. mannitol

    D. torsemide

11. Carbonic anhydrase inhibitors must be used with caution in pregnant women and are classified as:

    A. category D

    B. category C

    C. category B

    D. category A

12. Which of the following diuretics is most commonly used to decrease intracranial pressure?

    A. mannitol

    B. spironolactone

    C. amiloride

    D. trichlormethiazide

13. The generic name of Osmoglyn® is which of the following?

    A. isosorbide

    B. mannitol

    C. glycerin

    D. acetazolamide

14. The basic functional unit of the kidney is the:

    A. renal corpuscle

    B. glomerulus

    C. renal cortex

    D. nephron

15. A capillary network of renal corpuscles is called:

    A. Bowman's capsule

    B. Henle tubule

    C. proximal convoluted tubule

    D. glomerulus

Matching

Generic Name

_____ 1. acetazolamide

_____ 2. mannitol

_____ 3. indapamide

_____ 4. ethacrynic acid

_____ 5. chlorthalidone

_____ 6. furosemide

_____ 7. spironolactone

Trade Name

A. Lasix®

B. Aldactone®

C. Hygroton®

D. Edecrin®

E. Osmitrol®

F. Lozol®

G. Diamox®

Critical Thinking

A 25-year-old male patient is admitted to the intensive care unit following a car-train collision. The patient sustained a depressed skull fracture and is on a ventilator. Two days after surgery, there are obvious signs of increasing intracranial pressure. The nurse administers mannitol (Osmitrol®) intravenously over 30 minutes. The patient's wife asks his physician to explain why her husband needs this drug.

1. What explanation should the physician offer?

2. If the patient shows symptoms of intracranial bleeding, what would be the explanation that the physician should give for discontinuing the drug?

Anticoagulant Drugs

OBJECTIVES

After completing this chapter, the reader should be able to:

1. Explain the terms *hemostasis, aggregation,* and *thrombophlebitis.*
2. Describe the mechanism of action of heparin.
3. Discuss the uses and adverse effects of anticoagulant therapy.
4. Explain factors that usually predispose an individual to the development of a thrombus.
5. List three common coagulation disorders.
6. Describe the mechanism of action of thrombolytic drugs.
7. Explain the indications for use of antiplatelet drugs.
8. Identify oral anticoagulant agents and their indications.
9. Explain thrombocytopenia and thrombolytics.
10. Discuss the role of vitamin K in the process of clotting.

GLOSSARY

Aggregation – the clumping together of platelets to form a clot

Alopecia – loss of hair from anywhere on the body, sometimes until complete baldness is reached

Anticoagulants – agents used to prevent the formation of a blood clot

Antiplatelet agents – drugs that inhibit normal platelet function, usually by reducing their ability to aggregate and inappropriately form blood clots

Blood coagulation – the process of clotting

Embolism – obstruction of a blood vessel by a plug (embolus)

Fibrin – a protein formed from fibrinogen that forms a net-like structure that allows a blood clot to organize and anchor itself to a blood vessel wall

Fibrinogen – a blood clotting factor responsible for forming fibrin. Without fibrinogen and fibrin, blood would not be able to form the clots necessary to stop bleeding

Fibrinolysis – the enzymatic destruction of fibrin. Once a clot has stopped blood loss and injured blood vessels have healed, fibrin has no further purpose. Enzymes in the blood dissolve the remaining fibrin so normal blood flow can be restored through the injured area

Hemostasis – a process that stops bleeding in a blood vessel

Heparin – a potent anticoagulant naturally obtained from the liver and lungs of domestic animals; in humans, it is usually found in basophils or mast cells

Mast cells – large cells found in connective tissue that contain many biochemicals, including histamine; mast cells are involved in inflammation secondary to injuries and infections, and are sometimes implicated in allergic reactions

Phlebothrombosis – clotting in a vein without primary inflammation

Prothrombin – a glycoprotein formed and stored in the parenchymal cells of the liver and present in the blood; a deficiency of prothrombin leads to impaired blood coagulation

Thrombin – an enzyme formed from prothrombin and thromboplastin in plasma during the clotting process. Thrombin causes fibrinogen to change to fibrin

Thrombocytopenia – decrease in the number of platelets in circulating blood

Thrombogenic – substances causing blood clots

Thrombolytics – drugs designed to dissolve blood clots that have already formed within a blood vessel

Thrombophlebitis – venous inflammation with thrombus formation

Thromboplastin – a lipoprotein that functions in the extrinsic pathway of blood coagulation, activating factor X

Thrombosis – the formation of a clot

Thrombus – an aggregation of platelets, fibrin, clotting factors, and the cellular elements of the blood attached to the interior wall of a vein or artery, sometimes occluding the lumen of the vessel

Venous stasis – injury to the veins causing loss of proper function of the vein and impairing the ability of blood flow to return to the heart

von Willebrand's disease – the most common hereditary bleeding disorder, caused by a deficiency of von Willebrand factor in the blood; though there are several different types, this disease is signified by abnormal bleeding, easy bruising, and skin rash

OVERVIEW

The ability of blood to clot in response to injury is essential to protection of the body from unnecessary blood loss. Clotting disorders impair this ability of the body to protect itself. Excessive blood loss can lead to shock and ultimately death if left untreated. In this circumstance, drugs may be administered to aid the clotting process.

There are other instances in which clots may form and travel through the venous system, becoming lodged in a vessel and causing a blockage of blood flow. This can cause tissue damage and may also cause the death of the individual if the blockage occurs in the vessels of the lungs or the heart. Drugs that can dissolve or prevent clots from forming may be given to alleviate or prevent this type of event. Hemophilia is an inherited disorder in which the blood does not clot properly. It most commonly affects males and is signified by bleeding and bruising that may occur after even slight injuries. Hemophilia is treated by administering clotting factors or medications that temporarily increase clotting factors in the blood.

BLOOD COAGULATION

Blood coagulation (clotting) is of the utmost importance in protecting the body from undue blood loss. It is well known that people with blood clotting disorders, such as hemophilia, live at high risk; their lives can be terminated abruptly by a minor injury, such as slight bruising. In a healthy person, such injuries would often pass unnoticed.

On the other end of the spectrum, many individuals suffer from problems related to the formation of intravascular clots (thrombi). This can lead to blockage of the smaller blood vessels in the body and, consequently, tissue ischemia. A common cause of such clot formation is **venous stasis** (injury to the veins causing loss of proper function of the vein and impairing the ability of blood flow to return to the heart), due to inactivity such as occurs in prolonged bed rest.

A **thrombus** is related to a blood embolus, which is a fragment of a blood clot that occludes a vessel. The clot may have been formed due to procedures such as surgery. In this case, a fragment of a natural clot escapes into the

Key Concept

Not all emboli are blood clots. They can be derived from various materials, such as fat, amniotic fluid, and even air.

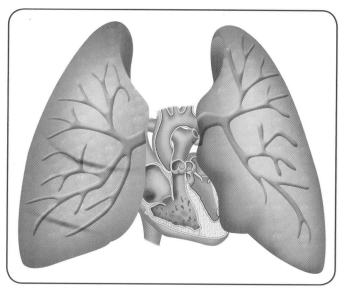

Figure 15-1 Pulmonary embolism.

Key Concept

The circulating clotting factors are produced primarily in the liver. Vitamin K, a fat-soluble vitamin, is required for the synthesis of most clotting factors. Calcium ions are essential for many steps in the clotting process.

circulation and blocks a major vessel. For example, blockage of one of the pulmonary arteries results in a pulmonary embolism (Figure 15-1).

Hemostasis is the spontaneous arrest of bleeding from a damaged blood vessel. The normal vascular endothelial cells and circulating blood platelets are not **thrombogenic** (causing blood clots) unless blood vessels or platelets are damaged by cuts or injury. Hemostasis or blood clotting occurs as a result of the following steps:

- The immediate response of a blood vessel to injury is vasoconstriction or vascular spasm due to the release of serotonin. In small blood vessels, this decreases blood flow and allows a platelet plug to form.

- Blood platelets release **thromboplastin** (a substance that causes clotting) at the site of the injury. Thromboplastin and calcium react with **prothrombin** (a plasma protein produced by the liver) to create **thrombin**.

- The thrombin then changes **fibrinogen** (a plasma protein) into **fibrin** (gel-like threads) which layers over the site of the injury like mesh. This fibrin sheath traps blood cells and plasma and forms a clot (Figure 15-2).

COAGULATION DISORDERS

Thrombophlebitis refers to the development of a thrombus in a vein where inflammation is present. The platelets adhere to the inflamed site, and a thrombus develops. In **phlebothrombosis**, a thrombus forms spontaneously in a vein without prior inflammation, although inflammation may develop

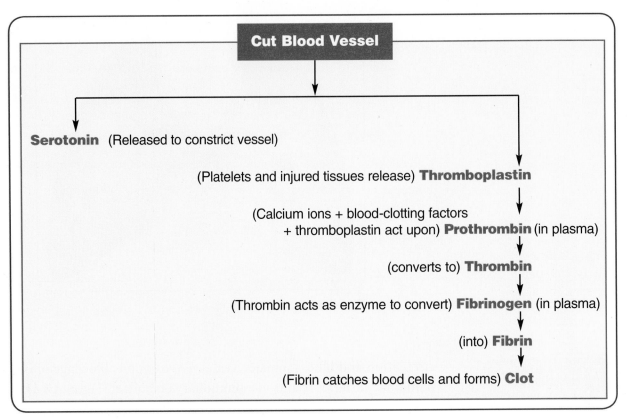

Figure 15-2 Blood clotting process.

secondarily in response to **thrombosis**. The clot is less firmly attached in this case, and its development is asymptomatic or silent. Several factors usually predispose an individual to the development of a thrombus:

- The first group of factors involves stasis of blood or sluggish blood flow, which is often present in people who are immobile.

- The second factor involves injury to the endothelial lining of the blood vessels, which may have arisen from trauma, chemical injury, intravenous injection, or inflammation.

- The third factor involves increased blood coagulability, which may result from dehydration, cancer, pregnancy, or increased platelet adhesion.

Spontaneous bleeding or excessive bleeding following minor tissue trauma often indicates a blood clotting disorder. Excessive bleeding has many causes:

- **Thrombocytopenia** may be caused by acute viral infections in children and in adults when platelets are destroyed by HIV infection and certain drugs.

- Chemotherapy, radiation treatments, and cancers such as leukemia also reduce platelet count.

- Vitamin K deficiency may cause a decrease in prothrombin and fibrinogen levels.

- Liver disease reduces the available proteins and vitamin K, and thus, interferes with the production of clotting factors in the liver.

- Inherited defects, such as hemophilia, cause bleeding disorders resulting from a deficiency of one of the clotting factors (factor VIII).

ANTICOAGULANT DRUGS

Anticoagulants are drugs that reduce the ability of blood to clot. Anticoagulants are often mistakenly called blood thinners. These drugs do not dissolve clots that have already formed. Anticoagulants are used to prevent new clots from forming. They include heparin and warfarin. Heparin may be administered intravenously to patients at risk for thrombus formation, and warfarin is given orally. These drugs are considered "high alert" and must be used very carefully, since they may cause significant patient harm. In inpatient settings, injected heparin is commonly used. After a few days, anticoagulation is maintained commonly by oral warfarin. After discharge, oral warfarin usually continues. Anticoagulants are contraindicated with over-the-counter (OTC) products such as acetylsalicylic acid (aspirin or ASA), and herbal supplements such as fish oil capsules, St. John's wort, and CoQ10 should be used with caution.

Heparin

Heparin is a potent anticoagulant naturally obtained from the liver and lungs of domestic animals. In humans, it is usually found in basophils or **mast cells**. Heparin preparations are available as heparin sodium and the low- and high-molecular-weight heparins (fractionated heparins). Problems with heparin and its packaging have prompted FDA recalls and many lawsuits over its use. Contaminants in the drug have caused severe injury and death in a number of patients. Confusing packaging has led to overdoses in infants and children, in some cases also leading to injury or death. The antidote for heparin is protamine sulfate. Examples of anticoagulants are listed in Table 15-1.

Mechanism of Action

Heparin prevents the conversion of fibrinogen to fibrin, and inactivates several of the factors needed for blood clotting. Heparin can be inactivated by hydrochloric acid in the stomach, and must not be administered orally. Therefore, it is given either subcutaneously or through intravenous infusion. The onset of action for intravenous heparin is immediate, whereas subcutaneous heparin may take up to an hour for maximum therapeutic effect.

TABLE 15-1   Anticoagulants

Generic Name	Trade Name	Route of Administration	Average Adult Dosage
Direct Thrombin Inhibitors			
bivalirudin **(bih-val-ih-ROO-din)**	Angiomax®	IV	0.75 mg/kg bolus followed by 1.75 mg/kg/h for 4 h
dabigatran **(dah-bih-GAH-tran)**	Pradaxa®*	PO	Patients with creatinine clearance > 30 mL/min: 150 mg bid; severe renal impairment: 75 mg bid
lepirudin **(leh-PEER-roo-din)**	Refludan®	IV	0.4 mg/kg bolus followed by 0.15–16.5 mg/kg/h for 2–10 days
Indirect Thrombin Inhibitor			
heparin sodium, (preservative-free heparin lock flush solution) **(HEH-pah-rin SOH-dee-um)**	Hep-Lock U/P®	IV Infusion, SC	IV: 5000–40,000 units/day; SC: 15,000–20,000 units bid
Xanthine Derivative			
pentoxifylline **(pen-tok-SIH-fil-leen)**	Trental®	PO	400 mg tid
Direct Factor Xa Inhibitor			
rivaroxaban **(rih-vah-ROK-sah-ban)**	Xarelto®**	PO	15 mg bid with food, for first 21 days; then 20 mg once daily with food, for remaining treatment
Vitamin K₁ Inhibitor			
warfarin sodium **(WAR-fah-rin SOH-dee-um)**	Coumadin®	PO, IV	Usual dose: 2–10 mg/day
Low-Molecular-Weight (fractionated) Heparins (LMWHs)*			
dalteparin sodium **(dal-TEH-pah-rin SOH-dee-um)**	Fragmin®	SC	For the first 30 days, give 200 units/kg once daily (max: 18,000 units/day); Months 2–6: give 150 units/kg once daily
enoxaparin **(eh-nok-sah-PAH-rin)**	Lovenox®	SC	30 mg bid for 10–14 days
tinzaparin sodium **(tin-ZAH-pah-rin SOH-dee-um)**	Innohep®	SC	175 units/kg daily for at least 6 days

*This drug carries the following Black Box Warning: "Discontinuing Pradaxa in patients without adequate continuous anticoagulation increases risk of stroke."

**This drug carries the following Black Box Warning: "(A) Premature discontinuation of Xarelto increases the risk of thrombotic events, (B) spinal/epidural hematoma."

***All three of the low-molecular-weight heparins sold in the United States carry the following Black Box Warning: "Epidural or spinal hematomas may occur in patients who are anticoagulated with LMWHs or heparinoids and are receiving neuraxial anesthesia or undergoing spinal puncture. These hematomas may result in long-term or permanent paralysis."

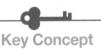

Key Concept

Garlic is an herb that has been shown to decrease the aggregation (stickiness) of platelets, thus producing an anticoagulant effect.

Indications

Heparin and heparin substitutes are used prophylactically for deep vein thrombosis, pulmonary embolism, or atrial embolism. Heparin is also indicated in patients with atrial fibrillation and heart valve replacement surgery. Low-molecular-weight heparins (LMWHs) have become the drugs of choice for many clotting disorders such as coronary occlusion, acute myocardial infarction, and peripheral arterial embolism. After the initiation of anticoagulant therapy with heparin, oral anticoagulants can be started immediately. After about 48 hours, the heparin can be withdrawn, as the oral anticoagulants take this time to exert their effect.

Adverse Effects

Spontaneous bleeding is the major complication of heparin administration. Skin rashes, pruritus, burning sensations of the feet, hypertension, fever, chills, headache, and chest pain occur in some patients. Hypersensitivity reactions may cause bronchospasms and an anaphylactic reaction. The LMWHs may produce fewer adverse effects than other types of heparin.

Contraindications and Precautions

Heparin preparations are contraindicated in patients with a history of hypersensitivity to this agent, active bleeding hemophilia, open wounds, or severe thrombocytopenia. LMWHs should be avoided in patients with hypersensitivity to the drug and in those with thrombocytopenia or active bleeding. Heparin preparations are used with caution in patients with a history of alcoholism or allergy (asthma, hives, hay fever, eczema); and during menstruation, pregnancy (category C), especially the last trimester, and in the immediate postpartum period. Heparin therapy requires caution in the elderly, patients who work in hazardous occupations, and those with cerebral embolism. There is no need to shake heparin since this can cause unwanted, excessive air bubbles to develop and interfere with dosage. A few air bubbles are safe, however, because of the subcutaneous administration.

Drug Interactions

Use of heparin with other anticoagulants may increase anticoagulant effects to a dangerous level. Use with caution in patients who take salicylates such as aspirin.

Warfarin

Warfarin is the mainstay of long-term anticoagulant therapy and is one of the original drugs of the coumarin group. The goal of warfarin therapy is to administer the lowest effective dose to maintain the target *international normalized ratio (INR)*. The earliest changes in INR are usually seen 24 to 36 hours after administration. Administration of a loading dose may require prolonged hospitalization secondary to significant rises in the INR, along with administration of vitamin K (which is its antidote). Once the INR has maintained a therapeutic level for at least two days, the supplemental anticoagulants may be discontinued. Newer drugs such as Pradaxa® and Xarelto® do not require use of the INR.

Mechanism of Action

Warfarin is structurally similar to vitamin K, which is involved in the synthesis of prothrombin in the liver. Therefore, warfarin indirectly interferes with blood clotting by depressing hepatic synthesis of vitamin K-dependant coagulation factors II, VII, IX, and X.

Indications

Warfarin is used as a prophylaxis and for the treatment of deep vein thrombosis, pulmonary embolism, and treatment of atrial fibrillation with **embolism**. Warfarin is also prescribed as an adjunct in the treatment of coronary occlusion and cerebral transient ischemic attacks, and as a prophylactic in patients with prosthetic cardiac valves.

Adverse Effects

In the correct and individualized dosage, warfarin is almost devoid of adverse effects not related to its anticoagulant action. **Alopecia** and sustained erection are the only ones of any consequence, but these are rare. Adverse effects such as nausea and dizziness occur with similar frequency to those caused by a **placebo**.

Contraindications and Precautions

Warfarin is contraindicated in patients with a known hypersensitivity to this drug, bleeding tendencies, vitamin C or K deficiency, hemophilia, clotting factor deficiency, active bleeding, open wounds, and active peptic ulcer. Warfarin should be avoided in patients with severe hepatic and renal disease, pericarditis with acute myocardial infarction, and recent surgery of brain, spinal cord, or eye.

Warfarin is used cautiously in debilitated patients, older adults, and patients with alcoholism, allergic disorders, or psychosis. Warfarin should be used with caution in patients with hepatic and renal insufficiency, diarrhea, fever, and pancreatic disorders.

Drug Interactions

Cholestyramine can decrease warfarin absorption, thus reducing its effects. Colestipol and sucralfate have also been reported to interfere with warfarin absorption, but only to a minor degree.

Acetohexamide, acetaminophen, and allopurinol may enhance the anticoagulant effects of warfarin.

ANTIPLATELET DRUGS

Platelets play a key role in hemostasis and thrombus formation. Platelets adhere to thrombin, collagen, and various other substances. **Antiplatelet agents** are prescribed to suppress **aggregation** (clumping) of platelets. A number of drugs may be used to stop thrombi in arteries, rather than in veins (i.e., using anticoagulants). The most commonly used antiplatelet drug is aspirin. It has been proven effective for preventing myocardial infarctions and strokes. Other medications that may be used as antiplatelet drugs include glycoprotein antagonists, ticlopidine, and abciximab (Table 15-2).

Mechanism of Action

Eptifibatide and tirofiban are two of the newest glycoprotein antagonists that have received approval by the FDA. These agents are used to delay clotting

TABLE 15-2 | **Antiplatelet Drugs**

Generic Name	Trade Name	Route of Administration	Average Adult Dosage
aspirin (acetylsalicylic acid) **(AS-pih-rin or AS-prin), (ah-see-tihl-sah-lih-SIH-lik AH-sid)**	Bayer Aspirin®, many others	PO	80 mg daily–650 mg bid
dipyridamole **(dy-pih-RIH-dah-mol)**	Persantine®	PO	75–100 mg qid
prasugrel **(PRAH-soo-grel)**	Effient®	PO	Loading dose: 60 mg; then 10 mg/day
ticagrelor **(ty-KAH-greh-lor)**	Brilinta®	PO	Loading dose: 180 mg; then 90 mg bid
Adenosine Diphosphate (ADP) Receptor Blockers			
clopidogrel bisulfate **(klo-PIH-doh-grel by-SUL-fayt)**	Plavix®	PO	75 mg daily
ticlopidine **(ty-KLOH-pih-deen)**	Ticlid®	PO	250 mg bid
Glycoprotein IIB/IIIA Receptor Blockers			
abciximab **(ab-SIK-sih-mab)**	ReoPro®	IV	0.25 mg/kg initial bolus over 5 min; then 10 mcg/min for 12 h
eptifibatide **(ep-tih-FIH-bah-tyd)**	Integrilin®	IV	180 mcg/kg initial bolus over 1–2 min; then 2 mcg/kg/min for 24–72 h
tirofiban hydrochloride **(ty-roh-FY-ban hy-droh-KLOR-ryd)**	Aggrastat®	IV	0.4 mcg/kg/min for 30 min; then 0.1 mcg/kg/min for 12–24 h

by altering platelet aggregation and are prescribed in conjunction with heparin and aspirin. Other antiplatelet agents have the same mechanism of action as these new drugs.

Indications

Ticlopidine prevents platelet aggregation, which reduces risk of thrombotic stroke in patients who have experienced stroke precursors. Abciximab is an antiplatelet drug used with heparin and aspirin to prevent coronary vessel occlusion in patients undergoing percutaneous transluminal coronary angioplasty or atherectomy. Clopidogrel is an antiplatelet agent used in patients who have recently had myocardial infarction or stroke.

Adverse Effects

The primary side effects associated with glycoprotein antagonists are bleeding and thrombocytopenia (a decrease in blood platelet levels). Adverse effects of ticlopidine include neutropenia (a decrease in white blood cells), thrombocytopenia, and bleeding. The adverse effects of clopidogrel include fatigue, arthralgic pain, headache, dizziness, hypertension, edema, and risk of bleeding.

Contraindications and Precautions

Antiplatelet drugs are contraindicated in patients with hypersensitivity to these drugs or those who have neutropenia, thrombocytopenia, bleeding ulcer, or uncontrolled hypertension. Antiplatelets should be avoided in patients with recent major surgery or trauma, intracranial bleeding within six months, renal dialysis, and aneurysm.

Antiplatelet drugs are used cautiously in patients with severe liver and renal impairment. These agents should be given with caution to patients at risk for bleeding from trauma, surgery, or gastrointestinal bleeding, and in pregnancy (category B).

Drug Interactions

Aspirin has drug interactions with anticoagulants, hypoglycemic agents, uricosuric agents, spironolactone, alcohol, corticosteroids, pyrazolone derivatives, nonsteroidal anti-inflammatory drugs (NSAIDs), urinary alkalinizers, phenobarbital, phenytoin, and propranolol. Ticlopidine potentiates the effect of aspirin and NSAIDs; it also should not be used along with antacids, cimetidine, digoxin, theophylline, phenobarbital, phenytoin, or propranolol. No direct drug information is available about eptifibatide; however, its adverse effects on the body are well documented. Tirofiban, when used in combination with heparin and aspirin, has been associated with an increase in bleeding. Formal drug interaction studies with abciximab have not been conducted, although an increase in bleeding when abciximab is used concurrently with heparin, other anticoagulants, thrombolytics, and antiplatelet agents has been documented. Use of clopidogrel with NSAIDs has caused increased gastrointestinal blood loss, and it should be used with caution in patients taking aspirin, heparin, or warfarin.

THROMBOLYTIC DRUGS

Thrombolytics are agents that dissolve existing clots. Administration of thrombolytic agents, such as tissue plasminogen activator, urokinase, or streptokinase, is capable of dissolving an arterial clot, such as a clot in a coronary artery in a patient with an acute myocardial infarction. These agents also are able to dissolve clots in various access devices.

The body normally regulates fibrinolysis such that unwanted fibrin clots are removed, whereas fibrin present in wounds is left to maintain hemostasis. The steps of fibrinolysis are shown in Figure 15-3.

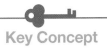

Key Concept

Alteplase with herbal supplements (ginkgo) may increase thrombolytic effects.

Mechanism of Action

Thrombolytic agents break down fibrin clots by converting plasminogen to plasmin (fibrinolysis). Plasmin is an enzyme that breaks down the fibrin of a blood clot.

Indications

Thrombolytic drugs are used to treat acute myocardial infarction, pulmonary embolism, acute ischemic cerebrovascular accident, deep vein thrombosis, and coronary thrombosis, and to clear clots in arteriovenous cannulas and blocked intravenous catheters. Table 15-3 lists the major thrombolytic drugs.

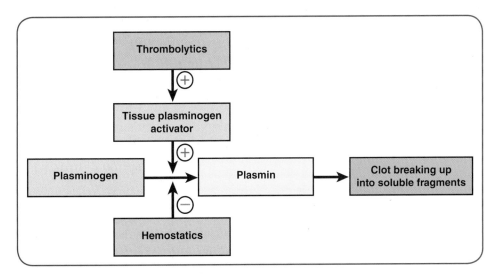

Figure 15-3 Process of fibrinolysis.

TABLE 15-3	Thrombolytic Drugs		
Generic Name	Trade Name	Route of Administration	Average Adult Dosage
alteplase recombinant **(AL-teh-plays ree-KOM-bih-tant)**	Activase®	IV	Initial: 60 mg; then infuse 20 mg/h over next 2 h
anistreplase **(ah-NIS-treh-plays)**	Eminase®	IV	30 units over 2–5 min
reteplase recombinant **(REH-teh-plays ree-KOM-bih-nant)**	Retavase®	IV	10 units over 2 min; repeat dose in 30 minutes
streptokinase **(strep-toh-KY-nays)**	Streptase®	IV	250,000–1.5 million units over 60 minutes
tenecteplase **(teh-NEK-teh-plays)**	TNKase®	IV	30–50 mg infused over 5 seconds
urokinase **(yoo-roh-KY-nays)**	Kinlytic®	IV	Loading dose: 4400 international units at a rate of 90 mL/h over 10 min; followed by continuous infusion of 4400 units/kg/h at a rate of 15 mL for 12 h

Adverse Effects

Bleeding is the most common adverse effect of thrombolytic drugs, often because of percutaneous trauma or spontaneous bleeding from the gastrointestinal tract. Other adverse effects include unstable blood pressure, ventricular dysrhythmias, itching, and nausea.

Contraindications and Precautions

Thrombolytic drugs are contraindicated in patients with known hypersensitivity, active bleeding, or a history of recent trauma, recent intracranial surgery, or stroke. The patient must be monitored carefully for signs of bleeding every 15 minutes for the first hour of therapy and every 30 minutes thereafter.

Thrombolytic drugs should be used cautiously in patients who have recently undergone major surgery, or those who have hypertension and diabetic retinopathy. Thrombolytic drugs are used with caution in pregnancy (category C) with the exception of urokinase (category B).

Drug Interactions

Thrombolytic drugs along with aspirin, dipyridamole, or an anticoagulant may increase the risk of bleeding.

HEMOPHILIA DRUGS

Hemophilia is usually an inherited blood clotting disorder that results in prolonged bleeding. There are several types of hemophilia, and the most serious concern with this disease is deep internal bleeding and bleeding into joints. All forms are X-linked disorders. Hemophilia A, or *classic hemophilia*, is caused by a deficiency of clotting factor VIII. It is the most common form, affecting 1 in 5000 males. Hemophilia B is caused by a deficiency of clotting factor IX, and affects 1 in 30,000 males. A less common form of hemophilia may be caused by new genetic mutations. The rarest form is *acquired hemophilia*, which occurs when antibodies form that attack the blood clotting factors. This type may occur in males or females.

Though incurable, hemophilia can be treated, based on the form of the disease that exists. For mild hemophilia A, treatment may involve slow injection of the hormone desmopressin to stimulate release of sufficient clotting factor to stop bleeding. For moderate to severe hemophilia or hemophilia B, a clotting factor derived from donated human blood or a genetically engineered recombinant clotting factor is injected. For hemophilia C, plasma infusions are used in the United States to stop bleeding, but in Europe, clotting factor XI is used. Overall, regular preventive infusions of clotting factors may help prevent bleeding. Antifibrinolytics may also be prescribed. Hemophilia drugs are listed in Table 15-4.

Mechanism of Action

For the drugs that are not clotting factor replacements, the mechanisms of action differ. Aminocaproic acid works by inhibiting fibrinolysis. Though not completely understood, desmopressin shortens the prolonged activated partial thromboplastin time and bleeding time, probably by increasing factor VIII and von Willebrand factor. It also enhances platelet adhesion to blood vessel walls. Tranexamic acid competitively inhibits activation of plasminogen, reducing conversion of plasminogen to plasmin, and also directly inhibits plasmin activity.

Indications

Aminocaproic acid is used to enhance hemostasis when fibrinolysis contributes to bleeding. Desmopressin is indicated for patients with hemophilia A, with factor VIII coagulant activity levels greater than 5%. It is also indicated for mild to moderate classic **von Willebrand's disease** (type 1) with factor VIII levels greater than 5%. Tranexamic acid is indicated for short-term use (2–8 days) to reduce or prevent hemorrhage, and reduce need for replacement therapy. It can also be used for excessive bleeding in relation to menstruation, surgery, or trauma.

TABLE 15-4	Drugs Used to Treat Hemophilia		
Generic Name	**Trade Name**	**Route of Administration**	**Average Adult Dosage**
aminocaproic acid **(ah-MEE-noh-kah-proh-ik AH-sid)**	Amicar®	PO	1000 mg (in oral tablets) or 20 mL (oral solution) administered in first hour, followed by continuing rate of 1000 mg (tablets) or 5 mL (solution) per hour, for 8 h, or until bleeding has been controlled
antihemophilic factor **(an-ty-hee-moh-FIL-lik FAK-tor)**	Xyntha®	IV	20–100 international units per dL or percentage of normal q8–24h, for 1–4 days, prn
antihemophilic factor/von Willebrand factor **(an-ty-hee-moh-FIL-lik FAK-tor / vawn WIL-leh-brand FAK-tor)**	Alphanate®	IV	0.50 international unit/kg, based on raising clotting factors in plasma 20%–50%, usually bid over several days
anti-inhibitor coagulant complex **(AN-ty in-HIH-bih-tor koh-AG-yoo-lent KOM-pleks)**	Autoplex-T® (this formulation only to be used in patients with inhibitors to factor VIII), Feiba-VH®	IV	25–100 international units/kg, based on severity of hemorrhage, repeated in 6 h, prn
coagulation factor VIIa **(koh-ag-yoo-LAY-shun FAK-tor 8a)**	NovoSeven®	IV	90 mcg/kg q2h by bolus, prn
coagulation factor IX complex **(koh-ag-yoo-LAY-shun FAK-tor 9 KOM-pleks)**	Konyne®	IV	30–40 international units/kg to maintain plasma levels of 15%–80%, prn
coagulation factor IX recombinant **(koh-ag-yoo-LAY-shun FAK-tor 9 ree-KOM-bih-nant)**	Benefix®, Rixubis®	IV	1 international unit/kg, prn
desmopressin **(des-moh-PREHS-sin)**	DDAVP Injection®	IV	4 mcg/mL at 0.3 mcg/kg, over 15–30 min
tranexamic acid **(trah-nek-ZAH-mik AH-sid)**	Cyklokapron®	IV	10 mg/kg, along with clotting factor replacement therapy; may increase to bid or qid, prn, for 2–8 days

Adverse Effects

Aminocaproic acid may cause general edema, headache, and malaise. Serious adverse effects may include bradycardia, hypotension, peripheral ischemia, thrombosis, agranulocytosis, coagulation disorder, leukopenia, thrombocytopenia, myopathy, convulsions, intracranial hypertension, stroke, and pulmonary embolism. Desmopressin only causes infrequent adverse effects, which may include headache, local swelling or burning pain, changes in blood pressure, and rarely, thrombotic events. Tranexamic acid may cause gastrointestinal disturbances, hypotension, and rarely, thromboembolic events.

Contraindications and Precautions

Aminocaproic acid is contraindicated if there is evidence of an active intravascular clotting process. It must not be used in the presence of disseminated intravascular coagulation without concomitant heparin. Desmopressin is contraindicated if there is known hypersensitivity to this drug or any of its components. It should be used with caution in patients with coronary artery insufficiency, hypertensive cardiovascular disease, fluid and electrolyte imbalances, cystic fibrosis, and predisposition to thrombus formation. Tranexamic acid is contraindicated in patients with defective color vision, subarachnoid hemorrhage, and active intravascular clotting. It should be used in reduced dosages if there is renal insufficiency, and with caution if there is upper urinary tract bleeding, history of thromboembolic disease, concurrent use of factor IX complex concentrates or anti-inhibitor coagulant concentrates, or if the patient has disseminated intravascular coagulation. It should be used with caution in women who are lactating.

Drug Interactions

Aminocaproic acid has no significant drug interactions. Doses of desmopressin of 0.3 mcg/kg, or larger, should be used with similar agents only with careful patient monitoring. Tranexamic acid has no significant drug interactions.

SUMMARY

Anticoagulants are used to treat deep venous thrombosis by disrupting the coagulation process and the formation of fibrin. The most potent anticoagulants include heparin and warfarin. Antiplatelet agents suppress clumping of platelets to stop thrombi from forming in arteries. Thrombolytics dissolve existing clots by breaking down fibrin and converting plasminogen to plasmin. All these agents are important to help avoid blood clotting problems in the body, which can lead to a variety of conditions, including tissue ischemia, various embolisms, and stroke.

EXPLORING THE WEB

Visit **www.heart.org**

- Search for "anticoagulants" and review related articles to further enhance your understanding of these drugs.

Visit **www.medicinenet.com**

- Choose a disorder or drug type discussed in this chapter, and search for it. What additional information or research is available related to this topic?

Visit **www.webmd.com**

- From the "Health A-Z," index choose "H," then "Heart Disease." Look for articles related to the topics covered in this chapter. What additional information is available?

REVIEW QUESTIONS

Multiple Choice

1. Anticoagulants are used prophylactically for all of the following conditions or disorders, *except:*

    A. prevention of thrombus in pulmonary embolus

    B. hypothyroidism

    C. deep vein thrombosis

    D. atrial fibrillation

2. Which of the following is an antagonist of warfarin?

    A. vitamin D

    B. vitamin A

    C. vitamin K

    D. niacin

3. The spontaneous arrest of bleeding from a damaged blood vessel is called:

    A. hematoma

    B. hemosiderosis

    C. hemostasis

    D. hemostatic

4. The onset of action for intravenous heparin is:

    A. immediate

    B. an hour

    C. three days

    D. one week

5. Which of the following is a major complication of heparin administration?

    A. hypertension

    B. hypersensitivity reaction

    C. bronchospasms

    D. bleeding

6. Ticlid® (ticlopidine) is a drug that includes which of the following groups of drugs?

   A. thrombolytics

   B. anticoagulants

   C. antiplatelets

   D. hemostatics

7. Which of the following anticoagulants have become the drugs of choice for many clotting disorders?

   A. low-molecular-weight heparins

   B. high-molecular-weight heparins

   C. warfarin

   D. vitamin K

8. Which of the following agents is used to suppress aggregation of platelets?

   A. heparin

   B. aspirin

   C. warfarin

   D. protamine sulfate

9. Which of the following is an example of thrombolytic drugs?

   A. protamine sulfate

   B. plasminogen activator

   C. warfarin

   D. heparin

10. Which of the following is the most common adverse effect of thrombolytics?

    A. constipation

    B. hypertension

    C. vomiting

    D. bleeding

11. Which of the following anticoagulant agents is used to treat von Willebrand's disease?

    A. desmopressin

    B. dalteparin

    C. enoxaparin

    D. bivalirudin

12. Which of the following is not an antiplatelet drug?

    A. dipyridamole

    B. aspirin

    C. desmopressin

    D. ticagrelor

13. Which of the following anticoagulants is naturally obtained from the livers and lungs of domestic animals?

    A. dalteparin

    B. heparin

    C. enoxaparin

    D. tinzaparin

14. Warfarin is structurally similar to:

    A. vitamin B_6

    B. vitamin D

    C. vitamin E

    D. vitamin K

15. Thrombolytic agents break down fibrin clots by converting plasminogen to:

    A. plasmin

    B. glycoprotein

    C. thrombin

    D. tissue plasminogen activator

Fill in the Blank

1. Thrombophlebitis refers to the development of a clot in a vein where _____.

2. Anticoagulants are drugs that reduce the ability of _____.

3. After initiation of anticoagulant therapy with heparin, _____can be started immediately.

4. The major complication of heparin administration is _____.

5. Warfarin is structurally similar to _____.

6. The most commonly used antiplatelet drug is _____.

Matching

Match the first column (generic names) with the second column (trade names):

_____1. urokinase

_____2. streptokinase

_____3. anistreplase

_____4. alteplase recombinant

A. Activase®

B. Eminase®

C. Kinlytic®

D. Streptase®

Critical Thinking

George is 99 years old. He has had multiple disorders and taken many different medications in his life. His skin is very thin, and only a little pressure to his skin can cause bleeding. Some of his regular medications include antidepressants, antihypertensive drugs, and baby aspirin for his heart condition.

1. What do you think are the causes of bleeding from the skin?

2. What can George's physician suggest to prevent his bleeding?

3. What medications should George stop taking because they may increase the likelihood of bleeding?

CHAPTER 16

Drug Therapy for Allergies and Respiratory Disorders

OBJECTIVES

After completing this chapter, the reader should be able to:

1. Identify basic anatomical structures of the respiratory system.
2. Discuss chemical mediators.
3. Compare histamines and antihistamines.
4. List three popular asthma medications.
5. Identify the chemical mediators that are important in asthma.
6. Discuss the uses and general drug actions of the bronchodilators in asthma.
7. Explain the indications for use of mast cell stabilizers and the mechanism of action.
8. Discuss different types of mucolytics and expectorants.
9. Explain how decongestants work and identify serious adverse effects.
10. Discuss drugs used for smoking cessation.

GLOSSARY

Allergic rhinitis – inflammation of the nasal mucosa that is due to the sensitivity of the nasal tissue to an allergen

Allergy – a state of hypersensitivity induced by exposure to a particular antigen

Antigen – a substance that is introduced into the body and induces the formation of antibodies

Antihistamines – drugs that counteract the action of histamine

Antitussives – agents that relieve or prevent coughing

Asthma – a chronic inflammatory disorder of the airways of the respiratory system

Bronchiectasis – destruction and widening of the large airways

Bronchodilators – agents that relax the smooth muscle of the bronchial tubes

Chemical mediators – substances released by mast cells and platelets into interstitial fluid and blood; these substances include histamines, leukotrienes, serotonin, and prostaglandins

Chronic obstructive pulmonary disease (COPD) – a group of common chronic respiratory disorders that are characterized by progressive tissue damage and obstruction in the airways of the lungs

Cystic fibrosis – a genetic disorder affecting the exocrine glands, causing thick mucus to obstruct the bronchioles in the lungs

Dry powder inhalers (DPIs) – devices used to deliver medication in the form of micronized powder into the lungs

Emphysema – the destruction of the alveolar walls and septae, which leads to large, permanently inflated alveolar air spaces

Expectorants – agents that promote the removal of mucous secretions from the lung, bronchi, and trachea, usually by coughing

Glucocorticoids – steroid hormones that can bind with the cortisol receptor and trigger similar effects; they are also potent and consistently effective anti-inflammatory agents used for relief of many conditions, including chronic asthma

Histamine – a chemical substance naturally found in all body tissues that protects the body from factors in the environment that produce allergic and inflammatory reactions

Leukotriene modifiers – a relatively new class of drugs designed to prevent asthma and allergic reactions before they occur by either inhibiting leukotriene production or preventing leukotrienes from binding to cellular receptors

Leukotrienes – substances that contribute to the inflammation associated with asthma

Mast cell stabilizers – substances that work to prevent allergy cells (called mast cells) from breaking open and releasing chemicals that help cause inflammation; they work slowly over time

Metered dose inhaler (MDI) – a hand-held pressurized device used to deliver medications for inhalations

Mucolytic – destroying or dissolving the active agents that make up mucus

Septae – walls of the bronchioles

Xanthine derivatives – substances that are effective for relief of bronchospasm in asthma, chronic bronchitis, and emphysema

OVERVIEW

The respiratory system provides the mechanisms for transporting oxygen from the air into the blood, and for removing carbon dioxide from the blood. Oxygen is essential for cell metabolism, and the respiratory system is the only means of acquiring oxygen. Carbon dioxide is a waste material resulting from cell metabolism.

The respiratory system consists of two anatomical areas: the upper and lower respiratory tracts. In addition, the pulmonary circulation, the muscles required for ventilation, and the nervous system (which plays a role in controlling respiratory function) are integral to the function of the respiratory system.

ANATOMY REVIEW

- The upper respiratory system consists of the nasal cavity, sinuses, and pharynx. The lower respiratory system consists of the larynx, trachea, bronchi, bronchioles, alveoli, and lungs (Figure 16-1).

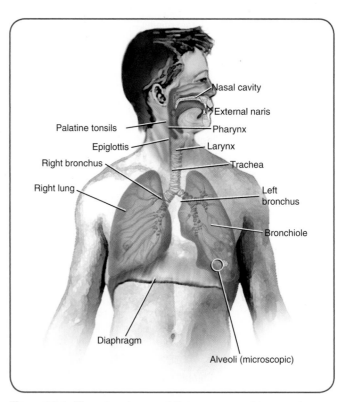

Figure 16-1 The structures of the upper and lower airways.

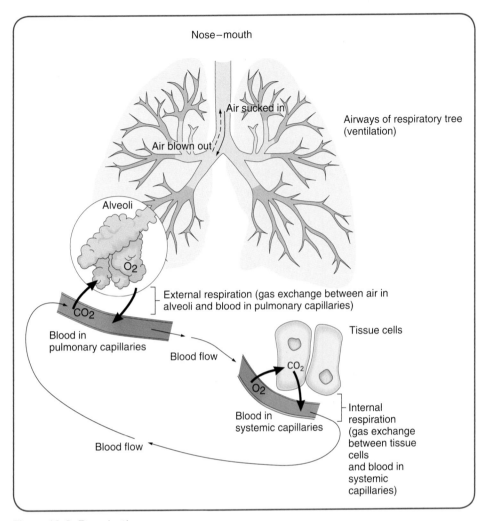

Figure 16-2 Respiration.

- The respiratory system exchanges oxygen and carbon dioxide in the body through respiration.

- There are three types of respiration: external respiration is breathing or ventilation, internal respiration is the exchange of oxygen and carbon dioxide between the cells and capillaries, and cellular respiration is the use of oxygen to release energy stored in nutrient molecules (Figure 16-2).

- Figure 16-3 outlines the functions of each of the structures that make up the respiratory system.

ALLERGIES

An **allergy** is a state of hypersensitivity induced by exposure to a particular **antigen** (a substance that, when introduced into the body, induces the formation of antibodies), resulting in harmful immunological reactions on

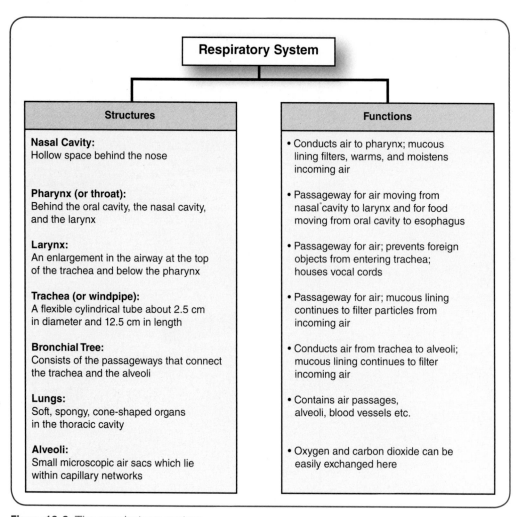

Figure 16-3 The respiratory system.

subsequent exposures. The term *allergy* is usually used to refer to hypersensitivity to an environmental antigen. There are varieties of allergic reactions such as allergic rhinitis, allergic conjunctivitis, allergic asthma, and allergic dermatitis. This chapter focuses on respiratory disorders and drug therapy, including discussion of allergic rhinitis and allergic asthma.

CHEMICAL MEDIATORS

Allergies result in an inflammatory process in the nasal passages and airways. The inflammatory process is basically the same regardless of the cause of the allergic response. The severity of the inflammation may vary with the specific situation. The inflammation may result in tissue injury, which damages cells. Mast cells and platelets release **chemical mediators**, such as histamines and leukotrienes into the interstitial fluid and blood. The chemical mediators that are mostly involved with allergies and asthma include histamines and leukotrienes, which are discussed below.

Histamines

Histamine is a chemical substance naturally found in all the body tissues that protects the body from factors in the environment that produce allergic and inflammatory reactions. The greatest concentration of histamine is in the basophils, platelets, and mast cells in the skin, lungs, and gastrointestinal tract. The mast cells are the principal sites of storage. Histamine has several functions, including:

1. Dilation of capillaries, which increases capillary permeability and results in hypotension

2. Contraction of most smooth muscle of the bronchial tree, which may cause wheezing and difficulty breathing

3. Increased stomach acid secretion

4. Initiation of allergic reactions

5. Acceleration of the heart rate

There are two types of histamines in the body. One causes allergic reactions in the respiratory tract and interacts with H_1 receptors on cells, and the other works on the gastrointestinal tract and interacts with H_2 receptors on cells (see Chapter 17). Histamine causes dilation and increased permeability of capillaries. It is one of the first mediators of an inflammatory response. Antihistamine drugs inhibit this immediate, transient response. Both H_1 and H_2 receptors mediate the contraction of vascular smooth muscle. Histamine has also been postulated to be a neurotransmitter in the central nervous system. The H_1 receptor may be blocked with antihistamine drugs.

Leukotrienes

Leukotrienes contribute to the inflammation associated with asthma. They are bronchoconstrictive substances released during asthma and inflammation. Leukotrienes (slow-reacting substances of anaphylaxis [SRS-A]) are substances that produce effects similar to those of histamine. These substances cause smooth muscle contraction and increased vascular permeability. Leukotrienes appear to be important in the later stages of the inflammation associated with asthma. They stimulate slower and more prolonged responses than do histamines.

ALLERGIC REACTION

An allergic reaction occurs when the immune system reacts to a foreign substance. The body attempts to get rid of the substance, be it an allergen from the environment or a medication. In the case of an allergic reaction to a medication, the body's response is harmful and may cause serious symptoms. Common allergic reactions include nausea, diarrhea, vomiting, headache, and light-headedness. Other symptoms include anxiety, hives, palpitations, shortness of breath, rash, swelling, and wheezing. The most common allergies caused by natural environmental allergies include dust, pollen, and pet dander. The most common medications that cause allergic reactions include anticonvulsants, barbiturates, iodine, anesthetics, and antibiotics (including sulfa medications).

Anaphylactic Shock

Anaphylactic shock is an allergic reaction that may be life threatening. Its onset is sudden, severe, and involves the entire body. Anaphylactic shock causes a massive release of histamine and other substances, which cause airway constriction (making breathing very difficult), abdominal cramping, vomiting, and diarrhea. Common causes of anaphylactic shock include foods, medications, insect stings, and allergies to latex. Foods that are most likely to cause this condition include nuts, fish, milk, and eggs. Individuals who have food allergies or asthma are believed to be more likely to develop anaphylactic reactions. The most common insect stings in the United States include bees, yellow jackets, hornets, wasps, and ants. Anaphylactic reactions often begin with tingling sensations, itching, metallic taste sensation, hives, sensation of warmth, symptoms of asthma, swelling of the mouth and throat, a drop in blood pressure, or loss of consciousness. These types of reactions are usually treated with epinephrine, followed by antihistamines and steroids.

Allergic Rhinitis

> **Medical Terminology**
> **Review**
>
> **rhinitis**
> rhin- = nose
> -itis = inflammation
> inflammation of the nose

Allergic rhinitis is inflammation of the mucous membranes in the nose, throat, and airways that is due to the sensitivity of the tissue to an antigen, also called an allergen. The nasal mucosa is rich with mast cells (large cells that contain a wide variety of biochemicals, including histamine). These cells, along with basophils (a type of white blood cell), recognize environmental agents as they try to enter the body. Individuals with allergic rhinitis have numerous mast cells. Allergic rhinitis is usually associated with watery nasal discharge and itching of the nose and eyes, caused by a localized sensitivity reaction to house dust, animal dander, or an antigen, commonly pollen. The condition may be seasonal. It is commonly known as "hay fever." Allergic rhinitis is caused by histamine release, while nonallergic rhinitis is often a symptom of the common cold.

ANTI-ALLERGIC AGENTS

The therapeutic goals of treating allergic rhinitis are to prevent its occurrence and to relieve symptoms. Drugs used to prevent or treat allergic rhinitis include antihistamines (H_1-receptor antagonists), intranasal steroids, and mast cell stabilizers. Antihistamines and common over-the-counter (OTC) antihistamine combinations will be focused on here. Mast cell stabilizers and steroids are discussed later in this chapter.

H₁-Receptor Antagonists

H_1-receptor antagonists (**antihistamines**) are commonly used for the treatment of allergies. These drugs relieve the symptoms of runny nose, sneezing, and itching of the eyes, nose, and throat as seen in allergic rhinitis. Table 16-1 shows various H_1-receptor antagonists. Antihistamines are often combined with decongestants and antitussives in OTC sinus and cold medicines. Table 16-2 shows examples of combination OTC drugs.

TABLE 16-1	First- and Second-Generation H₁-Receptor Antagonists		
Generic Name	**Trade Name**	**Route of Administration**	**Average Adult Dosage**
First-Generation Agents			
azatadine **(ah-ZAH-tah-deen)**	Optimine®	PO	1–2 mg bid–tid prn
azelastine hydrochloride **(ah-zeh-LAS-teen hy-droh-KLOR-ryd)**	Astelin®	Intranasal	2 sprays per nostril bid
brompheniramine maleate **(brom-feh-NY-rah-meen MAH-lee-ayt)**	Veltane®	PO	4–8 mg tid–qid (max: 40 mg/day)
chlorpheniramine maleate **(klor-feh-NEER-ah-meen MAL-lee-ayt)**	Chlor-Trimeton®	PO	2–4 mg tid–qid (max: 24 mg/day)
clemastine fumarate **(kleh-MAS-teen FYOO-mah-rayt)**	Tavist®	PO	1.34 mg bid (max: 8.04 mg/day)
cyproheptadine hydrochloride **(sy-pro-HEP-tah-deen hy-droh-KLOR-ryd)**	Periactin®	PO	4 mg tid or qid (max: 0.5 mg/kg/day)
dexbrompheniramine maleate and pseudoephedrine **(deks-brom-feh-NY-rah-meen MAL-lee-ayt and soo-doh-eh-FEH-dreen)**	Drixoral®	PO	6 mg bid
dexchlorpheniramine maleate **(deks-klor-feh-NEER-ah-meen MAL-lee-ayt)**	Dexchlor®	PO	2 mg q4–6h (max: 12 mg/day)
diphenhydramine hydrochloride **(dy-fen-HY-drah-meen hy-droh-KLOR-ryd)**	Benadryl®	PO	25–50 mg tid–qid (max: 300 mg/day)
promethazine hydrochloride **(pro-MEH-thah-zeen hy-droh-KLOR-ryd)**	Phenergan®	PO	12.5 mg/day (max: 50 mg/day)
tripelennamine hydrochloride **(try-peh-LEN-nah-meen hy-droh-KLOR-ryd)**	PBZ-SR®	PO	25–50 mg q4–6h (max: 600 mg/day)
triprolidine hydrochloride **(try-PROH-lih-deen hy-droh-KLOR-ryd)**	Actidil®	PO	2.5 mg bid or tid

continued on next page

Table 16-1 continued

Second-Generation Agents			
cetirizine hydrochloride **(seh-TEER-ih-zeen hy-droh-KLOR-ryd)**	Zyrtec®	PO	5–10 mg/day
desloratadine **(des-loh-RAH-tah-deen)**	Clarinex®	PO	5 mg/day
fexofenadine hydrochloride **(fek-soh-FEH-nah-deen hy-droh-KLOR-ryd)**	Allegra®	PO	60 mg bid or 180 mg once daily
loratadine **(loh-RAH-tah-deen)**	Claritin®	PO	10 mg/day

TABLE 16-2	OTC Combination Antihistamine Drugs	
Antihistamine	**Decongestant**	**Trade Name**
chlorpheniramine **(klor-feh-NEER-ah-meen)**	phenylephrine **(fen-nihl-EF-freen)**	Actifed® Cold and Allergy tablets
chlorpheniramine	pseudoephedrine **(soo-doh-eh-FEH-dreen)**	Actifed® Cold and Sinus caplets
diphenhydramine **(dy-fen-HY-drah-meen)**	phenylephrine	Benadryl® Allergy/Cold caplets
chlorpheniramine	pseudoephedrine	Chlor-Trimeton® Allergy-Decongestant tablets
brompheniramine **(brom-feh-NY-rah-meen)**	phenylephrine	Dimetapp® Cold and Allergy Elixir
dexbrompheniramine **(deks-brom-feh-NY-rah-meen)**	pseudoephedrine	Drixoral® Allergy and Sinus Extended Release tablets
chlorpheniramine	pseudoephedrine	Sinutab® Sinus Allergy tablets
diphenhydramine	phenylephrine	Sudafed® PE Nighttime*
chlorpheniramine	pseudoephedrine	Triaminic® Cold/Allergy
chlorpheniramine	pseudoephedrine	Tylenol® Allergy Sinus caplets

*Sudafed is sold behind the counter and requires identification to purchase.

Mechanism of Action

The primary action of antihistamines is to block the effect of histamine at H_1-receptors, thus blocking histamine release.

Indications

H_1-receptor antagonists are used to treat minor symptoms of various allergic conditions and the common cold, such as runny nose and sneezing, and for the prevention of motion sickness, vertigo, and reactions to blood or plasma in susceptible patients.

Adverse Effects

Common adverse effects of H_1-receptor antagonists include dry mouth, dizziness, headache, urinary retention, nausea, vomiting, sedation, hypotension, and a decrease in the number of white blood cells.

Contraindications and Precautions

H_1-receptor antagonists are contraindicated in patients with hypersensitivity to these agents, prostatic hypertrophy, glaucoma, and gastrointestinal obstructions. H_1-receptor antagonists should be used cautiously in patients with asthma or hyperthyroidism.

Drug Interactions

Use of H_1-receptor antagonists with central nervous system (CNS) depressants such as opioids or alcohol will cause increased sedation. Some OTC cold preparations (e.g., diphenhydramine) may increase anticholinergic adverse effects. Monoamine oxidase inhibitors (MAOIs) may cause a hypertensive crisis.

ASTHMA

Asthma is a chronic inflammatory disorder of the airways of the respiratory system (Figure 16-4). It is characterized by wheezing and shortness of breath resulting from constriction of the bronchioles. Asthma is most commonly classified as allergic, exercise-induced, or caused by infections of the respiratory tract. Symptoms include breathlessness, cough, wheezing, and chest tightness. The airway becomes inflamed with edema and mucous plugs, and hyperactivity of the bronchial tree adds to the symptoms.

During asthmatic attacks, when bronchiole constriction and increased secretions are present, bronchodilators are used for relief. Anti-inflammatory drugs, such as glucocorticoids, leukotriene inhibitors, and cromolyn, may be prescribed for relief of symptoms. The majority of medications for asthma are administered by inhalation. Anti-asthma medications can be divided into two categories: long-term control (or *controller* medications) and quick-relief medications (also called bronchodilators).

For safety, asthmatic patients should learn how to manage their disease and its complications, as well as limit exposure to irritants that will trigger asthma attacks. Since symptoms alone are not always sufficient to measure respiratory status, patients learn how to use peak flow meters. These meters measure the peak expiratory flow rate (PEFR) from a patient's lungs. They should be used two times per day with the results of each usage written down so that results over time can be discussed with the patient's physician.

Medical Terminology Review

bronchiole
bronchi- = air tube
-ole = small; little; minute
small tube in the airway

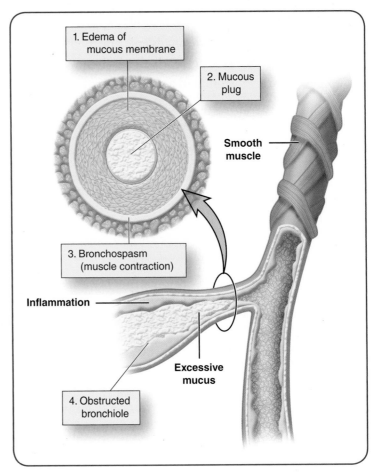

1. Edema of mucous membrane

2. Mucous plug

Smooth muscle

3. Bronchospasm (muscle contraction)

Inflammation

Excessive mucus

4. Obstructed bronchiole

Figure 16-4 Acute asthmatic episode.

ANTI-ASTHMA AGENTS

There are various groups of medications used in the treatment of asthma, including bronchodilators, anti-inflammatory drugs, leukotriene modifiers (antagonists), and mast cell stabilizers.

Bronchodilators

Bronchodilators are agents that widen the diameter of the bronchial tubes. They are used to rapidly relieve the acute bronchospasm of asthmatic attack. Bronchodilators include beta-adrenergic agonists and xanthenes (theophylline). Beta-adrenergic drugs are the most commonly prescribed bronchodilators. Table 16-3 lists bronchodilators for asthma.

Beta-Adrenergic Drugs

Beta-adrenergic drugs work as both cardiac and respiratory agonists. They are commonly referred to simply as beta-blockers. These drugs or hormones act through the sympathetic nervous system. Their effects include increased

TABLE 16-3   Bronchodilators Used for Asthma

Generic Name	Trade Name	Route of Administration	Average Adult Dosage
Anticholinergics			
ipratropium bromide (ih-prah-TROH-pee-um BROH-myd)	Atrovent®	PO	2 inhalations by MDI qid (max: 12 inhalations/day)
ipratropium bromide and albuterol sulfate (ih-prah-TROH-pee-um BROH-myd and al-BYOO-teh-rahl SUL-fayt)	Combivent®	PO	2 inhalations q6h (max: 12 inhalations/day)
tiotropium bromide (ty-oh-TROH-pee-um BROH-myd)	Spiriva®	PO	2 inhalations of the powder contents of 1 capsule/day using Handihaler device
Beta-Agonists/Sympathomimetics			
albuterol (al-BYOO-teh-rahl)	Proventil®, Ventolin®	PO	2–4 mg tid–qid
epinephrine bitartrate (eh-pih-NEH-frin by-TAR-trayt)	AsthmaHaler®	PO	Inhalation aerosol: 160–200 mg (1 inhalation) once. An additional inhalation may be used after at least 1 min.
formoterol fumarate (for-MOH-teh-rahl FYOO-mah-rayt)	Foradil®	PO	1–2 inhalations by DPI q4h up to 5 days
isoproterenol hydrochloride (eye-soh-proh-TEH-reh-nahl hy-droh-KLOR-ryd)	Isuprel®	IV	0.01–0.02 mg prn
levalbuterol hydrochloride (leh-val-BYOO-teh-rahl hy-droh-KLOR-ryd)	Xopenex®	Nebulizer	0.63 mg tid–qid
metaproterenol sulfate (meh-tah-proh-TEH-reh-nahl SUL-fayt)	Alupent®, Metaprel®	PO, Inhalation	MDI: 2–3 inhalations q3–4h (max: 12 inhalations/day); PO: 20 mg q6–8h
pirbuterol acetate (per-BYOO-teh-rahl AH-seh-tayt)	Maxair®	Inhalation	2 inhalations by MDI qid (max: 12 inhalations/day)
salmeterol xinafoate (sal-MEH-teh-rahl zih-NAH-foh-ayt)	Serevent Diskus®	Inhalation	2 inhalations of aerosol by MDI bid
terbutaline sulfate (ter-BYOO-tah-leen SUL-fayt)	Terbutaline Sulfate Tablets®, Terbutaline Sulfate Injection®	PO, SC	PO: 2.5–5 mg tid at 6 hour intervals; SC: 0.25 mL, may be repeated in 15 to 30 min (max. dose is 0.5 mg within 4 hours)
Methylxanthines			
aminophylline (ah-mih-NAW-fil-leen)	Truphylline®	PO, IV	PO: 6.3 mg/kg once; IV: 6 mg/kg over 30 min
theophylline (thee-AW-fil-leen)	Elixophyllin®	PO, IV	PO: 5 mg/kg in divided doses, q6h; IV: Loading dose: 5 mg/kg

heart rate, dilation of bronchial tubes in the lungs, and reduction of the force and rate of uterine contractions during labor.

Drugs with primarily beta$_1$-agonist activity act mainly on the heart, increasing heart rate and raising blood pressure. Those with primarily beta$_2$-agonist activity act mainly on the lungs and uterus. Consequently, drugs that stimulate the beta$_2$ receptors produce bronchodilation. They are used to treat asthma and premature labor. Epinephrine (which is normally secreted from the adrenal gland) and isoproterenol are two potent beta-receptor stimulators.

Mechanism of Action   The main action of beta-agonist drugs is on the smooth muscle of the bronchial tree and on the heart. A typical medication is isoproterenol, which may be taken orally or by injection. Beta$_2$-receptor drugs are the most effective medications to reduce acute bronchospasms and exercise-induced asthma. These agents provide bronchodilation by stimulating the beta$_2$ receptors in the smooth muscle of the lung. Epinephrine and ephedrine are nonselective adrenergic agents, and naturally occurring catecholamine may be obtained from animal adrenal glands or prepared synthetically.

Indications   Epinephrine is used for the temporary relief of bronchospasm. Beta$_2$-receptor agonists are used in acute asthmatic attacks and congestion. Salmeterol is preferred for prophylaxis and maintenance therapy for asthma or bronchospasm. Salmeterol is the only long-acting beta$_2$-adrenergic agonist available in the United States, and is indicated for long-term prevention of asthma symptoms and the prevention of exercise-induced bronchospasm. Salmeterol should not be used in place of anti-inflammatory therapy or to treat acute bronchospasm.

Adverse Effects   Adverse effects of beta$_2$ agonists include dizziness, headache, tremor, palpitations, and sinus tachycardia. Common adverse effects of epinephrine and ephedrine include insomnia, tachycardia, nervousness, and anorexia. The cardiotoxic effects have led to the discovery and use of more specific respiratory agents that do not cause tachycardia or nervousness.

Contraindications and Precautions   Beta$_2$-adrenergic agents are contraindicated in patients with hypersensitivity to these drugs, or during pregnancy (category C) and lactation.

Drug Interactions   Salmeterol generally does not interact with other drugs. Other beta$_2$ agonists may have drug interactions with anesthetics, digitalis, ergotamine, and MAOIs.

Xanthine Derivatives

This group of drugs is chemically related to caffeine, which dilates bronchioles in the lungs. **Xanthine derivatives** are effective for the relief of bronchospasm in several diseases (see Table 16-3).

Medical Terminology Review

bronchospasm
broncho- = air tube
-spasm = narrowing; contraction
narrowing of the bronchioles or airways

Mechanism of Action Xanthine derivatives relax the smooth muscles of the bronchial tree and stimulate cardiac muscle and the CNS. Methylxanthine is the base of xanthine derivatives that must be converted to theophylline. Theophylline provides mild bronchodilation in asthmatics. This drug may also have important anti-inflammatory properties and enhances mucociliary clearance. Theophylline is available for oral administration in standard or sustained-release formulas with forms that last up to 24 hours. It is also available in an IV formulation.

Indications Xanthine agents are used for the prevention and treatment of bronchial asthma and for the treatment of emphysema and bronchitis. Theophylline has a narrow therapeutic range and is not used as commonly today as in the past, because the beta$_2$-adrenergic agents are safer and more effective.

Adverse Effects Adverse effects include tachycardia, insomnia, nervousness, headache, and nausea. Patients with hyperthyroidism, acute pulmonary edema, convulsive disorders, and heart disease cannot use xanthine derivatives. Adverse effects of theophylline at therapeutic doses include insomnia, upset stomach, aggravation of dyspepsia, and urination difficulties in elderly men with prostatism. Dose-related toxicities are common and include nausea, vomiting, tachyarrhythmias, headache, seizures, hyperglycemia, and hypokalemia.

Contraindications and Precautions Xanthine derivatives are contraindicated in individuals with known hypersensitivity, seizure disorders, uncontrolled arrhythmias, peptic ulcers, and hyperthyroidism. These drugs should be used cautiously in patients older than 60 years or those who have cardiac disease, hypertension, congestive heart failure, hypoxemia, or liver dysfunctions. These agents are used during pregnancy (category C) and lactation with caution.

Drug Interactions Xanthine drugs can produce drug interactions with caffeine, cimetidine, fluoroquinolones, antibiotics, rifampin, phenobarbital, and phenytoin.

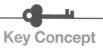

Key Concept

Observe and report early signs of possible toxicity from xanthine derivatives, which may include: anorexia, nausea, vomiting, dizziness, shakiness, restlessness, abdominal discomfort, and marked hypotension.

Anti-Inflammatory Drugs

Many anti-inflammatory agents are used to reduce the incidence of asthma attacks. Glucocorticoids, leukotriene inhibitors, and mast cell stabilizers are commonly used (Table 16-4).

Glucocorticoids

Glucocorticoids are the most potent and consistently effective anti-inflammatories that are currently available. They are the drugs of choice for chronic asthma. Three devices are commonly used for inhalation administration: metered dose inhalers, nebulizers, and dry powder inhalers. Drug administration with a **metered dose inhaler (MDI)** is often accomplished with one

TABLE 16-4	Anti-Inflammatory Medications Used for Asthma		
Generic Name	Trade Name	Route of Administration	Average Adult Dosage
Glucocorticoids			
beclomethasone dipropionate **(beh-kloh-MEH-thah-zohn dy-proh-PY-oh-nayt)**	Beconase AQ®, Vancenase®	Oral inhalation	1–2 inhalations by MDI tid–qid
budesonide **(byoo-DEH-soh-nyd)**	Pulmicort Turbuhaler®	Oral inhalation	1–2 inhalations by MDI (200 mcg/inhalation)
flunisolide **(floo-NIH-soh-lyd)**	AeroBid®	Oral inhalation	2–3 inhalations by MDI bid–tid
fluticasone propionate **(floo-TIH-kah-zohn proh-PY-oh-nayt)**	Flovent®, Flonase®	Oral inhalation (Flovent®), Nasal spray (Flonase®	(Flovent®): 2 inhalations by MDI (44 mcg each) bid, (Flonase®): 2 sprays (50 mcg) each in each nostril once daily (max daily dosage is 200 mcg).
triamcinolone acetonide **(try-am-SIH-noh-lohn ah-SEH-toh-nyd)**	Azmacort®	Oral inhalation	2 inhalations by MDI tid–qid
Leukotriene Modifiers (Antagonists)			
montelukast **(mon-teh-LOO-kast)**	Singulair®	PO	10 mg/day in the evening
zafirlukast **(zah-fer-LOO-kast)**	Accolate®	PO	20 mg bid 1 h before or 2 h after meals
zileuton **(zy-LOO-ton)**	Zyflo®	PO	600 mg qid
Mast Cell Stabilizers			
cromolyn sodium **(KROH-moh-lin SOH-dee-um)**	Intal®	Oral inhalation	1 inhalation by MDI qid
nedocromil sodium **(neh-DOK-roh-mil SOH-dee-um)**	Tilade®	Oral inhalation	2 inhalations by MDI qid

or two puffs from a hand-held pressurized device (Figure 16-5). After inhalation, the patient must rinse his or her mouth out and gargle with water.

Dry powder inhalers (DPIs) deliver medication in the form of micronized powder into the lungs. An example of a medication that is available in DPI form is albuterol. DPIs are breath-activated and are easier to use than MDIs. A nebulizer uses a small machine that converts a solution into a mist. The mist droplets are inhaled through either a facemask or a mouthpiece.

Quick-relief asthma medicines are also referred to as "rescue inhalers." They are usually given via nebulizers or MDIs. Examples of these medicines

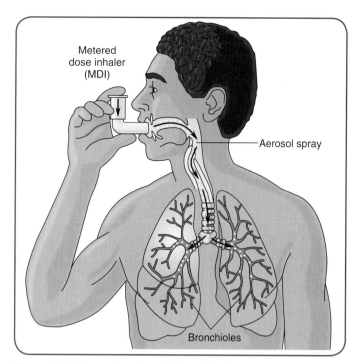

Figure 16-5 Use of metered dose inhaler.

include Proventil® and Atrovent®. Some oral steroids such as prednisone and prednisolone also are utilized in rescue inhalers.

Systemic glucocorticoids are used to treat status asthmaticus, and inhaled glucocorticoids are used for maintenance therapy. Inhaled glucocorticoids are the most effective means of controlling asthma. Combined preparations containing a glucocorticoid and a long-acting bronchodilator are considered useful in limiting the amount of the glucocorticoid needed to control asthma.

Mechanism of Action Glucocorticoids enter target cells where they have anti-inflammatory, immunosuppressive, and salt-retaining effects.

Indications Inhaled glucocorticoids are preferred for the long-term control of asthma and are first-line agents for patients with persistent asthma. Dosages for inhaled glucocorticoids vary depending on the specific agent and delivery device (see Table 16-4). Systemic glucocorticoids are most effective for long-term asthma therapy. Long-term use of inhaled glucocorticoids in children is not recommended because these agents may suppress growth and suppress the adrenal glands for production of hormones.

Adverse Effects Adverse reactions to corticosteroid inhalation include nasal irritation and dryness, headache, nausea, epistaxis, dizziness, hoarseness, and cough.

Contraindications and Precautions Local (inhaled) glucocorticoids are contraindicated in patients with hypersensitivity to the drugs and lactation. These drugs should be used cautiously in patients who are receiving

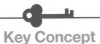

Key Concept

Inhaled glucocorticoids may cause broncho-spasm, requiring their use to be discontinued and an alternate treatment started.

concomitant systemic oral steroids, and in those with active tuberculosis, viral infections, and recurrent epistaxis. Glucocorticoids should be used with caution in pregnancy (category C for oral forms, and category B for inhaled). Safety and efficacy in children younger than six years of age is not established.

Drug Interactions The therapeutic and toxic effects of glucocorticoids are increased if taken concurrently with troleandomycin. Effects of anticholin-esterases are decreased if taken concurrently with corticotropin; profound muscular depression is possible.

Leukotriene Modifiers (Antagonists)

Leukotriene modifiers are a class of biologically active compounds that occur naturally in leukocytes and produce allergic and inflammatory reactions similar to those of histamine. They are thought to play a role in the development of allergic and autoallergic diseases such as asthma, rheumatoid arthritis, inflammatory bowel disease, and psoriasis.

Mechanism of Action Leukotriene antagonists such as zafirlukast (Accolate®) block the bronchoconstriction, mucous production, and inflammation that occur with asthma. Zafirlukast was the first medication in this new anti-inflammatory class. A newer drug is called zileuton (Zyflo®). It is rapidly absorbed through oral administration. Montelukast (Singulair®) is the latest addition to this class of drugs. Montelukast acts as a bronchodilator, respiratory stimulant, and leukotriene receptor antagonist. This medication should be given at night for maximum effectiveness.

Indications Leukotriene modifiers are used for prophylaxis and chronic asthma in adults and children older than 12 years. Zafirlukast is prescribed as maintenance therapy for patients with chronic asthma. Montelukast is prescribed prophylactically for asthma attacks (see Table 16-4).

Adverse Effects Zafirlukast is a safer drug and has few adverse effects compared to other leukotriene modifiers. However, rare but occasionally severe cases of liver injury have been linked to zafirlukast. Adverse effects of zileuton include liver toxicity and dyspepsia. The main adverse effects of montelukast are headaches and gastrointestinal symptoms.

Contraindications and Precautions The leukotriene modifiers are contraindicated in patients with history of hypersensitivity to these medications. Montelukast is contraindicated in severe asthma attacks, bronchoconstriction due to asthma, or status asthmaticus. Montelukast should be avoided during lactation. Zileuton and zafirlukast are contraindicated in patients with active liver disease and during lactation and pregnancy. The leukotriene modifiers should be used cautiously in patients with hepatic insufficiency. Safety and effectiveness in children younger than 12 years have not been established.

Drug Interactions Leukotriene modifiers may double theophylline levels and increase toxicity. They increase the hypoprothrombinemic effects of warfarin. These agents may increase levels of beta-blockers (especially propranolol) and lead to hypotension and bradycardia.

Mast Cell Stabilizers

The two **mast cell stabilizers** that are available for the prophylaxis of asthma include cromolyn sodium and nedocromil. They are used to prevent asthma symptoms and improve airway function in patients with mild persistent asthma or exercise-induced asthma (see Table 16-4).

Mechanism of Action Mast cell stabilizers suppress the release of substances that cause bronchoconstriction and inflammation from the mast cells in the respiratory tract.

Indications Cromolyn is the drug of choice as a prophylactic for moderate allergic asthma, especially in children, because of its safety and efficacy. It is also used to reduce the symptoms of seasonal allergic attacks. Mast cell stabilizers are used in combination with other drugs in the treatment of allergic disorders and in the prevention of exercise-induced bronchospasm.

Adverse Effects Adverse effects of mast cell stabilizers include nausea, fatigue, headache, dizziness, hypotension, and an unpleasant taste.

Contraindications and Precautions Mast cell stabilizers are contraindicated in patients with a known hypersensitivity, coronary artery disease or history of arrhythmias, dyspnea, and acute asthma, and during pregnancy (category B) and lactation. Safe use in children younger than six years of age is not determined. Mast cell stabilizers should be used cautiously in patients with renal or hepatic dysfunction.

Drug Interactions There are no clinically important drug interactions with cromolyn.

DECONGESTANTS

The common cold generally involves a runny nose, sneezing, nasal congestion, coughing, sore throat, headache, and many other symptoms. There are over one billion colds in the United States every year. Colds occur mostly during the winter or during rainy seasons. People are most contagious during the first two to three days of the cold, and usually not contagious at all by days seven to ten. Certain cold viruses can also cause the patient to experience muscle aches, postnasal drip, and decreased appetite. Complications of the common cold include bronchitis, pneumonia, ear infection, sinusitis, and aggravation of asthma.

Nasal congestion and a runny nose are primarily associated with the first stage of inflammation, vasodilation, and increased capillary permeability.

TABLE 16-5	Drugs Used to Treat Nasal Congestion		
Generic Name	Trade Name	Route of Administration	Average Adult Dosage
Anticholinergic			
ipratropium bromide (**ih-prah-TRO-pee-um BROH-myd**)	Atrovent®	Nasal	2 sprays in each nostril tid–qid for only 4 days
Sympathomimetics			
naphazoline hydrochloride (**na-FAH-zoh-leen hy-droh-KLOR-ryd**)	Privine®	Intranasal	2 drops q3–6h
oxymetazoline (**ok-see-meh-TAH-zoh-leen**)	Afrin®, Neo-Synephrine®	Intranasal	2–3 sprays bid for up to 3–5 days
pseudoephedrine hydrochloride (**soo-doh-eh-FEH-dreen hy-droh-KLOR-ryd**)	Sudafed®	PO	60 mg q4–6h
tetrahydrozoline hydrochloride (**teh-trah-hy-DRAW-zoh-leen hy-droh-KLOR-ryd**)	Tyzine®	Intranasal	2–4 drops or sprays q3h
xylometazoline (**zy-loh-meh-TAH-zoh-leen**)	Otrivin®	Intranasal	1–2 sprays bid

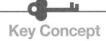

Key Concept

Chicken soup may actually help you fight off a cold. The heat, fluid, and salt found in chicken soup may help you fight off the viral infection that is a cold.

Decongestants cause vasoconstriction of nasal mucosa and reduce congestion or swelling. These agents are available in both oral and nasal preparations. Table 16-5 shows decongestant agents.

Mechanism of Action

The most effective way of alleviating the symptoms of nasal congestion is to induce vasoconstriction through stimulation of alpha receptors of the sympathetic nervous system that are affiliated with the nasal vasculature. Therefore, decongestants are alpha agonists.

Indications

The most common uses for decongestants are the relief of nasal congestion due to infection or allergy, and inflammation in the eyes. They are also used to relieve respiratory distress of bronchial asthma, chronic bronchitis, and emphysema.

Adverse Effects

Decongestants should only be used by order of a physician for those patients with glaucoma, prostate cancer, and heart disease. Decongestants may increase blood glucose levels in patients with diabetes mellitus. Warnings on the labels of OTC preparations instruct patients with hypertension, diabetes mellitus, ischemic heart disease, and hyperthyroidism about possible adverse effects involved in the use of decongestants. They may cause tachycardia, insomnia, nervousness, restlessness, blurred vision, and nausea or vomiting. Although ephedrine is still legal in many applications, except dietary supplements, the drug is being phased out of the market due to its toxicities. The purchasing of ephedrine or pseudoephedrine is currently limited and monitored, and regulations vary between states.

Contraindications and Precautions

Decongestants are contraindicated in patients with hypersensitivity to these agents, glaucoma, hypertrophy of prostate, certain types of heart disease, or diabetes mellitus. Decongestants should be avoided in patients with hyperthyroidism and hemorrhagic stroke.

Decongestants are used cautiously in patients with ischemic heart disease. The safe use of decongestants during pregnancy (category C) and lactation is not established.

Drug Interactions

Nasal decongestants such as ephedrine or pseudoephedrine may cause severe hypertension with MAOIs such as furazolidone. They may also decrease vasopressor response with reserpine, methyldopa, and urinary acidifiers.

ANTITUSSIVES, EXPECTORANTS, AND MUCOLYTICS

Coughing is a reflex response to irritation of the bronchial mucosal layer, such as that seen in inflammatory conditions. The cough reflex has an important role in clearing the lungs of excessive mucous and other secretions. **Antitussives** are agents that suppress coughing. **Expectorants** promote the removal of mucous secretions from the lungs, bronchi, and trachea, usually by coughing. These medications are available OTC and by prescription. Expectorant and mucolytic drugs include acetylcysteine, guaifenesin, and dornase alfa (Table 16-6).

Mechanism of Action

Expectorants are also **mucolytic** (destroying or dissolving the active agents that make up mucus). In many cases, expectorants are added to other drugs, such as antitussives, decongestants, and antihistamines, to help remove mucus. Acetylcysteine is a mucolytic agent that decreases the viscosity of mucus. It is also an antidote to acetaminophen hepatotoxicity. Guaifenesin is safer and more effective mucolytic.

Indications

Specific expectorants, including acetylcysteine and dornase alfa, are indicated for the treatment of cystic fibrosis. These agents are able to reduce the risk of respiratory infections. Drug effects are seen within three to seven days of starting the medication.

Medical Terminology Review

mucolytic
muco- = mucus
-lytic = breaking down
agent to break down mucus

TABLE 16-6	Antitussive, Expectorant, and Mucolytic Drugs		
Generic Name	Trade Name	Route of Administration	Average Adult Dosage
Opioid Antitussives			
codeine (C-II)	(generic only)	PO	10–20 mg q4-6h prn (max: 120 mg/24h)
hydrocodone bitartrate (C-III) **(hy-droh-KOH-dohn by-TAR-trayt)**	Hycodan®, others	PO	5–10 mg q4-6h prn (max: 15 mg/dose)
Nonopioid Antitussives			
benzonatate **(ben-ZOH-nah-tayt)**	Tessalon®	PO	100 mg tid prn up to 600 mg/day
dextromethorphan **(deks-troh-meh-THOR-fan)**	Benylin®	PO	10–20 mg q4h or 30 mg q6–8h
Expectorant			
guaifenesin **(gwy-FEH-neh-sin)**	Robitussin®, others	PO	200–400 mg q4h (max: 2.4 g/day)
Mucolytics			
acetylcysteine **(ah-see-til-SIS-teen)**	Mucomyst®	PO	Inhalation by MDI: 1–10 mL of 20% solution q4-6h or 2–20 mL of 10% solution q4–6h
dornase alfa **(DOR-nays AL-fah)**	Pulmozyme®	PO	Inhalation by nebulizer: 1 ampule (2.5 mg)/day

Adverse Effects

The common adverse effects of antitussives include dizziness, drowsiness, nausea, and vomiting. Acetylcysteine may cause bronchospasm and a burning sensation in the upper respiratory passage.

Contraindications and Precautions

The contraindications and precautions for these agents are not significant.

Drug Interactions

By inhibiting platelet function, guaifenesin may increase the risk of hemorrhage in patients receiving heparin therapy. There are no significant drug interactions listed for acetylcysteine or dornase alfa.

CHRONIC OBSTRUCTIVE PULMONARY DISEASE

Chronic obstructive pulmonary disease (COPD) is a group of common chronic respiratory disorders that are characterized by progressive tissue damage and obstruction in the airways of the lungs. Emphysema, chronic

TABLE 16-7	Comparisons Between Emphysema and Chronic Bronchitis	
Characteristic	**Emphysema**	**Chronic Bronchitis**
Etiology (cause)	Smoking, genetics	Smoking, air pollution
Location	Alveoli	Bronchi
Cough and dyspnea	Some coughing, marked dyspnea	Early, constant cough; some dyspnea
Cyanosis (bluish skin)	No	Yes
Sputum	Little	Large amounts

bronchitis, and chronic asthma are some examples. Other conditions, such as **cystic fibrosis** (a genetic disorder affecting the exocrine glands, causing thick mucus to obstruct the bronchioles in the lungs), and **bronchiectasis** may lead to similar obstructive effects. Table 16-7 compares the characteristics of emphysema and chronic bronchitis.

Emphysema

Emphysema is the destruction of the alveolar walls and **septae**, which leads to large, permanently inflated alveolar air spaces (Figure 16-6). Cigarette smoking is implicated in most cases of emphysema. However, a genetic factor contributes to the early development of the disease in nonsmokers.

Avoidance of respiratory irritants and cessation of smoking may slow the progress of emphysema. Immunization against influenza and pneumonia is essential.

Key Concept

Electronic cigarettes are also known as "e-cigarettes." They are battery-operated devices that deliver nicotine along with flavorings and various chemicals in vapor instead of smoke. They are promoted as being safer than traditional cigarettes, cigars, or pipes. Though they do offer less of the toxic chemicals that come from burning tobacco leaves, known carcinogens such as formaldehyde and acetaldehyde are still present. Testing has not yet proven their overall safety levels, but users can be exposed to potentially toxic levels of nicotine when refilling e-cigarettes.

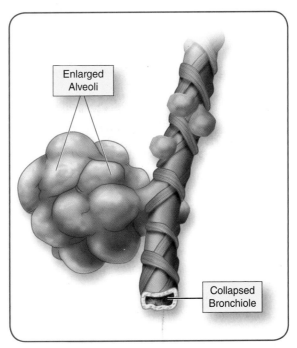

Enlarged Alveoli

Collapsed Bronchiole

Figure 16-6 Alveoli and bronchioles affected by emphysema.

Chronic Bronchitis

Chronic bronchitis involves significant changes in the bronchi resulting from constant irritation from smoking or exposure to industrial pollution. The effects are irreversible and progressive.

Individuals with chronic bronchitis usually have a history of cigarette smoking or of living in an urban or industrial area, particularly in geographical locations where smog is common. In some cases, asthma is an associated condition.

DRUGS FOR SMOKING CESSATION

Key Concept

Cigarette smoking, along with the aging process, can reduce the strength of the immune system in elderly individuals, which is a predisposing factor for various conditions and infections.

Cigarette contains chemical compounds that affect most of the organs of the human body. Cigarette smoking causes cancers of the mouth, pharynx, larynx, lungs, esophagus, pancreas, kidney, bladder, and cervix. It also may cause leukemia and may increase the risk of heart disease, lung disease, or stroke. Cigarette smoking can cause the lungs to develop emphysema, chronic bronchitis, and bacterial pneumonia.

The benefits of smoking cessation include better health and a longer life. The most commonly used drugs for smoking cessation are listed in Table 16-8.

Various products and dosage forms are available for smoking cessation. Nicotine replacement therapy (NRT) includes several transdermal patches

TABLE 16-8	Drugs for Smoking Cessation		
Generic Name	Trade Name	Route of Administration	Average Adult Dosage
bupropion hydrochloride **(byoo-PROH-pee-on hy-droh-KLOR-ryd)**	Zyban®	PO	75–100 mg tid
nicotine polacrilex **(NIH-koh-teen poh-LAH-crih-leks)**	Nicorette Gum®	PO	2–4 mg q1–2h prn (max: 24 pieces/day)
nicotine polacrilex	Nicotrol Inhaler®	Nasal	Inhalation: 4 mg prn (max: 64 mg/day)
nicotine polacrilex	Commit lozenge®	PO	4 mg q1–2h prn
nicotine polacrilex	Nicotrol NS®	Nasal	1–2 sprays per nostril per hour (max: 40 sprays per nostril per day)
nicotine polacrilex	Nicotrol®, Nicoderm CQ®	Topical	7–21 mg/day (transdermal patch)
varenicline	Chantix®	PO	Days 1–3: Take one 0.5 mg tablet/day; Days 4–7: Take one 0.5 mg tablet bid (morning and evening); Days 8–end of treatment: Take one 1 mg tablet bid (morning and evening)

Key Concept

Patients using Zyban « registered symbol » or Chantix « reg. symbol » must be monitored for signs of suicidal thought and depression. Both drugs carry black box warnings concerning these and other potential changes in behavior that have been linked to their use.

(Habitrol®, Nicoderm®, Nicotrol®, and Prostep®), a gum (Nicorette®), and a spray (Nicotrol NS®). Bupropion (Zyban®), an antidepressant, is the first non-nicotine drug for smoking cessation. It is available in tablet form and can be used alone or with the nicotine patch. Some nicotine inhalers may be used in combination with fluoxetine for smoking cessation. It is suspected that certain antidepressants such as fluoxetine, when added to NRT, might improve abstinence rates.

NRT is thought to be useful and beneficial for tobacco users who want to quit their addiction. NRT products are intended to help patients stop smoking while dealing with withdrawal symptoms and cravings that result from ceasing the habit. For most people, this therapy is considered to be completely safe. According to a Cochrane review, former smokers using nicotine replacement therapy are 1.5 to 2 times more likely to stop smoking than patients who try to stop using any other methods.

Mechanism of Action

The neurochemical mechanism of the antidepressant effect of bupropion is not understood; it is chemically unrelated to other antidepressant agents. It is a weak blocker of neuronal uptake of serotonin and norepinephrine, and inhibits the reuptake of dopamine to some extent.

Indications

Bupropion is used for treatment of depression. It also aids in smoking cessation.

Adverse Effects

Adverse effects of nicotine, nicotine polacrilex, and nicotine transdermal systems include headache, dizziness, light-headedness, insomnia, irritability, tachycardia, palpitations, hypertension, nausea, salivation, vomiting, cough, hiccups, and hoarseness.

Contraindications and Precautions

Products containing nicotine are contraindicated during pregnancy or lactation, in patients with known hypersensitivity, heart or blood vessel disease, high blood pressure, diabetes mellitus, overactive thyroid, skin rash or irritation, stomach ulcers, pheochromocytoma, dental problems, mouth sores, sore throat, jaw pain, or temporomandibular joint disorder. Precautions include the regular monitoring of the patient's health by his or her physician during use of smoking cessation drugs, and keeping these products away from children and pets because they can cause severe harm if ingested.

Drug Interactions

Bupropion may increase the risk of adverse effects with levodopa and toxicity with MAOIs. It also increases the risk of seizures with drugs that lower seizure threshold, including alcohol.

SUMMARY

The exchange of oxygen and carbon dioxide in the lungs is one of the most important tasks of physiology, as it supplies oxygen at the cellular level in body tissue. Oxygen is essential to sustain life. Therefore, the respiratory tract is necessary for the inspiration of oxygen and the expiration of carbon dioxide. Respiratory system disorders such as allergic asthma and chronic obstructive pulmonary disease (COPD) are common in the United States. Antihistamines are used to relieve allergic reactions throughout the body, but they are also used commonly in patients with respiratory tract disorders to relieve rhinorrhea and allergic bronchitis.

Cough-suppressing preparations are indicated for nonproductive coughs. If the cough is productive, suppression is not available, and an expectorant may be used to assist in expelling the secretions.

Bronchodilators induce smooth muscle relaxation, which eases breathing. They are used to treat asthma, COPD, and chronic bronchitis. Epinephrine and beta$_2$ agonists are indicated in acute asthma. Leukotriene agonists (new on the market), such as albuterol and mast cell stabilizer (cromolyn), are used for exercise-induced asthma. Glucocorticoids are administered by inhalation.

EXPLORING THE WEB

Visit **http://familydoctor.org**

- Search for "decongestants." What information is available to further aid in your understanding of this type of drug?

Visit **www.aafa.org**, **www.nhlbi.nih.gov, and www.lung.org**.

- Review information on the different types of asthma and allergies. Do a search for some of the other disorders covered in this chapter. Bookmark these sites for future reference.

REVIEW QUESTIONS

Multiple Choice

1. Which of the following substances may cause allergic rhinitis?

    A. epinephrine

    B. chlorpheniramine

    C. hydrocodone

    D. histamine

2. Adverse reactions to corticosteroid inhalation include:

    A. cough, hoarseness, and headache

    B. cough, diarrhea, and dyspepsia

    C. pulmonary edema, convulsive disorders, and hypothyroidism

    D. pulmonary edema, convulsive disorders, and hyperthyroidism

3. Which of the following drugs is an expectorant?

   A. ephedrine

   B. adrenaline

   C. acetylcysteine

   D. bupropion

4. Which of the following is a trade name for guaifenesin?

   A. Tussionex®

   B. Robitussin®

   C. Benadryl®

   D. Tessalon®

5. Which of the following is indicated for cessation of smoking tobacco?

   A. bupropion

   B. diazepam

   C. salmeterol

   D. albuterol

6. Which of the following is the brand name of bupropion?

   A. Habitrol®

   B. Zyban®

   C. Nicotrol®

   D. Prostep®

7. Dextromethorphan is classified as:

   A. an opioid cough suppressant

   B. a xanthine derivative

   C. a nonsteroid contraceptive

   D. a nonopioid cough suppressant

8. Another name for allergic rhinitis is:

   A. contact dermatitis

   B. hay fever

   C. yellow fever

   D. photosensitivity

9. Which of the following is/are considered the drug(s) of choice for chronic asthma?

   A. theophylline

   B. albuterol

   C. antihistamines

   D. glucocorticoids

10. The initial stimulus for cough probably arises from which of the following parts of the respiratory system?

    A. bronchial mucosa

    B. pharynx

    C. mouth

    D. nasal cavities

11. Which of the following is a trade name of fluticasone?

    A. Flonase®

    B. Pulmicort®

    C. Singulair®

    D. Tilade®

12. Which of the following agents is an opioid?

    A. guaifenesin

    B. hydrocodone

    C. albuterol

    D. aminophylline

13. Leukotrienes are part of a class of biologically active compounds that occur naturally in which of the following body cells?

    A. white blood cells

    B. red blood cells

    C. platelets

    D. mast cells

14. Which of the following agents would increase bronchial secretions?

    A. theophylline

    B. cromolyn

    C. hydrocodone

    D. acetylcysteine

15. The destruction of the alveolar walls and septae that leads to permanently inflated alveolar air spaces is called:

    A. chronic bronchitis

    B. asthma attack

    C. emphysema

    D. bronchiectasis

Fill in the Blank

1. Cromolyn is one of the mast cell stabilizers and the drug of choice as a prophylactic for moderate _____, especially in _____.

2. The leukotriene modifiers are used for prophylaxis and chronic asthma in _____.

3. Xanthine derivatives are indicated for treatment of:

   a. _____

   b. _____

   c. _____

4. Zileuton® is one of the leukotriene modifiers that may cause _____.

5. Anaphylactic shock causes a massive release of _____.

Matching

Generic Name

_____1. terbutaline

_____2. pirbuterol

_____3. ephedrine bitartrate

_____4. albuterol

_____5. salmeterol

Trade Name

A. Serevent®

B. AsthmaHaler®

C. Proventil®

D. Maxair®

E. Brethaire®

Critical Thinking

A 75-year-old man went to the emergency department with a complaint of shortness of breath, coughing, sputum production, and fever. The physician ordered a chest x-ray and blood tests. The patient had a history of cigarette smoking for 30 years. After the various tests, the physician diagnosed this patient with emphysema and pneumonia.

1. Name the major predisposing factors for emphysema and pneumonia at this patient's age.

2. With this patient's history of cigarette smoking, what other complications may he have?

3. If the patient is advised to stop smoking, name the available drugs that help a person to stop smoking.

CHAPTER 17

Drug Therapy for Gastrointestinal Disorders

OBJECTIVES

After completing this chapter, the reader should be able to:

1. Explain the mechanisms of action and therapeutic effects of antacids.
2. Identify the major classes of drugs used to treat peptic ulcers.
3. Describe the use of H₂-receptor antagonists in the treatment of peptic ulcers.
4. Define proton pump inhibitor agents and their indications.
5. Explain the treatment for the bacterium *Helicobacter pylori*.
6. Identify the common adverse effects of major laxative, antidiarrheal, and antiemetic drugs.
7. Name the five major classifications of laxatives.
8. Identify the most effective antidiarrheal agents.
9. Explain adsorbent agents and their indications.
10. Describe the mechanism of action of bulk-forming agents.

GLOSSARY

Adsorbent agents – drugs with the ability to adsorb gases, toxins, and bacteria

Antacids – drugs that neutralize hydrochloric acid and raise gastric pH, thus inhibiting pepsin (a gastric enzyme)

Antiemetics – drugs that stop vomiting

Bulk-forming laxatives – natural or synthetic polysaccharide derivatives that absorb water to soften the stool and increase bulk to stimulate peristalsis

Calcium carbonate – a substance that causes acid rebound, which may delay ulcer-related pain relief and ulcer healing

Chemical digestion – the alteration of food into different forms through chemicals and enzymes

Emetic – a drug that induces vomiting

Emollient laxatives – substances that act as surfactants by allowing absorption of water into the stool

Helicobacter pylori – a bacterial species that is associated with several gastroduodenal diseases

Histamine H₂-receptor antagonists – drugs that block the action of histamine on parietal cells in the stomach, decreasing acid production

Lubricant laxative – a substance, such as mineral oil, that works by increasing water retention in the stool to soften it

Mechanical digestion – the breakdown of large food particles into smaller pieces by physical means

Peptic ulcer – a lesion located in either the stomach (gastric ulcer) or the duodenum (small intestine)

Saline laxatives – substances that create an osmotic effect to increase water content and stool volume

Stimulant laxatives – substances that stimulate bowel mobility and increase secretion of fluids in the bowel

Stool softeners – substances that decrease the consistency of stool by reducing surface tension

Zollinger-Ellison syndrome – peptic ulceration with gastric hypersecretion and tumor of the pancreatic islets

OVERVIEW

The digestive system, sometimes called the gastrointestinal tract, alimentary tract, or gut, consists of a long hollow tubule. The digestive tract secretes substances used in the process of digestion into the canal. The growth of the body depends upon the consumption, absorption, and metabolism of food. This system also involves the elimination of waste. The digestive system is subject to many disorders, some of which are very common. Numerous drugs are used to treat these varying conditions.

ANATOMY REVIEW

- The digestive system consists of the mouth, pharynx, esophagus, stomach, small intestine, large intestine, rectum, and anus (Figures 17-1 and 17-2).

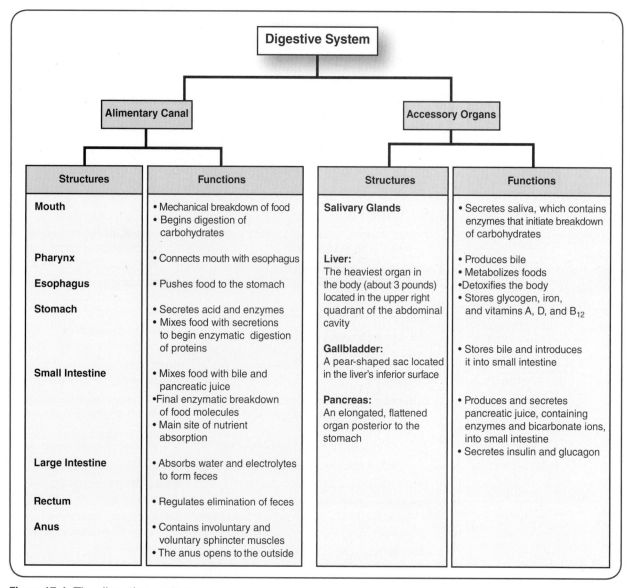

Figure 17-1 The digestive system.

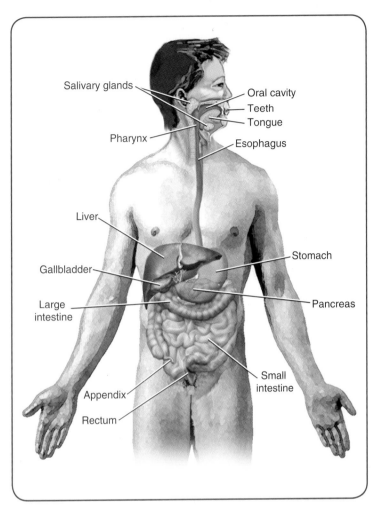

Figure 17-2 Structures of the digestive system.

- There are several accessory organs of the digestive system; these include the salivary glands, liver, gallbladder, and pancreas (see Figure 17-1).

- The role of the digestive tract is to change food into forms the body can use and to eliminate waste.

- There are two forms of digestion: **Mechanical digestion** breaks large food particles into smaller pieces such as by chewing. **Chemical digestion** is the alteration of the smaller food particles by substances such as digestive enzymes, bile, and acids.

- Nutrients from the digestive tract are absorbed into the bloodstream by moving across the lining of the digestive tract.

ACID PEPTIC DISEASES

Peptic ulcer refers to a lesion located in either the stomach (gastric ulcer) or the duodenum (small intestine) (Figure 17-3). In general, ulcers occur whenever there is an increase in acid secretion or a decrease in mucosal resistance.

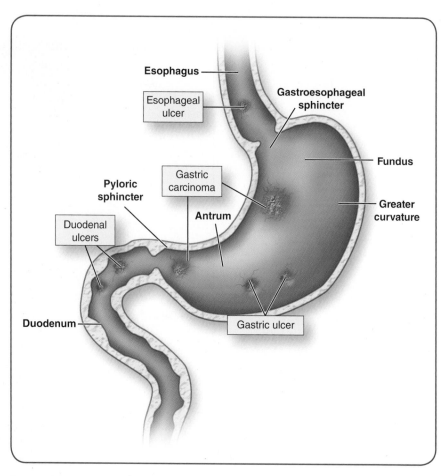

Figure 17-3 Sites of peptic ulcers.

Mucosal injury in the acid peptic diseases includes gastric ulcer, duodenal ulcer, and gastroesophageal reflux disease (GERD), which are mediated by gastric acid. Hydrochloric acid is secreted by parietal cells in the body of the stomach. It is regulated by adjacent endocrine hormones, such as gastrin, or by histamine, somatostatin, and prostaglandin E_2. Gastrin is a relatively weak stimulant of the parietal cells. It acts primarily to cause the release of histamine, which is the most potent stimulus of acid secretion, and acts as the common mediator. Histamine antagonists inhibit acid secretion that is stimulated by gastrin and acetylcholine, as well as histamine. There are a number of causes of peptic ulcer, including:

- Family history
- Smoking tobacco
- Alcohol
- Coffee
- Stress
- Infection with *Helicobacter pylori* (*H. pylori*)

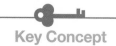

Key Concept

Gastroesophageal reflux disease (GERD) involves the periodic flow of gastric contents into the esophagus.

- Blood group O
- Anti-inflammatory drugs (aspirin, nonsteroidal anti-inflammatory drugs [NSAIDs], and glucocorticoids)

A wide variety of prescription and over-the-counter (OTC) medications are available for the treatment of peptic ulcer. These drugs include antacids, H_2-receptor antagonists, proton pump inhibitors, and antibiotics. Antibiotics treat peptic ulcers caused by *H. pylori*.

Antacids

There are differences in the types of antacids, in terms of their formulation, neutralizing capacity, duration of action, side effects, and cost. These must be considered when choosing an antacid for therapeutic use. Antacids are OTC drugs. The most common antacids are shown in Table 17-1. The most widely used antacids are sodium bicarbonate, calcium carbonate, aluminum hydroxide, and magnesium hydroxide.

Mechanism of Action

Antacids neutralize hydrochloric acid and raise gastric pH, thus inhibiting pepsin (a gastric enzyme). Antacids reduce the concentration and total load of acid in the gastric contents. By increasing gastric pH, antacids also inhibit pepsin activity. In addition, they strengthen the gastric mucosal barrier.

TABLE 17-1	Common Antacids		
Generic Name	**Trade Name**	**Route of Administration**	**Average Adult Dosage**
aluminum hydroxide **(ah-LOO-mih-num hy-DROK-syd)**	Amphojel®	PO	600 mg tid–qid
calcium carbonate **(KAL-see-um KAR-boh-nayt)**	Tums®	PO	0.5–2 g bid–tid
calcium carbonate with magnesium hydroxide **(KAL-see-um KAR-boh-nayt with mag-NEE-see-um hy-DROK-syd)**	Mylanta Gel-caps®, Rolaids®	PO	2–4 capsules or tablets prn
magnesium hydroxide and aluminum hydroxide **(mag-NEE-see-um hy-DROK-syd and ah-LOO-mih-num hy-DROK-syd)**	Maalox®, Mylanta®	PO	5–15 mL liquid or 2–4 tablets
magaldrate **(MAH-gal-drayt)**	Riopan®	PO	480–1080 mg (5–10 mL) or 1–2 tablets daily
sodium bicarbonate (baking soda); aspirin, and citric acid **(SOH-dee-um by-KAR-boh-nayt [BAY-king SOH-dah]; AS-prin, and SIH-trik AH-sid)**	Alka Seltzer®	PO	300 mg–2 g/day

Indications

These agents are used widely for the relief of heartburn, dyspepsia, and medical treatment of peptic ulcer. The primary role of antacids in the management of acid peptic disorders is the relief of pain. Nonsystemic antacids (magnesium or aluminum substances) are preferred to systemic antacids such as sodium bicarbonate for intensive ulcer therapy because they avoid the risk of alkalosis. Liquid antacid forms have a greater buffering capacity than tablets. However, tablets are more convenient to carry. Antacid mixtures such as aluminum hydroxide with magnesium hydroxide provide more even, sustained action than single-agent antacids, and permit a lower dosage of each compound.

Adverse Effects

Constipation can occur in patients using calcium carbonate- and aluminum-containing antacids. Diarrhea is a common adverse effect of magnesium- and sodium-containing antacids. If diarrhea occurs, the patient may alternate the antacid mixture with aluminum hydroxide. Hypophosphatemia and osteomalacia can occur with long-term use of aluminum hydroxide, but these conditions can also occur with short-term use in severely malnourished patients, such as alcoholics. Calcium carbonate usually is avoided because it causes acid rebound, hypercalcemia, vomiting, metabolic alkalosis, confusion, and renal calculi. It may also delay pain relief and ulcer healing.

Contraindications and Precautions

Antacids are contraindicated in patients with severe abdominal pain of unknown cause and during lactation. Sodium bicarbonate is contraindicated in patients with hypertension, congestive heart failure, severe renal disease, and edema. It should not be used for ulcer therapy. All antacids should be used cautiously in elderly patients and renally impaired patients. Chronic administration of calcium carbonate-containing antacids should be avoided because of hypercalcemia. Calcium carbonate- and magnesium-containing antacids should be used cautiously in patients with severe renal disease.

Drug Interactions

Because antacids alter gastric pH and affect absorption of ingested substances, they have a high potential for drug interactions. To ensure consistent absorption and therapeutic efficacy, orally administered drugs should be given 30 to 60 minutes before antacids. These agents bind with tetracycline and inhibit its absorption, reducing its therapeutic efficacy. Antacids may destroy the coating of enteric-coated drugs, leading to premature drug dissolution in the stomach. Antacids may interfere with the absorption of many drugs, including cimetidine, ranitidine, digoxin, isoniazid, iron products, anticholinergics, and phenothiazines.

Medical Terminology Review

hypophosphatemia
hypo- = under, below, less than normal
phosphat = phosphate
-emia = blood condition
having lower than normal phosphate levels in the blood

osteomalacia
osteo = bone
malacia = softening
softening of the bone

hypercalcemia
hyper = over, above, more than normal
calc = calcium
emia = blood condition
having excess amounts of calcium in the blood

Prostaglandin E$_1$ Analog

Prostaglandin analogs are used in the treatment of acid peptic diseases, including peptic ulcer. The endogenous prostaglandins include the prostaglandin E analogs. They act by regulating mucosal blood flow, proliferation and restoration of epithelial cells, function of mucosal immunocytes, and secretion of mucus, bicarbonate, and basal acid. The only prostaglandin analog approved by the FDA for the prevention of NSAID-induced ulcer disease is misoprostol (Cytotec®). It is a synthetic prostaglandin E$_1$ analog.

Mechanism of Action

Misoprostol enhances mucosal defense mechanisms while inhibiting gastric acid secretion. Its protective actions occur by increasing bicarbonate and mucous production, and decreasing pepsin levels during basal conditions.

Indications

Misoprostol is used in the prevention of aspirin- and other NSAID-induced gastric ulcers in patients with a high risk of gastric ulcer complications, such as geriatric patients with debilitating disease, or in those with a history of ulcer.

Adverse Effects

The most common adverse effects of misoprostol include abdominal pain, diarrhea, flatulence, nausea, vomiting, dyspepsia, headache, and uterine cramping. Though diarrhea is usually self-limiting, it may be severe.

Contraindications and Precautions

Misoprostol is contraindicated in patients with an allergy to prostaglandins, during lactation, and during pregnancy. This drug may cause diarrhea in nursing infants. Misoprostol carries a Black Box Warning against use in pregnant women, and is in pregnancy category X. This is because it stimulates uterine contractions, which may endanger pregnancy.

Drug Interactions

The major drug interaction with misoprostol occurs with dinoprostone, a prostaglandin E$_2$ drug used in labor. Moderate drug interactions occur with quinapril, hydrochlorothiazide, acetaminophen, aspirin, famotidine, simethicone, diphenhydramine, lidocaine, and many others. There are also minor drug interactions with a large variety of drugs.

Histamine H$_2$-Receptor Antagonists

As discussed in Chapter 16, there are two types of histamine receptors: H$_1$ and H$_2$. The second of these mediates the acid secretion from gastric parietal cells and is inhibited by the H$_2$-receptor-blocking drugs. These drugs may be preferred to other antiulcer agents because of their convenience and lack of effect on gastrointestinal motility. H$_2$-receptor antagonists are listed in Table 17-2.

TABLE 17-2	H_2-Receptor Antagonists		
Generic Name	Trade Name	Route of Administration	Average Adult Dosage
cimetidine (sy-MEH-tih-deen)	Tagamet®	PO	300–400 mg qd–bid
famotidine (fah-MOH-tih-deen)	Pepcid®, Pepcid AC®	PO	40 mg hs
nizatidine (ny-ZAH-tih-deen)	Axid®, Axid AR®	PO	150 mg bid or 300 mg hs
ranitidine hydrochloride (rah-NIH-tih-deen hy-droh-KLOR-ryd)	Zantac®	PO, IV	PO: 100–150 mg bid or 300 mg at bedtime; IV: 50 mg q6–8h; 150–300 mg/24 h by continuous infusion

Mechanism of Action

Cimetidine was the first H_2-receptor antagonist approved for clinical use. It blocks the H_2 receptor on the parietal cells of the stomach, thus decreasing gastric acid secretion.

Indications

Histamine H_2-receptor antagonists are used to promote healing of gastric and duodenal ulcers, and hypersecretory states such as **Zollinger-Ellison syndrome**. Prototypes of H_2-receptor antagonists include cimetidine, famotidine, nizatidine, and ranitidine. They are a remarkably safe group of drugs.

Cimetidine is available OTC for the treatment of acute gastric ulcer, duodenal ulcer, and GERD. It is also used in the treatment of Zollinger-Ellison syndrome. Ranitidine is five to ten times more potent than cimetidine and requires a less-frequent dosing schedule. It is an H_2-receptor antagonist indicated for the short-term treatment of duodenal ulcers and the management of hypersecretory conditions such as Zollinger-Ellison syndrome. The pharmacokinetic profile of ranitidine is similar to that of cimetidine.

Famotidine is the most potent H_2-receptor antagonist. After a 40-mg dose, mean nocturnal gastric acid secretion is reduced by 94% for up to 10 hours. It is recommended for the short-term treatment of mucosal ulcers of the gastrointestinal tract. Famotidine is absorbed incompletely. It should be used in a lower dosage and at longer dosing intervals in patients with severe renal insufficiency.

The newest H_2-receptor antagonist, nizatidine, may be used to treat and prevent recurrence of duodenal ulcers. It is also used for gastric ulcers and gastroesophageal reflux. More than 90% of an oral dose is excreted in the urine within 12 hours, and 60% as unchanged drug. Therefore, it should be used at reduced dosage in patients with severe renal insufficiency.

Adverse Effects

The list of adverse reactions for these drugs is long, but the incidence is low. Among the adverse effects associated with all four drugs are headache, dizziness, malaise, myalgia, nausea, diarrhea, constipation, rashes, pruritus, and impotence. Adverse effects, such as unusual bleeding, fever, sore throat, hallucinations, or skin rash should be reported promptly, and the therapy must be discontinued.

Contraindications and Precautions

Histamine H_2 antagonists should be avoided in patients with a known hypersensitivity, and during lactation or pregnancy. These agents are used cautiously in patients with hepatic or renal dysfunction. Cimetidine is used with caution in patients with diabetes mellitus. Histamine H_2 antagonists are used cautiously in elderly patients because they may cause confusion, and a dosage reduction may be needed. Cimetidine, famotidine, and ranitidine are pregnancy category B drugs, while nizatidine is a pregnancy category C drug. All of these drugs should be used cautiously during pregnancy and lactation.

Drug Interactions

Cimetidine increases the risk of decreased white blood cell counts with anti-metabolites and alkylating agents. It also increases serum levels and risk of toxicity of warfarin-type anticoagulants, phenytoin, beta-adrenergic blocking agents, alcohol, quinidine, lidocaine, theophylline, chloroquine, and diazepam.

Nizatidine increases serum salicylate levels with aspirin. Ranitidine also increases the effects of warfarin and toxicity of lidocaine. Ranitidine decreases the effectiveness of diazepam and its clearance.

Proton Pump Inhibitors

The final common pathway in gastric acid secretion is the proton pump adenosine triphosphatase. The physiological essence of this enzyme is the exchange of hydrogen ions for potassium ions. Thus, hydrogen is secreted by the parietal cell into the gastric lumen in exchange for potassium. Proton pump inhibitors should be taken before meals, as they are more potent when taken orally prior to food. They are also absorbed more effectively in the morning.

Mechanism of Action

Proton pump inhibitors or gastric pump inhibitors inhibit H^+ and K^+ ions, which generate gastric acids.

Indications

Proton pump inhibitors are widely used in the short-term therapy of duodenal and gastric ulcers. Proton pump inhibitor agents are also used in the treatment of GERD, gastric ulcer, and for long-term treatment of pathological hypersecretory conditions such as Zollinger-Ellison syndrome. Examples of proton pump inhibitors are shown in Table 17-3.

TABLE 17-3	Proton Pump Inhibitors		
Generic Name	Trade Name	Route of Administration	Average Adult Dosage
dexlansoprazole (deks-lan-SOH-prah-zohl)	Dexilant®	PO	30-60 mg/day for 4–8 weeks
esomeprazole magnesium (eh-soh-MEH-prah-zohl)	Nexium®	PO	20–40 mg/day
lansoprazole (lan-SOH-prah-zohl)	Prevacid®	PO	15–60 mg/day for 4 weeks
omeprazole (oh-MEH-prah-zohl)	Prilosec®	PO	20 mg once daily for 4–8 weeks
pantoprazole sodium (pan-TOH-prah-zohl)	Protonix®	PO	40 mg/day
rabeprazole sodium (rah-BEH-prah-zohl)	AcipHex®	PO	20 mg/day for 4 weeks

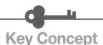

Key Concept

Goals of drug therapy for peptic ulcer include the relief of symptoms, promotion of ulcer healing, and prevention of reoccurrences.

Omeprazole is used in the treatment of acid peptic disorders. It is approved for the short-term treatment of duodenal ulcers, severe gastroesophageal reflux, and hypersecretory conditions. It is also effective in the prevention of NSAID ulcers and their complications. The antisecretory effect of omeprazole occurs within one hour, with maximum effect occurring within two hours.

Lansoprazole suppresses gastric acid formation in the stomach. Lansoprazole is indicated for the short-term treatment of acute duodenal ulcer, gastric ulcer, and erosive esophagitis. It is most effective given 30 to 60 minutes before a meal. Like other proton pump inhibitors, it is very effective in healing acid peptic disease.

Adverse Effects

Proton pump inhibitors have numerous adverse effects, but they occur infrequently. Headache, diarrhea, abdominal pain, dizziness, rash, and constipation are seen with nearly the same frequency as with the H_2 blockers.

Adverse reactions to omeprazole include headache, diarrhea, abdominal pain, nausea, dizziness, vomiting, and constipation. It is contraindicated for long-term use in patients with GERD, duodenal ulcers, and in lactating women.

Adverse effects of lansoprazole are fatigue, dizziness, headache, nausea, diarrhea, constipation, anorexia, or increased appetite.

Contraindications and Precautions

Proton pump inhibitors are contraindicated in long-term use for GERD and duodenal ulcers. They are also contraindicated in patients with hypersensitivity to these agents and children younger than two years, and during pregnancy (categories B and C). Lansoprazole should be avoided in patients with severe hepatic impairment.

Proton pump inhibitors are used with caution in patients with dysphasia, metabolic or respiratory alkalosis, and hepatic disease, and during pregnancy. Safety and efficacy in children younger than 18 years of age are not established.

Drug Interactions

Omeprazole increases serum levels and potentially increases the toxicity of benzodiazepines, phenytoin, and warfarin. This agent shows decreased absorption with sucralfate (these drugs should be given at least 30 minutes apart).

Lansoprazole decreases serum levels if taken concurrently with sucralfate. It decreases serum levels of ketoconazole and theophylline. Rabeprazole increases serum levels and potentially increases the toxicity of benzodiazepines when taken concurrently.

Treatment for *Helicobacter pylori* with Ulcer

Peptic ulcer disease is believed to be caused by high gastric secretion. *H. pylori* is found in 75% of duodenal ulcers. In chronic peptic ulcer, it has been found that eradication of the bacterium prevents ulcer relapse in about 95% of the cases. There is also a relationship between *Helicobacter* infection and adenocarcinoma of the stomach. Treatments for peptic ulcer patients usually include antacids, H$_2$-receptor antagonists, or proton pump inhibitors, but other drugs are added as necessary. For the eradication of *H. pylori* and healing of duodenal and gastric ulcers in drug therapy, special antibiotics must be added. These antibiotics include amoxicillin (Amoxil®), clarithromycin (Biaxin®), tetracycline (Achromycin®), and metronidazole (Flagyl®). Bismuth products must also be added, such as bismuth subsalicylate (Pepto-Bismol®) and ranitidine bismuth citrate. Bismuth compounds are highly effective when combined with proton pump inhibitors or antibiotics, or both. Eradication rates with these combinations are greater than 80%. Adverse effects of bismuth products include neurotoxicity, dark stools, black hairy tongue, bleeding headache, diarrhea, and abdominal pain. Also, in children, the use of these products is connected to Reye's syndrome. For the treatment of *H. pylori* with ulcer, antisecretory agents (proton pump inhibitors) should be included. Therefore, combination drugs for *H. pylori* infections should be used as follows:

- Helidac® (bismuth, metronidazole, tetracycline)
- Prevpac® (amoxicillin, clarithromycin, lansoprazole)
- Tritec® (bismuth, ranitidine)

Key Concept

Peptic ulcers are most commonly caused by the use of NSAIDs or are due to a *H. pylori* infection.

The goals of treatment of active *H. pylori*–associated ulcers are to relieve dyspeptic symptoms, to promote ulcer healing, and to eradicate *H. pylori* infection.

PANCREATIC DISORDERS

The pancreas plays an extremely important role in digestion and secretes digestive enzymes. The main pancreatic enzymes include lipase, amylase, chymotrypin, and trypsin. These enzymes aid in the digestion of fats, carbohydrates, and proteins. Fat digestion is compromised if pancreatic enzyme secretions are insufficient. The most common cause of pancreatic insufficiency is chronic pancreatitis.

Pancreatic Enzyme Replacement Therapy

Pancreatic enzyme replacements include pancreatin and pancrelipase (Table 17-4). These agents may be obtained from beef or pork pancreas, which contains the necessary enzymes to digest fats, proteins, and carbohydrates. Pancrelipase is preferred because it has more enzyme activity.

Mechanism of Action

Pancreatic enzyme replacement therapy works similarly to the way pancreatin and pancrelipase work normally in the body. These enzymes hydrolyze triglycerides to fatty acids and glycerol, proteins to oligopeptides, and starches to oligosaccharides and maltose.

Indications

Pancrelipase is used as replacement therapy in the symptomatic treatment of malabsorption syndrome due to cystic fibrosis, chronic pancreatitis, pancreatectomy, gastrointestinal bypass surgery, and cancer of the pancreas.

TABLE 17-4	Pancreatic Enzyme Replacements		
Generic Name	**Trade Name**	**Route of Administration**	**Average Adult Dosage**
pancreatin (pan-KREE-ah-tin)	Entozyme®	PO	1–3 capsules with each meal, and 1 capsule with each snack as directed by physician; may be swallowed whole with or without fluid, or contents may be sprinkled into food or drink
pancrelipase (pan-kree-LY-pays)	Cotazym®, Pancrease®, Viokase®	PO	1–3 capsules or tablets, or 1–2 packets of powder 1–2 h before, during, or 1 h after meals, with an extra dose taken with any food eaten between meals

Adverse Effects

In the recommended dosage, pancrelipase is free of adverse effects. Serious adverse effects of replacement therapy of pancreatic enzymes are rare. Common adverse effects include nausea, vomiting, anorexia, diarrhea, cramping, and hyperuricemia.

Contraindications and Precautions

Pancreatic enzyme replacement therapy is contraindicated in patients with a known history of allergy to hog protein or enzymes. These agents should be avoided in patients suffering from esophageal strictures, in those with pancreatitis, and during pregnancy (category C). Pancreatic enzyme replacement therapy should be used in lactating women with caution.

Drug Interactions

Pancreatic enzyme replacement therapy may decrease the absorption of iron.

GALLSTONE-SOLUBILIZING AGENTS

The gallbladder is a hollow organ located next to the liver that acts as the storage place for bile. Bile is formed in the liver to aid in digestion. The bile is then stored in the gallbladder to be released into the intestines as food passes.

A gallstone is a solid mass that forms in the gallbladder or the bile duct (Figure 17-4). Gallstones are usually formed by the combination of cholesterol and calcium compounds. They can produce intense pain when they block the bile duct. Gallstone-solubilizing agents include ursodiol and chenodiol. Only ursodiol is sold in the United States.

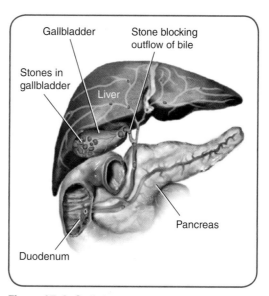

Figure 17-4 Gallstones.

Mechanism of Action

Ursodiol is a naturally occurring bile acid that is made by the liver and secreted in bile. It blocks the liver enzyme that produces cholesterol, and thereby decreases production of cholesterol by the liver and the amount of cholesterol in bile. It also reduces the absorption of cholesterol from the intestine. By decreasing the concentration of cholesterol in bile, it prevents the formation and promotes the dissolution of cholesterol-containing gallstones.

Indications

Ursodiol is used to prevent cholesterol gallstones from forming during rapid loss of weight. It is also used to dissolve cholesterol gallstones that do not contain calcium and are less than 2 cm in diameter. It is also used to treat primary biliary cirrhosis.

Adverse Effects

The most common adverse effects are rash, itching, nausea, vomiting, stomach pain, back pain, constipation, and diarrhea.

Contraindications and Precautions

Contraindications include hypersensitivity to ursodiol, bile acids, or any component of the formulation, high cholesterol, radiopaque substances, bile pigment stones, stones greater than 20 mm in diameter, and allergy to bile acids.

Gallstone-solubilizing agents should be used with caution in patients with a nonvisualizing gallbladder and those with chronic liver disease. Ursodiol is not recommended for use in children.

Drug Interactions

Aluminum-containing antacids, cholestyramine, and colestipol reduce the absorption of ursodiol and therefore reduce its action.

DIARRHEA

Diarrhea is the manifestation of many illnesses. Its etiology includes infections (bacterial, viral, fungal, and parasitic), irritable bowel syndrome, inflammatory bowel disease (ulcerative colitis and Crohn's disease), toxins (food poisoning), drugs, and other causes. Treatment should be directed to the underlying cause.

Irritable bowel syndrome (IBS) is a common disorder that affects the large intestine, causing cramping, abdominal pain, bloating, gas, diarrhea, and constipation. It is a chronic condition requiring long-term management. To manage IBS, dietary changes include elimination of high-gas foods, gluten, and certain sugars. Medications include fiber supplements, antidiarrheals, anticholinergics, antispasmodics, antidepressants, and antibiotics.

Inflammatory bowel disease (IBD), which comprises ulcerative colitis and Crohn's disease, involves chronic inflammation of the digestive tract. It causes severe diarrhea, pain, fatigue, and weight loss. Ulcerative colitis causes chronic inflammation and ulcers in the large intestine and rectum. Crohn's disease often spreads deep into affected tissues and may also involve the small intestine. For IBD, medications include antiinflammatories, immunosuppressants, antibiotics, antidiarrheals, analgesics, iron supplements, vitamin B_{12} injections, calcium and vitamin D supplements, and improved enteral nutrition or parenteral nutrition therapy. Table 17-5 lists medications used for IBS and IBD.

TABLE 17-5 | **Drugs Used to Treat Irritable Bowel Syndrome and Inflammatory Bowel Disease**

Generic Name	Trade Name	Route of Administration	Average Adult Dosage
adalimumab **(ay-dah-LIM-yoo-mab)**	Humira®	SC	160 mg initially on day 1, given as four 40-mg injections in one day or as two 40-mg injections per day for 2 consecutive days, followed by 80 mg 2 weeks later (day 15); 2 weeks later (day 29), continue with dose of 40 mg every other week
alosetron hydrochloride **(ah-LO-seh-tron hy-droh-KLOH-ryd)**	Lotronex®	PO	Start at 0.5 mg bid, stopping if constipation occurs; may be restarted at 0.5 mg qd, but then stop completely if constipation recurs
atropine, hyoscyamine, phenobarbital, scopolamine **(AT-ro-peen, hy-oh-SY-ah-meen, fee-no-BAR-bih-tol, sko-PO-lah-meen)**	Donnatal Extentabs®	PO	1 tablet q12h; if necessary, 1 tablet q8h
budesonide **(byoo-DEH-so-nyd)**	Entocort EC®	PO	9 mg once daily in a.m. for up to 8 weeks; repeated 8 week courses can be given for recurring episodes
chlordiazepoxide, clidinium **(klor-dy-ah-zeh-POK-zyd, kiln-DIN-ee-um)**	Librax®	PO	Dose should be smallest effective amount; initial dose should not exceed 2 capsules per day, increased gradually prn
dicyclomine **(dy-SY-klo-meen)**	Bentyl®	PO, IM	PO: 20 mg qid; after 1 week, may increase to 40 mg qid prn; IM: 10–20 mg qid for 1–2 days when oral medication cannot be taken
infliximab **(in-FLIK-zih-mab)**	Remicade®	IV induction	5 mg/kg at 0, 2, and 6 weeks, followed by maintenance of 5 mg/kg q8 wk

continued on next page

Table 17-5 continued

lubiprostone (loo-bih-PROS-tohn)	Amitiza®	PO	8 mcg bid with food and water
mesalamine (meh-SAL-ah-meen)	Asacol®	PO	Two 400 mg tablets tid with or without food (total daily dose 2.4 g), for 6 weeks
sulfasalazine (sul-fah-SAL-ah-zeen)	Sulfazine®	PO	3–4 g/day in evenly divided doses

Antidiarrheals

It is occasionally necessary to use antidiarrheals for convenience, or for conditions for which there is no primary treatment. The most commonly used antidiarrheals are anticholinergics, opioid narcotics, meperidine congeners (diphenoxylate), and loperamide. Opioid antidiarrheals are the most effective drugs for controlling diarrhea. Selected agents used to treat diarrhea are shown in Table 17-6.

Mechanism of Action

The mechanism of action for anticholinergics and opioid narcotics is discussed in Chapters 7 and 22.

Indications

Antidiarrheal agents are used to treat diarrhea, a symptom of bowel disorders, and not the disorder itself. The management of diarrhea depends on finding the underlying cause, replacing water and electrolytes as needed, reducing cramping, and reducing the passage of stools. Diarrhea is usually

TABLE 17-6	Drugs Used to Treat Diarrhea			
Generic Name	**Trade Name**	**Route of Administration**	**Average Adult Dosage**
bismuth subsalicylate (BIS-muth sub-sah-lih-SY-layt)	Pepto-Bismol®	PO	2 tablets qid with 2 additional antibiotics for 10–14 days
camphorated opium tincture (C-III) (KAM-foh-ray-ted OH-pee-um TINK-chur)	Paregoric®	PO	5–10 mL after loose stool, q2h up to qid prn
difenoxin with atropine (dy-feh-NOK-sin with AH-troh-peen)	Motofen®	PO	1–8 mg/day
diphenoxylate with atropine (dy-fen-OK-sih-layt with AH-troh-peen)	Lomotil®	PO	1–2 tablets or 5–10 mL tid–qid
loperamide (loh-PEH-rah-myd)	Imodium®	PO	4 mg as a single dose, then 2 mg after each diarrhea episode

self-limiting and resolves without further effects. Diarrhea in children may become a medical emergency in as little as 24 hours because of the loss of electrolytes.

Adverse Effects

Adverse effects of antidiarrheal drugs commonly include nausea, vomiting, anorexia, constipation, drowsiness, sedation, euphoria, headache, dizziness, drowsiness, and rash. Diphenoxylate is a narcotic-related agent that has no analgesic activity, but causes sedation and euphoria. Generally, this drug is combined with atropine (an anticholinergic drug), which may produce dry mouth.

Contraindications and Precautions

Antidiarrheal drugs are contraindicated in patients with pseudomembranous colitis, abdominal pain of unknown origin, or obstructive jaundice. These agents should be avoided in children younger than two years.

Antidiarrheals are used with caution in patients with severe liver impairment or IBD. They should be used cautiously in pregnant women (category B).

Drug Interactions

Concurrent use of antidiarrheals with a monoamine oxidase inhibitor increases the risk of a hypertensive crisis. Antidiarrheals may cause an additive central nervous system depression when given with antihistamines, sedatives, hypnotics, alcohol, and narcotics.

GAS RETENTION

The production of excessive gas necessitates relief of gastric and intestinal distention. Gas retention is caused by air swallowing, peptic ulcer, dyspepsia, irritable bowel disease, and diverticulitis. Other factors for production of gas in the gastrointestinal tract include gas-forming foods such as beans, onions, and cabbage, or after gastroscopy, and bowel radiography.

Antiflatulents

Medications for excessive gas, or to prevent formation of gas in the gastrointestinal tract, include some antacids or carminatives (substances that stimulate the expulsion of gas from the tract, and also increase muscle tone, thereby stimulating peristalsis), that are available as OTC drugs. Simethicone is the most common active ingredient used, in such trade names as Phazyme®, Mylanta®, and Gas-X®. Simethicone disperses in the gastrointestinal tract, and prevents the formation of gas pockets in the tract. For infants and children, *simethicone oral drops* are administered to relieve symptoms of extra gas caused by swallowing air, infant formulas, and certain foods. Simethicone works by breaking up gas bubbles in the gastrointestinal tract.

Mechanism of Action

The actual mechanism of action for antiflatulents is unknown, but the predominant theory is that these agents reduce the surface tension of small air bubbles trapped in the gastrointestinal tract. This allows them to coalesce into larger bubbles, which are more easily eliminated than the smaller ones.

Indications

Antiflatulents are used to prevent the formation of gas in the gastrointestinal tract. Gas retention is a problem in conditions of air swallowing, diverticulitis (inflammation of the colon), peptic ulcer, IBD, and dyspepsia. Another use of antiflatulents is to relieve gas following gastroscopy and bowel radiography.

Adverse Effects

Antiflatulents are generally safe and have no side effects.

Contraindications and Precautions

Antiflatulents are contraindicated in patients with a known hypersensitivity to any component of these drugs. Charcoal should be used in pregnant women with caution (category C).

Drug Interactions

There are no reported drug interactions with antiflatulents.

CONSTIPATION

Constipation is the difficult or infrequent passage of stool. Normal stool frequency ranges from two to three times daily to two to three times per week. Since constipation is a symptom rather than a disease, medical evaluation should be undertaken in patients who develop constipation.

Laxatives

Laxatives are drugs that either accelerate fecal passage or decrease fecal consistency. They work by promoting one or more of the mechanisms that cause diarrhea. Because of the wide availability and marketing of OTC laxatives, there is a potential that an appropriate diagnosis will not be sought. Table 17-7 shows the most commonly used laxatives.

Mechanism of Action

Laxatives are divided into several categories as a function of their mechanisms of action, including bulk-forming, saline or osmotic, stimulant, lubricant, and stool softeners (also called emollient laxatives). Laxatives should not be taken if nausea, vomiting, or abdominal pain is present.

TABLE 17-7	Commonly Used Laxatives		
Generic Name	Trade Name	Route of Administration	Average Adult Dosage
Bulk-Forming			
methylcellulose **(meh-thil-SEL-yoo-lohs)**	Citrucel®	PO	500–6000 mg/day
polycarbophil **(paw-lee-KAR-boh-fil)**	Equalactin®, FiberNorm®	PO	1 g qid prn (max: 6 g/day)
psyllium hydrophilic muciloid **(SIL-lee-um hy-droh-FIH-lik MYOO-sih-loyd)**	Metamucil®	PO	1–2 tsp in 8 oz water up to qid
Saline or Osmotic			
glycerin **(GLIH-seh-rin)**	Fleet Babylax®, Glycerol®	Rectal	1 suppository or 5–15 mL enema (inserted high into rectum and retained for 15 min)
lactulose **(LAK-too-lohs)**	Cephulac®	PO	30–60 mL/day prn
magnesium citrate **(mag-NEE-zee-um SY-trayt)**	Citrate of Magnesia®	PO	1000–6000 mg/day
magnesium hydroxide **(mag-NEE-zee-um hy-DROK-syd)**	Phillips' Milk of Magnesia®	PO	15 mL hs
sodium biphosphate / sodium phosphate **(SOH-dee-um by-FOS-fayt / SOH-dee-um FOS-fayt)**	Fleet Enema®	PO	133 mL/day
sorbitol **(SOR-bih-tol)**	Sorbitol systemic®	PO, Rectal	PO: 30–150 mL/day Rectal: 120 mL (25% to 30% solution) once
Stimulant			
bisacodyl **(bih-sah-KOH-dil)**	Dulcolax®	PO, Rectal	PO: 5–15 mg prn; Rectal: 1 suppository
castor oil **(KAS-tor OYL)**	Emulsoil®, Purge®	PO	15–60 mL/day prn
cascara sagrada **(kas-KAH-rah sah-GRAH-dah)**	Cascara Sagrada® (fluid extract)	PO	0.5–1.5 mL/day
Lubricant			
mineral oil **(MIH-neh-ral OYL)**	Kondremul®	PO	2–15 tsp/day

continued on next page

Table 17-7 continued

Stool Softeners (Emollient Laxatives)

docusate calcium **(DOK-yoo-sayt KAL-see-um)**	Surfak®	PO, Rectal	PO: 50–500 mg/day; Rectal: 50–100 mg added to enema fluid
docusate potassium **(DOK-yoo-sayt poh-TAH-see-um)**	Dialose®	PO, Rectal	PO: 1–3 capsules/day; Rectal: 1 suppository
docusate sodium **(DOK-yoo-sayt SOH-dee-um)**	Colace®	PO, Rectal	PO: 1–4 tablets or capsules/day; Rectal: 200 to 283 mg administered as an enema, once or twice.

> ### Key Concept
>
> All bulk-forming agents must be given with at least 8 oz of water to minimize the possible constipation experienced by some patients.

Bulk-forming laxatives are natural or synthetic polysaccharide derivatives that absorb water to soften the stool and increase bulk, which stimulates peristalsis. Bulk-forming laxatives work in both the small and large intestines. The onset of action of these agents is slow, usually occurring between 12 and 72 hours.

Saline laxatives (or *osmotic laxatives*) create an *osmotic* effect that increases the water content and volume of the stool. This increased volume results in distention of the intestinal lumen, causing increased peristalsis and bowel motility. The onset of action varies depending on the effect and dosage form. Rectal formulations such as enemas or suppositories have an onset of action of 5 to 30 minutes, whereas oral preparations work within 3 to 6 hours.

Stimulant laxatives work in the small and large intestine to stimulate bowel motility and increase the secretion of fluids into the bowel. The oral preparations usually have an onset of action within 6 to 10 hours. Rectal preparations usually have an onset of action within 30 to 60 minutes.

Mineral oil, which is a **lubricant laxative**, works in the colon to increase water retention and soften the stool. Mineral oil has an onset of action of between 6 and 8 hours.

Stool softeners decrease the consistency of stools by reducing the surface tension. Stool softeners permit easier penetration and mixing of fats and fluids with the fecal mass. This results in a softer, more easily passed stool. Docusate (Colace®) acts as a detergent and stool softener. It usually takes one to three days to be effective. Stool softeners have a wide margin of safety and few potential adverse reactions. Stool softeners are combined with laxatives in such medications as Peri-Colace® and Doxidan® to soften stools while enhancing stool evacuation (see Table 17-7). They are also known as **emollient laxatives**, and are not considered the drugs of choice for severe acute constipation. They are more useful for preventing constipation.

Indications

Laxatives are used prophylactically in patients who should avoid straining during defecation, and for treatment of constipation associated with hard, dry stools. They are prescribed for short-term relief of constipation. Certain laxatives are indicated to empty the large intestine for rectal and bowel examinations. Emollient laxatives are particularly useful in patients who must avoid straining to pass hard stools, such as patients who have had a recent myocardial infarction or rectal surgery.

Adverse Effects

Stool softeners have a wide margin of safety and few potential adverse reactions. High doses or prolonged use of laxatives may cause diarrhea and a loss of water and electrolytes. Serious adverse effects include abdominal pain, perianal irritation, fainting, and weakness.

Contraindications and Precautions

Laxatives are contraindicated in patients with a known hypersensitivity, acute appendicitis, intestinal obstruction, fecal impaction, and acute hepatitis. Laxatives should be used cautiously in patients with rectal bleeding, in pregnant women (category C), and during lactation. Magnesium hydroxide is used with caution in patients with renal impairment.

Drug Interactions

Mineral oil may impair gastrointestinal tract absorption of fat-soluble vitamins (A, D, E, and K).

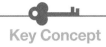

Key Concept

Specialized laxatives are used to prepare patients for colonoscopies. The preferred preparations contain polyethylene glycol, and are known as "PEG preps." These laxatives draw water out of the intestinal lining and also contain sodium and potassium to replace lost electrolytes. They provide extreme cleansing of the colon and rectum.

VOMITING

The causes of vomiting include infectious diseases that can directly irritate vomiting centers to inhibit impulses going to the stomach. Certain drugs, radiation, and chemotherapy may irritate the gastrointestinal tract or stimulate the chemoreceptor trigger zone and vomiting center in the brain (medulla). After surgery, particularly abdominal surgery, nausea and vomiting are common. The main neurotransmitters that produce nausea and vomiting include dopamine, serotonin, and acetylcholine. Persistent vomiting may cause dehydration, imbalance of electrolytes, metabolic alkalosis, and arrhythmias, which in turn, may precipitate further vomiting.

Emetics

An **emetic** is a drug that induces vomiting. Emetics such as apomorphine, morphine, and digitalis may act directly by stimulation of the medulla oblongata, or they may act reflexively by irritant action on the gastrointestinal tract (e.g., copper sulfate, mustard, sodium chloride, and zinc sulfate).

Key Concept

A nasogastric tube is a safer and more efficient tool for emptying the stomach than the use of emetics.

Mechanism of Action

The emetic known as ipecac induces vomiting by stimulating the chemoreceptors of the vomiting reflex, and by the irritation of the gastric mucosa. Approximately 80% to 90% of people taking the medication begin vomiting within 20 to 30 minutes.

In most cases, ipecac is not absorbed because it is removed in vomitus. The effects of ipecac are stopped with activated charcoal.

Indications

Emetics are drugs used to promote vomiting, usually in cases of poisoning or drug overdose. The nearest poison control center should be called prior to using these medications. Syrup of ipecac is the OTC drug used to bring about vomiting and should be included in any home emergency kit.

Adverse Effects

There are no serious adverse effects to ipecac. The only problem associated with use of any emetic is the aspiration of stomach contents.

Contraindications and Precautions

Emetics should not be used in patients who are unconscious or semi-comatose, or in whom coma is expected imminently. These agents should not be used in patients with severe heart disease or advanced pregnancy. They are contraindicated in poisoning caused by corrosive or petroleum products. Safe use in pregnancy has not been established (category C).

Drug Interactions

Drug interactions with emetic drugs are rare. Other medications should not be taken with syrup of ipecac, as the rapid onset of vomiting will not allow enough time for the other medications to be absorbed.

Antiemetics

Antiemetics are used to prevent or relieve nausea and vomiting that are associated with many different disorders. Table 17-8 shows the most commonly used antiemetics.

Mechanism of Action

The mechanism of action of antiemetics is largely unknown, except that they help to relax the portion of the brain that controls the muscles that cause vomiting. Some of these agents, such as prochlorperazine, depress the center of vomiting in the medulla.

Indications

Several classes of drugs used as antiemetics are discussed in other chapters of this book. These agents are used for the treatment of drug overdose and

Key Concept

The administration of ipecac should be followed by a full 8-oz glass of water to promote vomiting. If vomiting does not occur in 30 minutes, another dose may be given.

Key Concept

The misuse of ipecac syrup has occurred in persons with eating disorders, such as bulimia, which may result in ipecac toxicity (muscle weakness and cardiotoxic effects).

TABLE 17-8 | Common Antiemetic Agents

Generic Name	Trade Name	Route of Administration	Average Adult Dosage
Antihistamines and Anticholinergics			
cyclizine hydrochloride **(SY-klih-zeen hy-droh-KLOR-ryd)**	Marezine®	PO	50 mg q4–6h
dimenhydrinate **(dy-men-HY-drih-nayt)**	Calm-x®, Dramamine®	PO	50–100 mg q4–6h
meclizine hydrochloride **(MEH-klih-zeen hy-droh-KLOR-ryd)**	Antrizine®, Bonamine®	PO	25–50 mg/day
scopolamine **(skoh-PAW-lah-meen)**	Transderm-Scop®, Transderm-V®	Transdermal	1 patch q72h starting 12 h before anticipated travel
Corticosteroids			
dexamethasone **(dek-sah-MEH-thah-zohn)**	Decadron®	PO	0.25–4 mg bid–qid
methylprednisolone sodium succinate **(meh-thil-pred-NIH-soh-lohn SO-dee-um SUK-sih-nayt)**	Solu-Medrol®	PO	2–60 mg/day in divided doses
Dopamine Antagonists			
droperidol **(droh-PEH-rih-dol)**	Inapsine®	IM, IV	2.5 mg; additional doses of 1.25 may be given
metoclopramide hydrochloride **(meh-toh-KLOH-prah-myd hy-droh-KLOR-ryd)**	Reglan®	IM, IV	10–20 mg near end of surgery
promethazine hydrochloride **(pro-MEH-thah-zeen hy-droh-KLOR-ryd)**	Phenergan®, Prometh®	PO, IM, IV	12.5–25 mg q4–6h prn
Sedatives			
diazepam **(dy-AH-zeh-pam)**	Diastat®, Valium®	PO, IM, IV	2–30 mg/day
lorazepam **(loh-RAH-zeh-pam)**	Ativan®	IV	1–1.5 mg prior to chemotherapy
Serotonin Receptor Antagonists			
dolasetron mesylate **(doh-lah-SEH-tron MEH-sih-layt)**	Anzemet®	PO	100 mg/day 1 h prior to chemotherapy
granisetron **(grah-nih-SEH-tron)**	Kytril®	IV	10 mcg/kg 30 min prior to chemotherapy

continued on next page

Table 17-8 continued

ondansetron hydrochloride **(on-DAN-seh-TRON** **hy-droh-KLOR-ryd)**	Zofran®	PO	4 mg tid prn (0.25 mg); 30 min prior to chemotherapy
palonosetron **(pah-loh-NOH-seh-tron)**	Aloxi®	IV	0.25 mg infused over 30 sec (30 min prior to chemotherapy)
Neurokinin Receptor Antagonist			
aprepitant **(ah-PREH-pih-tant)**	Emend®	PO	125 mg 1 h prior to chemotherapy

for certain poisonings. They are also prescribed for conditions that are associated with vomiting, postchemotherapy, for motion sickness, and during pregnancy.

Phenothiazines are the largest group of drugs used for severe nausea and vomiting. Prochlorperazine is the most commonly prescribed antiemetic medication in this group.

Adverse Effects

Since drowsiness is common to most of the antiemetics, patients should be cautioned not to drive or operate hazardous machinery while taking these drugs. Dose-related anticholinergics adverse effects, such as dry mouth, constipation, and tachycardia, are common.

Contraindications and Precautions

Antiemetics are contraindicated in patients with hypersensitivity to these drugs. They are also contraindicated in children younger than two years of age, and during pregnancy (category C). Antiemetics are used with caution in children, pregnant women, and dehydrated patients.

Drug Interactions

Antiemetics may have differing drug interactions based on their types. For example, serotonin antagonists usually have no drug interactions, while dopamine is affected by antiemetics, which are antagonistic. Prochlorperazine interacts with alcohol to increase central nervous system depression. Antacids and antidiarrheals inhibit absorption of this agent.

> **Key Concept**
>
> Transdermal scopolamine is a 72-hour patch that is placed behind the ear.

ADSORBENTS

Adsorbent agents have the ability to adsorb gases, toxins, and bacteria. Only certain materials that possess chemical adsorptive properties lend themselves effectively to detoxification and to the adsorption of gases resulting from abnormal intestinal fermentation. Such substances are kaolin and activated charcoal. Many of the nonsystemic antacids may serve as internal protectives and adsorbents. Antacids commonly are combined with kaolin or other adsorbents.

Mechanism of Action

These agents adsorb bacterial toxins that might be implicated in causing diarrhea or adsorb toxic substances swallowed into the gastrointestinal tract by inhibiting gastric adsorption. Adsorbents work by increasing the viscosity of the gut contents, and forming sludge.

Indications

Adsorbents are used for acute treatment of poisoning, primarily as an emergency antidote in many forms of poisoning. They are the emergency treatment of choice for virtually all drugs and chemicals. Charcoal capsules are also used for the relief of flatulence and the discomfort of abdominal gas.

Adverse Effects

Adverse effects include vomiting (related to rapid ingestion of high doses), constipation, diarrhea, and black stools.

Contraindications and Precautions

Adsorbents are contraindicated in patients with suspected obstructive bowel lesion and pseudomembranous colitis. These agents should not be used for more than two days without medical direction. Safety during pregnancy (category C) or lactation is not established. Adsorbents should be used cautiously in infants or children younger than three years, and in elderly patients.

Drug Interactions

Adsorbents such as activated charcoal can inactivate syrup of ipecac and laxatives. Adsorbents decrease the effectiveness of other medications.

SUMMARY

The functions of the gastrointestinal tract include digestion, storage, food absorption, and waste elimination. Several varieties of drugs are used to treat disorders of the gastrointestinal system, including antacids, H_2-receptor antagonists, proton pump inhibitors, antidiarrheals, laxatives, antiemetics, and adsorbents. Gastric ulcer, duodenal ulcer, and GERD are accompanied by increased secretion of hydrochloric acid, for which antacids, prostaglandin E_1 analogs, H_2-receptor antagonists, and proton pump inhibitors should be used. Peptic ulcer, which may be caused by *H. pylori* bacteria, should be treated with the combination of special antibiotics, bismuth products, and proton pump inhibitor drugs. There are several different laxative drugs that either accelerate fecal passage or decrease fecal consistency. Antiemetics are used to prevent or relieve nausea and vomiting. Adsorbents are used primarily as emergency antidotes in many forms of poisoning.

EXPLORING THE WEB

Visit *http://digestive.niddk.nih.gov*

- Search for additional information about the digestive diseases and disorders discussed in this chapter. Enhance your understanding of the function of the digestive system and the drug therapies used to treat disorders of the digestive system.

Visit *http://familydoctor.org*

- Search for OTC remedies to relieve gastrointestinal symptoms.

Visit *www.medicalnewstoday.com*

- Search for the various types of drugs discussed in this chapter. Is there new information about or research being done on these types of drugs?

REVIEW QUESTIONS

Multiple Choice

1. Gastrin is released from the stomach and acts primarily to release:
   A. histamine
   B. pepsin
   C. pancreatic enzymes
   D. all of the above

2. The generic name of Amphojel® is:
   A. magaldrate
   B. sodium bicarbonate
   C. aluminum hydroxide
   D. calcium carbonate

3. Sodium bicarbonate is contraindicated in patients with:
   A. congestive heart failure
   B. severe renal disease
   C. hypertension
   D. all of the above

4. Which of the following H_2-receptor antagonists was the first drug approved for clinical use?
   A. famotidine
   B. nizatidine
   C. ranitidine
   D. cimetidine

5. The generic name of Axid® is:

   A. cimetidine

   B. nizatidine

   C. famotidine

   D. ranitidine

6. Which of the following types of laxatives is particularly useful in patients who have recently had rectal surgery to avoid straining to pass hard stools?

   A. lubricant

   B. emollient

   C. saline

   D. stimulant

7. Which of the following is the generic name of Dulcolax®?

   A. bisacodyl

   B. docusate

   C. senna

   D. cascara sagrada

8. For eradication of *Helicobacter pylori* with ulcer, you should combine:

   A. bismuth products and proton pump inhibitors

   B. antibiotics, bismuth, and proton pump inhibitors

   C. proton pump inhibitors and antibiotics

   D. antibiotics and bismuth products

9. The generic name of Tagamet® is:

   A. ranitidine

   B. nizatidine

   C. famotidine

   D. cimetidine

10. Chronic administration of calcium carbonate-containing antacids may cause:

    A. hyperparathyroidism

    B. hypercalcemia

    C. hypertension

    D. hyperglycemia

11. Activated charcoal is used therapeutically for which of the following purposes?

    A. increased effectiveness of other medications

    B. decreased blood glucose level

    C. relief of vomiting and diarrhea

    D. relief of flatulence and the discomfort of abdominal gas

12. Which of the following agents is used for treatment of vomiting after chemotherapy?

    A. mineral oil

    B. scopolamine patch

    C. senna

    D. magnesium citrate

13. The trade name of diphenoxylate with atropine is:

    A. Imodium®

    B. Furoxone®

    C. Lomotil®

    D. Motofen®

14. Which of the following is an adverse effect of antiflatulents?

    A. coma

    B. vomiting

    C. headache

    D. generally none

15. Cytotec® carries a Black Box Warning against use in pregnant women, and is in pregnancy category:

    A. D

    B. X

    C. A

    D. C

Matching

Generic Name	Trade Name
_____1. lansoprazole	A. Pepcid®
_____2. cimetidine	B. Axid®
_____3. omeprazole	C. AcipHex®
_____4. ranitidine	D. Tagamet®
_____5. rabeprazole sodium	E. Prevacid®
_____6. famotidine	F. Zantac®
_____7. nizatidine	G. Prilosec®

Fill in the Blank

1. What are the indications for antacids?

   _____

2. What is the mechanism of action of H_2-receptor antagonists?

   _____

3. What are the most serious adverse effects of mineral oil laxatives?

   _____

Critical Thinking

A 45-year-old male patient was diagnosed with gastritis caused by *Helicobacter pylori*. He exhibited symptoms of this disorder for more than 15 months, and did not take any medications or see any physicians before this visit.

1. List medications that may be used to treat this disorder.

2. If this disorder remains untreated, what would the probable consequences be?

3. Explain why *H. pylori*, rather than other microorganisms, is a focus of drug therapy for patients with ulcers of the stomach.

CHAPTER 18

Hormonal Therapy for Endocrine Gland Disorders

OBJECTIVES

After completing this chapter, the reader should be able to:

1. Explain the location of the major endocrine glands and their hormone secretion.
2. Define the term *hormone* and list the hormones that are secreted from the anterior pituitary gland.
3. Describe the effect of thyroxine on the body organs.
4. Compare and contrast the roles of calcitonin and parathyroid hormone.
5. Compare and contrast the functions of the pancreatic hormones.
6. Explain diabetes mellitus.
7. Name some risk factors for development of diabetes mellitus in older adults.
8. Identify the different types of insulin.
9. Explain the primary functions of the adrenal cortex.
10. Explain the key factors in behavior modification for diabetes.

GLOSSARY

Acromegaly – a chronic metabolic condition in adults, caused by oversecretion of growth hormones by the pituitary gland

Adrenocorticotropic hormone (ACTH) – a hormone from the anterior pituitary gland that stimulates the growth of the adrenal gland cortex and the secretion of corticosteroids

Adrenogenital syndrome – congenital adrenal hyperplasia; a group of disorders involving steroid hormone production in the adrenal glands, leading to a deficiency of cortisol; also called *adrenal virilism*

Androgen – the generic term for any natural or synthetic compound, usually a steroid hormone, that stimulates or controls the development of masculine characteristics by binding to androgen receptors

Antidiuretic hormone (ADH) – a hormone released by the pituitary gland when the body is low on water, causing the kidneys to conserve water, but not salt, by concentrating the urine and reducing urine volume; also called *vasopressin*

Antithyroid drug – a chemical agent that lowers the basal metabolic rate by interfering with the formation, release, or action of thyroid hormones

Calcitonin (CT) – a hormone produced primarily by the parafollicular cells of the thyroid gland

Conn's syndrome – a disease of the adrenal glands involving excess production of the hormone aldosterone

Cushing's syndrome – a disease caused by the excessive body production of cortisol; it can also be caused by excessive use of cortisol or other steroid hormones

Diabetes mellitus – a complex disorder of carbohydrate, fat, and protein metabolism caused by lack of or inefficient use of insulin in the body; classified as type 1 (insulin-dependent diabetes mellitus [IDDM]), or type 2 (non-insulin-dependent diabetes mellitus [NIDDM])

Dwarfism – a condition of lack of growth of the arms and legs in proportion to the head and trunk; it may be caused by over 200 medical disorders, including achondroplasia, kidney disease, genetic

OUTLINE (*cont.*)

conditions, and problems with hormones or metabolism

Epiphyses – the ends of long bones that are originally separated from the main bone by a layer of cartilage, becoming unified through ossification

Galactorrhea – abnormal secretion of breast milk in men, or in women who are not breastfeeding an infant

Gigantism – an abnormal condition characterized by excessive size and stature; it is caused by hypersecretion of growth hormone before puberty

Glucagon – a hormone produced in the pancreas that increases blood sugar

Graves' disease – an autoimmune disorder that involves overactivity of the thyroid gland (hyperthyroidism)

Growth hormone (GH) – a peptide hormone and protein secreted by the anterior pituitary gland in response to growth hormone-releasing hormone (GHRH)

Hirsuitism – excessive hair growth on the face, abdomen, breasts, and back

Hormones – chemical messengers that serve as signals to target cells; they are produced by nearly every organ system and type of tissue

Hyperactive – abnormally and easily excitable or exuberant

Hypercalcemia – an excessive amount of calcium in the blood

Hyperpituitarism – a condition that results in the excess secretion of hormones from the pituitary gland

Hyperprolactinemia – increased levels of prolactin in the blood, often linked to a pituitary adenoma

Hyperthyroidism – a condition of excessive amounts of thyroxine

Hypoactive – abnormally inactive

Hypothalamus – the part of the brain that lies below the thalamus; it regulates body temperature, certain metabolic processes, and other autonomic activities

Hypothyroidism – a deficiency disease that causes cretinism (mental and physical retardation) in children

Insulin – a hormone secreted by the pancreas that regulates carbohydrate and fat metabolism, especially the conversion of glucose to glycogen

Lugol's solution – Lugol's iodine; a solution of iodine often used as an antiseptic, disinfectant, or starch indicator, to replenish iodine deficiency, to protect the thyroid from radioactive materials, and for emergency disinfection of drinking water

Luteinizing hormone (LH) – a hormone secreted by the anterior lobe of the pituitary gland that is necessary for proper reproductive function

Mineralocorticoids – steroid hormones that influence salt and water balance; they are released from the adrenal cortex

Myxedema – condition of thyroid insufficiency or resistance to thyroid hormone

Negative feedback system – a method by which regulation of hormones is achieved; release occurs in response to concentration in the blood

Oxytocin (OT) – a hormone that also acts as a neurotransmitter in the brain; in women, it is released during labor and lactation

Parathyroid hormone (PTH) – a hormone secreted by the parathyroid glands that increases the levels of calcium in the blood; also called *parathormone*

Prolactin (PRL) – a hormone that is primarily associated with lactation; it is secreted from the anterior pituitary gland

Spermatogenesis – the process by which male gametes develop into mature spermatozoa

Steroids – numerous naturally occurring or synthetic fat-soluble organic compounds that include sterols, bile acids, adrenal hormones, sex hormones, digitalis compounds, and certain vitamin precursors

Thyroid-stimulating hormone (TSH) – a hormone secreted by the anterior lobe of the pituitary gland that controls the release of thyroid hormone and is necessary for the growth and function of the thyroid gland

Thyroxine (T_4) – the major hormone secreted by the follicular cells of the thyroid gland

OVERVIEW

The endocrine system consists of specialized cell clusters, glands, hormones, and target tissues. The glands and cell clusters secrete hormones and chemical transmitters in response to stimulation from the nervous system and other sites. Together with the nervous system, the endocrine system regulates and integrates the body's metabolic activities, and maintains internal homeostasis. Each target tissue has receptors for specific hormones. Hormones connect with the receptors, and the resulting hormone-receptor complex triggers the target cell's response.

The overactivity or underactivity of a gland is the malfunction that most commonly causes endocrine disease. If a gland secretes an excessive amount of its hormone, it is **hyperactive**. When a gland fails to secrete its hormone or secretes an inadequate amount, it is **hypoactive**.

ANATOMY REVIEW

- The major glands of the endocrine system include the pituitary, pineal, thyroid, parathyroid, thymus, adrenals, pancreas, and the gonads (Figure 18-1).

- Endocrine glands secrete **hormones**, or chemical messengers, directly into the bloodstream. These hormones coordinate and direct activities of specific target cells or organs.

- Each gland releases a specific hormone or hormones and generates specific effects (Table 18-1).

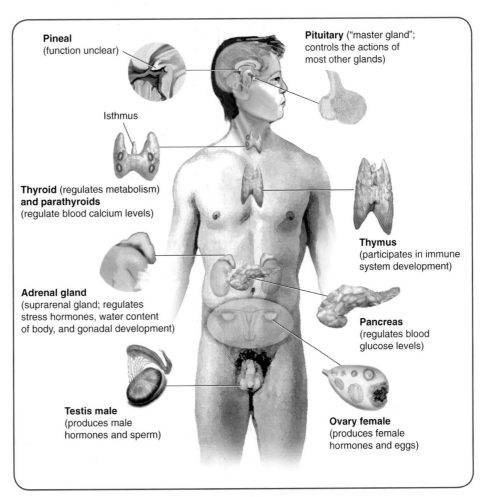

Figure 18-1 Location of the endocrine glands.

TABLE 18-1	Sources and Effects of Major Hormones	
Source	**Hormone**	**Primary Effects**
Hypothalamus	Hypothalamic-releasing hormones	Stimuli to anterior pituitary to release specific hormone; decrease release of specific hormone by anterior pituitary
Pituitary – anterior lobe (adenohypophysis)	Growth hormone (GH, somatotropin)	Stimulates synthesis of protein
	Adrenocorticotropic hormone (ACTH)	Stimulates secretion of (primarily) cortisol from adrenal cortex
	Thyroid-stimulating hormone (TSH)	Stimulates thyroid gland
	Follicle-stimulating hormone (FSH)	In women: stimulates ovarian follicle growth and estrogen secretion; in men: stimulates sperm production
	Luteinizing hormone (LH)	In women: stimulates ovum maturation and ovulation; in men: stimulates testosterone secretion
Pituitary – posterior lobe (neurohypophysis)	Prolactin (PRL)	Stimulates milk production during lactation
	Antidiuretic hormone (ADH, or vasopressin)	Increases kidney reabsorption of water
	Oxytocin	Stimulates uterine contractions after delivery; stimulates milk ejection during lactation
Pancreas – beta cells of islets of Langerhans	Insulin	Transports glucose and other substances into cells; lowers blood glucose levels
Pancreas – alpha cells	Glucagon	Increases blood glucose level; glycogenolysis in the liver
Parathyroid gland	Parathyroid hormone (PTH)	Increases blood calcium levels by stimulating bone demineralization; increases absorption of serum calcium in kidneys and digestive tract
Thyroid gland	Calcitonin	Decreases calcium release from bones to lower blood calcium levels
	Thyroxine (T_4) and triiodothyronine (T_3)	Increase cellular metabolic rates
Adrenal cortex	Aldosterone	Increases water and sodium kidney reabsorption
	Cortisol	Decreases immune response; is anti-inflammatory; has a catabolic effect on tissues; stress response
Adrenal medulla	Norepinephrine	Generalized vasoconstriction
	Epinephrine	Stress response; increases force and rate of heart contraction; bronchodilation; vasodilation in skeletal muscle; visceral and cutaneous vasoconstriction

HORMONAL REGULATION

Hormones are secreted only as needed by the body and organs. When the concentration of a particular hormone in the body reaches a particular level, the gland that secretes the hormone will stop secretion of the hormone until the concentration of the hormone in the body drops below a particular level and it is triggered to release more. For example, insulin is secreted when the blood glucose level rises. This type of control is called a **negative feedback system**.

ROLE OF THE HYPOTHALAMUS IN THE ENDOCRINE SYSTEM

> **Medical Terminology Review**
>
> **hypothalamus**
> hypo- = low; under; beneath
> -thalamus = gray matter deeply situated in the forebrain
> structure deep to the gray matter of the forebrain
> **corticotrophin**
> cortico- = stimulating the cortex
> -tropin = hormone
> a hormone that stimulates the cortex

The **hypothalamus** of the brain is the main integrative center for the endocrine and autonomic nervous systems. The hypothalamus helps control some endocrine glands by neural and hormonal pathways. Neural pathways connect the hypothalamus to the posterior pituitary gland. Neural stimulation of the posterior pituitary causes the secretion of two effector hormones: antidiuretic hormone (also known as vasopressin) and oxytocin.

The hypothalamus also exerts hormonal control at the anterior pituitary gland, by releasing and inhibiting hormones and factors, which arrive by a portal system. Hypothalamic hormones stimulate the pituitary glands to synthesize and release trophic hormones. These hormones include corticotropin (also called adrenocorticotropic hormone), thyroid-stimulating hormone, and gonadotropins, such as luteinizing hormone and follicle-stimulating hormone. Secretion of trophic hormones stimulates the adrenal cortex, thyroid gland, and gonads. Hypothalamic hormones also stimulate the pituitary gland to release or inhibit the release of effector hormones, such as growth hormone and prolactin (Figure 18-2).

HORMONES

Hormones are natural chemical substances secreted into the bloodstream from the endocrine glands that regulate and control the activity of an organ or tissues in another part of the body. The synthesis and secretion of many hormones are controlled by other hormones or changes in the concentration of essential chemicals or electrolytes in the blood. Drugs and diseases can modify hormone secretion as well as specific hormone effects at target organs. Some hormones affect nearly all the tissues of the body, but the action of others is restricted to a few tissues or organs. The majority of hormones, such as thyroxine, epinephrine, parathyroid hormone, insulin, and glucagon, are proteins. Several other groups of hormones, such as those

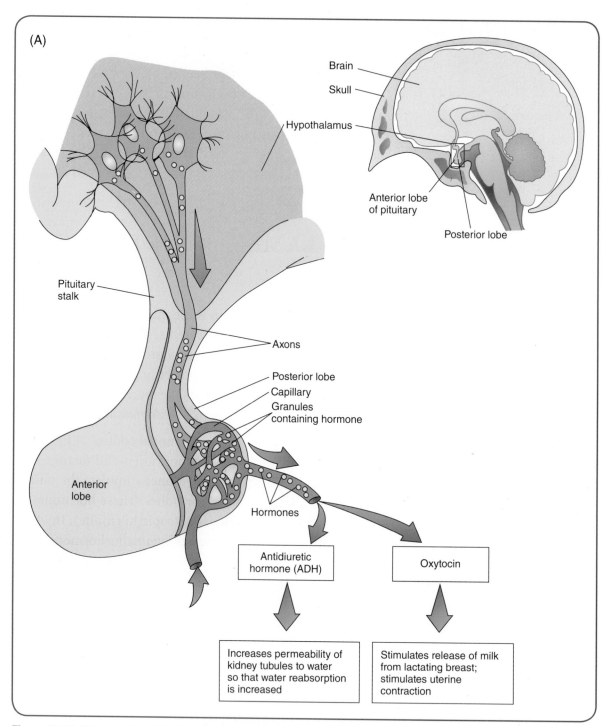

Figure 18-2A The relationship between the hypothalamus and (A) the posterior lobe of the pituitary gland; (B) the anterior lobe of the pituitary gland.

produced by the adrenal cortex and the gonads, are **steroids**. A list of major hormones and endocrine glands is provided in Table 18-1. Hormones from the various endocrine glands work together to regulate vital processes of the body that include the following:

1. Secretions in the digestive tract

2. Energy production

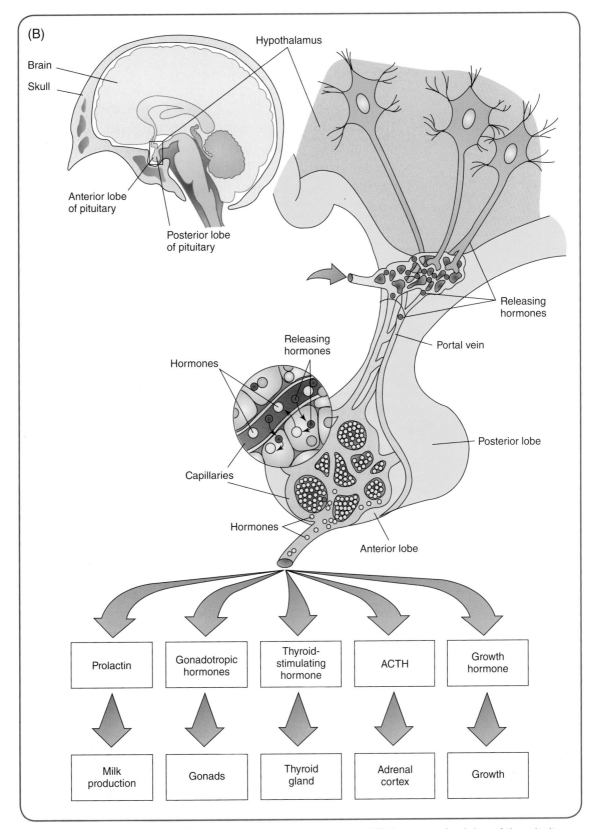

Figure 18-2B The relationship between the hypothalamus and (A) the posterior lobe of the pituitary gland; (B) the anterior lobe of the pituitary gland.

3. Composition and volume of extracellular fluid

4. Adaptation and immunity

5. Growth and development

6. Reproduction and lactation

The inactivation of hormones occurs enzymatically in the blood, liver, kidneys, or target tissues. Hormones are secreted primarily in the urine and, to a lesser extent, in bile. In medicine, hormones generally are used in three ways: (1) for replacement therapy; (2) for pharmacological effects beyond replacement; and (3) for endocrine diagnostic testing.

Growth Hormone

Growth hormone (GH) is secreted by the anterior pituitary gland in response to growth hormone-releasing hormone (GHRH). Its secretion is controlled in part by the hypothalamus. Growth hormone is a peptide hormone and protein that promotes protein synthesis in all cells, increased fat mobilization, and the use of fatty acids for energy. Growth effects depend on the presence of thyroid hormone, insulin, and carbohydrates. It is prescribed for **dwarfism**, a condition in which the growth of long bones is abnormally decreased by an inadequate production of GH. Somatropin is a recombinant form of human GH. In children and adults, it is prescribed for the treatment of GH deficiency. Adverse effects include myalgia, joint pain, and peripheral edema. Octreotide (Sandostatin®) is a GH inhibitor used to treat acromegaly. Pegvisomant (Somavert®) is a GH antagonist that is approved for the treatment of acromegaly when patients have had an inadequate response to surgery or radiation therapy.

Adrenocorticotropic Hormone

Adrenocorticotropic hormone (ACTH) is another hormone from the anterior pituitary gland that stimulates the growth of the adrenal gland cortex and the secretion of corticosteroids. Under normal conditions, a diurnal rhythm occurs in ACTH secretion, with an increase beginning after the first few hours of sleep and reaching a peak at the time a person awakens. ACTH is used generally for diagnostic testing, and not for therapeutic purposes. The adverse effects include insomnia, delayed wound healing, increased susceptibility to infection, and acne.

Thyroid-Stimulating Hormone

Thyroid-stimulating hormone (TSH) is a substance secreted by the anterior lobe of the pituitary gland that controls the release of thyroid hormone and is necessary for the growth and function of the thyroid gland. It stimulates the thyroid gland to increase the uptake of iodine and increase the synthesis and release of thyroid hormones. Thyroid-stimulating hormone is prescribed for hypothyroidism and diagnostic tests.

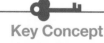

Key Concept

Many of the drugs used to alter pituitary function are proteins that cannot be administered orally. They must be injected, although some may be administered intranasally.

Follicle-Stimulating Hormone

Follicle-stimulating hormone (FSH) is a gonadotropin that stimulates the growth and maturation of follicles in the ovary and promotes **spermatogenesis** (the process by which male gametes develop into mature spermatozoa) in the male. It is secreted by the anterior pituitary gland. The ovarian follicle produces estrogen, which reaches a high level before ovulation and suppresses release of FSH. In males, FSH maintains the integrity of the seminiferous tubules and influences all the stages of sperm production. It may be used to treat some conditions. One form is derived from the urine of postmenopausal women.

Luteinizing Hormone

Luteinizing hormone (LH) is secreted by the anterior lobe of the pituitary gland and is necessary for proper reproductive function. In females, an acute rise of LH triggers ovulation. In males, where LH is also called interstitial cell-stimulating hormone, it stimulates the production of testosterone.

Prolactin

Prolactin (PRL) is a hormone that is primarily associated with lactation. It is secreted from the anterior pituitary gland. Prolactin release is stimulated by thyrotropin-releasing factor. In adults, **hyperprolactinemia** and **galactorrhea** can result from adenomas that secrete excessive prolactin. In hyperprolactinemia, bromocriptines such as cabergoline (Dostinex®) and pergolide (Permax®) may reduce serum prolactin concentrations.

Antidiuretic Hormone

Antidiuretic hormone (ADH) is released when the body is low on water, and causes the kidneys to conserve water, but not salt, by concentrating the urine and reducing urine volume. Antidiuretic hormone is also called *vasopressin*. It also raises blood pressure by inducing vasoconstriction. This hormone is released from the hypothalamus and stored in the posterior lobe of the pituitary gland. There are several vasopressin receptor antagonists, such as conivaptan (Vaprisol®) and tolvaptan (Samsca®), that are used to offset fluid retention caused by excessive production of vasopressin, which may be linked to hyponatremia or acute heart failure.

Oxytocin

Oxytocin (OT) also acts as a neurotransmitter in the brain. In women, it is released during labor and lactation. It is also released by both sexes during orgasm. Oxytocin is mostly manufactured by the hypothalamus and is stored in the posterior pituitary gland. Oxytocin greatly stimulates uterine contractions and is administered intravenously to induce or reinforce labor. Atosiban (Tractocile®, Antocin®) is an oxytocin receptor antagonist that is used in other countries as a *tocolytic*, which is a drug used to treat preterm labor.

Thyroxine

Thyroxine (T4) is the major hormone secreted by the follicular cells of the thyroid gland. It is involved in controlling metabolic body processes and influencing physical development.

Calcitonin

Calcitonin (CT) is produced primarily by the parafollicular cells of the thyroid gland. Calcitonin participates in calcium and phosphorus metabolism. In many ways, it counteracts the effects of parathyroid hormone.

Parathyroid Hormone

Parathyroid hormone (PTH), also called parathormone, is secreted by the parathyroid glands and increases the levels of calcium in the blood. Parathyroid hormone reduces the uptake of phosphate in the proximal tubules of the kidney, meaning that more phosphate is excreted through the urine.

Glucocorticoids

Glucocorticoids are steroid hormones that can bind with the cortisol receptor and trigger similar effects. They are released from the adrenal cortex. Cortisol (hydrocortisone) is the most important human glucocorticoid. It regulates or supports a variety of important cardiovascular, metabolic, immunological, and homeostatic functions. Mifepristone (Korlym®, Mifeprex®) is a competitive inhibitor of glucocorticoid receptors that has been used to treat Cushing's syndrome.

Mineralocorticoids

Mineralocorticoids are steroid hormones that influence salt and water balance. They are released from the adrenal cortex. The primary endogenous mineralocorticoid is aldosterone, which acts on the kidneys to provide active reabsorption of sodium and passive reabsorption of water. This eventually results in an increase of blood pressure and blood volume. Besides aldosterone, other mineralocorticoids include the aldosterone precursor known as *deoxycorticosterone*, and the drug of choice for replacement therapy after an adrenalectomy, *fludrocortisone*.

Androgens

Androgen is the generic term for any natural or synthetic compound, usually a steroid hormone, which stimulates or controls the development of masculine characteristics by binding to androgen receptors. They are released from the adrenal cortex. Androgens are also the original anabolic steroids. The primary and most well known androgen is testosterone.

Medical Terminology Review

glucocorticoids
gluco- = glucose; glucagon; sugar
-corticoids = steroid hormones
steroid hormones released in response to sugar levels in the blood

Epinephrine

Epinephrine (adrenaline) is produced by the medulla of adrenal glands, and is a "fight or flight" hormone that is released when danger threatens. It increases heart rate and stroke volume, dilates the pupils, constricts arterioles in the skin and gut, and dilates arterioles in the leg muscles. It is commonly used to treat cardiac arrest and other cardiac dysrhythmias.

Norepinephrine

Norepinephrine (noradrenaline) is released from the medulla of the adrenal glands and is also a central nervous system and sympathetic nervous system neurotransmitter. It supports the "fight or flight" response, increasing heart rate, triggering the release of glucose, and increasing skeletal muscle readiness.

Glucagon

Glucagon is a hormone that is very important for carbohydrate metabolism. It is synthesized and secreted by the alpha cells of the pancreas. Glucagon helps maintain the level of glucose in the blood by causing the liver to release glucose through a process known as glycogenolysis. This release prevents the development of hypoglycemia.

Insulin

Insulin is a hormone that regulates carbohydrate and fat metabolism. It is synthesized and released by the beta cells of the pancreas. Insulin is used medically to treat some forms of diabetes mellitus. Most insulin produced each day is produced during the digestion of meals. Insulin therapy often requires frequent blood glucose checking by the patient.

Insulin may be administered using syringes, injection pens, insulin pumps, and inhalers. Inhalation insulin uses only short-acting insulin, and is given in combination with a long-acting insulin to treat type 1 diabetes. Short, intermediate, mixed, and long-acting insulins may be injected using syringes and injection pens. Lantus insulin (insulin glargine) is a newer, ultra-long-acting type of insulin, administered by injection once per day. Its activity begins in a little more than one hour, and lasts for about 24 hours, without any peaks in its effectiveness.

> **Key Concept**
>
> Glucagon is used in emergency situations for severe hypoglycemia in diabetic patients. In type 1 diabetes, an unintended excessive dose of injected insulin or oral glucose-lowering medications may lead to severe hypoglycemia, meaning that glucagon may be needed immediately to counteract the condition.

ALTERATIONS IN THE FUNCTION OF THE PITUITARY GLAND

Hyperpituitarism can result from damage to the anterior lobe of the pituitary gland or from inadequate secretion of hormones. The most noticeable result of hyperpituitarism is the effect of excessive amounts of GH. The condition produces excessive growth (a "giant") if the hypersecretion of GH

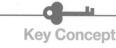

Key Concept

Regular monitoring of height, weight, and blood glucose levels is essential for a patient taking somatotropin.

Medical Terminology Review

somatotropin
somato- = body
-tropin = hormone
hormones involved in regulating body functions

occurs before puberty, which is called **gigantism**. If the excessive production of GH occurs after puberty, it can result in **acromegaly** (overdevelopment of the bones of the head, face, and feet). Treatment of these two conditions includes surgery, radiation, and medication therapy. Growth hormone insufficiency during childhood causes **dwarfism**.

Diabetes insipidus is a disease that results from a deficiency of ADH. In the absence of ADH, water is not reabsorbed by the kidneys and is excreted in the urine. Excessive water loss can quickly lead to dehydration. Whenever possible, the underlying cause of diabetes insipidus must be corrected. ADH is used in the treatment of diabetes insipidus.

Growth Hormone Replacement

Growth hormone replacement therapy may be used to treat many different conditions, including Turner's syndrome, chronic renal failure, intrauterine growth retardation, and severe idiopathic short stature; to maintain muscle mass in AIDS patients; and for patients with short bowel syndrome.

Mechanism of Action

Although still widely debated, it is believed that the mechanism of action of GH is similar to that of tryptophan, which is released by increased levels of serotonin at night.

Indications

The main indication for replacement of GH is growth failure in children. Treatment is prolonged and may cause a six-inch growth in height. Special agents used for hormone therapy of the pituitary gland are listed in Table 18-2.

Adverse Effects

The side effects of GH therapy include headache, increased blood glucose levels, and muscle weakness. Other adverse effects include swelling at the injection site, myalgia, hypercalciuria, and hyperglycemia.

Contraindications and Precautions

Growth hormones such as somatrem and somatropin are contraindicated in patients with closed **epiphyses** (the ends of long bones that are originally separated from the main bone by a layer of cartilage, becoming unified through ossification), underlying progressive intracranial tumor, and diabetic retinopathy. These hormones should be avoided in patients during chemotherapy, radiation therapy, untreated hypothyroidism, and obesity. Growth hormones are also contraindicated in pregnancy (category B or category C, depending on the brand).

Growth hormones should be used cautiously in patients with diabetes mellitus or family history of the disease, sleep apnea, lactation, and hypothyroidism.

TABLE 18-2	Drugs Used in Hormone Therapy of the Pituitary Gland		
Generic Name	**Trade Name**	**Route of Administration**	**Average Adult Dosage**
Anterior Pituitary Gland			
Growth Hormone			
sermorelin (ser-moh-REH-lin)	Geref®	SC	30 mcg/kg/day
somatropin (soh-mah-TROH-pin)	Humatrope®	SC	0.006 mg/kg/day (0.018 international units/kg/day)
somatrem (SOH-mah-trem)	Protropin®	IM, SC	0.18 mg/kg/wk, divided into equal doses
Growth Hormone Inhibitors			
octreotide (OK-tree-oh-tyd)	Sandostatin®	SC, IV	Initial: 50 mcg; 100–600 mcg/day in 2–4 divided doses
pegvisomant (peg-VIH-soh-mant)	Somavert®	SC	Initial: 40 mg; Maint: 10–30 mg/day
Adrenocortical Hormones			
corticotropin (kor-tih-koh-TROH-pin)	Acthar®, ACTH-80®	IM, SC	IM: 80–120 units/day; SC: 10–25 units in 500 mL D5W infused over 8 h
cosyntropin (koh-sin-TROH-pin)	Cortrosyn®	IM, IV (diagnostic agent)	0.25 mg
Posterior Pituitary Gland			
conivaptan (koh-NY-vap-tan)	Vaprisol®	IV	20 mg in 100 mL of 5% dextrose over 30 minutes
desmopressin acetate (des-moh-PRES-sin AH-seh-tayt)	DDAVP®, Stimate®	PO, IV, SC, Nasal spray	PO: 0.2–0.4 mg/day; IV/SC: 0.3 mcg/kg/min preoperatively, may repeat in 48 h prn; Nasal spray: 10 mcg bid
vasopressin (VAH-soh-pres-sin)	Pitressin®	IM, SC	5–10 units bid–tid

Drug Interactions

Depending on dosage, anabolic steroids, androgens, estrogens, and thyroid hormones may interact with growth hormones.

ALTERATIONS IN THE FUNCTION OF THE THYROID GLAND

Hypothyroidism is a deficiency disease that causes cretinism (mental and physical retardation) in children. It is usually due to a deficiency of iodine in the mother's diet during pregnancy. Hypothyroidism in adults results from hypothalamic pituitary or thyroid insufficiency or resistance to thyroid hormone, which is called **myxedema**. The disorder can progress to hyposecretion of thyroid hormone. Hypothyroidism is more common in women than in men in the United States. Hyposecretion of thyroid hormones may also be caused by lack of iodine in the diet, surgical removal of the thyroid, radiation therapy to the thyroid, or pituitary dysfunction. Thyroid hormones are approved for supplement or replacement needs of hypothyroidism. Thyroid hormones are usually initiated in small doses until adequate response is reached. Long-term use of thyroxine may cause osteoporosis or progressive loss of bone mass in postmenopausal women. Thyroxine is contraindicated in patients who have had a myocardial infarction. Table 18-3 shows common drugs used for disorders of the thyroid gland.

TABLE 18-3	Drugs Used in Hormone Therapy of the Thyroid Gland		
Generic Name	Trade Name	Route of Administration	Average Adult Dosage
Natural Thyroid Replacement			
desiccated thyroid (T_3, T_4) **(DEH-sih-kay-ted THY-royd)**	Armour Thyroid®	PO	None; it is based on natural production of the hormone per patient
Synthetic Thyroid Replacement			
levothyroxine sodium (T_4) **(leh-voh-thy-ROK-sin SOH-dee-um)**	Levothroid®, Synthroid®	PO	100–400 mcg/day
liothyronine sodium (T_3) **(ly-oh-THY-roh-neen SOH-dee-um)**	Cytomel®	PO	25–75 mcg/day
liotrix (T_3, T_4) **(LY-oh-triks)**	Thyrolar®	PO	12.5–30 mcg/day
Antithyroid Preparations			
potassium iodide **(poh-TAS-see-um EYE-oh-dyd)**	Pima®, Lugol's Solution®	PO	50–250 mg tid for 10–14 days before surgery
methimazole **(meh-THIH-mah-zohl)**	Tapazole®	PO	5–15 mg tid
propylthiouracil systemic (PTU) **(proh-pil-thy-oh-YOO-rah-sil)**	(generic only)	PO	300–450 mg/day divided q8h
sodium iodide I¹³¹ **(ray-dee-oh-AK-tiv EYE-oh-dyn)**	(generic only)	PO	148–370 megabecquereles (MBq), or 4–10 millicuries (mCi)
Calcitonin			
calcitonin (salmon) **(kal-sih-TOH-nin)**	Fortical®, Calcimar®	IM/SC, Nasal spray	IM/SC: 100 international units/day, may decrease to 50–100 international units/day; Nasal spray: 200 international units/day

Hyperthyroidism is a condition of excessive amounts of thyroxine. This condition stimulates cellular metabolism and increases respiration and body temperature. Hyperthyroidism causes nervousness and tremors (e.g., shakiness of the hands).

Graves' disease is an example of hyperthyroidism. This disease is far more common in women than in men, and usually affects young women. Signs of Graves' disease include exophthalmos and goiter (see Figure 18-3). Graves' disease can sometimes be treated with medication that inhibits the synthesis of thyroxine or by administration of radioactive iodine, which destroys the thyroid gland. Removal of the thyroid gland, however, may be necessary. If the gland is removed, hormonal supplements must be given. With partial removal of the thyroid gland, the remaining portion still secretes hormones.

Hypothyroidism Agents

Hypothyroidism can be easily treated using thyroid hormone; the most effective thyroid replacement hormone is synthetically made. Treatment involves regular visits to the physician to assess correct dosage. Symptoms usually begin to improve within one week, and usually disappear within a few months. Infants and children with hypothyroidism must always be treated. Also, it is important to understand that older adults and patients who are in poor health may require more time to respond to medications that treat hypothyroidism. Examples of medications used for hypothyroidism include levothyroxine, which is listed in Table 18-3.

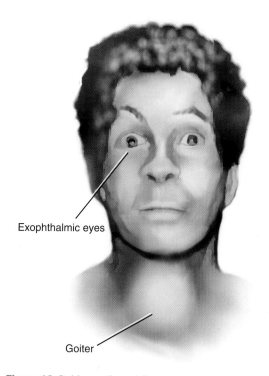

Exophthalmic eyes

Goiter

Figure 18-3 Hyperthyroidism.

Antithyroid Agents

An **antithyroid drug** is a chemical agent that lowers the basal metabolic rate by interfering with the formation, release, or action of thyroid hormones. A variety of compounds are known as antithyroid drugs. Iodine thyroid products (iodide ions), radioactive iodine, methimazole, and propylthiouracil are the drugs of choice for antithyroid therapy. These medications can cross the placenta and stop fetal thyroid development. They also pass through breast milk to affect the infant. Selected medication used as drugs for the thyroid gland are shown in Table 18-3.

Radioactive Iodine

Radioactive iodine is a radioactive isotope of iodine used in diagnostic radiology and radiotherapy. It is used particularly for the treatment of some thyroid conditions. Most radioactive iodine is excreted in urine, but small amounts may be found in sputum, perspiration, feces, and vomitus.

Mechanism of Action Destructive radiation (beta rays) is emitted by the trapped isotope, which effectively destroys thyroid cells without appreciably damaging surrounding tissue.

Indications Radioactive isotopes of iodine, particularly sodium iodide I^{131} are commonly used for the diagnosis and treatment of hyperthyroidism. When administered orally or intravenously, I^{131} is rapidly taken up and stored by the thyroid gland.

Adverse Effects The extent of thyroid damage can be predetermined by carefully selecting the proper dosage of isotope. Low dosages are used diagnostically and pose a minimal risk to thyroid tissue, although high dosages can effectively destroy all thyroid function, resulting in hypothyroidism.

Contraindications and Precautions The antithyroid drugs are contraindicated in the last trimester of pregnancy (category D) and during lactation. These agents are also contraindicated with concurrent administration of sulfonamides or coal tar derivatives such as aminopyrine or antipyrine. Antithyroid agents must be used with caution in patients with infection, bone marrow depression, and impaired liver function. These drugs are also used cautiously in patients with concomitant administration of anticoagulants or other drugs known to cause agranulocytosis.

Drug Interactions Iodine interacts with selenium and possibly with vanadium. Amiodarone, potassium iodide, or sodium iodide can reverse the efficacy of thyroid hormones.

Iodine Thyroid Products

These drugs have been shown to be useful in treatment of mild hyperthyroidism, particularly in young patients. Prior to the introduction of the thioamides in the 1940s, iodides were major antithyroid agents; today, they are rarely used as sole therapies.

Mechanism of Action Iodine ion (**Lugol's solution**) inhibits the synthesis of the active thyroid hormones T_3 and T_4 and inhibits the release of these hormones into blood circulation.

Indications Iodides may be used in several different forms. The most popular are Lugol's solution (strong iodine solution), which contains 5% iodine and 10% potassium iodide, and saturated solution of potassium iodide (SSKI). Iodides are used as adjunctive therapy with antithyroid drugs in preparation for thyroidectomy, treatment of thyrotoxic crisis, or neonatal thyrotoxicosis.

Adverse Effects Lugol's solution may cause hypothyroidism, hyperthyroidism, goiter (enlargement of the thyroid), rashes, and swelling of the salivary glands.

Contraindications and Precautions Potassium iodide is contraindicated in patients with hypersensitivity to iodine. This agent should be avoided in patients with hyperthyroidism, hyperkalemia, and acute bronchitis, and during pregnancy (category D) and lactation.

Potassium iodide should be used cautiously in patients with renal impairment, cardiac disease, pulmonary tuberculosis, and Addison's disease.

Drug Interactions Lugol's solution can increase the risk of hypothyroidism if taken concurrently with lithium. Potassium-sparing diuretics, potassium supplements, and angiotensin-converting enzyme inhibitors increase the risk of hyperkalemia.

Methimazole

Methimazole is an antithyroid agent that is about 10 times more potent than propylthiouracil.

Mechanism of Action Methimazole inhibits the synthesis of thyroid hormones by the coupling of iodine. This agent crosses the placental barrier and is concentrated by the fetal thyroid.

Indications Methimazole has emerged as an effective drug for controlling hyperthyroidism. It is also used prior to surgery or radiotherapy of the thyroid.

Adverse Effects Observation of patients using methimazole has shown that adverse effects are not common. Some patients may develop a mild skin rash, and agranulocytosis has developed in a small number of patients. In very rare instances, methimazole may affect the central nervous system, causing headache, depression, drowsiness, vertigo, and neuritis.

Contraindications and Precautions Methimazole is contraindicated during lactation and pregnancy (category D). This drug should be used cautiously with other drugs known to cause agranulocytosis.

Drug Interactions Methimazole increases theophylline clearance and decreases effectiveness if given to hyperthyroid patients. This agent alters the effects of oral anticoagulants. It increases the therapeutic effects and toxicity of digitalis glycoside, metoprolol, and propranolol when hyperthyroid patients become euthyroid.

Propylthiouracil

Propylthiouracil (PTU) is a chemically related antithyroid drug and is a major drug for the treatment of thyrotoxicosis.

Mechanism of Action Propylthiouracil inhibits the synthesis of thyroid hormones, partially inhibiting the peripheral conversion of T_4 to T_3.

Indications Propylthiouracil is used for treatment of hyperthyroidism, iodine-induced thyrotoxicosis, and hyperthyroidism associated with thyroiditis. It is also used to establish euthyroidism prior to surgery or radioactive iodine treatment.

Adverse Effects Propylthiouracil may cause neuritis, vertigo, drowsiness, depression, and headache. Other adverse effects include skin rash, skin pigmentation, loss of hair, nausea, vomiting, loss of taste, hepatitis, or nephritis. The most dangerous complication of PTU is agranulocytosis, an infrequent but potentially fatal adverse effect.

Contraindications and Precautions Propylthiouracil is contraindicated in the last trimester of pregnancy (category D) and during lactation. The drug should be avoided with concurrent administration of sulfonamides or coal tar derivatives such as aminopyrine or antipyrine. It is used cautiously in patients with infection, liver dysfunction, and bone marrow depression.

Drug Interactions Propylthiouracil increases the risk of oral bleeding. The other side effects of PTU are similar to methimazole.

> **Medical Terminology Review**
>
> **thyroiditis**
> thyroid- = thyroid gland
> itis = inflammation; disease of inflammation of the thyroid gland

> **Key Concept**
>
> The cross-sensitivity between PTU and methimazole is about 50%; therefore, switching drugs in patients with severe reactions is not recommended.

ALTERATIONS IN THE FUNCTION OF THE PARATHYROID GLAND

A deficiency of PTH may occur in some patients for a variety of reasons, ranging from a congenital absence of the parathyroid glands to surgery involving the thyroid gland. Such a deficiency results in a reduction of serum calcium levels, elevated phosphate levels, and a wide array of symptoms, including increased neuromuscular irritability and psychiatric disorders.

The treatment of hypoparathyroidism focuses on the replenishment of calcium stores to reverse the patient's hypocalcemia. Therefore, administration of calcium salts, particularly calcium chloride and calcium gluconate, is indicated.

Vitamin D is also commonly used in patients with hypoparathyroidism to promote calcium absorption from the gastrointestinal tract and to further stabilize a patient's condition.

An overactive parathyroid gland secretes too much PTH, which raises the level of circulating calcium above normal. This condition is called **hypercalcemia**. Much of the calcium comes from bone resorption and increased absorption of calcium by the kidneys and the gastrointestinal system. As the calcium level rises, the phosphate level falls.

With the loss of calcium bones are weakened. They tend to bend, become deformed, and fracture spontaneously. Excessive amounts of calcium cause the development of kidney stones because calcium forms insoluble compounds. Calcium deposited within the walls of the blood vessels makes them hard. Calcium deposits may also be found in the stomach and lungs.

Therapy for hyperparathyroidism often includes surgery. However, phosphate supplementation or potent diuretics, such as furosemide (Lasix®), may be administered to promote increased excretion of excess calcium. Calcitonin may also be used in the treatment of hypercalcemia.

ALTERATIONS IN THE FUNCTION OF THE ADRENAL GLANDS

Overactivity of the adrenal cortex can take different forms, depending on which group of hormones is secreted in excess. **Cushing's syndrome** develops from an excess of glucocorticoids, the hormones that raise the blood sugar level. In excess, they cause hyperglycemia. The patient with Cushing's syndrome retains salt and water, resulting in hypertension and atherosclerosis, which develops as a result of excess circulating lipids.

Conn's syndrome is another form of hyperadrenalism. In this disease, aldosterone is secreted in excess. This causes retention of sodium and water and an abnormal loss of potassium in the urine. Hypertension develops as a result of the salt imbalance and water retention. Muscles become weak to the point of paralysis.

Adrenogenital syndrome is another form of hyperadrenalism, also called *adrenal virilism*. In this condition, androgens (male hormones) are secreted in excess. If this excessive secretion occurs in children, it stimulates premature sexual development. The sex organs of a male child greatly enlarge, and in a female, the clitoris enlarges, a male distribution of hair develops, and the voice deepens.

Excessive androgen secretion in a woman causes masculinization (adrenal virilism). Hair develops on the face, a condition called **hirsuitism**, and the hairline recedes. The breasts diminish in size, the clitoris enlarges, and ovulation and menstruation cease.

Addison's disease results when the adrenal glands fail to produce corticosteroids and aldosterone. Decreased adrenal hormones may also occur if the

Medical Terminology
Review

virilism
viril(e)- = having male characteristics
-ism = state; condition; quality a condition in which male characteristics develop

adrenal glands are destroyed by cancer or infection, or inhibited by chronic use of steroid hormones, such as prednisone.

With aldosterone deficiency, the patient is unable to retain salt and water. The kidneys are unable to concentrate urine and eventually dehydration ensues. Severe dehydration can ultimately lead to shock. Cortisol deficiency leads to low blood glucose levels, impaired protein and carbohydrate metabolism, and generalized weakness.

Treatment with Glucocorticoids

Prolonged use of glucocorticoids may suppress the pituitary gland, causing the body to cease producing its own hormones. If hormone therapy is used for extended periods of time, it cannot be stopped abruptly. Instead, and a step-down dosage should be used to taper gradually the amount of drug the patient is receiving.

Mechanism of Action

Cortisone enters target cells, where it has anti-inflammatory and immuno-suppressive effects.

Indications

Adrenal corticosteroids are used as replacement therapy in patients with adrenal insufficiency, such as Addison's disease. In this condition, administration of both mineralocorticoids and glucocorticoids may be required. Glucocorticoids are also used to treat rheumatic, inflammatory, allergic, neoplastic, and other disorders as supportive therapy with other medications. These agents are of value in decreasing some instances of cerebral edema. Certain skin conditions are often markedly improved with the use of topical or systemic glucocorticoids. Probably the most common use of these agents is in the treatment of arthritic and rheumatic disorders. Table 18-4 lists glucocorticoids and corticosteroid inhibitors.

Adverse Effects

Certain side effects may appear during the first week of treatment with glucocorticoids. They include euphoria, suicidal depression, psychoses, anorexia, hyperglycemia, increased susceptibility to infections, and acne. Chronic glucocorticoid therapy may cause additional side effects such as diabetes mellitus, glaucoma, cataracts, osteoporosis, and edema.

Glucocorticoids must be used cautiously in patients with congestive heart failure, hypertension, liver failure, and renal failure.

Contraindications and Precautions

Glucocorticoids are contraindicated in patients with emotional instability or psychotic tendencies, hyperlipidemia, diabetes mellitus, hypothyroidism, osteoporosis, and peptic ulcer.

TABLE 18-4	Glucocorticoids and Corticosteroid Inhibitors			
Generic Name	**Trade Name**	**Route of Administration**	**Average Adult Dosage**	
Glucocorticoids				
betamethasone acetate **(beh-tah-MEH-thah-zohn AH-seh-tayt)**	Celestrone®	PO, IM, IV, Topical	PO: 0.6–7.2 mg/day; IM/IV: 0.5–9 mg/day as sodium phosphate; Topical: Apply thin film bid	
cortisone acetate **(kor-tih-zohn AH-seh-tayt)**	Cortone®	PO, IM	20–300 mg/day in 1 or more divided doses; try to reduce periodically by 10–25 mg/day to lowest effective dose	
dexamethasone **(dek-sah-MEH-thah-zohn)**	Decadron®	PO, IM	PO: 0.25–4 mg bid–qid; IM: 8–16 mg q1–3 wk or 0.8–1.6 mg intralesional q1–3 wk	
methylprednisolone **(meh-thil-pred-NIH-soh-lohn)**	Medrol®	PO	5–60 mg/day in single or divided doses	
prednisone **(PRED-nih-zohn)**	Prelone® Aristocort®	PO	0.1–0.15 mg/kg/day	
triamcinolone **(try-am-SIH-noh-lohn)**	Kenacort®	PO, IM, SC	4–48 mg qd–bid	
Corticosteroid Inhibitors				
Glucocorticoid Antagonist				
mifepristone	Korlym®	PO	300 mg/day with a meal	
Mineralocorticoid Antagonist				
spironolactone	Aldactone®	PO	100 mg/day, which may be divided into 2 daily doses (max: 400 mg/day)	

Drug Interactions

Increased therapeutic and toxic effects of cortisone occur if taken concurrently with troleandomycin. Cortisone decreases the effects of anticholinesterases if taken concurrently with corticotropin, and profound muscular depression is possible. Steroid blood levels are decreased if cortisone is taken concurrently with phenytoin, phenobarbital, or rifampin. Decreased serum levels of salicylates are seen if these drugs are taken concurrently with cortisone.

Treatment with Mineralocorticoids

Treatment with the primary mineralocorticoid (aldosterone) results in the renal tubule retaining sodium and losing potassium. Aldosterone is utilized in treating Addison's disease, which is a deficiency of adrenocortical secretions.

Treatment with Androgens

Androgen therapy is used for a variety of conditions, depending on gender. Androgens are primarily used to treat prostate cancer, breast cancer, and menopausal conditions. They are also often used illegally to build muscle mass.

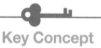

Key Concept

Addison's disease is a deficiency of all the hormones that are secreted from the adrenal cortex, which include cortisol, aldosterone, and androgens.

ALTERATIONS IN THE FUNCTION OF THE PANCREAS

The most important disease involving the endocrine pancreas is **diabetes mellitus**, a disorder of carbohydrate metabolism that involves an insulin deficiency, insulin resistance, or both. Diabetes, if untreated or uncontrolled, leads to hyperglycemia. Severe hyperglycemia and ketoacidosis may produce diabetic coma or unconsciousness, which requires much higher doses of insulin.

Diabetes mellitus is a complex disorder of carbohydrate, fat, and protein metabolism caused by lack of or inefficient use of insulin in the body. The two general classifications for diabetes mellitus are type 1, or insulin-dependent diabetes mellitus (IDDM), and type 2, or non-insulin-dependent diabetes mellitus (NIDDM). Table 18-5 compares type 1 and type 2 diabetes.

Treatment with Insulin

Normally, insulin is used for the treatment of patients with type 1 diabetes if the pancreas does not produce enough insulin. Insulin needs may vary every 6 to 8 hours. Normal fasting insulin levels range from 80 to 100 mg/dL. Insulin preparations are available from three different species, including cows, pigs, and humans. Human insulin now is produced by chemical conversion from porcine insulin and by *Escherichia coli*, into which the human genes for insulin have been inserted. The recombinant product has the same physiological properties as insulin from beef or pork but is much less likely to cause allergic reactions. Insulins are classified based on their time of pharmacological action as short acting, intermediate acting, and long acting. Most diabetic patients require a combination of short- and long-acting insulin. Table 18-6 shows varieties of insulins and their properties.

Key Concept

The most significant diagnostic sign of type 1 diabetes mellitus is sustained hyperglycemia. A fasting blood glucose level of 126 mg/dL or greater on at least two separate occasions is diagnostic for diabetes.

TABLE 18-5	General Differences Between Type 1 and Type 2 Diabetes	
	Type 1	**Type 2**
Age at onset	Preadolescence (juvenile onset)	After age 30 years (adult onset)
Onset	Acute	Insidious
Body weight	Thin	Obese
Hereditary factors	Family history	Present in immediate family
Treatment	Insulin replacement	Diet or oral hypoglycemic agents or insulin replacement
Hypoglycemia or ketoacidosis	Often	Less common

TABLE 18-6	Insulin Preparations		
Preparation	Trade Name	Onset of Action	Duration of Action
Short-Acting Insulin			
Insulin (regular) **(IN-soo-lin)**	Novolin®, Humulin R®	30–60 min, 15 min	6–8 h, 6–8 h
Prompt insulin zinc suspension	Semilente®	60–90 min	12–16 h
Intermediate-Acting Insulin			
Isophane insulin (NPH) **(EYE-soh-fayn IN-soo-lin)**	Novolin N®, Humulin N®	2 h	18–24 h
Insulin zinc suspension (lente) **(LEN-tay)**	Humulin L®, Novolin L®	60–150 min	18–24 h
Long-Acting Insulin			
Protamine zinc insulin suspension **(PROH-tah-meen)**	PZI®	4–8 h	36 h
Extended insulin zinc suspension	Ultralente®, Humulin U®	4–8 h	36 h

Key Concept

Hypoglycemic reactions may occur at any time, but most commonly occur when insulin is at its peak activity.

Medical Terminology Review

ketoacidosis
keto- = ketone; ketone group
acid = having a pH below 7.0
-osis = condition; process; action
a condition of metabolic acidosis caused by high concentrations of ketone bodies

Special Consideration

Patients who will be using insulin must be instructed on the rotation method of taking their medication. Insulin is absorbed more rapidly in the arm or thigh, especially with exercise. The abdomen is used for a more consistent absorption. Glucose levels should be checked according to physician instructions. All insulin should be checked for expiration date and clearness. Insulin should not be given if it appears cloudy. Vials should not be shaken but rotated in between the hands to mix contents.

If regular insulin is to be mixed with NPH or lente insulin, the regular insulin should be drawn into the syringe first. Unopened vials should be stored in the refrigerator and freezing should be avoided. The vial in use can be stored at room temperature. Vials should not be put in glove compartments, suitcases, or trunks. It is imperative that the physician be called if any adverse reactions to the medications are observed.

Mechanism of Action

The primary action of insulin is to promote the entry of glucose into cells.

Indications

Insulin is used to control hyperglycemia in the diabetic patient and for the emergency treatment of acute ketoacidosis. It may be administered intravenously or subcutaneously. Regular insulin is also available as Humulin 70/30 (a mixture of 70% isophane insulin and 30% regular insulin) or as Humulin 50/50 (a mixture of 50% of both isophane and regular insulin).

Adverse Effects

The most dangerous adverse effect of insulin therapy is hypoglycemia. The other adverse effects include tachycardia, sweating, drowsiness, and confusion. If severe hypoglycemia is not immediately treated with glucose, convulsions, coma, and death may occur.

Contraindications and Precautions

Insulin is contraindicated in patients with hypersensitivity to insulin animal protein. It is also contraindicated during episodes of hypoglycemia. Insulin should be used with caution in patients with insulin-resistant hyperthyroidism or hypothyroidism, during lactation, in older adults, during pregnancy (category B), and in those with renal or hepatic impairment.

Drug Interactions

Alcohol, anabolic steroids, monoamine oxidase inhibitors, and salicylates may potentiate hypoglycemic effects. Dextrothyroxine, corticosteroids, and epinephrine may antagonize hypoglycemic effects. Herbals such as garlic and ginseng may potentiate the hypoglycemic effects of insulin.

Oral Antidiabetic Agents

Type 2 diabetic patients are treated with oral antidiabetics (oral hypoglycemic medications) and diet. The first oral antidiabetic agents were the sulfonylureas, which act by stimulating pancreatic production of more insulin. The five classes of oral hypoglycemic medications used in the treatment of type 2 diabetes are sulfonylureas, alpha-glucosidase inhibitors, biguanides, meglitinides, and thiazolidinediones. The alpha-glucosidase inhibitors act by slowing digestion of complex carbohydrates. Biguanides act by decreasing sugar production in the liver, increasing amounts of sugar that are absorbed by muscle cells, and by decreasing the body's need for insulin. Meglitinides act by quickly increasing the amount of insulin produced by the pancreas. They do not remain in the body long, so they must be taken just before a meal, or during a meal. Thiazolidinediones act by lowering insulin resistance in muscle and fat, and by reducing glucose produced by the liver. Table 18-7 shows some examples of oral hypoglycemic agents and their duration of action.

Mechanism of Action

Oral hypoglycemic agents stimulate the pancreas to secrete more insulin and increase the sensitivity of insulin receptors in target tissues.

Indications

Oral hypoglycemic agents are indicated for the treatment of uncomplicated type 2 diabetes in patients whose diabetes cannot be controlled by diet or

TABLE 18-7   Oral Hypoglycemic Agents

Generic Name	Trade Name	Route of Administration	Average Adult Dosage
Sulfonylureas			
First-Generation			
acetohexamide **(ah-see-toh-HEK-sah-myd)**	Dymelor®	PO	250 mg–1.5 g/day
chlorpropamide **(klor-PROH-pah-myd)**	Diabinese®	PO	100–250 mg/day (with breakfast)
tolazamide **(toh-LAH-zah-myd)**	Tolinase®	PO	100–1000 mg qd–bid
tolbutamide **(tol-BYOO-tah-myd)**	Orinase®	PO	250 mg–3 g/day in 1–2 divided doses
Second-Generation			
glimepiride **(gly-MEH-pih-ryd)**	Amaryl®	PO	Initial: 1–2 mg/day with breakfast; may increase to maint. dose of 1–4 mg qd (max: 8 mg/day)
glipizide **(GLIH-pih-zyd)**	Glucotrol®, Glucotrol XL®	PO	2.5–5 mg qd–bid
glyburide **(GLY-byoo-ryd)**	DiaBeta®, Glynase®	PO	1.25–5 mg with breakfast
Alpha-Glucosidase Inhibitors			
acarbose **(AH-kar-bohs)**	Precose®	PO	Start with 25 mg tid (with meals)
miglitol **(MIH-glih-tol)**	Glyset®	PO	25 mg tid at the start of each meal
metformin hydrochloride **(met-FOR-min hy-droh-KLOR-ryd)**	Glucophage®	PO	500–850 mg/day
Meglitinides			
nateglinide **(nah-TEH-glih-nyd)**	Starlix®	PO	60–120 mg tid
repaglinide **(ree-PAH-glih-nyd)**	Prandin®	PO	0.5–4.0 mg bid–qid
Thiazolidinediones			
pioglitazone hydrochloride **(py-oh-GLIH-tah-zohn hy-droh-KLOR-ryd)**	Actos®	PO	15–30 mg/day
rosiglitazone maleate **(roh-zih-GLIH-tah-zohn MAH-lee-ayt)**	Avandia®	PO	2–4 mg qd–bid

continued on next page

Table 18-7 continued

Combination Drugs			
glipizide/metformin **(GLIH-pih-zyd/met-FOR-min)**	Metaglip	PO	2.5 mg glipizide/250 mg metformin per day
glyburide/metformin **(GLY-byoo-ryd/met-FOR-min)**	Glucovance®	PO	1.25–5 mg glyburide/250–500 mg metformin qd–bid
rosiglitazone maleate/metformin **(roh-zih-GLIH-tah-zohn MAH-lee-ayt/met-FOR-min)**	Avandamet®	PO	1–4 mg rosiglitazone maleate/500 mg metformin per day

exercise only. The second-generation agents offer the advantages of a long duration of action and fewer side effects. Consequently, first-generation drugs are rarely used today. Of the first-generation agents, tolazamide has advantages similar to those of the second-generation drugs.

Adverse Effects

Adverse effects include nausea, vomiting, headache, blurred vision, sedation, confusion, anxiety, nightmares, and tachycardia.

Contraindications and Precautions

Oral hypoglycemic agents are contraindicated in patients who are receiving sulfonamide or thiazide-type diuretics, who are hypersensitive to the agents, and who have acidosis, severe burns, or severe diarrhea. These agents should be used cautiously in patients with high fevers, severe infections, hyperthyroidism, or kidney function impairment.

Drug Interactions

Oral hypoglycemic medications have the potential to interact with a number of drugs; thus, the patient should always consult with a health care practitioner before adding a new medication or herbal supplement. Ingestion of alcohol will result in distressing symptoms that include headache, nausea, abdominal pain, and flushing.

Behavior Modification for Diabetes

Because diabetes is a lifelong disorder, education of the patient and the family is probably the most important obligation of the physician who provides initial care. This disease is markedly affected on a daily basis by fluctuations in environmental stress, exercise, diet, and the presence of infections. Therefore, the best people to monitor and manage the disease are the patients themselves and their families.

SUMMARY

The endocrine system provides a means of chemical communication between body parts. The anterior pituitary gland controls activities of the thyroid, adrenals, and sex glands. It also stimulates growth, development, and tissue repair. The pituitary is called the master gland for these reasons. Pituitary activity is governed by the hypothalamus in the brain.

Hyperpituitarism causes an excess of growth hormone (GH). This condition, if present before puberty, results in gigantism. In an adult, excessive production of GH leads to acromegaly.

Severe hypopituitarism impedes growth and development in a child, causing dwarfism. Glands that depend on stimulation by the anterior pituitary are the thyroid, adrenal, and sex glands. The posterior pituitary gland releases vasopressin, also called antidiuretic hormone (ADH), and oxytocin. Insufficiency of ADH causes diabetes insipidus.

The rate of metabolism is controlled by the thyroid gland. An enlargement of this gland is called a goiter. Hyperthyroidism, which is an excess of thyroxine, accelerates heart and respiratory activity, increases metabolic rate, and raises body temperature. A congenital lack of thyroxine results in cretinism (mental and physical retardation). Myxedema is a disease of severe hypothyroidism in an adult.

Hormones of the adrenal cortex are essential to life. Aldosterone regulates salt balance and cortisol affects the metabolism of nutrients. The sex hormones estrogen and androgen are also produced by this gland. Hypoactivity of the adrenal cortex is called Addison's disease.

Hyperactivity of the adrenal cortex causes different diseases, depending on which hormones are in excess amounts. Cushing's syndrome results from an excess of cortisol, and Conn's syndrome results from excessive aldosterone. Precocious puberty and adrenal virilism develop from too much androgen secretion.

Parathyroid hormone (PTH) regulates the level of circulating calcium and phosphate. Hyperactivity of the parathyroid glands causes hypercalcemia. The high level of calcium comes primarily from bone resorption that weakens the bones. Hypoparathyroidism reduces the level of calcium in the blood, which results in tetany. Hormones of the pancreas, insulin, and glucagon control blood glucose level. Lack of insulin causes an increase in blood glucose level, the condition called diabetes mellitus.

Hypoglycemia, an abnormally low blood glucose level, results from excess insulin. This condition can develop in the diabetic patient from an overdosage of insulin.

With the loss of calcium, the bones are weakened. They tend to bend, become deformed, and fracture spontaneously. Excessive calcium causes the formation of kidney stones because calcium forms insoluble compounds. Calcium deposited within the walls of the blood vessels makes them hard. It may also be found in the stomach and lungs.

The therapy for hyperparathyroidism often includes surgery. However, phosphate supplementation or potent diuretics, such as furosemide (Lasix®), may be administered to promote an increase in the excretion of excess calcium. Calcitonin may also be used to treat hypercalcemia.

EXPLORING THE WEB

Visit **www.endocrineweb.com**

- Look for additional readings and information of the various endocrine glands and the disorders that may occur when they malfunction.

Visit **www.nlm.nih.gov/medlineplus**

- Search for articles related to the topics addressed in this chapter.

Visit **http://pituitary.org**

- Review the FAQs and disorders discussed at this site to further your understanding of the function of the pituitary gland.

REVIEW QUESTIONS

Multiple Choice

1. Which of the following is secreted from the pancreas?

   A. prolactin

   B. growth hormone

   C. glucagon

   D. calcitonin

2. Another name for vasopressin is:

   A. testosterone

   B. cortisol

   C. prolactin

   D. antidiuretic hormone

3. FSH and LH are released from which of the following organs?

   A. hypothalamus

   B. pituitary

   C. ovaries

   D. pancreas

4. Which of the following is a protein?

   A. testosterone

   B. androgen

   C. growth hormone

   D. cortisol

5. Which of the following hormones is stored in posterior parts of the pituitary gland?

   A. oxytocin

   B. growth hormone

   C. prolactin

   D. cortisol

6. The glucocorticoid hormones are under the control of:

   A. LH

   B. TSH

   C. ACTH

   D. FSH

7. Which of the following is a side effect of corticosteroids (glucocorticoids)?

   A. increased susceptibility to infections

   B. hypotension

   C. weight loss

   D. hypertrophy of the adrenal cortex

8. Which of the following is the trade name of methimazole?

   A. Cytomel®

   B. Tapazole®

   C. Propyl-Thyracil®

   D. Celestrone®

9. Glucophage® is the trade name of:

   A. metformin

   B. miglitol

   C. glimepiride

   D. glipizide

10. Which of the following agents is used for the diagnosis and treatment of hyperthyroidism?

    A. thyroxin

    B. sodium iodide

    C. parathyroid hormone

    D. phenytoin

11. Propylthiouracil (PTU) is chemically related to which of the following drugs?

    A. Antineoplastic drugs

    B. Antithyroid drugs

    C. Antiparathyroid drugs

    D. Antidiuretic drugs

12. The mechanism of action of oral hypoglycemic medications is to:

    A. increase insulin production in the pancreas

    B. decrease insulin secretion from the pancreas

    C. release insulin into the bloodstream

    D. stimulate insulin release from the pancreas

13. All of the following include intermediate-acting insulin, *except*:

    A. NPH (Humulin®)

    B. Lente®

    C. Humulin N®

    D. Ultralente®

14. Which of the following is the trade name of chlorpropamide?

    A. Diabinese®

    B. Dymelor®

    C. Tolinase®

    D. Glucotrol®

15. Which of the following is the most serious adverse effect of insulin?

    A. hyperthermia

    B. hyperthyroidism

    C. hyperglycemia

    D. hypoglycemia

Matching

_____ 1. Adrenal cortex

_____ 2. Thyroid

_____ 3. Neurohypophysis

_____ 4. Beta cells of pancreas

_____ 5. Alpha cells of pancreas

_____ 6. Adrenal medulla

_____ 7. Anterior lobe of pituitary

A. Prolactin

B. Glucagon

C. Norepinephrine

D. Aldosterone

E. Insulin

F. Oxytocin

G. Calcitonin

Critical Thinking

A 43-year-old woman is experiencing chills, weight gain, and a general feeling of weakness, as well as an enlarged thyroid gland. Her physician diagnoses her with hypothyroidism.

1. List the most common causes of hypothyroidism.

2. Explain the common treatments for this condition.

3. If the patient were to refuse treatment, what would be the consequence?

Hormones of the Reproductive System and Contraceptives

OBJECTIVES

After completing this chapter, the reader should be able to:

1. Explain the relationship between the anterior pituitary gland and the ovaries.
2. Describe the classes of sex hormones in both males and females.
3. Explain the regulation of the menstrual cycle.
4. Describe four indications for prescribing estrogens.
5. Discuss common adverse effects accompanying the use of estrogens.
6. Describe four indications for progestational drugs.
7. Describe the contraindications and precautions of oral contraceptives.
8. Explain four indications for androgens.
9. Discuss the therapeutic uses of anabolic drugs.
10. List five common sexually transmitted diseases and define them.

GLOSSARY

Amenorrhea – the absence of a menstrual period in a woman of reproductive age

Estrogen – a substance capable of producing sexual receptivity in female individuals

Follicle-stimulating hormone (FSH) – a hormone synthesized and secreted by gonadotropes in the anterior pituitary gland; in females, it stimulates the maturation of Graafian follicles; in males, it is critical for spermatogenesis

Gonadotropes – cells in the anterior pituitary gland that produce the gonadotropins known as luteinizing hormone and follicle-stimulating hormone

Gonadotropin-releasing hormone (GnRH) – a hormone that stimulates the release of follicle-stimulating hormone and luteinizing hormone from the anterior pituitary gland

Graafian follicles – matured and grown ovarian follicles; these egg-containing tubes grow and develop between puberty, sexual maturation, and menopause

Hypogonadism – a condition of little or no production of sex hormones, usually due to poor function or inactivity of either the testes or the ovaries

Hypoprothrombinemic – relating to a decreased amount of prothrombin factor II in the circulating blood

Progesterone – a hormone secreted primarily by the ovarian cells in the corpus luteum at the time of ovulation during the female reproductive years

Testosterone – a hormone that stimulates the development of the male secondary sex characteristics, which include sexual maturity, libido, hair growth, deepening of the voice, and skeletal muscle development; it also initiates the production of sperm, and enhances the functional capacity of the penis and accessory sex organs

OVERVIEW

The female and male reproductive systems are controlled by a small number of hormones, particularly those secreted by the hypothalamus and the anterior pituitary glands. These hormones can be supplemented with natural or synthetic hormones to achieve therapeutic goals ranging from the prevention of pregnancy to milk production or even replacement therapy.

ANATOMY REVIEW

- The female reproductive system is composed of two ovaries, two fallopian tubes, the uterus, and the vagina (Figure 19-1).

- The male reproductive system is composed of two testes, seminal ducts, glands, and the penis (Figure 19-2).

- The functions of the reproductive system are to create new life through reproduction and to manufacture hormones responsible for the development of reproductive organs and secondary sex characteristics (Figure 19-3).

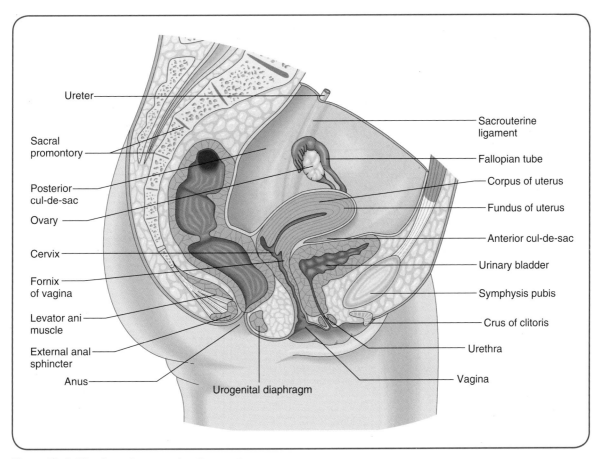

Figure 19-1 The female reproductive system.

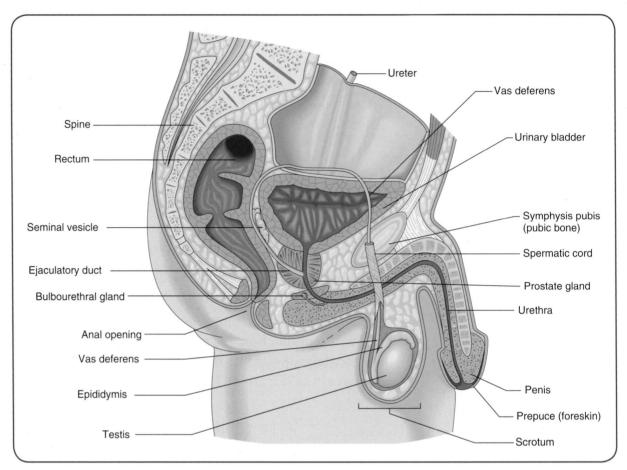

Figure 19-2 The male reproductive system.

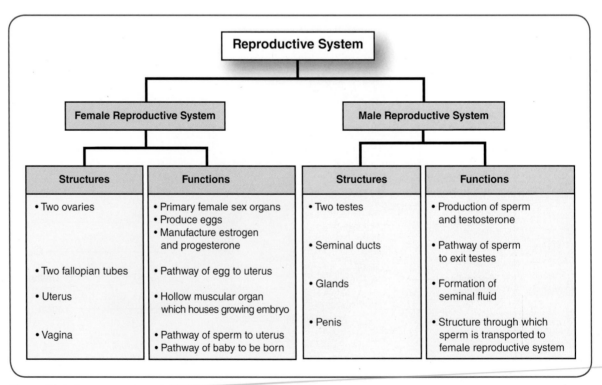

Figure 19-3 The reproductive system.

GONADAL HORMONES

Three main classes of steroid hormones are produced by gonadal tissues: estrogenic, progestational, and androgenic. The ovary is the primary site for synthesis and secretion of **estrogen** and **progesterone** hormones in women. The menstrual cycle is regulated by the production of hypothalamic **gonadotropin-releasing hormone (GnRH)**, which stimulates the release of follicle-stimulating hormone (FSH) and luteinizing hormone (LH) from the anterior pituitary gland (Figure 19-4).

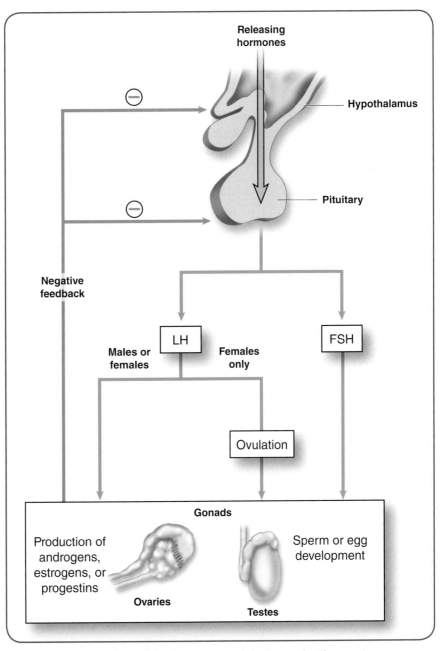

Figure 19-4 Regulation of the hormones of the reproductive system.

Follicle-stimulating hormone (FSH) is a hormone synthesized and secreted by gonadotropes (cells that produce protein hormones) in the anterior pituitary gland. In women, FSH stimulates the maturation of the Graafian follicles (maturing ovarian follicles, which are actually egg-containing tubes). In men, it is critical for spermatogenesis. In men and postmenopausal women, the principal source of estrogen is adipose tissue, in which the level of estrogens is regulated in part by the availability of androgenic precursors from the adrenal cortex. The most important androgenic hormone produced by the testes in men is testosterone, although the adrenal cortex also produces some androgenic hormones in both men and women. Both FSH and LH also regulate testosterone production by specific cells in the testes that control spermatogenesis and the development of primary and secondary sexual characteristics in men.

ORAL CONTRACEPTIVES

Oral contraceptives are hormone medications for the prevention of pregnancy. An oral contraceptive is commonly referred to as "the pill." Oral contraceptives include estrogens and progestins, or a combination of them, to prevent ovulation.

Estrogens

Estrogens are substances capable of producing sexual receptivity in female individuals. Estrogen is involved in the development and maintenance of the female reproductive system and secondary sex characteristics. Naturally occurring estrogens include estrone, estradiol, and estriol. They are found in the blood of both males and females. Most naturally occurring estrogens are not effective when administered orally, because they are rapidly inactivated by the liver. However, their chemical derivatives, such as ethinyl estradiol and mestranol, are only slowly inactivated by the liver and may be administered orally. Both the natural estrogens and their derivatives may be administered by the intramuscular or subcutaneous route.

Mechanism of Action

Estrogen binds to intracellular receptors that stimulate DNA and RNA to synthesize proteins responsible for effects of estrogen.

Indications

Estrogens are used for a variety of conditions, including the treatment of amenorrhea, dysfunctional uterine bleeding, and hirsuitism, as well as the palliative treatment of prostate cancer. Though generally contraindicated in patients with breast cancer, estrogens can be used for palliative treatment of postmenopausal women who have inoperable, progressive breast cancer.

Estrogens are also used in primary ovarian failure, atrophic vaginitis, **hypogonadism**, and atrophic urethritis. They are sometimes used for the relief of menopausal symptoms and for the prevention of osteoporosis. The beneficial effects of estrogen therapy on irritability, depression, anxiety, memory, and insomnia are more unpredictable. It is not clear whether estrogen administration can prevent arteriosclerotic cardiovascular disease, but recently, estrogens have been found to be of value in maintaining healthy cardiac status of some women during early menopause. Overall, studies have shown mixed results. There is a choice of compounds for estrogenic therapy. Major estrogens are listed in Table 19-1.

Adverse Effects

The most common adverse effects of estrogen therapy are nausea, vomiting, breast swelling, fluid retention (weight gain), hypertension, and thromboembolic disorders. Other adverse effects include leg cramps, intolerance to contact lenses, spotting, changes in menstrual flow, dysmenorrhea, and amenorrhea.

Contraindications and Precautions

Estrogens should not be used in patients who have a sensitivity to any of the ingredients, or in those who are pregnant, have breast cancer, or have undiagnosed abnormal uterine bleeding, thrombophlebitis, and thromboembolic disorders.

| TABLE 19-1 | **Major Estrogens** |

Generic Name	Trade Name	Route of Administration	Average Adult Dosage
estradiol **(es-trah-DY-ol)**	Estrace®, Estraderm®	PO, Transdermal patch	PO (Estrace): 0.45–2 mg twice weekly
			Transdermal patch (Estraderm): 0.45–2 mg qd in a cyclical regimen (21 days on, 7 days off)
estrogen, conjugated **(ES-troh-jen, KON-joo-gay-ted)**	Premarin®	PO	0.3–1.25 mg qd in a cyclical regimen (21 days on, 7 days off)
estropipate **(es-troh-PY-payt)**	Ogen®, Ortho-Est®	PO	0.75–6 mg qd in a cyclical regimen (21 days on, 7 days off)
estradiol cypionate **(es-trah-DY-ol sih-PY-oh-nayt)**	Dep-Gynogen®, Depogen®	IM	1–5 mg q3–4 wk
estradiol valerate **(es-trah-DY-ol VAH-leh-rayt)**	Delestrogen®, Valergen®	PO	0.45–2 mg/day in a cyclical regimen (21 days on, 7 days off)
ethinyl estradiol **(EH-thih-nil es-trah-DY-ol)**	Estinyl®	PO	0.02–0.05 mg qd in a cyclical regimen (21 days on, 7 days off)

Drug Interactions

Barbiturates, phenytoin, and rifampin decrease estrogen effects by increasing estrogen metabolism. The **hypoprothrombinemic** effects of oral anticoagulants may be decreased due to interaction with estrogen, resulting in increased levels of prothrombin factor II in the blood. Estrogen may also interfere with the effects of bromocriptine and cause toxicity of cyclosporine.

Progesterone

Progesterone is secreted primarily by the ovarian cells in the corpus luteum at the time of ovulation during the female reproductive years. The corpus luteum secretes progesterone only during the last two weeks of the menstrual cycle. The greatest amount is secreted during the week after ovulation has taken place. Progesterone is responsible for the changes in the uterine endometrium during the second half of the menstrual cycle, the development of the maternal placenta after implantation, and the development of the mammary glands. Progesterone also causes an increase in the viscosity of cervical secretions, which impedes the movement of sperm. Progesterone in high doses suppresses the pituitary release of LH and the hypothalamic release of GnRH, thus preventing ovulation. Progesterone also decreases uterine motility. A synthetic form of progesterone produced by a chemical modification is needed because the natural type of hormone would be inactivated by the liver. These synthetic preparations are called progestins.

Mechanism of Action

Progesterone changes the uterine lining (endometrium) from a proliferative structure to a secretory one. If fertilization does not take place, the corpus luteum diminishes in size, progesterone and estrogen production drop, and menstruation follows.

Indications

Progesterone is used in the treatment of irregular uterine bleeding and is combined with estrogen in the treatment of amenorrhea. It is also used in cases of infertility and threatened or habitual abortion. Progesterone is indicated in the treatment of endometriosis and premenstrual syndrome. It is also used as an emergency contraceptive.

Adverse Effects

Common adverse effects include migraine headache, dizziness, lethargy, mental depression, and insomnia. Thromboembolic disorder and pulmonary embolism may occur with administration of progesterone.

Contraindications and Precautions

Progesterone is contraindicated in patients with thrombophlebitis, liver disease, breast cancer, reproductive organ cancer, undiagnosed vaginal bleeding,

Key Concept

Progesterone can cause changes in vision, ptosis, diplopia, and retinal vascular lesions.

missed periods, and a hypersensitivity to the medication or any of its ingredients. Use during pregnancy and breastfeeding is not recommended. This agent must be used cautiously in patients with previous ectopic pregnancy, venereal disease, or unresolved abnormal Pap smear. Additionally, progesterone should be used cautiously in patients with anemia, diabetes mellitus, asthma, seizure disorders, cardiac or kidney dysfunction, impaired liver function, or a history of psychic depression. Table 19-2 shows the most commonly used progestins.

Drug Interactions

Ketoconazole may inhibit progesterone metabolism. Barbiturates, carbamazepine, phenytoin, and rifampin may alter contraceptive effectiveness.

Estrogen and Progesterone Combinations

Combinations of estrogens and progestins may be used as oral contraceptives in women. This method is nearly 100% effective in preventing pregnancy when used as directed. Oral contraceptives contain various amounts of estrogen and progestins. The estrogen inhibits ovulation by suppressing the normal secretion of FSH. The progestin inhibits pituitary secretion of LH, causes changes in the cervical mucus that makes it unfavorable to penetration by the sperm, and alters the nature of the endometrium.

Mechanism of Action

Fixed combinations of estrogen and progestin produce contraception by preventing ovulation and rendering reproductive tract structures hostile to sperm penetration and zygote implantation.

TABLE 19-2	**Most Commonly Used Progestins**		
Generic Name	**Trade Name**	**Route of Administration**	**Average Adult Dosage**
levonorgestrel (emergency contraceptive) **(leh-vo-nor-JES-trel)**	Plan B®	PO	One tablet as soon as possible within 72 h after unprotected intercourse, or suspected contraceptive failure; second tablet taken 12 h later
medroxyprogesterone acetate **(meh-drok-see-pro-JES-teh-rohn AH-seh-tayt)**	Provera®, Depo-Provera®	PO, SC	PO: 5–10 mg/day; SC: one injection every 3 months
norethindrone acetate **(nor-EH-thin-drohn AH-seh-tayt)**	Aygestin®	PO	2.5–10 mg/day for 5–10 days
progesterone **(pro-JES-teh-rohn)**	Progest®	PO, IM	PO: 400 mg hs for 10 days; IM: 5–10 mg for 6–8 consecutive days

Indications

The use of estrogen-progestin combinations in a cyclical fashion generally results in the inhibition of conception without preventing menstruation. Most oral contraceptives are taken daily for 20 to 21 days, starting on the fifth day after menstrual bleeding begins. Also available are oral contraceptives with 28-day pill cycles, wherein a pill is taken every day of the cycle so that once started, the pill is not stopped. In the 28-day pill cycle, an inactive pill is taken during the week of menstruation, whereas with the 20- to 21-day pill there is a week without medication, and this is when menstruation takes place. The use of oral contraceptives containing only a progestin has been advocated as a means of reducing some of the risk associated with their use. These products, which are sometimes referred to as "minipills," are generally taken continuously rather than cyclically. Because they contain no estrogen, they do not suppress ovulation. Table 19-3 shows the most commonly used contraceptive agents.

Depot-medroxyprogesterone acetate (Depo-Provera®) is an injectable long-acting progestin that is approved for contraceptive use in the United States. There has been extensive worldwide experience with this method over the past three decades. The medication is given as a deep intramuscular injection of 150 mg every three months and has a contraceptive efficacy of 99.7%. It has been proven safe and is relatively inexpensive. Many women find this method more convenient than the use of daily oral contraceptives.

TABLE 19-3	**Commonly Used Contraceptive Agents**		
Generic Name	Trade Name	Route of Administration	Average Adult Dosage
Monophasic Agents			
ethinyl estradiol/ drospirenone **(EH-thih-nil es-trah-DY-ol / droh-SPY-rih-nohn)**	Yasmin®	PO	0.03 mg ethinyl estradiol with 3 mg drospirenone taken cyclically (21 days on, 7 days off)
ethinyl estradiol/ ethynodiol **(EH-thih-nil es-trah-DY-ol / eh-thih-no-DY-ol)**	Zovia®, Demulen®	PO	0.035 mg or 0.05 mg ethinyl estradiol with 1 mg ethynodiol diacetate taken cyclically (as above)
ethinyl estradiol/ levonorgestrel **(EH-thih-nil es-trah-DY-ol / leh-voh-nor-JES-trel)**	Alesse®, Nordette®	PO	0.02 mg ethinyl estradiol with 0.10 mg levonorgestrel taken cyclically (as above)
ethinyl estradiol/ norelgestromin **(EH-thih-nil es-trah-DY-ol / no-rel-JES-troh-min)**	Ortho-Evra®	Transdermal patch	0.75 mg ethinyl estradiol with 6 mg norelgestromin; apply 1 patch for 21 days followed by a 7-day interval with no patch
ethinyl estradiol/ norethindrone (various strengths) **(EH-thih-nil es-trah-DY-ol / nor-EH-thin-drohn)**	Ovcon®, Loestrin®	PO	0.035 mg ethinyl estradiol with varying amounts of norethindrone taken cyclically (21 days on, 7 days off)

Table 19-3 continued

mestranol/ norethindrone **(MEH-strah-nol / nor-EH-thin-drohn)**	Necon 1/50®, Ortho-Novum1/50®	PO	0.05 mg mestranol with 1 mg norethindrone taken cyclically (as above)
mifepristone **(my-feh-PRIS-tohn)**	Mifeprex®	PO	Day 1: three 200-mg tablets as a single dose; patient must see physician 2 days after ingestion; if termination of pregnancy not confirmed, an additional two tablets are required, followed in 14 days by another physician visit for confirmation
Biphasic Agents			
ethinyl estradiol/ norethindrone **(EH-thih-nil es-trah-DY-ol / nor-EH-thin-drohn)**	Nelova 10/11®	PO	First 10 tablets contain 0.035 mg ethinyl estradiol and 0.5 mg norethindrone; next 11 pills contain 0.035 mg ethinyl estradiol and 1 mg norethindrone; taken cyclically (21 days on, 7 days off)
Triphasic Agents			
ethinyl estradiol/ levonorgestrel **(EH-thih-nil es-trah-DY-ol / leh-voh-nor-JES-trel)**	Triphasil®, Tri-Levlen®	PO	First 6 tablets contain 0.03 mg ethinyl estradiol and 0.05 mg levonorgestrel; next 5 tablets contain 0.04 mg ethinyl estradiol and 0.075 mg levonorgestrel; final 10 tablets contain 0.03 mg ethinyl estradiol and 0.125 mg levonorgestrel; taken cyclically (as above)
ethinyl estradiol/ norgestimate **(EH-thih-nil es-trah-DY-ol / nor-JES-tih-mayt)**	Ortho Tri-cyclin®	PO	In this product, the amount of ethinyl estradiol remains constant at 0.035 mg per tablet, while the norgestimate increases from0.18 mg per tablet to 0.25 mg; taken cyclically (as above)
Estrophasic Agents			
ethinyl estradiol/ norethindrone acetate **(EH-thih-nil es-trah-DY-ol / nor-EH-thin-drohn AH-seh-tayt)**	Estrostep Fe®	PO	In this product, the amount of ethinyl estradiol changes from 0.02 to 0.03 and then to 0.035 mg per tablet, while the norethindrone acetate remains constant at 1 mg per tablet; taken cyclically (as above)
Progestin-only Agents			
norethindrone **(nor-EH-thin-drohn)**	Ortho Micronor®, Nor-QD®	PO	1 tablet of 0.35 mg/day (each package lasts 28 days with no stoppage in between packages)

continued on next page

Table 19-3 continued

norgestrel (nor-JES-trel)	Ovrette®	PO	0.75 mg/day
Long-Acting Agents			
etonogestrel **(ee-toh-no-JES-trel)**	Implanon®	Implant	One implant inserted subdermally in upper arm (inner side of non-dominant arm, 3–4 inches above medial epicondyle of humerus)
ethinyl estradiol, etonogestrel **(EH-thih-nil eh-STRAH-dy-ol, eh-toh-no-JES-trel)**	NuvaRing®	Vaginal ring	Insert into vagina; leave in place for 3 weeks, then remove for 1-week break; new ring inserted 1 week after last ring was removed
intrauterine progesterone contraceptive system **(in-trah-YOO-teh-rin pro-JES-teh-rohn kon-trah-SEP-tiv SIS-tem)**	Progestasert®	IUD	38 mg IUD inserted by a health care professional; lasts for 12 months
levonorgestrel intrauterine system **(lee-voh-nor-JES-trel)**	Mirena®	Insert (by trained health care provider)	52 mg inserted into uterine cavity during first 7 days of menstrual cycle, or immediately after first trimester abortion
medroxyprogesterone **(meh-drok-see-pro-JES-teh-rohn)**	Depo-Provera®	IM	150 mg/mL q13 wk

Adverse Effects

The classic adverse effects associated with birth control drugs are nausea, weight gain, and breast tenderness, which result from the progesterone they contain. Other adverse effects include fluid retention, irregular vaginal bleeding, and skin discoloration. The most serious adverse effects of oral contraceptives include heart attack, stroke, hypertension, or other forms of thromboembolic disease. Table 19-4 summarizes the dose-related effects of oral contraceptives.

Contraindications and Precautions

Contraceptives are contraindicated in pregnancy (category X), lactation, and missed abortion. These agents should be avoided in individuals with a familial or personal history of or existence of breast cancer. Patients with diabetes mellitus, hypertension, or hypercholesterolemia (increased blood cholesterol levels) should not take contraceptive agents. Before the use of any hormonal type of contraception, the patient should have a complete history and physical examination performed. The patient should be informed of the precautions, warnings, and adverse effects. Smoking increases the risk of serious adverse effects on the heart and blood vessels from oral contraceptive use. The risk increases with age and heavy smoking (15 or more cigarettes per day), and is quite marked in women older than 35 years of age.

TABLE 19-4	Dose-Related Adverse Effects of Oral Contraceptives
Estrogen Excess	**Progestin Excess**
Nausea	Increased appetite
Hypertension	Weight gain
Breast tenderness	Fatigue
Edema	Acne
Migraine headache	Hair loss
	Depression
Estrogen Deficiency	**Progestin Deficiency**
Early or mid-cycle bleeding	Late breakthrough bleeding
Increased spotting	Amenorrhea
Hypomenorrhea	Hypermenorrhea

Drug Interactions

Several drugs interact with oral contraceptive agents. Some commonly prescribed drugs in this category are phenytoin, phenobarbital (and other barbiturates), primidone, carbamazepine, and rifampin. Women taking these drugs should use another means of contraception for maximum safety.

DRUGS USED DURING LABOR AND DELIVERY

Generally, two types of medications are used during labor and delivery: uterine stimulants and uterine relaxants.

Uterine Stimulants

Uterine stimulants cause contractions of the myometrium during labor and delivery. Many agents are capable of stimulating the smooth muscle of the uterus, but a few are selective, to be used for the myometrium. These agents are known as oxytocic substances, and include oxytocin (Pitocin®), nifedipine (Adalat CC®, Procardia®), magnesium sulfate, and misoprostol (Cytotec®).

Mechanism of Action

Oxytocin injection, by direct action on the myometrium, produces phasic contractions characteristic of normal delivery. It also promotes milk ejection (letdown) reflex in nursing mothers, thereby increasing flow (not volume) of milk.

Indications

Oxytocic agents are used to initiate or improve uterine contraction at term only in carefully selected patients and only after the cervix is dilated and presentation of the fetus has occurred. These agents are also indicated to relieve pain from breast engorgement and control of postpartum hemorrhage and promotion of postpartum uterine involution. Oxytocic agents are often used to induce labor in cases of maternal diabetes, preeclampsia, and eclampsia.

Adverse Effects

Oxytocic agents may stimulate contractions of the uterus and cause fetal trauma from rapid pushing (forward) through the pelvis. This can result in fetal death. Adverse effects of these agents may result in anaphylactic reactions, postpartum hemorrhage, edema, fetal bradycardia, maternal cardiac arrhythmias, and hypertensive episodes.

Contraindications and Precautions

Oxytocic agents are contraindicated in patients with hypersensitivity to them. These agents should be avoided in cases of unfavorable fetal position or presentations that are undeliverable without conversion before delivery, fetal distress in which delivery is not imminent, prematurity, placenta previa, and previous surgery of the uterus or cesarean section. Oxytocic drugs should be used with caution in patients receiving concomitant cyclopropane anesthesia or vasoconstrictive drugs.

Drug Interactions

Oxytocic drugs may interact with vasoconstrictors and cause severe hypertension. Oxytocic agents with clopropane anesthesia cause hypotension, maternal bradycardia, and other types of arrhythmias.

Uterine Relaxants

Uterine relaxants are prescribed in the management of preterm labor. These agents decrease uterine contraction and prolong the pregnancy with the goal of allowing the fetus to develop to full term. Two agents are currently used as uterine relaxants: terbutaline (Brethine®) and nifedipine (Adalat®, Procardia®).

Mechanism of Action

Uterine relaxants preferentially stimulate beta$_2$-receptors in uterine smooth muscle, reducing intensity and frequency of uterine contractions.

Indications

Uterine relaxants are used to delay preterm labor in pregnancies of greater than 20 weeks' gestation.

Adverse Effects

Uterine relaxants often alter fetal and maternal heart rates and maternal blood pressure. Common adverse effects of these drugs include nausea, vomiting, nervousness, restlessness, headache, and palpitations.

Key Concept

Herbal supplements such as ephedra and mahuang may interact with oxytocic drugs, causing hypertension.

Key Concept

The major drugs used to slow down or speed up labor include oxytocin (Pitocin®), nifedipine (Adalat CC® or Procardia®), magnesium sulfate, and misoprostol (Cytotec®). For postpartum bleeding, methylergonovine maleate (Methergine®) may be administered.

Contraindications and Precautions

Uterine relaxants are contraindicated in patients with hypersensitivity, antepartum hemorrhage, eclampsia, or asthma, and in pregnancies of less than 20 weeks' gestation. Uterine relaxants should be used cautiously in patients receiving concomitant potassium-depleting diuretics and in those with cardiac disease.

Drug Interactions

Uterine relaxants interact with corticosteroids and may precipitate pulmonary edema. These agents are less effective when given with a beta-adrenergic blocking drug such as propranolol.

DRUGS USED IN THE TREATMENT OF SEXUALLY TRANSMITTED DISEASES

Sexually transmitted diseases (STDs) commonly include gonorrhea, chlamydia, syphilis, genital herpes and warts, and trichomoniasis. All of these diseases are spread by sexual contact. Overall, STDs are on the increase, attributable to more people engaging in premarital sex, higher divorce rates, and increased numbers of sexual partners. Failure to use barrier methods of contraception is a common factor that leads to infection with STDs. Other infections, such as hepatitis B and HIV, can also be spread through sexual contact.

Many STDs are asymptomatic, and a person may be unaware that he or she is carrying a disease. In addition, certain infections may be transmitted from an infected woman to her fetus or newborn. Recurrent infections due to a lack of immunity to many STDs occur frequently, and an individual may have more than one STD at a given time. Table 19-5 lists common STD infections, their causes, and treatments.

TABLE 19-5	Common Sexually Transmitted Diseases	
Infection	**Cause**	**Cure or Treatment**
Chlamydia	Bacterium: *Chlamydia trachomatis*	Antimicrobial therapy such as azithromycin; to eradicate, retesting is necessary
Genital herpes	Virus: Herpes simplex type 2 (HSV-2)	No cure; treatment with antiviral drugs such as oral acyclovir, which reduces activity and shedding
Genital warts	Virus: Human papillomavirus (HPV)	Rarely cured; warts can be removed
Gonorrhea	Bacterium: *Neisseria gonorrhoeae*	Antibacterial drugs such as penicillin or ceftriaxone plus doxycycline; there are some drug-resistant strains; to eradicate, retesting is necessary
Syphilis	Bacterium: *Treponema pallidum*	Penicillin G (long-acting); to eradicate, retesting is necessary
Trichomoniasis	Protozoan: *Trichomonas vaginalis*	Antimicrobial drugs such as metronidazole

MALE SEX HORMONES

The hypothalamus, anterior pituitary gland, and testes secrete hormones that control the reproductive functions of males. These hormones initiate and maintain the production of sperm cells, and oversee the development and maintenance of male secondary sex characteristics.

The hypothalamus secretes GnRH, which enters blood vessels that lead to the anterior pituitary gland, resulting in release of LH and FSH. Luteinizing hormone in males, also called interstitial cell-stimulating hormone (ICSH), promotes development of testicular interstitial cells, which in turn secrete male sex hormones. Follicle-stimulating hormone stimulates the supporting cells of the seminiferous tubules to respond to the effects of the male sex hormone testosterone.

Androgens are secreted mainly in the interstitial tissue of the testes in the male, and secondarily in the adrenal glands of both sexes. Androgens include testosterone and androsterone. Inadequate production of androgens in the male may be due to pituitary malfunction. Testosterone stimulates the development of the male secondary sex characteristics, initiates the production of sperm, and enhances the functional capacity of the penis and accessory sex organs.

Mechanism of Action

Synthetic steroid compounds with both androgenic and anabolic activity control development and maintenance of secondary sexual characteristics (Table 19-6).

TABLE 19-6 **Male Hormones**

Generic Name	Trade Name	Route of Administration	Average Adult Dosage
Androgens			
fluoxymesterone **(floo-ok-see-MEH-steh-rohn)**	Halotestin®	PO	Males: hypogonadism 2.5–20 mg/day; females: breast cancer, 10–40 mg/day in divided doses
methyltestosterone **(meh-thil-tes-TOS-teh-rohn)**	Android®	PO	Males: 10–50 mg/day or via buccal tablets, 5–25 mg/day; Females: 50–200 mg/day or via buccal tablets, 25–100 mg/day
testosterone cypionate (in oil) **(tes-TOS-teh-rohn sih-PY-oh-nayt)**	Depo-Testosterone®	IM	Males: 50–200 mg/dose; Females: 200–400 mg/dose
testosterone enanthate **(tes-TOS-teh-rohn eh-NAN-thayt)**	Delatest®	IM	50–400 mg q2–4 wk

Table 19-6 continued

testosterone gel **(tes-TOS-teh-rohn JEL)**	Androgel®	Topical	5–10 mg/day applied to any area of skin
testosterone transdermal system **(tes-TOS-teh-rohn trans-DER-mal SIS-tem)**	Androderm®	Transdermal	One system applied per day
Anabolic Steroids			
nandrolone decanoate **(NAN-droh-lohn deh-kah-NO-ayt)**	(generic only)	IM	50–200 mg q1–4 wk
oxandrolone **(ok-ZAN-droh-lohn)**	Oxandrin®	PO	2.5 mg bid–qid up to 4 weeks (max: 20 mg/day)
oxymetholone **(ok-see-MEH-thoh-lohn)**	Anadrol-50®	PO	1–5 mg/kg/day
stanozolol **(stah-no-ZOH-lol)**	Winstrol®	PO	2 mg tid to 4 mg qid for 5 days; may reduce to 2 mg daily or every other day
Androgen Hormone Inhibitor			
finasteride **(fih-NAH-ster-ryd)**	Proscar®	PO	5 mg/day

Indications

Male sex hormones are used for replacement therapy in androgen deficiency, for the treatment of hypogonadism and cryptorchidism, and for palliative treatment of certain metastatic breast carcinomas in women. Androgen replacement therapies are listed as Schedule III drugs.

Adverse Effects

Adverse effects of male hormones in males include gynecomastia, excessive frequency and duration of penile erection, oligospermia, hirsuitism, male pattern baldness, acne, increased or decreased libido, headache, anxiety, and depression. In females, adverse effects include amenorrhea, menstrual irregularities, inhibition of gonadotropin secretion, and virilization (deepening of the voice, clitoral enlargement, increased growth of facial and body hair, and male type baldness).

Contraindications and Precautions

Male hormones are contraindicated in patients with known hypersensitivity to any of their ingredients, in women during pregnancy and lactation, and in men with cancer of the breast or suspected cancer of the prostate. These agents are also contraindicated in patients with pituitary insufficiency, a history of myocardial infarction, hypercalcemia, prostatic hyperplasia, hepatic dysfunction, nephrosis, and in infants and young children. They should be used with caution in elderly patients, in diabetic patients, in those who have hypertension, coronary artery disease, renal disease, hypercholesterolemia and gynecomastia, and in prepubertal males.

Drug Interactions

Testosterone may decrease insulin requirements, and it may interact with oral anticoagulants and potentiate hypoprothrombinemia.

ANABOLIC STEROIDS

A number of compounds derived from or closely related to testosterone may exhibit considerable anabolic effects without causing significant androgenic effects. The anabolic agents, or steroids, are employed to promote weight gain in underweight individuals. Under U.S. federal law, as well as the law of most states, anabolic androgenic steroids are classified as controlled substances. They are illegal for use, possession, or distribution without a licensed and viable medical purpose.

> **Key Concept**
>
> The use of anabolic steroids by young athletic individuals to promote an increase in muscle mass and strength is a real and dangerous problem. The abuse of anabolic steroids has caused death in young, healthy persons.

Mechanism of Action

The anabolic steroids are synthetic agents chemically similar to the androgens. These drugs promote tissue-building processes.

Indications

The anabolic steroids are prescribed for management of anemia of renal insufficiency and control of metastatic breast cancer in women.

Adverse Effects

Common adverse effects of anabolic steroids include muscle cramps, nausea, vomiting, diarrhea, anorexia, and abdominal fullness. Jaundice, hepatocellular neoplasms, an increased risk of atherosclerosis, excitation, and insomnia are the most serious adverse effects with prolonged use. Virilization in women is also the most common reaction associated with the use of anabolic steroids, especially when higher doses are used. Acne occurs often in all age groups in both sexes.

Contraindications and Precautions

Anabolic steroids are contraindicated in patients with known hypersensitivity, serious cardiac disorder, or liver impairment, and in men with prostate cancer or enlargement. These agents should not be used during pregnancy (category X) and lactation. Anabolic steroids should be used cautiously in benign prostatic hypertrophy and in patients with a history of myocardial infarction.

Drug Interactions

Anabolic steroids may interact with anticoagulants and increase their effects. These agents may decrease insulin and sulfonylurea requirements.

ANDROGEN HORMONE INHIBITORS

Androgen hormone inhibitors such as finasteride (Propecia®, Proscar®) are synthetic substitutes that are known as antiandrogens.

Mechanism of Action

Finasteride prevents the conversion of testosterone into the potent steroid 5-alpha dihydrotestosterone in the prostate gland.

Indications

Finasteride is used in the treatment of benign prostatic hypertrophy. Androgen inhibitors are also used for the prevention of male pattern baldness in men with early signs of hair loss.

Adverse Effects

The adverse effects of finasteride are usually mild. In some patients, the adverse effects may be impotence, decreased libido, and a decreased volume of ejaculate.

Contraindications and Precautions

Finasteride is contraindicated in patients with hypersensitivity to these agents, in pregnant women (category X), and during lactation. These agents should be used cautiously in patients with liver dysfunction.

Drug Interactions

Finasteride may antagonize the gastrointestinal motility effects of metoclopramide.

SUMMARY

In females, the ovaries are the primary sites for synthesis and secretion of estrogen and progesterone hormones in women. These two hormones are under the influence of FSH and LH from the anterior pituitary gland and the hypothalamus. They produce ova and form endocrine secretions that initiate and maintain the secondary female sex characteristics. Estrogens can be used for the treatment of amenorrhea, dysfunctional uterine bleeding, hirsuitism, palliative treatment of breast cancer and prostate cancer, for relief of menopausal symptoms, and for the prevention of osteoporosis. Progesterone is used in irregular uterine bleeding, infertility, threatened or habitual abortion, endometriosis, premenstrual syndrome, and combined with estrogen for the treatment of amenorrhea.

The hypothalamus, anterior pituitary gland, and testes secrete hormones that control the reproductive functions of males. Male sex hormones include testosterone and androsterone. Male sex hormones are used for replacement therapy in androgen deficiency, for the treatment of hypogonadism and cryptorchidism, and for palliative treatment of certain metastatic breast carcinomas in women.

EXPLORING THE WEB

Visit **www.ahealthyme.com**

- Search for information on drugs used during labor.

Visit **www.healthline.com**

- Search for additional information on sex hormones.

Visit **www.healthywomen.org**

- From the health topics menu choose topics discussed in this chapter and research additional information to further your understanding of the chapter topics.

Visit **www.nlm.nih.gov/medlineplus**

- Search for information on anabolic steroids, oral contraceptives, or both. What additional information can you find on these topics?

REVIEW QUESTIONS

Multiple Choice

1. FSH and LH are released from which of the following organs?
   A. hypothalamus
   B. pituitary
   C. ovaries
   D. pancreas

2. Which of the following is the trade name of medroxyprogesterone?
   A. Gesterol®
   B. Provera®
   C. Norlutate®
   D. Norlutin®

3. Progesterone is produced in the corpus luteum, which is located in the:
   A. kidneys
   B. ovaries
   C. uterus
   D. testes

4. Which of the following agents is used for the treatment of amenorrhea, dysfunctional uterine bleeding, and hirsuitism?

    A. progesterone

    B. testosterone

    C. oxytocin

    D. estrogen

5. Which of the following hormones is a uterine stimulant?

    A. prolactin

    B. estrogens

    C. oxytocin

    D. insulin

6. Estrogen is contraindicated in which of the following conditions or diseases?

    A. breast cancer

    B. amenorrhea

    C. hirsuitism

    D. prostate cancer

7. Which of the following is the most serious adverse effect of progesterone?

    A. lethargy

    B. mental depression

    C. diplopia

    D. pulmonary embolism

8. All of the following are adverse effects of testosterone in males, *except:*

    A. penile erection

    B. gynecomastia

    C. thromboembolic disorder

    D. oligospermia

9. Which of the following is an indication for use of anabolic steroids?

    A. pernicious anemia

    B. megaloblastic anemia

    C. renal insufficiency anemia

    D. prostatic hypertrophy

10. Which of the following hormones is responsible for the changes in the uterine endometrium during the second half of the menstrual cycle?

    A. progesterone

    B. estrogen

    C. estrogen and progesterone

    D. testosterone

11. Which of the following is an example of an androgen hormone inhibitor?

    A. medroxyprogesterone (Provera®)

    B. fluoxymesterone (Halotestin®)

    C. finasteride (Propecia®)

    D. methyltestosterone (Virilon®)

12. Gonadotropin-releasing hormone is secreted from which of the following?

    A. ovaries

    B. hypothalamus

    C. anterior pituitary

    D. posterior pituitary

13. All of the following are adverse effects of estrogens, *except:*

    A. weight gain

    B. deepening of the voice

    C. intolerance to contact lenses

    D. amenorrhea

14. Which of the following is a trade name of progesterone?

    A. Norlutin®

    B. Norlutate®

    C. Provera®

    D. Progest®

15. All of the following statements are correct about minipills, *except:*

    A. they contain no estrogen

    B. they are taken cyclically

    C. they do not suppress ovulation

    D. they are taken continuously

Fill in the Blank

1. Young athletes often use anabolic steroids to promote an increase in_____.

2. Androgens are secreted mainly in the _____ tissue of the testes in the male.

3. Inadequate production of androgens in the male may be due to _____ malfunction.

4. The use of estrogen-progestin combinations in a cyclical fashion generally results in the inhibition of _____ without preventing menstruation.

5. Estrogens are used for the treatment of amenorrhea, dysfunctional uterine bleeding and hirsuitism, as well as the palliative treatment of _____ and _____.

6. Follicle-stimulating hormone (FSH) is released from the _____ and gonadotropin-releasing hormone (GnRH) is released from the _____.

7. Depo-Provera® is a long-acting _____.

Critical Thinking

A 16-year-old male patient has been prescribed testosterone cypionate (Depo-Testosterone®) to treat hypogonadism (failure of the sexual organs to develop normally).

1. Why does this patient need this hormone?

2. How should the physician explain the effects of this hormone to the patient?

3. What are the common adverse effects of male hormones such as testosterone cypionate?

Pharmacology for Disorders Affecting Multi-Body Systems

Vitamins, Minerals, and Nutritional Supplements

OBJECTIVES

After completing this chapter, the reader should be able to:

1. Identify characteristics that differentiate vitamins from other nutrients.
2. Describe the functions of common vitamins and minerals.
3. Classify vitamins and minerals.
4. Explain trace elements and their major effects on the body.
5. Define pernicious anemia, keratomalacia, osteomalacia, and cheilosis.
6. Describe the role of vitamin and mineral therapies in the treatment of deficiency disorders.
7. Explain the rationale behind food labeling.
8. Describe the purposes of additives in foods and supplements.
9. Explain the major complication of total parenteral nutrition therapy.
10. Define pharma food.

GLOSSARY

Ataxia – loss of the ability to coordinate muscular movement

Beriberi – a deficiency disease caused by deficiency of thiamine, characterized by neurological symptoms, cardiovascular abnormalities, and edema

Cachexia – weight loss, wasting of muscle, loss of appetite, and general debility that can occur during a chronic disease

Calcium (Ca) – the fifth-most abundant element in the human body, present mainly in the bones

Carotenoids – any of a class of yellow to red pigments, including the carotenes and xanthophylls, found in many plants

Cheilosis – fissures on the lips caused by deficiency of riboflavin

Chloride (Cl) – involved in the maintenance of fluid and the body's acid-base balance

Copper (Cu) – important because it is part of a coenzyme involved in the synthesis of hemoglobin; also a component of several important enzymes in the body, and essential to good health

Cretinism – arrested physical and mental development with dystrophy of bones and soft tissues due to congenital lack of thyroid secretion

Cyanocobalamin – a water-soluble substance that is the common pharmaceutical form of vitamin B_{12}; involved in the metabolism of protein, fats, and carbohydrates, and also in normal blood formation and neural function

Electrolytes – compounds, particularly salts, that when dissolved in water or another solvent, dissociate into ions and are able to conduct an electric current

Enteral nutrition (EN) – feeding by tube directly into the patient's digestive tract

Fluoride (F) – a mineral that strengthens tooth enamel and acts as a coenzyme for one or more enzyme systems; it is introduced into drinking water or applied directly to the teeth to prevent tooth decay

Food additive – any substance that becomes part of a food product

Hemolysis – the destruction or dissolution of red blood cells, with release of hemoglobin

Hyperalimentation (total parenteral nutrition) – also known as *TPN*, this treatment is used to supply complete nutrition to patients, through an infusion pump, when the enteral route cannot be used; all needed nutrients are injected into the body intravenously

Hypervitaminosis – an abnormal condition resulting from excessive intake of toxic amounts of one or more vitamins, especially over a long period

Hypomagnesemia – an abnormally low level of magnesium in the blood

Hypovitaminosis – a condition related to the deficiency of one or more vitamins; it differs from avitaminosis, which is any disease caused by chronic or long-term vitamin deficiency or by a metabolic defect

Intrinsic factor – a substance secreted by the gastric mucous membrane that is essential for the absorption of vitamin B_{12} in the intestines

Iodine (I) – an essential micronutrient of the thyroid hormone (thyroxine)

Iron (Fe) – a common metallic element essential for the formation of hemoglobin and myoglobin, as well as the transfer of oxygen to the body tissues

Keratomalacia – a condition, usually in children with vitamin A deficiency, characterized by softening, ulceration, and perforation of the cornea

Magnesium (Mg) –important for the function of many enzyme systems, and the second-most abundant ion of the intracellular fluids in the body

Malabsorption – inability of the body to take in nutrients

Menadione – a water-soluble injectable form of the product of vitamin K_3

Minerals – inorganic substances occurring naturally in the earth's crust having characteristic chemical compositions

Osteomalacia – a disease in which the bone softens and becomes brittle

Pellagra – a disease caused by a deficiency of niacin and protein in the diet, characterized by skin eruptions, digestive and nervous system disturbances, and eventual mental deterioration

Pharma food – a system of receiving nourishment by breathing in nutritional microparticles

Phosphorus (P) – an element that is essential for the metabolism of protein, calcium, and glucose; it aids in building strong bones and teeth, and helps in the regulation of the body's acid-base balance

Potassium (K) – the major electrolyte in intracellular fluids, helping to regulate neuromuscular excitability and muscle contraction

Rickets – a deficiency disease resulting from a lack of vitamin D or calcium and from insufficient exposure to sunlight, characterized by defective bone growth and occurring mostly in children

Sodium (Na) – one of the most important elements in the body, involved in acid-base balance, water balance, transmission of nerve impulses, and contraction of muscles

Sulfur (S) – an element necessary to all body tissues and found in all body cells

Vitamin A (retinol) – a fat-soluble vitamin essential for skeletal growth, maintenance of normal mucosal epithelium, reproduction, and visual acuity

Vitamin B complex – a pharmaceutical term applied to drug products containing a mixture of the B vitamins, usually B_1 (thiamine), B_2 (riboflavin), B_3 (nicotinamide), and B_6 (pyridoxine)

Vitamin B_1 (thiamine) – a water-soluble, crystalline compound of the B complex, essential for normal metabolism and health of the cardiovascular and nervous systems

Vitamin B_2 (riboflavin) – one of the heat-stable components of the B complex, it is involved as a coenzyme in the oxidative processes of carbohydrates, fats, and proteins

Vitamin B_3 (niacin or nicotinic acid) – contains parts of two enzymes that regulate energy metabolism and is essential for a healthy skin, tongue, and digestive system

Vitamin B_5 (pantothenic acid) – a member of the vitamin B complex that is widely distributed in plant and animal tissues and may be an important element in human nutrition

Vitamin B_6 (pyridoxine) – a water-soluble vitamin that is part of the B complex and acts as a coenzyme essential for the synthesis and breakdown of amino acids

Vitamin B_7 (biotin) – a water-soluble B complex vitamin that aids in fatty acid production, and in the oxidation of fatty acids and carbohydrates

Vitamin B_9 (folic acid) – essential for cell growth and the reproduction of red blood cells

Vitamin B_{12} (hydroxycobalamin) – a water-soluble vitamin involved in the metabolism of protein, fats, and carbohydrates; it aids in hemoglobin synthesis, is essential for normal functioning of all cells, and is important in energy metabolism; the pharmaceutical form is known as *cyanocobalamin*

Vitamin C (ascorbic acid) – a water-soluble vitamin that is essential for the formation of collagen and fibroid tissue for teeth, bones, cartilage, connective tissue, and skin

Vitamin D (calciferol) – a fat-soluble vitamin chemically related to steroids that is essential for the normal formation of bones and teeth and important for the absorption of calcium and phosphorus from the gastrointestinal tract

Vitamin E (tocopherol) – a fat-soluble vitamin essential for normal reproduction, muscle development, resistance of erythrocytes to hemolysis, and various other biochemical functions

Vitamin K – essential for the synthesis of prothrombin in the liver

Vitamins – organic compounds essential in small quantities for physiological and metabolic functioning of the body

Xerophthalmia – extreme dryness of the conjunctiva resulting from an eye disease or from a systemic deficiency of vitamin A

Zinc (Zn) – a trace element that is essential several body enzymes, growth, glucose tolerance, wound healing, and taste acuity

OVERVIEW

Vitamins and minerals are required for maintenance of normal body function and, more important, they are essential for life. The body cannot synthesize all the necessary vitamins and minerals, and thus relies on outside sources to provide daily requirements. The vitamins and minerals the body needs come primarily from the foods we eat or from supplements. Vitamins are considered "natural substances" and food additives rather than drugs. However, niacin and vitamin K may also be used as drugs to effect cholesterol reduction and blood clotting.

The vitamin, mineral, and supplement business is a multimillion-dollar industry in the United States. Some health conditions are greatly benefited by the use of nutritional supplements, and specific vitamins and minerals are prescribed when needed to correct deficiency states. Pharmacy technicians are asked many questions about foods and nutrition, including specific questions about products or supplements clients may be considering for purchase, and the amount of these supplements or products to ingest.

VITAMINS

Vitamins are organic compounds essential in small quantities for physiological and metabolic functioning of the body. With few exceptions, vitamins cannot be synthesized by the body and must be obtained from the diet or dietary supplements. No one food contains all the vitamins. Vitamin deficiency diseases produce specific symptoms that are usually alleviated by the administration of the appropriate vitamin. Vitamins are classified according to their fat or water solubility, their physiological effects, or their chemical structures. They are designated by alphabetic letters and chemical or other specific names. The fat-soluble vitamins are A, D, E, and K; the B complex and C vitamins are water-soluble.

An abnormal condition resulting from excessive intake of toxic amounts of one or more vitamins, especially over a long period, is called **hypervitaminosis**. Serious effects may result from overdoses of fat-soluble vitamins A, D, E, or K, but adverse reactions are less likely with the water-soluble B and C vitamins, except when taken in megadoses. **Hypovitaminosis** may occur due to a deficiency of one or more vitamins. Examples of diseases or conditions caused by hypovitaminosis include avitaminosis, **beriberi**, malnutrition, scurvy (scorbutus), **rickets**, and night blindness.

Fat-Soluble Vitamins

Each of the fat-soluble vitamins A, D, E, and K has a distinct and separate physiological role. For the most part, they are absorbed with other lipids, and efficient absorption requires the presence of bile and pancreatic juice. They are transported to the liver, and stored in various body tissues. They are not normally excreted in the urine. Table 20-1 provides a summary of the fat-soluble vitamins, sources, functions, and deficiencies or toxicities.

Vitamin A

Vitamin A (retinol) is one of the fat-soluble vitamins and is essential for skeletal growth, maintenance of normal mucosal epithelium, and visual acuity. Normal stores can last up to one year but are rapidly depleted by stress. Vitamin A has essential roles in the development of vision, bone growth,

TABLE 20-1	Fat-Soluble Vitamins		
Name	**Sources**	**Functions**	**Deficiency/Toxicity**
Vitamin A (retinol)	*Animal:*	Maintenance of vision in dim light	*Deficiency:*
	Liver	Maintenance of mucous membranes and healthy skin	Night blindness
	Whole milk	Growth and development of bones	Xerophthalmia
	Butter	Reproduction	Respiratory infections
	Cream	Healthy immune system	Cessation of bone growth
	Cod liver oil		
	Plants:		*Toxicity:*
	Dark green leafy vegetables		Birth defects
	Deep yellow or orange fruit		Anorexia
	Fortified margarine		Enlargement of liver
			Bone pain
Vitamin D (calciferol) (*kal-SIH-feh-rol*)	*Animal:*	Regulation of absorption of calcium and phosphorus	*Deficiency:*
	Eggs	Building and maintenance of normal bones and teeth	Rickets
	Liver	Prevention of tetany	Osteomalacia
	Fortified milk		Osteoporosis
	Fortified margarine		Poorly developed teeth and bones
	Oily fish		Muscle spasms
	Plants:		*Toxicity:*
	None		Kidney stones
	Sunlight		Calcification of soft tissues
Vitamin E (tocopherol) (*toh-KOH-pheh-rol*)	*Animal:*	Antioxidant	*Deficiency:*
	None	Considered essential for protection of cell structure, especially of red blood cells	Destruction of red blood cells

continued on next page

Table 20-1 continued

Plants:		Toxicity:
Green and leafy vegetables		No toxicity has been reported
Margarines		
Salad dressing		
Wheat germ and wheat germ oils		
Vegetable oils		
Nuts		

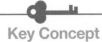

Medical Terminology
Review

xerophthalmia
xer- = dry
ophthalm = related to the eye or eyeball
-ia = condition
excessive dryness of the conjunctiva and cornea

Key Concept

Xerophthalmia is the major cause of blindness among young children in most developing countries.

the maintenance of epithelial tissue, the immunological process, and normal reproduction. Retinol is not found in plant products but fortunately most plants contain substances called **carotenoids**, which act as provitamins and can be converted into retinol in the intestinal wall and liver. The principal carotenoid in plants is beta-carotene, which gets its name from carrots. Deficiency leads to atrophy of epithelial tissue, resulting in **keratomalacia**, **xerophthalmia**, night blindness, growth retardation (in children), and lessened resistance to infection of the mucous membranes. Plasma vitamin A concentrations are reduced in patients with cystic fibrosis, alcohol-related cirrhosis, hepatic disease, and proteinuria. Plasma vitamin A concentrations are elevated in patients with chronic renal disease.

Toxicity can result from taking only ten times the reference daily intake (RDI) of vitamin A for several months. Note that RDI has replaced the *recommended daily allowance* or *RDA*, and represents the daily dietary intake level of a nutrient considered sufficient to meet the requirements of 97% to 98% of healthy individuals in each life-stage and gender group. The RDI also includes tolerable upper intake levels that warn against excessive intake of nutrients such as vitamin D, which can be harmful in large amounts. A nutrient's RDI is calculated in milligrams or grams.

Symptoms of toxicity are varied and can include excessive peeling of the skin, hyperlipidemia, hypercalcemia, and hepatotoxicity. Ultimately, death can result. An acute dose of about 200 mg can cause immediate toxicity, resulting in increased cerebrospinal pressure. This can cause severe headache, blurring of vision, and the bulging of the fontanelles in infants. The use of vitamin A is contraindicated in hypervitaminosis A or hypersensitivity. Its oral use is contraindicated in malabsorption syndrome. Also, vitamin A is not to be administered intravenously.

Vitamin D

Vitamin D (calciferol) is a fat-soluble vitamin that is chemically related to steroids, and essential for the normal formation of bones and teeth as well

osteoporosis
osteo- = bone
oporo = cavity; porousness
-sis = state; condition
porous state of bones

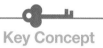

Key Concept

Inadequate exposure to sunlight and low dietary intake are usually necessary for the development of clinical vitamin D deficiency.

as the absorption of calcium and phosphorus from the gastrointestinal tract. Ultraviolet rays activate a form of cholesterol in an oil of the skin and convert it to a form of the vitamin, which is then absorbed. Vitamin D is considered a hormone. It is used for the prophylaxis and treatment of **rickets**, **osteomalacia**, and other hypocalcemic disorders (e.g., tetany) and hypoparathyroidism. Vitamin D_3 is the predominant form of vitamin D of animal origin. It is found in most fish-liver oils, butter, bran, and egg yolks. Deficiency of the vitamin results in rickets in children, the destruction of bony tissue, and osteoporosis. Hypervitaminosis D produces a toxicity syndrome that may result in hypercalcemia, **malabsorption** (which can lead to constipation), kidney stones, and calcium deposits on bones. Vitamin D therapy is contraindicated in hypercalcemia, malabsorption syndrome, and renal dysfunction, and in individuals with evidence of vitamin D toxicity or abnormal sensitivity to the effects of vitamin D. Vitamin D_2 is also called ergocalciferol.

Vitamin E

Vitamin E (tocopherol) is a fat-soluble vitamin that is essential for normal reproduction, muscle development, and resistance of erythrocytes to **hemolysis**. It is an intracellular antioxidant and acts to maintain the stability of polyunsaturated fatty acids.

Deficiency of vitamin E is rare, but can lead to anemia in infants, especially if premature. In adults, erythrocytes may have a shortened lifespan, which may result in muscle degeneration of vascular system abnormalities and kidney damage.

Vitamin E is relatively nontoxic, and it may cause problems only in the large-dosage range of about 300 mg/day (RDI is only 10 mg/day). In extremely high doses, interference with thyroid function and a prolonging of blood clotting time may occur. Sources of vitamin E include vegetable oils such as soybean, corn, cottonseed, and safflower, as well as nuts, seeds, and wheat germ.

Vitamin K

Vitamin K is essential for the synthesis of prothrombin in the liver. The naturally occurring forms, also called quinones, are vitamin K_1 (phylloquinone), which occurs in green plants, and vitamin K_2 (menaquinone), which is formed as the result of bacterial action in the intestinal tract. Water-soluble forms of vitamins K_1 and K_2 are also available. The fat-soluble synthetic compound, **menadione** (vitamin K_3), is about twice as potent biologically as the naturally occurring vitamins K_1 and K_2, on a weight basis.

In healthy adults, primary vitamin K deficiency is uncommon. Adults are protected from a lack of vitamin K because it is widely distributed in plant and animal tissues, the vitamin K cycle conserves the vitamin, and the microbiological flora of the normal gut forms menaquinone. However, vitamin K deficiency can occur in adults with marginal dietary intake if they undergo trauma or extensive surgery. Patients with biliary obstruction,

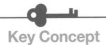

malabsorption, or liver disease also have a higher risk of vitamin K deficiency. Certain drugs, including anticonvulsants, anticoagulants, some antibiotics (particularly cephalosporins), salicylates, and megadoses of vitamin A or E can leave individuals vulnerable to vitamin K-related bleeding disease.

Vitamin K is used in the treatment of coagulation disorder and vitamin K deficiency. It is given prophylactically to infants to prevent hemorrhagic disease of the newborn. Natural vitamin K is stored in the body and is not toxic.

Water-Soluble Vitamins

Most of the water-soluble vitamins are components of essential enzyme systems. Many are involved in the reactions supporting energy metabolism. These vitamins are not normally stored in the body in appreciable amounts and are usually excreted in small quantities in the urine; thus, a daily supply is desirable to avoid depletion and interruption of normal physiological functions.

Vitamin B Complex

The **vitamin B complex** is a group of water-soluble vitamins that differ from each other structurally and in their biologic effects. Heat and prolonged cooking, especially cooking with water, can destroy B vitamins.

Vitamin B_1 Vitamin B_1 (thiamine) is a water-soluble component of the B vitamin complex that is essential for normal metabolism and the health of the cardiovascular and nervous systems. Thiamine plays a key role in the metabolic breakdown of carbohydrates. It is not stored in the body and must be supplied daily. Rich sources of vitamin B_1 are pork, organ meats, green leafy vegetables, legumes, sweet corn, egg yolks, corn meal, brown rice, yeast, and nuts. Other sources include fortified breads, pasta, cereals, whole grains (especially wheat germ), lean meats, fish, dried beans, peas, and soybeans. Deficiency of thiamine leads to the disease called beriberi, which has neurological, cardiovascular, and gastrointestinal symptoms. Thiamine toxicity can occur if very large doses are taken for long periods, and this can result in hepatotoxicity.

Vitamin B_2 Vitamin B_2 (riboflavin) is one of the heat-stable components of the B vitamin complex. It is essential for certain enzyme systems in the metabolism of fats and proteins and plays an important role in preventing some visual disorders, especially cataracts. Riboflavin is found in many food sources but can be destroyed through exposure to light.

Riboflavin deficiency is associated with inadequate consumption of milk and other animal products. It is common in patients with chronic diarrhea, liver disease, and chronic alcoholism. Deficiency of riboflavin produces **cheilosis** (fissures on the lips), glossitis (inflammation of the tongue), and seborrheic dermatitis (mainly of the face).

Vitamin B₃ Vitamin B₃ (niacin or nicotinic acid) contains parts of two enzymes that regulate energy metabolism. It is essential for a healthy skin, tongue, and digestive system. Severe deficiency results in **pellagra**, mental disturbances, various skin eruptions, and gastrointestinal disturbances. Pellagra may also occur during prolonged isoniazid therapy, and in cancer patients. Major sources of vitamin B₃ include lean meats, chicken, eggs, fish, cooked dried beans and peas, liver, nonfat or low-fat milk and cheese, soybeans, and nuts.

In large doses, nicotinic acid can lead to peptic ulcers, diabetes mellitus, cardiac dysrhythmias, and hepatic failure. High doses of nicotinic acid (100 mg and above) are available only by prescription, due to its adverse effects. The common adverse effects include flushing or redness of the face and neck, itching, headache, dizziness or lightheadedness, and diarrhea. Adverse effects include hives, stomach pain, loss of appetite, and jaundice.

Vitamin B₅ Vitamin B₅ (pantothenic acid) is a member of the vitamin B complex. The primary role of pantothenic acid is as a constituent of coenzyme A and as such it is essential in many areas of cellular metabolism, including fatty acid metabolism, synthesis of sex hormones, and functioning of the nervous system and adrenal glands.

As pantothenic acid is available in many plant and animal sources, it is very rare for individuals to have a deficiency of this vitamin. It is available generally in multivitamin preparations, and a diet rich in fruit, vegetable, cereal, or meat sources would ensure an adequate intake of pantothenic acid.

Vitamin B₆ Vitamin B₆ (pyridoxine) is a coenzyme essential for the synthesis and breakdown of amino acids, the conversion of tryptophan to niacin, the breakdown of glycogen to glucose, and the production of antibodies. Therefore, vitamin B₆ is important in the metabolism of blood, the central nervous system, and skin. It is used routinely in patients on isoniazid therapy to prevent the development of neuritis. There has been some success with its use in treating nausea of pregnancy, particularly when given parenterally, and orally in the suppression of lactation. Deficiency of pyridoxine is rare, because most foods contain vitamin B₆. However, deficiency may result from malabsorption, alcoholism, oral contraceptive use, and chemical inactivation by drugs (e.g., hydralazine and penicillamine). Vitamin B₆ deficiency may cause anemia, anorexia, neuritis, nausea, dermatitis, and depressed immunity. The ingestion of megadoses (2 to 6 g/day for 2 to 40 months) of pyridoxine may cause progressive sensory **ataxia**.

Vitamin B₇ Vitamin B₇ (biotin) is a water-soluble vitamin that is synthesized by intestinal flora; therefore, deficiency states are rare. Biotin functions in metabolism by means of biotin-dependent enzymes.

Vitamin B₉ Vitamin B₉ (folic acid) is essential for cell growth and the reproduction of red blood cells. It functions as a coenzyme with vitamins

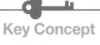

Key Concept

Pellagra is characterized by skin and mouth lesions, diarrhea, and loss of memory.

B_{12} and C in the breakdown of proteins and in the formation of nucleic acid and hemoglobin. It is also essential for fetal development, particularly of the neural tube. Deficiency causes anemia that may cause spina bifida in a fetus. It is also called *folacin*.

Vitamin B_{12}   Vitamin B_{12} (hydroxycobalamin) is often found as **cyanocobalamin** in pharmaceutical preparations. It is involved in the metabolism of protein, fats, and carbohydrates. It aids in hemoglobin synthesis, is essential for normal functioning of all cells, and is important in energy metabolism. Vitamin B_{12} is available in meat and animal protein foods. Its absorption is complex, occurring in the terminal portion of the small intestine (ileum), and requires **intrinsic factor** (a secretion of the stomach walls). Deficiency causes pernicious anemia and neurological disorders.

Vitamin B_{12} deficiency is caused by a lack of activated folic acid, which is essential for DNA synthesis and cell division. Lack of vitamin B_{12} can also affect the nervous system, causing numbness in the limbs, mood disturbances, and even hallucinations in severe deficiencies.

Patients who are suffering from vitamin B_{12} deficiency usually respond to massive doses of B_{12} every day, and then need weekly or biweekly intramuscular vitamin B_{12} injections. This vitamin B_{12} therapy must be continued for the remainder of the patient's life.

Vitamin C

Vitamin C (ascorbic acid) is essential for the formation of collagen tissue and for normal intercellular matrices in teeth, bone, cartilage, connective tissues, and skin. This is one of the most controversial vitamins, with some practitioners advocating up to 10 g or more per day. Smokers may need up to 150 mg per day. Anything over that is said merely to produce expensive urine. Ascorbic acid may protect the body against infections and help heal wounds. Therefore, ascorbic acid has multiple functions as either a coenzyme or co-factor. Its role in enhancing absorption of iron is well recognized. Deficiency causes scurvy, lowered resistance to infections, joint tenderness, dental caries, bleeding gums, delayed wound healing, bruising, hemorrhage, and anemia.

MINERALS AND ELECTROLYTES

Minerals are inorganic substances occurring naturally in the earth's crust that the body needs to help build and maintain body tissues for life functions. They are classified as major and trace elements.

Electrolytes are compounds, particularly salts, that when dissolved in water or another solvent dissociate into ions and are able to conduct an electric current. The concentrations of electrolytes differ in blood plasma and other tissues. Sodium, potassium, and chloride ions are electrolytes. Minerals help keep the body's water and electrolytes in balance.

Major Minerals

The major minerals are defined as those requiring an intake of more than 100 mg/day. The six major minerals are calcium, phosphorus, chloride, sodium, potassium, and magnesium.

Calcium (Ca) is the fifth-most abundant element in the human body and is present mainly in the bones. The body requires calcium ions for the transmission of nerve impulses, muscle contraction, blood coagulation, and cardiac functions. It is a component of extracellular fluid and of soft tissue cells.

Too much calcium will lead to cardiac failure (calcium chloride is included in the lethal injection given in judicial death sentences carried out in certain states of the United States). Too little calcium leads to tetany, which, if severe, can result in fatal muscular convulsions. Fortunately, both vitamin D and parathyroid hormone (PTH) can normally keep these levels constant, principally by mobilizing calcium from bone if hypocalcemia is present, and shunting it back into bone in hypercalcemia. Both hypocalcemia and hypercalcemia are due to factors involving either vitamin D or PTH. Benign hypercalcemia resulting from excessive absorption of calcium may cause calcification of soft tissues and renal damage.

Lack of calcium in the diet results in osteoporosis, a condition in which bone is less dense, and therefore, brittle and weak. The following factors enhance the absorption of calcium: adequate vitamin D, calcitonin, PTH, large quantities of calcium and phosphorus in the diet, and the presence of lactose. Abnormally high levels of ionized calcium in the extracellular fluid can produce muscle weakness, lethargy, and coma. Hypocalcemia can cause tetanic seizures and hypertension.

Phosphorus (P) is essential for the metabolism of protein, calcium, and glucose. It aids in building strong bones and teeth, and helps in the regulation of the body's acid-base balance. Nutritional sources are dairy foods, meat, egg yolks, whole grains, and nuts. A nutritional deficiency of phosphorus is rare, and is usually due to secondary factors. Phosphorus deficiency can occur when people abuse antacids containing aluminum compounds. Aluminum compounds combine with phosphates to produce aluminum complexes, which render the phosphates unavailable for absorption. Deficiency of phosphorus can cause weight loss, anemia, abnormal growth, muscular weakness, and bone pains. Anemia, **cachexia**, bronchitis, and necrosis of the mandible bone characterize chronic poisoning by phosphorus. Excessive doses of phosphorus may produce hypocalcemia in some cases.

Chloride (Cl) is involved in the maintenance of fluid and the body's acid-base balance. The most common metal chloride is sodium chloride (table salt). Chloride ions are needed for the production of hydrochloric acid in

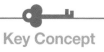

Key Concept

Soft tissue calcification may occur with intravenous administration of phosphate ions but is less likely to occur if the infusion is given slowly.

the stomach. Chloride is normally associated with sodium and potassium, which are involved in helping to maintain pressure balances between the various body compartments.

Sodium (Na) is one of the most important elements in the extracellular fluids. Sodium ions are involved in acid-base balance, water balance, transmission of nerve impulses, and contraction of muscles. Major dietary sources of sodium are table salt (sodium chloride), ketchup, mustard, cured meats and fish, cheese, and potato chips. Toxic levels may cause hypertension and renal disease. The kidney is the main regulator of sodium levels in body fluids. When environmental temperatures are high, and in high fever, the body loses sodium through sweat. A dietary deficiency of sodium and chloride ions is unknown.

There is a misconception that during hot weather, the intake of extra sodium as salt tablets is advisable. This may be helpful only in athletes and in people doing strenuous work. In these persons, it is probably better to encourage the consumption of low-fat milk and fruit juices, which contain sodium and potassium together in a more palatable form. Sodium chloride tablets can irritate the stomach.

Potassium (K) is the major electrolyte in intracellular fluids, helping to regulate neuromuscular excitability and muscle contraction. Sources of potassium in the diet are whole grains, meat, legumes, fruit, and vegetables. Potassium is important in glycogen formation, protein synthesis, and the correction of imbalances of acid-base metabolism, especially in association with the action of sodium and hydrogen ions. Potassium salts are very important as therapeutic agents but are extremely dangerous if used improperly. Potassium is also used to temporarily stop the heart in certain types of cardiac surgery. The kidney plays an important role in controlling secretion and absorption of potassium by the body tissues, especially in the muscles and the liver.

Potassium deficiency may result from increased renal excretion, which may be caused by diuretic therapy, large doses of anionic drugs, or renal disorders. Increased excretion of potassium may occur with the loss of gastrointestinal fluid through vomiting, diarrhea, surgical drainage, or chronic use of laxatives. Potassium loss through the skin is rare, but can result from perspiration during excessive exercise in a hot environment. Potassium deficiency can cause dysrhythmias, so it is important that patients taking certain diuretics also take some form of potassium supplement. Severe diarrhea can also cause hypokalemia. Potassium chloride is an irritant to the stomach mucosa, so tablets are enteric-coated. Another danger with potassium supplementation is hyperkalemia, which is just as serious as hypokalemia and may result in cardiac arrest.

Magnesium (Mg) is important for the function of many enzyme systems and is the second-most abundant ion of the intracellular fluids in the body. It helps to build strong bones and teeth, and aids in regulating the heartbeat.

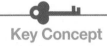

Key Concept

Drinking seawater leads to dehydration as the kidneys remove the extra salt by the excretion of essential body water

Key Concept

Administration of concentrated electrolytes must be carefully managed. If electrolytes are administered in excess of normal ranges, serious adverse events or even death may occur. Therefore, concentrated electrolytes should not be given as floor stock because of their potential for patient harm.

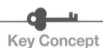

Key Concept

Consumption of a high-potassium diet, when possible, best treats diureticinduced hypokalemia. Foods that are high in potassium include fruit juices, bananas, whole grain cereals, and nuts.

It is stored in the bone and is excreted mainly by the kidneys. Renal excretion of magnesium increases during diuresis induced by ammonium chloride, glucose, and organic mercurials. Magnesium affects the central nervous, neuromuscular, and cardiovascular systems. Diarrhea, steatorrhea, chronic alcoholism, and diabetes mellitus can produce **hypomagnesemia**. Hypomagnesemia is often treated with administration of parenteral fluids containing magnesium sulfate or magnesium chloride. Excess magnesium (hypermagnesemia) in the body can slow the heartbeat or cause cardiac arrest. Hypermagnesemia is usually caused by renal insufficiency and is manifested by hypotension, muscle weakness, sedation, and confused mental state.

Sulfur (S) is necessary to all body tissues and is found in all body cells. It is necessary for metabolism. Sulfur is a component of some amino acids and is therefore found in protein-rich foods.

Trace Elements

Trace elements are not less important, but occur in very small amounts in the body. They include iron, iodine, zinc, fluoride, and copper. Trace elements are generally defined as those having a required intake of less than 100 mg/day. Trace elements are equally essential for their specific vital tasks.

Iron (Fe) is a common metallic element essential for the formation of hemoglobin and myoglobin. The major role of iron is to transfer oxygen to the body tissues. Inadequate supplies of iron to form hemoglobin, poor absorption of iron in the digestive system, or chronic bleeding can cause iron deficiency anemia. Iron exists in two ionic states, depending on its oxidative state: the ferrous (iron II) ion, or Fe^{2+}, and the ferric (iron III) ion, or Fe^{3+}. The ferrous ion is easily oxidized to the ferric ion, and antioxidants such as ascorbic acid help in the absorption of iron from the intestines. Iron is present in most meat, legumes, shellfish, and whole grains. Replacement iron may be supplied by ferrous sulfate (Feosol®), preferably the oral form. Iron dextran (Imferon®) is an injectable form of iron supplement. Milk and antacids should be avoided with iron consumption.

Iodine (I) is an essential micronutrient of the thyroid hormone (thyroxine). Almost 80% of the iodine present in the body is in the thyroid gland. Iodine deficiency can result in goiter or **cretinism**. Iodine is found in seafood, iodized salt, and some dairy products. Deficiencies are common in areas away from the sea, and where water levels of this element are inadequate. Iodine deficiency results in hypothyroidism and goiter. Excessive amounts of iodine can lead to similar conditions. Moderately high amounts of iodine in the diet can be bad for acne, so in areas where adequate amounts are obtainable in the diet, acne sufferers should avoid iodized salt. Iodine is used as a contrast medium for blood vessels in computed tomography (CT) scans. Radioisotopes of iodine are used in radioisotope-scanning procedures and in palliative treatment of cancer of the thyroid.

Key Concept

Patients should be made aware that iron may turn stools black, but that this effect is harmless. Iron preparations are best consumed on an empty stomach because this allows for maximum absorption. However, iron may be given with orange juice to assist in decreasing gastrointestinal symptoms.

Key Concept

Iodine poisoning can cause a brownish-colored staining of the mucous membranes.

Zinc (Zn) is essential for several body enzymes, growth, glucose tolerance, wound healing, and taste acuity. Nearly all functional units of the immune system are adversely affected by zinc deficiency. It is also used in numerous pharmaceuticals, such as zinc acetate, zinc oxide, zinc permanganate, and zinc stearate. The best sources are protein foods. Zinc deficiency is characterized by abnormal fatigue, decreased alertness, a decrease in taste and odor sensitivity, poor appetite, retarded growth, delayed sexual maturity, prolonged healing of wounds, and susceptibility to infection and injury. Excess zinc supplementation can be dangerous as it can cause an increase in copper excretion, leading to copper deficiency. Other problems with excessive zinc intake are atherosclerosis due to a rise in cholesterol and triglyceride levels, and gastric irritation. Megadoses can result in acute toxicity and can be fatal.

Fluoride (F) is probably the most controversial of the micronutrients, as it is added to many of the world's water supplies, and must therefore be consumed whether one wants to or not. There does not seem to be any doubt that, as a mineral, fluoride is an essential nutrient, not just to strengthen tooth enamel, but as a coenzyme for one or more enzyme systems. Unfortunately, many areas of the world have low fluoride concentrations in the soil and drinking water, causing people in these areas to become deficient in the element, resulting in an increase in dental caries. There is also evidence that fluoride can strengthen bones against osteoporosis.

> **Key Concept**
>
> The only food that contains significant amounts of fluoride is tea. The highest fluoride content is found in black and green teas, with less fluoride present in oolong or white teas. Herbal teas contain no fluoride.

Excessive amounts of fluoride are poisonous, and cause mottling of the teeth. Fluoride can also cause warts to become cancerous. Fluorine is the gas of which flouride is an ion.

Copper (Cu), like iron, is important for the synthesis of hemoglobin, because it is part of a coenzyme involved in its synthesis. Copper is also a component of several important enzymes in the body, and is essential to good health. Copper is mostly concentrated in the liver, heart, brain, and kidneys. Good sources of copper are liver, shellfish, nuts, and beans. Copper deficiency is rare. Copper toxicity may be seen in individuals with Wilson's disease (a rare, inherited disorder that causes accumulation of copper in the liver), and in primary biliary cirrhosis. In these patients, the buildup of copper in the tissue causes widespread tissue toxicity with multiple symptoms. The drug penicillamine (Cuprimine®) can bind to copper and remove it from the tissues for excretion.

FOOD LABELING

Food items and supplements must be labeled accurately and cannot be misleading. The Nutrition Labeling and Education Act of 1990 requires most packaged foods to include a list of a specified set of nutrition facts on the label. Setting of standards and enforcement for nutrition labeling are a

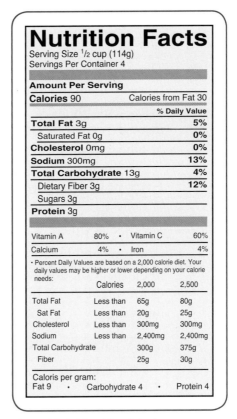

Figure 20-1 Nutrition label.

responsibility of the Food and Drug Administration (FDA). All the nutrition information on the label is based on the stated serving size. Larger packages, such as cereal boxes, often include additional information not required by law. In 2014, the FDA proposed changes to labeling, to provide more information to consumers about specific ingredients, such as added sugars. Figure 20-1 shows an example of a current food label with the minimum required facts.

FOOD ADDITIVES

Any substance that becomes part of a food product is called a **food additive**. Food additives can be included in a food intentionally, such as when salt or cinnamon is added for flavoring, or unintentionally, such as when a pesticide used to treat crops is accidentally incorporated into the plant (or when a drug given to an animal ends up in the food product supplied by the animal). One purpose of food additives is to maintain or improve nutritional value, such as the addition of vitamins and minerals to a food product. The surge in the addition of calcium to juices and other foods is an example of this function. Another purpose of additives is to maintain freshness in the food. Antioxidants added to foods processed with fat, such as potato chips, help to prevent the fat from becoming rancid, and preservatives help to prevent spoilage and changes in color, texture, and flavor of food. Additives also make food more appealing.

NUTRITIONAL CARE

The proper intake and assimilation of nutrients, especially for the hospitalized patient, is called nutritional care. The nutritional needs of a patient depend on the patient's condition. Nutritional requirements may be met through regular meals selected from menus developed for the ordered diet, by tube feeding, or by parenteral hyperalimentation.

Enteral Nutrition

Enteral nutrition (EN) is the delivery of nutrients through a gastrointestinal tube, or the ingestion of food orally. Enteral tube feeding maintains the structural and functional integrity of the gastrointestinal tract. It enhances the utilization of nutrients, and provides a safe and economical method of feeding. Enteral tube feedings are contraindicated in patients with the following:

- Diffused peritonitis (widespread peritonitis)
- Severe diarrhea
- Vomiting
- Intestinal obstruction that prohibits normal bowel function

Hyperalimentation (Total Parenteral Nutrition)

Hyperalimentation (total parenteral nutrition), or *TPN*, is used to meet the patient's nutritional requirements when the enteral route cannot accomplish this. Hyperalimentation, administered by using an infusion pump, is the treatment of choice for selected patients who are unable to tolerate and maintain adequate enteral intake. This type of nutrition is indicated for patients with severe gastrointestinal distress, poor absorption of nutrients, and for those who cannot eat. Examples of patients who may require TPN include those with AIDS, Crohn's disease, cancer, hyperemesis gravidarum, or severe diarrhea, and patients in whom the intestines have had to be surgically removed. Others for whom TPN may be indicated include comatose patients and premature neonates.

The TPN solution is able to supply all the calories, amino acids (proteins), dextrose (carbohydrates), lipids, electrolytes, vitamins, salts, and other essential nutrients needed for wound healing, immunocompetence, growth, and weight gain. The basic parenteral solution may contain amino acids, carbohydrates, lipids, vitamins, and minerals. It is administered by means of direct infusion in to a vein, most often over a 10- to 12-hour period. Two distinct routes are used, depending on the solution. The central venous route is used for hypertonic formulations such as dextrose concentrations that are greater than 10%. The peripheral venous route is used for hypotonic solutions, such as sodium chloride solutions that are 0.45% or less.

Parenteral nutrition (PN) should be started within one to three days after it is determined that enteral nutrition cannot be utilized. All patients receiving less than their targeted enteral feeding after two days should be considered for supplementary PN.

Careful compounding procedures are required for TPN solutions. There must be an accurate balance of all added ingredients so that the patient is not harmed. The supervising pharmacist should always double-check the calculations of ingredients in the mixture by the compounding pharmacy technician or pharmacist.

PHARMA FOOD

Pharma food is a system of receiving nourishment through breathing. All of us constantly ingest microparticles that are suspended in the air, such as the dust in every home. The idea behind pharma food is to convert this act—the ingestion of particles, which takes place in enclosed and outdoor urban areas—into a new form of nourishment. Pharma food is composed of a type of particle that is beneficial to the organism; these particles include (in general) vitamins, amino acids, minerals, and micronutrients. Once released, this volatile muesli of nutrients is inhaled, reaching its destination by the mouth. To enable the particles to reach the stomach and avoid inspiration into the lungs, an element called a saliva activator has been devised. It activates the salivary glands so that the inhaled particles adhere to saliva and are led to the stomach, where they are assimilated by the digestive system. Often, food products with pharmacological additives designed to improve health by lowering cholesterol or enhancing brain function are inhaled. Because of tough restrictions on advertising, pharma foods are not as popular as they could be, although there are continuing advances in their use.

Drugs, as well as foods, are also used in this manner. Inhaled lidocaine is now used as a treatment for asthma, which has led to a marked decline in use of steroids, the most popular type of treatment previously. Direct delivery of the lidocaine into the lungs in high concentrations results in minimal systemic exposure and toxicities, but it is not used much anymore. A similar therapy is the use of inhaled reformulated aztreonam to treat cystic fibrosis.

SUMMARY

No single food supplies all the nutrients needed by the body. Therefore, it is important to eat a variety of foods daily to meet all the nutrient needs of the body. Vitamins and minerals are essential in small quantities for physiological and metabolic functioning of the body. Vitamins include water- or fat-soluble substances. Minerals are inorganic substances occurring naturally in the earth's crust that the body needs to help build and maintain body tissues for life functions. Deficiency and toxicity of vitamins or minerals may cause specific conditions or disorders. Pharmacy technicians must be familiar with basic nutritional dietary standards and pathological conditions. In pharmacy practice, there are many questions that clients may ask about foods and nutrition.

EXPLORING THE WEB

Visit **http://ods.od.nih.gov**

- Explore the databases and various research that is being done on substances discussed in this chapter.

Visit **http://win.niddk.nih.gov**

- Look at the publications that are available. Review information and recommendations related to weight loss concerns.

Visit **www.eatright.org**

- Under the "Public" tab; click on "Food and Nutrition Topics" and review the content on vitamins, nutrients, and supplements. What foods provide the beneficial vitamins and minerals discussed in this chapter?

Visit **www.nal.usda.gov**

- Look for information on dietary supplements. What additional information is available?

Visit **www.nlm.nih.gov/medlineplus**

- Search for information on the vitamins and minerals discussed within this chapter.

REVIEW QUESTIONS

Multiple Choice

1. Which of the following vitamins is used for the patient with an overdose of warfarin?

   A. vitamin D

   B. vitamin K

   C. vitamin E

   D. vitamin A

2. Physicians should prescribe vitamin B_{12} for patients in which of the following situations?

   A. inadequate exposure to sunlight

   B. liver disease

   C. hemophilia

   D. pernicious anemia

3. Which of the following minerals should be restricted in patients who are complaining of weakness, dysrhythmias, and hypertension?

   A. magnesium

   B. aluminum

   C. sodium

   D. iron

4. The proper intake and assimilation of nutrients is known as:

   A. parenteral nutrition

   B. excretion

   C. nutritional insufficiency

   D. nutritional care

5. Severe deficiency of niacin (vitamin B_3) may result in:

   A. beriberi

   B. pellagra

   C. marasmus

   D. pernicious anemia

6. Which of the following types of feeding is more appropriate when a patient's gastrointestinal tract is not functioning?

   A. oral

   B. TPN

   C. enteral

   D. enema

7. An essential micronutrient of thyroid hormone (thyroxine) is:

   A. iron

   B. zinc

   C. iodine

   D. copper

8. Calcium deficiency may cause all of the following, *except*:

   A. rickets

   B. osteoporosis

   C. dwarfism

   D. osteomalacia

9. The Nutrition Labeling and Education Act of 1990 requires most packaged foods to list a specified set of:

   A. vitamin facts on the diet

   B. nutrition facts on the label

   C. mineral and vitamin facts on the diet

   D. nutritional deficiency data

10. All of the following describe the purposes of food additives, *except*:

    A. to make food more appealing

    B. to prevent misleading statements on the label

    C. to maintain nutritional value

    D. to main freshness in the food

11. A system of nourishing through breathing is known as:

    A. volatile muesli

    B. immune activation

    C. saliva activator

    D. pharma food

12. Which of the following minerals is able to help in the formation of hemoglobin and the transportation of iron to bone marrow?

    A. fluoride (F)

    B. copper (Cu)

    C. zinc (Zn)

    D. iodine (I)

13. Which of the following vitamins may protect the body against infections or help heal wounds?

    A. vitamin C

    B. vitamin B_{12}

    C. vitamin K

    D. vitamin E

14. All of the nutrition information on the label is based on which of the following?

    A. the amount of cholesterol

    B. the stated calories

    C. the stated serving size

    D. the amount of sodium

15. Which of the following is a food additive that occurs naturally?

    A. vitamin C

    B. aspartame

    C. partially hydrogenated vegetable oil

    D. mercury

Matching

_____ 1. vitamin B_2

_____ 2. vitamin B_3

_____ 3. vitamin B_5

_____ 4. vitamin B_9

_____ 5. vitamin B_{12}

A. folic acid

B. nicotinamide

C. hydroxycobalamin

D. pantothenic acid

E. riboflavin

Fill in the Blank

1. Vitamin K is an antagonist of _____.

2. The only food that contains significant amounts of fluoride is _____.

3. The drug penicillamine is able to remove _____ from the tissues for excretion in treatment of _____ disease.

4. Total parenteral nutrition may be administered through a(n) _____ so that nutrition can be precisely monitored.

Critical Thinking

A pharmacy technician named John, who has been working in this position for three years, goes to Seattle to visit his grandmother whom he hasn't seen for nearly ten years. While staying at her house, he notices that she has more than a dozen different types of vitamins and mineral supplements on her nightstand. He asks her if she takes all of these herself, and she answers, "Yes, I take all of them every day—they help me feel younger and give me more energy!" He finds out that she is also taking three to four different prescribed medications for hypertension and diabetes.

1. What should John's advice be to his grandmother?

2. Which vitamin or mineral supplements may have potential interactions with diabetes medications?

3. If John's grandmother were to take vitamins A and D in excess of the maximum daily requirements, what would be the symptoms of overdosage and toxicity from these vitamins?

Antineoplastic Agents

OBJECTIVES

After completing this chapter, the reader should be able to:

1. Identify the primary causes of cancer.

2. Explain the terms *benign, malignant, and neoplasm*.

3. Explain different phases of the cell cycle.

4. Describe chemotherapy and the types of antineoplastic drugs.

5. Explain the use of hormones as antineoplastic therapy.

6. Describe the first group of antineoplastic agents.

7. List the classes of mitotic inhibitors (plant alkaloids).

8. Explain the mechanism of drug action of antimetabolites and antitumor antibiotics.

9. Explain toxicity of antineoplastic agents.

10. List specific side effects of certain antineoplastic agents on particular organs or systems in the body.

GLOSSARY

Antimetabolite agents – drugs that prevent cancer cell growth by affecting its DNA production

Antineoplastic agents – drugs used to treat cancers or malignant neoplasms

Benign – cellular growth that is nonprogressive, and non–life-threatening

Carcinogens – any agent directly involved in or related to the promotion of cancer

Heterogeneous – consisting of a diverse range of different items

Malignant – cellular growth that is severe and becomes progressively worse, often becoming life-threatening

Metastasize – to spread from one part of the body to another

Mitotic inhibitors – drugs that block cell growth by stopping cell division

Neoplasm – a tumor; tissue that is composed of cells that grow in an abnormal way

Nitrosoureas – alkylating agents; they act by the process of alkylation to inhibit DNA repair

Palliation – treatment to relieve or reduce intensity of uncomfortable symptoms, but not to produce a cure

Radiation therapy – cancer treatment method whereby radiation is used to treat cancer, either before or after surgery

OVERVIEW

Medical Terminology
Review

neoplasm
neo- = new
-plasm = growth
new growth
metastasize
meta- = changing
-stasize = the state of
the process by which
something undergoes
change

A tumor, or **neoplasm**, arises from a single abnormal cell, which continues to divide indefinitely. The lack of growth controls, the ability to invade local tissue, and the ability to spread, or **metastasize**, are characteristics of cancer cells. These properties are not present in normal cells. Tumors are either **benign** (nonprogressive) or **malignant** (spreading). More than 100 different types of malignant neoplasms occur in humans. Malignant tumors are also referred to as *cancer*, and this disease category is second only to heart disease as a cause of death in the United States. Common sites for the development of malignant tumors are the skin, lungs, prostate, breasts, and large intestine (colon).

Cancer can be treated surgically, chemically, or with irradiation. A variety of chemical treatments are currently available, including specific drug combination regimens. Decisions about treatment are usually based on the type of cancer being treated and the stage of the cancer when diagnosed. This chapter discusses many of the chemotherapeutic treatments used in the treatment of cancer.

CHARACTERISTICS OF CANCER

The proliferation of neoplastic cells leads to the formation of masses called tumors. The terms **neoplasm** and *tumor* are used synonymously. However, it is very important to note that not all neoplasms form tumors. For example, leukemia is a malignant disease of the bone marrow, but the malignant cells are present in the circulating blood and thus do not form distinct masses.

Most tumors can be classified clinically as being either benign or malignant. Benign tumors have a limited growth potential and a good outcome, whereas malignant tumors grow uncontrollably and eventually kill the host.

Only malignant tumor cells have the capacity to metastasize. Benign tumors never metastasize and always remain localized. Metastasis involves a spread of tumor cells from a primary location to some other site in the body. The spread can occur through three main pathways:

- Through the lymphatics
- Via blood
- By seeding of the surface of body cavities

Key Concept

Chromosomal changes are common in cancer cells. The Philadelphia chromosome, the first chromosomal abnormality linked to a malignant disease in humans, was found in patients with chronic myelogenous leukemia. Causes of cancer development in humans may include exposure to chemicals, radiation, and viruses. Cancer is the second-most common cause of death in the United States, eclipsed only by cardiovascular disease.

The Cell Cycle

To understand cancer treatments, normal and malignant cell replication processes should be reviewed. This cell cycle may last from 24 hours to many days. The phases of the cell cycle consist of a first growth phase (G_1), synthesis (S_1), a second growth phase (G_2), mitosis (M), and a resting phase (G_0), shown in Figure 21-1.

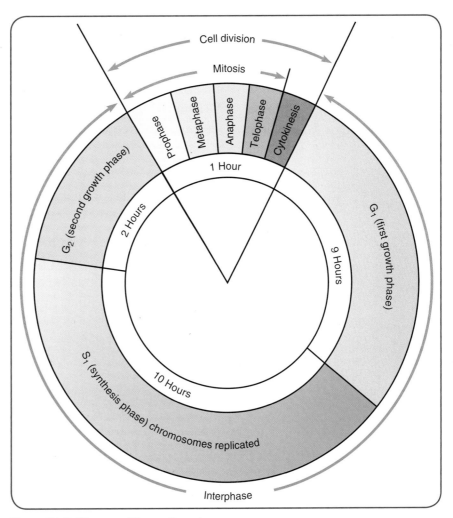

Figure 21-1 Stages of the cell cycle.

Causes of Cancer

The cause of most human cancers is unknown. Nevertheless, many potential agents (**carcinogens**) that result in the development of cancer have been identified, and the sources of many tumors have been explained (Table 21-1).

TABLE 21-1	Exposure to Carcinogens
Causes	**Cancer Sites**
Sunlight (UV radiation)	Skin cancer
Human papilloma viruses	Genital warts and cervical cancer
Inhalation carcinogens (3,4-benzpyrene); cigarette smoking	Lung cancer
Radiation	Thyroid and skin cancer
Metabolic liver carcinogens	Liver cancer
Metabolic excretory carcinogens	Bladder cancer
Metabolic carcinogens; nitrites and nitrates	Intestinal cancer

Treatment of Cancer

Cancer may be treated by using surgery, **radiation therapy**, and chemotherapy (drugs). Surgery is performed for the removal of a tumor that is localized in one area, or when the tumor is pressing on the airway, nerves, or other vital tissues. It remains the major form of treatment; however, irradiation is widely used as preoperative, postoperative, or primary therapy. Many malignant lesions are curable if detected in the early stage.

Radiation therapy is very effective in destroying tumor cells through nonsurgical means. Radiation therapy may follow surgery to kill any cancer cells that remain following the operation.

Anticancer drugs may be given to attempt a cure, for **palliation** (treatment to relieve or reduce intensity of uncomfortable symptoms, but not to produce a cure), or occasionally, as prophylaxis to prevent cancer from occurring. Chemotherapy is often combined with surgery and radiation to increase the probability of a cure. This chapter focuses on drug therapy for cancers.

ANTINEOPLASTIC AGENTS

Antineoplastic agents are used to treat cancers or malignant neoplasms. There are many types of drug therapies for the treatment of cancer. Antineoplastic agents are also called *chemotherapeutic agents*. They interrupt the development, growth, or spread of cancer cells. Antineoplastic agents are used for malignant tumors. Antineoplastic agents do not kill tumor cells directly, but interfere with cell replication (Figure 21-2). Each antineoplastic agent is effective at a specific stage in cell replication. It may inhibit DNA, RNA, or protein synthesis of cancer cells. Agents are most commonly given in combinations of two or more at a time. Many antineoplastic medications also have immunosuppressive properties that decrease the patient's ability to produce antibodies to attack infecting organisms. These medications are toxic to the body as a whole because they also destroy normal cells and decrease immunity.

The most common types of antineoplastic agents include antimetabolites, hormonal agents, special antibiotics, alkylating agents, and mitotic inhibitors (plant alkaloids). Antineoplastic agents require the following special care and handling:

- Preparation should take place only in restricted-access areas under biological safety cabinets

- Syringes and needles must have specialized fittings that are designed for use with these agents (for example, Luer-Lok™ fittings)

- Protective gowns must be worn during preparation

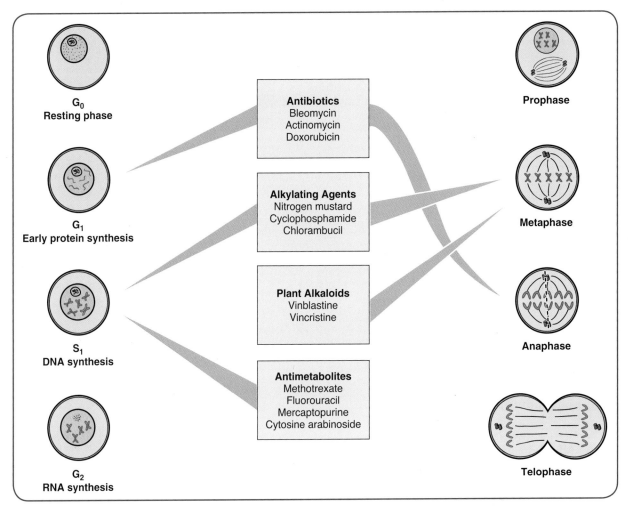

Figure 21-2 The effects of antineoplastic agents on various cell phases.

- Two pairs of protective gloves should be worn, and periodically changed

- A plastic face shield or splash goggles should be worn

- Training classes must be attended by all workers who will be handling antineoplastic agents

Antimetabolites

Antimetabolite agents prevent cancer cell growth by affecting its DNA production. They are only effective against cells that are actively participating in cell metabolism. The antimetabolite drugs are listed in Table 21-2.

The classes of antimetabolites include:

1. Folic acid antagonists: methotrexate

2. Purine analogs: mercaptopurine

3. Pyrimidine analogs: fluorouracil

Medical Terminology Review

Review

alkylating
alky(l)- = free radical
-lating = transfer
the transfer of free radicals

| TABLE 21-2 | Antimetabolites | | |

Antimetabolites

Generic Name	Trade Name	Route of Administration	Average Adult Dosage
Folic Acid Antagonists			
methotrexate sodium **(meh-thoh-TREK-sayt SOH-dee-um)**	Amethopterin®, Mexate®	PO	15–30 mg/day for 5 days
pemetrexed **(peh-meh-TREK-sed)**	Alimta®	IV	500 mg/m² on day 1 of each 21-day cycle
Purine Analogs			
cladribine **(KLAH-drih-been)**	Leustatin®	IV	0.09 mg/kg/day as a continuous infusion
clofarabine **(kloh-FAH-rah-been)**	Clolar®	IV	52 mg/m² over 2 h for 5 consecutive days
fludarabine phosphate **(floo-DAH-rah-been FOS-fayt)**	Fludara®	IV	25 mg/m² daily for 5 consecutive days
mercaptopurine (6-MP) **(mer-kap-toh-PYOO-reen)**	Purinethol®	PO	2.5 mg/kg/day
nelarabine **(neh-LAH-rah-been)**	Arranon®	IV	1500 mg/m² on days 1, 3, and 5; repeated every 21 days
pentostatin **(PEN-toh-stah-tin)**	Nipent®	IV	4 mg/m² every other week
thioguanine **(thy-oh-GWAH-neen)**	Tabloid®	PO	2 mg/kg/day
Pyrimidine Analogs			
capecitabine **(kah-peh-SY-tah-been)**	Xeloda®	PO	2500 mg/m²/day for 2 weeks
cytarabine **(sih-TAH-rah-been)**	Cytosar-U®	IV	200 mg/m² as a continuous infusion over 24 h
floxuridine **(floks-YOO-rih-deen)**	FUDR®	Intra-arterial	0.1–0.6 mg/kg/day as a continuous infusion
fluorouracil (5-FU) **(floo-roh-YOO-rah-sil)**	Adrucil®, Carac®	IV	12 mg/kg/day for 4 consecutive days
gemcitabine hydrochloride **(jem-SY-tah-been hy-droh-klor-ryd)**	Gemzar®	IV	1000 mg/m² every week

Mechanism of Action

Antimetabolites disrupt the metabolic functions of normal cells in the body. They interfere with the activity of enzymes and alter the DNA structure.

Indications

Antimetabolites are used in the treatment of a variety of neoplasms. Methotrexate is effective in the treatment of gestational choriocarcinoma and hydatidiform mole, as well as being immunosuppressant in kidney transplantation. Methotrexate is also used for acute and subacute leukemias and leukemic meningitis, especially in children. This drug is often indicated to treat severe psoriasis that is nonresponsive to other forms of therapy.

Mercaptopurine (6-MP) is used primarily for acute lymphocytic and myelogenous leukemia. Fluorouracil (5-FU) is used systemically as a single agent and in combination with other antineoplastics for palliative treatment of carefully selected patients with inoperable neoplasms of the breast, colon or rectum, stomach, pancreas, urinary bladder, ovary, cervix, and liver.

Adverse Effects

Antimetabolite agents may cause a wide variety of adverse effects. Common adverse effects include anorexia, nausea, vomiting, diarrhea, leukopenia, anemia, and thrombocytopenia. Some adverse effects of antimetabolites are dose-dependent, and may produce impaired liver function, hepatic necrosis, blurred vision, aphasia, and convulsions.

Contraindications and Precautions

Antimetabolite drugs are contraindicated in patients with anemia, thrombocytopenia, and poor nutrition. These agents are also contraindicated in patients with known hypersensitivity to these drugs, renal insufficiency, and during pregnancy (category D) or lactation.

Antimetabolite agents should be used with caution in patients with hepatic or renal impairment, active infection, or other debilitating disorders. These drugs should be avoided in patients with peptic ulcer, ulcerative colitis, and elderly patients.

Drug Interactions

Alcohol and other central nervous system (CNS) depressants may enhance CNS depression if taken with antimetabolites. Allopurinol may inhibit metabolism and increase toxicity of mercaptopurine.

Hormonal Agents

Hormonal agents are a class of **heterogeneous** compounds that have various effects on cells. These agents either block hormone production or block hormone action. Their action on malignant cells is highly selective. They are the least toxic of the anticancer medications. The most commonly used hormonal agents in cancer therapy are shown in Table 21-3.

Medical Terminology Review

leukopenia
leuko- = white
-penia = (blood cell) decrease
decrease in white blood cells

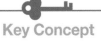

Key Concept

Administration of antimetabolite and other antineoplastic drugs in older adults may increase the risk of adverse effects. Therefore, a lower dosage is recommended for these patients, as well as those with renal impairment.

TABLE 21-3	Commonly Used Hormonal Agents		
Generic Name	Trade Name	Route of Administration	Average Adult Dosage
Hormones			
diethylstilbestrol (dy-eh-thil-stil-BEH-strol)	DES®, Stilbestrol®	PO	For prostate cancer: 500 mg tid; for palliation: 1–15 mg/day
ethinyl acetate (EH-thih-nil AH-seh-tayt)	Femring®	PO	For breast cancer: 10 mg tid; for palliation of prostate cancer: 1–2 mg tid
fluoxymesterone (floo-ok-see-MEH-steh-rohn)	Halotestin®	PO	10–40 mg tid
medroxyprogesterone acetate (meh-drok-see-proh-JEH-steh-rohn AH-seh-tayt)	Provera®, Depo-Provera®	IM	400–1000 mg q wk
megestrol acetate (meh-JEH-strol AH-seh-tayt)	Megace®	PO	40–160 mg bid–qid
prednisone (PRED-nih-zohn)	Deltasone®	PO	20–100 mg/m^2/day
testolactone (tes-toh-LAK-tohn)	Teslac®	PO	250 mg qid
testosterone (tes-TOS-teh-rohn)	Depo-Testosterone®	IM	200–400 mg q2–4 wk
Hormone Antagonists			
abarelix (ah-bah-REL-liks)	Plenaxis®	IM	100 mg on days 1, 15, and 29 and q4 wk thereafter
aminoglutethimide (ah-mee-noh-gloo-TEH-thah-myd)	Cytadren®	PO	250 mg bid–qid
anastrozole (ah-NAS-troh-zohl)	Arimidex®	PO	1 mg/day
bicalutamide (by-kah-LOO-tah-myd)	Casodex®	PO	50 mg/day
exemestane (ek-seh-MEH-stayn)	Aromasin®	PO	25 mg/day after a meal
flutamide (FLOO-tah-myd)	Eulexin®	PO	250 mg tid
goserelin acetate (goh-SEH-reh-lin AH-seh-tayt)	Zoladex®	SC	3.6 mg q28 days
letrozole (LEH-treh-zohl)	Femara®	PO	2.5 mg/day
leuprolide acetate (LOO-proh-lyd AH-seh-tayt)	Lupron®	SC, IM	SC: 1 mg/day; IM: 7.5 mg/month

Table 21-3 continued

nilutamide (ny-LOO-tah-myd)	Nilandron®	PO	300 mg/day for 30 days, then 150 mg/day
tamoxifen citrate (tah-MOK-sih-fen SIH-trayt)	Nolvadex®	PO	10–20 mg bid
toremifene citrate (toh-REH-mah-feen SIH-trayt)	Fareston®	PO	60 mg/day

Mechanism of Action

The precise action of hormones on malignant neoplasms is not known. However, these agents are able to counteract the effect of male or female hormones in hormone-dependent tumors.

Indications

Hormones and their antagonists have various uses in the treatment of malignant diseases. Steroids are especially useful in treating lymphomas, leukemias, and Hodgkin's disease. They are also used in conjunction with radiation therapy to reduce nausea, weight loss, and tissue inflammation caused by other antitumor drugs. Gonadal hormones are used in carcinomas of the reproductive tract and advanced breast cancer. For example, estrogen is given to a patient with testicular cancer or carcinoma of the prostate. Estrogen may also be administered to postmenopausal women with breast cancer. Androgens (male hormones) are prescribed in premenopausal women with breast cancer. Antiestrogens, such as tamoxifen, and anti-androgens are used to inhibit hormone production in advanced stages of breast cancer.

Adverse Effects

Major adverse effects include masculinization in female patients and feminization in male patients. Estrogen therapy may cause blood clots.

Contraindications and Precautions

Hormonal agents have a wide array of contraindications, including hypersensitivity to the agents. The use of hormonal agents must be avoided in patients with fungal infections, endometrial hyperplasia, or thromboembolic disease, and in children. They are ranked in a variety of categories if used during pregnancy and lactation (including categories C, D, and X).

Precautions for the use of hormonal agents include patients with hypertension, gallbladder disease, diabetes mellitus, heart failure, liver or kidney dysfunction, infections, nonspecific ulcerative colitis, diverticulitis, peptic ulcer, osteoporosis, and myasthenia gravis. Hormonal agents must be used with great caution in many other conditions.

Drug Interactions

Hormonal agents may cause drug interactions with many agents, including but not limited to carbamazepine, phenytoin, rifampin, corticosteroids, oral anticoagulants, barbiturates, amphotericin B, diuretics, ambenonium, neostigmine, and pyridostigmine. Hormonal agents may inhibit antibody response to vaccines and toxoids.

Antitumor Antibiotics

Several antibiotics of microbial origin are very effective in the treatment of certain tumors. They are used only to treat cancer, and are not used to treat infections. These antibiotics include bleomycin, doxorubicin, daunorubicin, idarubicin, mitomycin, and plicamycin (Table 21-4).

Mechanism of Action

The mechanism of action of antitumor antibiotics is the inhibition of DNA and RNA synthesis. Antitumor antibiotics attach to DNA, distorting its structure and preventing normal DNA-to-RNA synthesis.

Indications

Antitumor antibiotics are used for treating a few specific types of cancer. For example, plicamycin is used only for treatment of testicular cancer. The only indication for idarubicin is acute leukemia. Doxorubicin is the single most active agent against breast cancer.

Adverse Effects

The most serious adverse effects of antitumor antibiotics are low blood cell counts and congestive heart failure. Their common adverse effects include nausea, vomiting, diarrhea, fatigue, headache, and **alopecia** (hair loss). Bleomycin may cause pneumonitis, pulmonary fibrosis, and rash.

Contraindications and Precautions

Antitumor antibiotics are contraindicated in patients with known hypersensitivity, bleeding disorders, coagulation disorders, suppression of bone marrow, electrolyte imbalance, and chickenpox, herpes zoster, or other viral infections; in women of childbearing age; during pregnancy (various categories, including C and D) and lactation; and in infants younger than six months of age.

Precautions for use of antitumor antibiotics include patients with compromised hepatic, renal, or pulmonary function, and those with previous cytotoxic drug or radiation therapy, bone marrow depression, infections, gout, or obesity. There are many other precautions for these agents as well.

Drug Interactions

When bleomycin is given with cisplatin, there is an increased risk of bleomycin toxicity. Mitoxantrone, dactinomycin, mitomycin, and plicamycin

TABLE 21-4 | **Antitumor Antibiotics**

Generic Name	Trade Name	Route of Administration	Average Adult Dosage
bleomycin sulfate **(blee-oh-MY-sin SUL-fayt)**	Blenoxane®	SC, IM, IV	10–20 units/m² (1–2 times/wk)
dactinomycin **(dak-tih-no-MY-sin)**	Actinomycin D®, Cosmegen®	IV	500 mcg/day for a maximum of 5 days
daunorubicin citrate liposomal **(daw-noh-ROO-bih-sin SIH-trayt ly-poh-SOH-mal)**	DaunoXome®	IV	40 mg/m² q2 wk
daunorubicin hydrochloride **(daw-noh-ROO-bih-sin hy-droh-KLOR-ryd)**	Cerubidine®	IV	30–60 mg/m²/day for 3–5 days
doxorubicin hydrochloride **(dok-soh-ROO-bih-sin hy-droh-KLOR-ryd)**	Adriamycin®, Rubex®	IV	60–75 mg/m² as a single dose
doxorubicin liposomal **(dok-soh-ROO-bih-sin ly-poh-SOH-mal)**	Doxil®	IV	20 mg/m² q3 wk
epirubicin hydrochloride **(eh-pih-ROO-bih-sin hy-droh-KLOR-ryd)**	Ellence®	IV	100–120 mg/m² as a single dose
idarubicin **(eye-dah-ROO-bih-sin)**	Idamycin PFS®	IV	8–12 mg/m²/day for 3 days
mitomycin **(my-toh-MY-sin)**	Mutamycin®	IV	10–20 mg/m²/day as a single dose
mitoxantrone hydrochloride **(my-toh-ZAN-trohn hy-droh-KLOR-ryd)**	Novantrone®	IV	12–14 mg/m² q21 days
plicamycin **(plih-kah-MY-sin)**	Mithramycin®, Mithracin®	IV	25–30 mcg/kg/day for 3–4 days
valrubicin **(val-ROO-bih-sin)**	Valstar®	Intrabladder instillation	800 mg q wk for 6 weeks

increase bone marrow depression. There may be an increased risk of bleeding when plicamycin is used with aspirin, warfarin, heparin, or a nonsteroidal anti-inflammatory drug.

Alkylating Agents

Alkylating agents were the first group of antineoplastic agents. During World War I, chemical warfare was introduced using nitrogen mustard. Alkylating agents came to be used for cancer therapy as a result of observation of the effects of the mustard war gases on cell growth (Table 21-5).

TABLE 21-5	Alkylating Agents		
Generic Name	Trade Name	Route of Administration	Average Adult Dosage
Nitrogen Mustards			
chlorambucil (klor-AM-byoo-sil)	Leukeran®	PO	Initial: 0.1–0.2 mg/kg/day; Maint: 4–10 mg/day
cyclophosphamide (sy-kloh-FOS-fah-myd)	Cytoxan®	PO	Initial: 1–5 mg/kg/day; Maint: 1–5 mg/kg q7–10 days
estramustine sodium phosphate (ehs-trah-MUS-teen SOH-dee-um FOS-fayt)	Emcyt®	PO	14 mg/kg tid–qid
ifosfamide (eye-FOS-fah-myd)	Ifex®	IV	1.2 g/m^2/day for 5 days
mechlorethamine hydrochloride (meh-KLOH-reh-thah-meen hy-droh-KLOR-ryd)	Mustargen®	IV	6 mg/m^2 on days 1 and 8 for 28 days
melphalan (MEL-fah-lan)	Alkeran®	PO	6 mg/day for 2–3 weeks
Nitrosoureas			
carmustine (kar-MUH-steen)	Gliadel®	IV	150–200 mg/m^2 q6 wk
lomustine (LOH-muh-steen)	CeeNU®	PO	130 mg/m^2 as a single dose
streptozocin (strep-TOH-zoh-sin)	Zanosar®	IV	500 mg/m^2 for 5 consecutive days
Miscellaneous Agents			
busulfan (byoo-SUL-fan)	Myleran®	PO	4–8 mg/day
carboplatin (KAR-boh-plah-tin)	Paraplatin®	IV	360 mg/m^2 q4 wk
cisplatin (SIS-plah-tin)	Platinol®	IV	20 mg/m^2/day for 5 days
dacarbazine (dah-KAR-bah-zeen)	DTIC-Dome®	IV	2–4.5 mg/kg/day for 10 days
oxaliplatin (ok-ZAH-lih-plah-tin)	Eloxatin®	IV	85 mg/m^2 infused over 120 min once q2 wk
temozolomide (teh-moh-ZOH-lah-myd)	Temodar®	PO	150 mg/m^2/day for 5 consecutive days
thiotepa (thy-oh-TEH-pah)	Thioplex®	IV	0.3–0.4 mg/kg q1–4 wk

Mechanism of Action

Most alkylating agents interact with the process of cell division of cancer cells. Antineoplastic or cytotoxic action is primarily due to cross-linking of strands of DNA and RNA as well as inhibition of protein synthesis. These drugs bind with DNA, causing breaks and preventing DNA replication.

Indications

Alkylating agents are used to treat metastatic ovarian, testicular, and bladder cancers. They are also used for the palliative treatment of other cancers. The newer drugs in this category are **nitrosoureas**, lipid-soluble drugs used in treating brain tumors and testicular or ovarian cancers.

Adverse Effects

Major adverse effects of the alkylating agents include nausea, vomiting, anorexia, diarrhea, bone marrow suppression, hepatic and renal toxicity, and dermatitis. Other adverse effects of alkylating drugs include cataracts, anxiety, fever, skin rash, hypertension, tachycardia, dizziness, and insomnia. The alkylating agent busulfan may cause the adverse effect of gynecomastia.

Contraindications and Precautions

Alkylating agents are contraindicated in patients with known hypersensitivity, impaired renal function, myelosuppression, impaired hearing, history of gout and urate renal stones, hypomagnesia, Raynaud syndrome, and many more conditions; with concurrent administration with loop diuretics; and during pregnancy (various categories) and lactation. Safe use in children is not established for many of these agents.

Precautions include use in patients with previous cytotoxic drug or radiation therapy with other ototoxic and nephrotoxic drugs, hyperuricemia, electrolyte imbalances, hepatic impairment, and history of circulatory disorders. There are many other precautions for these agents as well.

Drug Interactions

Drug interactions with alkylating agents include aminoglycosides, amphotericin B, vancomycin, other nephrotoxic drugs, furosemide, barbiturates, phenytoin, chloral hydrate, and corticosteroids. There are other drug interactions with these various agents as well.

Mitotic Inhibitors

Mitotic inhibitors (plant alkaloids) are derived from plants. The primary plant alkaloids are vincristine and vinblastine. Teniposide is a close analog of etoposide and is active against acute leukemias in children. Topotecan is a semisynthetic plant alkaloid used for refractory ovarian cancer that may have activity against small-cell lung cancer. Examples of plant alkaloids are shown in Table 21-6.

Medical Terminology Review

myelosuppression
myelo- = bone marrow
-suppression = slowing of function
slowing of the production and function of the bone marrow

Medical Terminology Review

hyperuricemia
hyper- = more; excessive
uric = uric acid
-emia = blood condition
excessive uric acid in the blood

TABLE 21-6	Mitotic Inhibitors and Other Plant Products		
Generic Name	**Trade Name**	**Route of Administration**	**Average Adult Dosage**
Mitotic Inhibitors			
vinblastine sulfate **(vin-BLAH-steen SUL-fayt)**	Velban®	IV	3.7–18.5 mg/m^2 q wk
vincristine sulfate **(vin-KRIH-steen SUL-fayt)**	Oncovin®	IV	1.4 mg/m^2 q wk (max: 2 mg/m^2)
vinorelbine tartrate **(vin-oh-REL-been TAR-trayt)**	Navelbine®	IV	30 mg/m^2 q wk
Taxoids			
docetaxel **(doh-seh-TAK-sehl)**	Taxotere®	IV	60–100 mg/m^2 q3 wk
paclitaxel **(pak-lih-TAK-sehl)**	Taxol®	IV	135–175 mg/m^2 q3 wk
Topoisomerase Inhibitors			
etoposide **(ee-toh-POH-syd)**	VePesid®	IV	50–100 mg/m^2/day for 5 days
irinotecan hydrochloride **(eye-rih-noh-TEE-kan hy-droh-KLOR-ryd)**	Camptosar®	IV	125 mg/m^2 q wk for 4 weeks
teniposide **(teh-NIH-poh-syd)**	Vumon®	IV	165 mg/m^2 q3–4 days for 4 weeks
topotecan hydrochloride **(toh-poh-TEE-kan hy-droh-KLOR-ryd)**	Hycamtin®	IV	1.5 mg/m^2/day for 5 days

Mechanism of Action

Mitotic inhibitors may interfere with cell division, but the antineoplastic mechanism of these agents is unclear.

Indications

Mitotic inhibitor drugs are used in various cancers. For example, docetaxel is prescribed for breast cancer and non–small-cell lung cancer. Vinblastine is indicated for the treatment of Hodgkin's disease, lymphocytic lymphoma, testicular cancer, Kaposi's sarcoma, and breast cancer.

Vincristine is used in acute leukemia and combination therapy for various cancers. Paclitaxel is given to patients with ovarian or breast cancers, or those with AIDS-related Kaposi's sarcoma.

Adverse Effects

Common adverse effects of mitotic inhibitors include nausea, vomiting, diarrhea, fatigue, mental depression, and alopecia. Infection and peripheral neuropathy are also considered to be unwanted effects of mitotic inhibitors.

Contraindications and Precautions

Mitotic inhibitors are contraindicated in patients with known hypersensitivity to these drugs and should be avoided in patients with leukopenia or bacterial infection, and during pregnancy (category D) or lactation. Etoposide is contraindicated in patients with severe bone marrow depression, and in severe hepatic or renal impairment. Mitotic inhibitors should be used with caution in patients who have impaired kidney or liver function, gout, obstructive jaundice, or idiopathic thrombocytopenic purpura.

Drug Interactions

Mitotic inhibitors may interact with many drugs. For example, vincristine used with asparaginase may cause increased neurotoxicity secondary to decreased liver clearance of vincristine. When mitotic inhibitors are used with calcium channel blockers, they may increase accumulation of these agents in cells.

SUMMARY

A neoplasm is a tumor that occurs in response to abnormal cell division in the body. It may be benign or malignant. Only malignant tumors are capable of spreading to other organs or systems of the body. Treatment of the neoplasm depends on the progression of the tumor. Surgery, radiation therapy, chemotherapy, or immunotherapy may be indicated. Several agents are used for this purpose. Many antineoplastic medications also have immunosuppressive properties that decrease the patient's ability to produce antibodies to attack infecting organisms.

Common antineoplastic agents include antimetabolites, hormonal agents, specific antibiotics, alkylating agents, and mitotic inhibitors or plant alkaloids. In some cases, surgery and radiation therapy are also necessary. Toxicity and side effects of chemotherapy and radiation therapy are the major concerns associated with treatment of malignant tumors.

EXPLORING THE WEB

Visit the following websites for additional information on drug therapies used to treat cancer:

- **www.biochemweb.org** – Virtual Library of Biochemistry, Molecular Biology and Cell Biology
- **www.cancer.org** – American Cancer Society
- **www.cancer.gov** – National Cancer Institute
- **www.cdc.gov/niosh** – Centers for Disease Control and Prevention, National Institute for Occupational Safety and Health
- **www.mayoclinic.com** – Mayo Clinic

REVIEW QUESTIONS

Multiple Choice

1. The cell cycle consists of several phases, such as G_0, G_1, S_1, G_2, and M. Which of the following explains the G_0 phase?

   A. resting

   B. synthesis

   C. mitosis

   D. growth

2. Which of the following agents is an antimetabolite?

   A. cyclophosphamide

   B. fluorouracil

   C. mitomycin

   D. nitrogen mustard

3. Which of the following is an example of an antitumor antibiotic?

   A. vinorelbine

   B. topotecan

   C. bleomycin

   D. mercaptopurine

4. Mitotic inhibitors (plant alkaloids) include:

   A. mercaptopurine

   B. testolactone

   C. tamoxifen

   D. vincristine

5. Mercaptopurine may have drug interactions with which of the following agents?

   A. amoxicillin

   B. alcohol

   C. allopurinol

   D. estrogen

6. An adverse effect of methotrexate includes:

   A. anemia

   B. arthritis

   C. hypertension

   D. hyperthyroidism

7. Busulfan has some unusual side effects in addition to its bone marrow suppressive activity. Which of the following side effects are caused by busulfan?

   A. peptic ulcer

   B. testicular cancer

   C. gynecomastia

   D. gastrointestinal bleeding

8. Which of the following is the trade name of doxorubicin?

   A. Mutamycin®

   B. Adriamycin®

   C. Cosmegan®

   D. Blenoxane®

9. The route of administration for goserelin is:

   A. oral

   B. intramuscular

   C. intravenous

   D. subcutaneous

10. Most plant alkaloids may produce:

    A. nausea and vomiting

    B. internal bleeding

    C. hypertension

    D. gout

11. Which of the following antimetabolites is useful in maintenance therapy of children with acute leukemia or leukemic meningitis?

    A. fluorouracil (5-FU)

    B. methotrexate (MTX)

    C. mercaptopurine (6-MP)

    D. vincristine

12. Which of the following is the best drug that may be given to a patient with testicular cancer?

    A. tamoxifen

    B. estrogen

    C. progesterone

    D. megestrol

13. The term metastasize means to:

    A. arise

    B. divide

    C. spread

    D. occur

14. Hycamtin® is the trade name of which of the following agents?

    A. vincristine

    B. vinblastine

    C. vinorelbine

    D. topotecan

15. The single most active agent against breast cancer is:

    A. dactinomycin

    B. mitomycin

    C. doxorubicin

    D. bleomycin

Matching

_____ 1. Resting phase

_____ 2. Cell division

_____ 3. Synthesis

_____ 4. Second growth phase

_____ 5. First growth phase

A. G_1

B. S_1

C. G_2

D. M

E. G_0

Generic Names

_____ 1. vincristine

_____ 2. vinblastine

_____ 3. vinorelbine

_____ 4. paclitaxel

_____ 5. etoposide

Trade Names

A. VePesid®

B. Navelbine®

C. Oncovin®

D. Velban®

E. Taxol®

Critical Thinking

A biopsy revealed that a 45-year-old woman had breast cancer. She underwent surgery and her left breast was removed. Her physician ordered radiation therapy and chemotherapy as adjuvant therapies to the surgery.

1. If she were to refuse radiation or chemotherapy, what would be the likely consequence?

2. List the most common adverse effects of chemotherapy.

3. If the physician diagnosed that this patient had metastasis to her bones, which types of treatment should he recommend?

CHAPTER 22 — Analgesics

OBJECTIVES

After completing this chapter, the reader should be able to:

1. Identify the different types of analgesics.
2. Differentiate salicylates from nonsalicylate nonsteroid anti-inflammatory drugs.
3. Describe the uses and adverse effects of nonsalicylate analgesics.
4. List the dangers of aspirin use.
5. Explain the contraindications of aspirin use.
6. Describe the use of cyclooxygenase-2 inhibitors.
7. Explain the reason behind the use of narcotic analgesics.
8. Outline three narcotic antagonists.
9. Explain the major adverse effects of narcotic analgesics.
10. Describe the opioid receptors.

GLOSSARY

Acute pain – pain that is of sudden onset and brief course; can also mean "severe"

Agonist-antagonists – agents that can initiate or resist actions

Analgesic – a compound that relieves pain by altering perception without producing anesthesia or loss of consciousness

Bradykinin – a polypeptide that mediates inflammation, increases vasodilation, and contracts smooth muscle

Chronic pain – pain that is persistent or long term; can also mean "low intensity"

Cyclooxygenase inhibitors – drugs that prevent the action of one of two enzymes that have an essential role in the inflammatory process

Intracranial – within the cranium (skull)

Nonsteroidal anti-inflammatory drugs (NSAIDs) – drugs that have analgesic and antipyretic effects

Opioid – a natural or synthetic narcotic substance

Opioid agonists – drugs that can combine with opioid receptors to initiate drug actions

Opioid antagonists – drugs that oppose or resist the action of opioids

Pain – an unpleasant sensation associated with actual or potential tissue damage

Reye syndrome – an acquired encephalopathy of young children that follows an acute febrile illness; strongly associated with aspirin use

Salicylates – salts or esters of salicylic acid

OVERVIEW

Pain is a common problem and an unpleasant sensory experience that is associated with actual damage of tissue. **Pain** is the reaction of the central nervous system (CNS) to severe harmful stimuli. It may be an early warning system to prevent any further damage to the body. Pain stimuli may be caused by the process of inflammation or tissue injury. Pain may be described as mild, moderate, or severe; acute or chronic; dull or sharp; burning or piercing; and localized or generalized. **Acute pain** is severe pain with a sudden onset. **Chronic pain** lasts a long time or is marked by frequent reoccurrence. During an organ's injury or inflammation, different chemical substances are released. These substances include histamine, prostaglandins (hormone-like substances that control blood pressure, contract smooth muscle, and modulate inflammation), serotonin, and **bradykinin** (a polypeptide that mediates inflammation, increases vasodilation, and contracts smooth muscle). These chemical substances initiate an action potential along a sensory nerve fiber or sensitize pain receptors, enabling the pain signal to be transmitted. This chapter provides discussion of the various medicinal products used in the relief of pain.

ANALGESICS

> **Medical Terminology Review**
>
> **osteoarthritis**
> osteo- = bone
> arthr = joint
> -itis = inflammation
> inflammation of the bones affecting the joints

Pain-relieving (**analgesic**) drugs are currently available for all levels of painful stimuli. Analgesics may be classified as **opioid** (narcotic) or nonopioid medications. Many of these agents affect pain, fever, and inflammation, depending on their properties. Nonopioid analgesics, antipyretics, and anti-inflammatory drugs are used widely for minor aches and pains, headaches, malaise, rheumatoid arthritis, osteoarthritis, other forms of arthritis, gout, and other musculoskeletal disorders. The narcotic (opioid) analgesics are controlled substances used to treat moderate to severe pain.

Salicylates

Salicylates are the oldest of the nonopioid analgesics and nonsteroidal anti-inflammatory drugs (NSAIDs), which are discussed in detail below. They are still often used as analgesics (Table 22-1). The salicylates include aspirin (acetylsalicylic acid), which is the most commonly used. The salicylates may be combined with caffeine to increase their action. Anacin® and Excedrin® are examples of salicylates that are combined with caffeine. Caffeine can make some of these agents work more quickly or provide additional relief.

Mechanism of Action

The mechanism of action of salicylates is not fully understood. Major actions appear to be associated primarily with inhibiting the formation of prostaglandins involved in the production of inflammation, pain, and fever.

TABLE 22-1	Salicylates and Nonsalicylates		
Generic Name	**Trade Name**	**Route of Administration**	**Average Adult Dosage**
Salicylates			
aspirin (acetylsalicylic acid) **(AHS-pih-rin [ah-see-til-sah-lih-SIH-lik AH-sid])**	Bayer®, Ecotrin®	PO, Rectal	PO, Rectal: 325–650 mg q4h prn, up to 4 g/day
buffered aspirin **(BUF-ferd AHS-pih-rin)**	Ascriptin®	PO, Rectal	PO, Rectal: 325–650 mg q4h prn, up to 4 g/day
choline salicylate **(KOH-leen sah-LIH-sih-layt)**	Arthropan®	PO	870 mg q3–4h (max: 6 times/day)
diflunisal **(dy-FLOO-nih-sahl)**	Dolobid®	PO	500–1000 mg/day in 2 divided doses (max: 1.5 g/day)
magnesium salicylate **(mag-NEE-zee-um sah-LIH-sih-layt)**	Doan's Pills®, Mobidin®	PO	650 mg tid–qid up to 9.6 g/day in divided doses
salsalate **(SAL-sah-layt)**	Amigesic®	PO	325–3000 mg/day in divided doses
sodium salicylate **(SOH-dee-um sah-LIH-sih-layt)**	(generic only)	PO	325–650 mg q4h
sodium thiosalicylate **(SOH-dee-um thy-oh-sah-LIH-sih-layt)**	Rexolate®	IM	50–150 mg q4–6h
Nonsalicylates			
acetaminophen **(ah-see-tah-MIH-noh-fen)**	Tempra®, Tylenol®	PO	325–650 mg/day q4–6h or 1 g 3–4 times daily; max: 4 g/day

Indications

Salicylates are also prescribed as NSAIDs for patients with rheumatoid arthritis or osteoarthritis, and often for other inflammatory disorders. Aspirin is absorbed rapidly from the stomach and duodenum. It is used as an antipyretic, anti-inflammatory, and analgesic agent in a variety of conditions. Aspirin is indicated for the relief of pain from simple headache, minor muscular aches, and fever. When drug therapy is indicated for the reduction of a fever, it is one of the most effective and safest drugs. Because of its antiplatelet properties, aspirin may be useful in the prevention of coronary thrombosis by prolonging bleeding time, and to prevent blood clots in small arteries.

Adverse Effects

Common adverse effects of high doses of aspirin (in 70% of patients) include nausea, vomiting, diarrhea or constipation, dyspepsia, epigastric pain,

Medical Terminology Review

antipyretic
anti- = not
-pyretic = producing fever
fever-reducing

Key Concept

Salicylates must be used cautiously in children who have fever or are dehydrated, because they are particularly prone to intoxication from relatively small doses of these drugs. An allergic sensitivity to salicylates may cause a serious problem. Patients who have asthma, nasal polyps, or allergies must be very careful when they take these drugs to avoid potentially dangerous adverse effects.

Aspirin use should be avoided in infants and young children if they have flu-like illnesses, because it may cause the development of Reye syndrome.

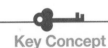

Key Concept

Some foods, such as prunes, paprika, raisins, and tea, contain salicylates, which can increase the risk of adverse effects.

bleeding, and ulceration in the stomach. Intolerance is relatively common with aspirin and includes rash, bronchospasm, rhinitis, edema, or an anaphylactic reaction with shock, which may be life threatening. Use of aspirin and other salicylates to control fever during viral infections in children and adolescents (e.g., influenza, common cold, and chickenpox) is associated with an increased incidence of **Reye syndrome**. Vomiting, hepatic disturbances, and encephalopathy characterize this illness. Salicylates that are combined with caffeine can, in very large doses, cause birth defects to a developing fetus. Caffeine, as used in some of these preparations, can make some kinds of heart disease worse.

Contraindications and Precautions

Salicylates are contraindicated in patients with known hypersensitivity and during pregnancy (category C), but aspirin during pregnancy is category D. The salicylates should be avoided in patients with bleeding disorders or peptic ulcers, or those receiving anticoagulant or antineoplastic drugs. The salicylates, particularly aspirin, are also contraindicated in patients with chickenpox and influenza.

Drug Interactions

Salicylates increase the risk of gastrointestinal (GI) ulceration with alcohol and corticosteroids. They also increase the risk of toxicity with carbonic anhydrase inhibitors and valproic acid. Ammonium chloride and other acidifying agents decrease renal elimination and increase the risk of salicylate toxicity. Anticoagulants increase the risk of bleeding. Antacids may decrease the effects of the salicylate. In order to prevent drug interactions, patients must be instructed by their physician and pharmacist about the use of NSAIDs with other over-the-counter (OTC) analgesics.

Acetaminophen

Another common nonopioid analgesic, acetaminophen, is available OTC and is found in most households.

Mechanism of Action

Like aspirin, acetaminophen has analgesic and antipyretic actions. It can be used with relative safety in age groups from young children through older adults. Unlike aspirin, it does not have anti-inflammatory actions. The mechanism of action may be inhibition of prostaglandin in the peripheral nervous system, which makes the sensory neurons less likely to receive the pain signal. Acetaminophen is recommended as a substitute for children with fever of unknown etiology.

Acetaminophen does not displace other drugs from plasma proteins; it causes minimal GI irritation. Acetaminophen has little effect on platelet adhesion and aggregation. It can be substituted for aspirin to treat mild to moderate pain or fever for selected patients who:

- Are intolerant to aspirin
- Have a history of peptic ulcer or hemophilia
- Are using anticoagulants
- Are at risk (viral infection) for Reye syndrome

Indications

Acetaminophen is used for fever reduction and the temporary relief of mild to moderate pain. Acetaminophen may be used as a substitute for aspirin when the latter is not tolerated or is contraindicated.

Adverse Effects

Acute acetaminophen poisoning may produce anorexia, nausea, vomiting, dizziness, chills, abdominal pain, diarrhea, hepatotoxicity, hypoglycemia, hepatic coma, and acute renal failure (rare). Chronic ingestion of acetaminophen may cause neutropenia, pancytopenia, leukopenia, and hepatotoxicity in alcoholics, as well as renal damage. For acetaminophen overdose, acetylcysteine (Acetadote®, Mucomyst®) is used.

Contraindications and Precautions

Acetaminophen is contraindicated in those with known hypersensitivity to this agent or phenacetin. Acetaminophen should not be used with alcohol.

Precautions include use in children younger than three years of age unless directed by a physician, and repeated administration to patients with anemia or hepatic disease. Cautious use is advised in arthritic or rheumatoid conditions affecting children younger than 12 years of age, and in patients with alcoholism, malnutrition, or thrombocytopenia. Safety during pregnancy (category B) or lactation is not established.

Drug Interactions

Cholestyramine may decrease acetaminophen absorption with chronic co-administration. Barbiturates, carbamazepine, phenytoin, and rifampin may increase the potential for chronic hepatotoxicity. Chronic, excessive ingestion of alcohol will increase the risk of hepatotoxicity.

Nonsteroidal Anti-Inflammatory Drugs

Most of the **nonsteroidal anti-inflammatory drugs (NSAIDs)** have analgesic and antipyretic effects. Little difference is seen between the effects of different NSAIDs, but some patients may respond better to one agent than to another. Anti-inflammatory effects may develop only after several weeks of treatment. Drug selection is generally dictated by the patient's ability to tolerate adverse effects. Aspirin, other salicylates, and newer drugs with

---

Medical Terminology Review

anticoagulant
anti- = not
-coagulant = an agent that causes clotting
an agent that will not cause clotting of the blood

Medical Terminology Review

thrombocytopenia
thrombo- = clot
cyto = cell (such as a platelet)
-penia = lack of
inability of the blood to clot

diverse structures are referred to as *nonsteroidal* anti-inflammatory drugs to distinguish them from the anti-inflammatory *corticosteroids*. The number of NSAIDs continues to increase. In addition to salicylate drugs, the NSAIDs available in the United States include indomethacin, meclofenamate, piroxicam, sulindac, tolmetin, celecoxib, and many more (Table 22-2).

TABLE 22-2	Nonsteroidal Anti-inflammatory Drugs (NSAIDs)		
Generic Name	**Trade Name**	**Route of Administration**	**Average Adult Dosage**
celecoxib (seh-leh-COK-sib)	Celebrex®	PO	100–200 mg bid prn
diclofenac sodium (dy-KLOH-feh-nak SOH-dee-um)	Voltaren®	PO	Osteoarthritis: 100–150 mg/day in divided doses; Rheumatoid arthritis: 150–200 mg/day in divided doses; Ankylosing spondylitis: 100–125 mg/day in divided doses
diflusinal (dy-FLOO-zih-nal)	(generic only)	PO	Initial: 1000 mg; Maint: 500 mg q12h
etodolac (ee-TOH-doh-lak)	Lodine®, Lodine XL®	PO	Acute pain: 200–400 mg q6–8h prn; Osteoarthritis: 600–1200 mg/day in 2–4 divided doses (max: 1200 mg/day or 20 mg/kg for patients who weigh less than 60 kg); Lodine XL®: 400–1000 mg once daily); Rheumatoid arthritis: 500 mg bid
fenoprofen calcium (fen-oh-PROH-fen KAL-see-um)	Nalfon®	PO	Rheumatoid arthritis and osteoarthritis: 300–600 mg tid–qid; Pain: 200 mg q4–8h
flurbiprofen (fler-bih-PROH-fen)	Ansaid®	PO	200–300 mg/day in divided doses
ibuprofen (eye-byoo-PROH-fen)	Advil®, Motrin®	PO	Arthritis disorders: 400–800 mg/day in divided doses (max: 3200 mg/day); Pain: 400 mg q4–6h; Dysmenorrhea: 400 mg q4h
indomethacin (in-doh-MEH-thah-sin)	Indocin®	PO	Anti-inflammatory and analgesic: 25–50 mg bid–tid (max: 200 mg/day); Acute painful shoulder: 75–150 mg/day in 3–4 divided doses
ketoprofen (kee-toh-PROH-fen)	Oruvail®	PO	Inflammatory disease: 75 mg tid or 50 mg qid (max: 300 mg/day) or 200 mg sustained release qd; Pain or dysmenorrhea: 25–50 mg q6–8 h
ketorolac tromethamine (kee-toh-ROH-lak troh-MEH-thah-meen)	Toradol®	PO, IM	PO: 10 mg q4–6 h prn (max: 40 mg/day); IM: 30–60 mg initially, followed by half of initial dose q6h prn
meclofenamate sodium (mek-loh-FEH-nah-mayt SOH-dee-um)	(generic)	PO	Rheumatoid arthritis: 200–400 mg/day in 3–4 doses; Pain: 50 mg q 4–6h (max: 400 mg/day); Dysmenorrhea: 100 mg tid.

Table 22-2 continued

mefenamic acid (**meh-feh-NAH-mik AH-sid**)	Ponstel®	PO	500 mg followed by 250 mg q6h prn (max: 1 wk of therapy)
meloxicam (**meh-LOK-sih-kam**)	Mobic®	PO	7.5–15 mg qd
naproxen sodium (**nah-PROK-sen SOH-dee-um**)	Aleve®, Anaprox®	PO	Pain, primary dysmenorrhea: 500 mg initially then 250 mg q6–8h; Arthritic disorders: 250–500 mg bid
oxaprozin (**ok-zah-PROH-zin**)	Daypro®	PO	600–1200 mg qd
piroxicam (**pih-ROK-sih-kam**)	Feldene®	PO	20 mg/day single dose or 10 mg bid
sulindac (**SOO-lin-dak**)	Clinoril®	PO	150–200 mg bid for 1–2 wks, then reduce dose (max: 400 mg/day)
tolmetin sodium (**TOHL-meh-tin SOH-dee-um**)	Tolectin®	PO	400 mg bid–tid (max: 2 g/day)

Mechanism of Action

The mechanism of action of NSAIDs is unknown. It may derive from irreversible inhibition of prostaglandin formation, which involves the conversion of arachidonic acid to prostaglandin by the enzyme cyclooxygenase (COX). This action is involved in the processes of pain and inflammation. Some experts believe that NSAIDs relieve fever by central action in the hypothalamus of the brain. In low doses, baby aspirin appears to affect blood clotting by inhibiting prostaglandin formation, which prevents synthesis of platelet-aggregating substances. This can help to prevent heart attacks and strokes. NSAIDs inhibit, in varying amounts, both cyclooxygenase-1 (COX-1) and cyclooxygenase-2 (COX-2).

Indications

NSAIDs are used for mild to moderate pain when opioids are not indicated. Most NSAIDs are used for inflammatory conditions such as arthritis, osteoarthritis, dysmenorrhea, and dental pain. NSAIDs are available OTC in lower dosages and by prescription in larger dosages. Aspirin and ibuprofen are available as inexpensive OTC drugs. Ibuprofen is available in many different formulations, including those designed for children.

Adverse Effects

Many NSAIDs are safe and produce adverse effects only at high doses. The most common adverse effects (at high doses) are GI distress, gastric ulcers, and GI bleeding. Other NSAIDs, such as the COX-2 inhibitors discussed in the following section, are being investigated for possible adverse effects.

Contraindications and Precautions

Nonsteroidal anti-inflammatory drugs are contraindicated in patients with known hypersensitivity to any NSAIDs. These drugs are also contraindicated in patients with nasal polyps, asthma, and angioedema. NSAIDs should be avoided during pregnancy and in patients with history of peptic ulcer, or renal or hepatic impairment. NSAIDs have Black Box Warnings since they may cause an increased risk of serious cardiovascular thrombotic events, myocardial infarction, and stroke, which can be fatal. They may also cause an increased risk of serious GI adverse events, including bleeding, ulceration, and perforation of the stomach or intestines, which can be fatal. NSAIDs should never be used right before or after a coronary artery bypass graft surgery.

Drug Interactions

NSAIDs should not be taken with other OTC analgesics such as acetaminophen, aspirin, or other NSAIDs. NSAIDs may result in harmful drug interactions if taken with alcohol and a wide variety of other medications. Use of NSAIDs with phenobarbital, antacids, and glucocorticoids may decrease their effects. Insulin, methotrexate, phenytoin, sulfonamides, and penicillin may increase the effects of NSAIDs.

Cyclooxygenase Inhibitors

The two main types of **cyclooxygenase inhibitors** (COX-1 and COX-2) have been found to have an essential role in the inflammatory process. Both are present in the synovial fluid of patients with arthritis. COX-2 is more specific for prostaglandin synthesis in response to an inflammatory event. It is thought to be primarily responsible for the desired anti-inflammatory, analgesic, and antipyretic effects, whereas COX-1 has a more extensive role in the body, including protection of the GI lining.

Although the U.S. Food and Drug Administration (FDA) approved the COX-2 inhibitors celecoxib (Celebrex®) and rofecoxib (Vioxx®) in 2000, rofecoxib was removed from the U.S. market after problems were reported in certain patients. A third inhibitor, meloxicam (Mobic®), has more recently been introduced. It actually inhibits both COX-1 and COX-2. The daily role of COX appears to be the synthesis of prostaglandins that contribute to normal homeostasis.

Mechanism of Action

These agents inhibit prostaglandin synthesis by selectively targeting specific COX enzymes. The COX-2 inhibitors have similar anti-inflammatory effects without the adverse GI effects that accompany COX-1 inhibitors.

Medical Terminology Review

angioedema
angio- = blood vessel
-edema = swelling caused by fluid
swelling of blood vessels

Key Concept

NSAIDs must be used cautiously with herbal supplements such as feverfew, which may increase the risk of bleeding.

Key Concept

Prostaglandins are derivatives of prostanoic acid. In the body, prostaglandins are principally synthesized from arachidonic acid (lipids) by the enzyme COX.

Indications

The FDA has approved celecoxib for the treatment of osteoarthritis, rheumatoid arthritis, primary dysmenorrhea, and acute pain. Rofecoxib, as mentioned, is off the market in the United States. Meloxicam, the newest COX inhibitor, has been approved by the FDA for the treatment of osteoarthritis.

Adverse Effects

The common adverse effects of COX-2 inhibitors include fatigue, flu-like symptoms, lower extremity swelling, and back pain. Dizziness, headache, hypertension, edema, heartburn, and nausea are also seen with the use of COX-2 inhibitors.

Contraindications and Precautions

COX-2 inhibitors are contraindicated in patients with known hypersensitivity to these agents, urticaria, asthma, or a history of anaphylactic reaction after taking NSAIDs or aspirin. COX-2 inhibitors are also contraindicated in elderly patients, during pregnancy (third trimester), and in lactating women. These drugs should be avoided in patients with renal disease or hepatic dysfunction.

COX-2 inhibitors should be used cautiously in patients with congestive heart failure, fluid retention, or hypertension.

Drug Interactions

COX-2 inhibitors diminish the effectiveness of angiotensin-converting enzyme inhibitors. Fluconazole increases concentrations of celecoxib. COX-2 inhibitors may increase lithium concentrations.

Narcotic Analgesics

Narcotic analgesics are derived from opium or opium-like compounds with potent analgesic effects associated with both significant alteration of mood and behavior, and potential for dependence and tolerance. The analgesic compounds of opium have been known for hundreds of years. Morphine is extracted from raw opium and may be altered chemically to produce the semisynthetic narcotics, such as hydromorphone, oxymorphone, oxycodone, and heroin. Synthetic narcotics are produced in laboratories, and have analgesic properties. Methadone, levorphanol, and meperidine are among the various narcotics listed in Table 22-3.

Mechanism of Action

The effects of natural opium alkaloids occur by binding to opioid receptors. These receptors are located in the CNS (brain and spinal cord). Narcotic agonist effects are identified with three types of opioid receptors: the mu, kappa, and delta receptors. Most of the currently used opioid analgesics act primarily at mu receptors. Opioid analgesics also act at kappa receptors in the brain responsible for spinal analgesia, miosis, and sedation.

Key Concept

Narcotic analgesics are classified as Schedule II drugs, except for heroin, which is classified as a Schedule I drug.

TABLE 22-3 | Opioids

Generic Name	Trade Name	Route of Administration	Average Adult Dosage
Opioid Agonists with Moderate Effects			
codeine **(C-II)** (KOH-deen)	(generic)	PO, SC, IM	15–60 mg qid
hydrocodone **(C-II in bulk quantities or as stand-alone product; C-III when in combination products with no more than 15 mg per dose unit)** (hy-droh-KOH-dohn)	Hycodan®	PO	5–10 mg q4–6h prn (max: 15 mg/dose)
oxycodone **(C-II)** (ok-see-KOH-down)	OxyContin®, Percolone®	PO	5–10 mg qid prn
Opioid Agonists with High Effects			
hydromorphone **(C-II)** (hy-droh-MOR-fohn)	Dilaudid®	PO, SC, IM, IV	PO: 2–4 mg q4–6h prn; SC/IM/IV: 0.75–2 mg q4–6h
levorphanol **(C-II)** (leh-VOR-fah-nol)	Levo-Dromoran®	PO	2–3 mg tid–qid prn
meperidine **(C-II)** (meh-PEH-rih-deen)	Demerol®	PO, SC, IM, IV	50–150 mg q3–4h prn
methadone **(C-II)** (MEH-thah-dohn)	Dolophine®, Methadose®	PO, SC, IM, IV	PO/SC/IM: 2.5–10 mg q3–4h prn; IV: 2.5–10 mg q8–12h prn
morphine **(C-II)** (MOR-feen)	Astramorph PF®, Duramorph®	PO	10–30 mg q4h prn
oxymorphone **(C-II)** (ok-see-MOR-fohn)	Numorphan®	PO, SC, IM	PO: 10–20 mg q4–6h prn; SC/IM: 1–1.5 mg q4–6h prn

Indications

Narcotic analgesics are used to manage moderate to severe acute and chronic pain after non-narcotic analgesics have failed. They are also used as preanesthetic medications. Narcotic analgesics are indicated to relieve dyspnea of acute left ventricular failure and pulmonary edema and pain of myocardial infarction. Opioid analgesics such as codeine and dextromethorphan are also useful as antitussive drugs. These agents may be given to treat severe diarrhea, intestinal cramping (camphorated tincture of opium), and persistent cough (codeine). Methadone is also used to treat opioid dependence.

Adverse Effects

The major adverse effect of opioid analgesics is respiratory depression, in which respiratory rate and depth decrease. The most common adverse effects include sedation, anorexia, nausea, vomiting, constipation, dizziness, light-headedness, and sweating. Agonist narcotic analgesics also have the following adverse effects on different systems:

- Gastrointestinal: dry mouth and biliary tract spasms

- Central nervous system: euphoria, pinpoint pupils, insomnia, tremor, agitation, and impairment of mental and physical tasks

- Cardiovascular: tachycardia, bradycardia, palpitations, and peripheral circulatory collapse

- Genitourinary: spasms of the ureters and bladder sphincter, urinary retention or hesitancy

Contraindications and Precautions

Narcotic analgesics are contraindicated in patients with known hypersensitivity, acute bronchial asthma, emphysema, or upper airway obstruction. Narcotic analgesics are also contraindicated in patients with head injury, increased **intracranial** pressure, convulsive disorders, and severe hepatic or renal dysfunction. Narcotic analgesics should be avoided during pregnancy or labor (they are ranked as category C drugs, except oxycodone which is ranked as a category B drug), because they prolong labor or produce respiratory depression in the neonate.

Narcotic analgesics should be used cautiously in patients with cardiac arrhythmias, toxic psychosis, emphysema, kyphoscoliosis, and severe obesity, and in very elderly patients.

Drug Interactions

Narcotic analgesics interact with several drugs, including CNS depressants such as alcohol, other opioids, general anesthetics, sedatives, and antidepressants such as monoamine oxidase inhibitors (MAOIs) and tricyclics. The action of opiates is increased if used with narcotic analgesics, and the risk of severe respiratory depression (and death) is also increased.

Opioid Antagonists

Opioid antagonists are agents that prevent the effects of **opioid agonists**. The opioid antagonist drugs have an affinity for a specific cell receptor and compete with opioid agonists to reach the opioid receptor site (Table 22-4).

Mechanism of Action

Pure opioid antagonists such as naloxone are able to block both mu and kappa receptors. The mechanism of action is not clearly delineated, but it appears that its competitive binding at opioid receptor sites reduces euphoria and drug cravings without supporting addiction.

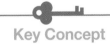

Key Concept

The use of narcotic analgesics is recommended during pregnancy only if the benefit to the mother outweighs the potential harm to the fetus.

Medical Terminology Review

kyphoscoliosis
kypho- = hunchback
-scoliosis = lateral and rotational spinal deformity
a deformity of the spinal column causing a hunchback appearance

Key Concept

Yohimbe (an herbal supplements) may increase the effects of morphine.

TABLE 22-4	Opioid Antagonists		
Generic Name	Trade Name	Route of Administration	Average Adult Dosage
nalmefene (NAL-meh-feen)	Revex®	SC, IM, IV	1 mg/mL concentration; nonopioid dependent: 0.5 mg/70 kg; opioid dependent: 0.1 mg/70 kg
naloxone (nah-LOK-sohn)	Narcan®	IV	0.4–2 mg, may be repeated q2–3 min up to 10 mg prn
naltrexone (nal-TREK-sohn)	ReVia®, Vivitrol®	PO	25 mg followed by another 25 mg in 1 h if no withdrawal response (max: 800 mg/day)

Indications

Opioid antagonists are used for complete or partial reversal of opioid effects in emergency conditions when acute opioid overdose is suspected. Administered intravenously, they begin to reverse opioid-initiated CNS and respiratory depression within minutes. Naloxone is the drug of choice when the nature of a depressant drug is not known and for the diagnosis of suspected acute opioid overdosage.

Adverse Effects

Opioid antagonists themselves have minimal toxicity. However, they reverse the effects of opioids and the patient may experience rapid loss of analgesia, increased blood pressure, nausea, vomiting, drowsiness, hyperventilation, and tremors.

Contraindications and Precautions

Opioid antagonists are contraindicated in respiratory depression due to nonopioid drugs. Safety during pregnancy or lactation is not established, other than during labor (category B).

Opioid antagonist drugs should be used with caution in neonates and children, and patients with cardiac irritability and known or suspected narcotic dependence.

Drug Interactions

Opioid antagonist drug interactions include a reversal of the analgesic effects of narcotic (opiate) agonists and **agonist-antagonists**.

MIGRAINE HEADACHES

Headache is a very common type of pain. There are many categories of headache associated with different causes, and some have specific locations and characteristics. The types of headache include:

- Headaches associated with congested sinuses.

- Headaches associated with muscle spasm and tension resulting from emotional stress that causes the neck muscles to contract to a greater degree, pulling on the scalp.

- Intracranial headaches resulting from increased pressure inside the skull.

- Migraine headaches, which are related to abnormal changes in blood flow and metabolism in the brain. There are many precipitating factors, including anxiety, atmospheric changes, bright or flashing lights, hormonal changes, stress, menstruation, hunger, certain dietary substances, lack of sleep, and heredity. The pain of a migraine headache is usually throbbing, quite severe, and sometimes incapacitating. Characteristically, these types of headaches begin unilaterally (on one side) in the temple area, but often spread to involve the entire head. Nearly one-third of patients can predict migraine onset because it is preceded by an "aura." This phenomenon includes visual disturbances appearing as flashing lights, zigzag lines, or temporary loss of vision. The pain is often accompanied by dizziness, nausea, abdominal pain, and fatigue. Migraine headaches may last up to 24 hours, and there is often a prolonged recovery period. The International Headache Society diagnosis of migraine headache is based on severity of pain and number of attacks (at least 5), lasting between 4 and 72 hours if untreated. Migraines are three times more common in women than in men. They affect more than 10% of people worldwide.

Treatment of Migraine Headaches

Treatment is difficult, although ergotamine may be effective if administered immediately after the onset of the headache. New forms of ergotamine are available as sublingual tablets, which provide a more readily available and rapid-acting treatment. Other drugs used for migraines are listed in Table 22-5.

Mechanism of Action

Antimigraine drugs include the ergot alkaloids and the triptans, which are both serotonin agonists. Serotonergic receptors (those that are related to the neurotransmitter serotonin) are found in the CNS, GI tract, and

TABLE 22-5 Drugs Used to Treat Migraine Headaches

Generic Name	Trade Name	Route of Administration	Average Adult Dosage
Ergot Alkaloids			
dihydroergotamine (dy-hy-droh-er-GOH-tah-meen)	D.H.E. 45®, Migranal®	SC, IM, IV	1 mg repeated at 1 h intervals to a total of 3 mg IM; or 2 mg SC/IV
ergotamine (er-GOH-tah-meen)	Ergomar®, Ergostat®	Sublingual	1–2 mg repeated q30 min until headache stops
ergotamine with caffeine (er-GOH-tah-meen with kah-FEEN)	Cafergot®, Ercaf®	PO	1–2 mg repeated q30 min until headache stops
Triptans			
almotriptan (al-moh-TRIP-tan)	Axert®	PO	6.25–12.5 mg repeated in 2 h prn
eletriptan (eh-leh-TRIP-tan)	Relpax®	PO	20–40 mg repeated in 2 h prn
frovatriptan (froh-vah-TRIP-tan)	Frova®	PO	2.5 mg repeated in 2 h prn
naratriptan (nah-rah-TRIP-tan)	Amerge®	PO	1–2.5 mg repeated in 4 h prn
rizatriptan (ry-zah-TRIP-tan)	Maxalt®	PO	5–10 mg repeated in 2 h prn or 5 mg with concurrent propranolol
sumatriptan (soo-mah-TRIP-tan)	Imitrex®	PO	25 mg for 1 dose
zolmitriptan (zol-mih-TRIP-tan)	Zomig®	PO	2.5–5 mg repeated in 2 h prn
Beta-Adrenergic Blockers			
atenolol (ah-TEH-noh-lol)	Tenormin®	PO	25–50 mg/day
metoprolol (meh-TOH-proh-lol)	Lopressor®	PO	50–100 mg 1–2 times daily
propranolol (pro-PRAH-noh-lol)	Inderal®	PO	80–240 mg/day in divided doses
timolol (TIH-moh-lol)	Blocadren®	PO	10 mg bid up to 60 mg/day in 2 divided doses
Calcium Channel Blockers			
nifedipine (nih-FEH-dih-peen)	Procardia®	PO	10–20 mg tid
nimodipine (ny-MOH-dih-peen)	Nimotop®	PO	60 mg q4h for 21 days; start therapy within 96 h of subarachnoid hemorrhage
verapamil (veh-RAH-pah-mil)	Isoptin®	PO	40–80 mg tid

cardiovascular system. These agents act by causing vasoconstriction of the cranial arteries. This vasoconstriction is moderately selective, and does not usually affect overall blood pressure.

Indications

The drugs of choice for treatment of migraine are often the triptans. Ergot alkaloids may be used to stop migraines. Prophylaxis includes various classes of drugs (such as beta blockers and calcium channel blockers) that are discussed in other chapters of this textbook.

Adverse Effects

Common adverse effects of ergot alkaloids include nausea, vomiting, abnormal pulse, weakness, and convulsive seizures. The adverse effects of triptans include warming sensations, dizziness, weakness, and tickling or prickling. The major adverse effects of triptans include coronary artery vasospasm, heart attack, and cardiac arrest.

Contraindications and Precautions

These agents are contraindicated in patients with recent myocardial infarction, a history of angina pectoris, diabetes, and high blood pressure. Because ergot alkaloids and triptans cause vasoconstriction of blood vessels, they should be used cautiously.

Drug Interactions

Ergot alkaloids and triptans may interact with several drugs. For example, an increased effect may occur when taken with MAOIs and selective serotonin reuptake inhibitors. Further vasoconstriction may occur.

SUMMARY

Non-narcotic analgesics are used to relieve pain without the possibility of resulting physical dependency. Non-narcotic analgesics include the salicylates, nonsalicylates (acetaminophen), and NSAIDs.

Salicylates are the oldest of the nonopioid analgesics and NSAIDs. They are still commonly used as analgesics. Aspirin is the most commonly used of these agents. Some of these analgesics are also used as anti-inflammatory and antipyretic drugs.

Adverse effects of salicylate drugs are common and include heartburn, nausea, vomiting, and GI bleeding. Acetaminophen may cause adverse reactions with chronic use or when the recommended dosage is exceeded.

New NSAIDs are available as analgesic, antipyretic, and anti-inflammatory agents. COX-2 inhibitors are more specific for prostaglandin synthesis in response to an inflammatory event. The FDA has approved the COX-2 inhibitors such as celecoxib and meloxicam.

Narcotic analgesics are controlled substances used to treat moderate to severe pain. Morphine is the most widely used drug in the management of chronic severe pain. Narcotic analgesics are classified as agonists and antagonists. One of the major adverse effects of agonist narcotic administration is respiratory depression.

Opioid antagonists are agents that prevent the effects of opioid agonists. These drugs have an affinity for opioid cell receptors and compete with opioid agonists to reach the receptor site.

A migraine headache is a very common type of pain. Various agents are used as antimigraine medications. The two major drug classes used for treating migraine headaches are ergot alkaloids and triptans. Other drugs used for this purpose include beta-adrenergic blockers, calcium channel blockers, and tricyclic antidepressants.

EXPLORING THE WEB

Visit www.fda.gov

- Search for the types of drugs discussed in this chapter. Look for safety information, advisories, patient education, and other relevant information.

Visit www.drugs.com

- Search for additional information on the drugs discussed within the chapter.

- You can also find drug information at **www.medicinenet.com** (click "Medications") or **www.nlm.nih.gov/medlineplus** (click on "Drugs and Supplements").

REVIEW QUESTIONS

Multiple Choice

1. Aspirin may be useful in the prevention of coronary thrombosis because of which of the following properties?

   A. thrombolytic

   B. antiarthritic

   C. anti-inflammatory

   D. antiplatelet

2. Celecoxib (Celebrex®) is classified as a:

   A. COX-1 and COX-2 inhibitor

   B. COX-1 inhibitor

   C. COX-2 inhibitor

   D. nonselective NSAID

3. Which of the following is a main contraindication of NSAIDs?

   A. rheumatoid arthritis

   B. corticosteroid sensitivity

   C. osteoarthritis

   D. allergy to aspirin

4. Which of the following terms is used for pain-relieving drugs?

   A. antitoxins

   B. antiemetics

   C. analgesics

   D. anaphylactics

5. Examples of nonsalicylate nonsteroidal anti-inflammatory drugs include:

   A. ibuprofen and indomethacin

   B. mefenamic acid and magnesium sulfate

   C. naproxen and neomycin

   D. piroxicam and lysergic acid

6. COX-2 is more specific for synthesis of which of the following in response to an inflammatory event?

   A. histamine

   B. prostaglandin

   C. heparin

   D. epinephrine

7. Which of the following classes of drugs are preferred for treating migraine headaches?

   A. tricyclic antidepressants

   B. NSAIDs

   C. beta-adrenergic blockers

   D. triptans

8. Which of the following drugs is used to treat opioid dependence?

   A. hydromorphone

   B. methadone

   C. oxycodone

   D. codeine

9. The main adverse effect of morphine is:

   A. diarrhea

   B. respiratory depression

   C. depression

   D. intestinal cramping

10. Narcotic analgesics are contraindicated in which of the following situations?

    A. moderate pain

    B. pulmonary edema

    C. persistent cough

    D. bronchial asthma

11. The trade name of ibuprofen is:

    A. Nalfon®

    B. Advil®

    C. Aleve®

    D. Actron®

12. Which of the following is considered an aspirin substitute?

    A. Indocin® (indomethacin)

    B. Celebrex® (celecoxib)

    C. Tylenol® (acetaminophen)

    D. Aleve® (naproxen)

13. If a patient has an allergy to aspirin, which of the following drugs may be used?

    A. sodium thiosalicylate injectable

    B. etolac

    C. acetaminophen

    D. allopurinol

14. Opioid analgesics may cause spinal analgesia, and which of the following?

    A. miosis and sedation

    B. physical dependence and psychosis

    C. euphoria and respiratory depression

    D. hyperventilation and tremors

15. Which of the following is an example of pure opioid antagonists?

    A. methadone

    B. oxycodone

    C. naloxone

    D. meperidine

Matching

_____ 1. Often used with aspirin or acetaminophen.

_____ 2. Competes with opioid agonists for reaching the opioid receptor site.

_____ 3. More addicting than codeine.

_____ 4. Extracted from raw opium.

_____ 5. Used for detoxification of opioid addiction.

A. morphine

B. methadone

C. oxycodone

D. hydrocodone

E. naloxone

Critical Thinking

A 58-year-old patient with a history of a recent myocardial infarction is on beta-blocker and anticoagulant therapy. The patient has a history of peptic ulcer (which is not bothering him currently). During a recent flare-up, he began taking aspirin because it helped control the pain that he experienced in his chest.

1. What recommendation would the pharmacist have for this patient?

2. If the patient takes aspirin, what major adverse effects could occur?

3. Name a drug that the pharmacist could advise the patient to take instead of aspirin.

OBJECTIVES

After completing this chapter, the reader should be able to:

1. Describe the various forms of microorganisms.
2. Compare the terms *bactericidal* and *bacteriostatic*.
3. Describe various mechanisms of action of antibacterial therapy.
4. Explain the indications and contraindications of antibiotics.
5. Describe the major side effects of antibacterial agents.
6. Understand the importance of drug interactions.
7. Explain the mechanisms of action for penicillins, cephalosporins, aminoglycosides, tetracyclines, macrolides, and quinolones.
8. Compare the effectiveness of penicillins with that of cephalosporins.
9. Explain the first line of antituberculosis drugs.
10. Describe the significant contraindications of rifampin and ethambutol.

GLOSSARY

Antibiotics – substances that are derived from a natural source rather than a synthetic source. They have the ability to destroy or interfere with the development of a living organism

Antimicrobials – anti-infective drugs that can kill or inhibit the reproduction of a microorganism. This is a very general term that can be applied to antibiotics, antifungals, and antivirals

Bacteria – small, one-celled microorganisms that lack a true nucleus or mechanism to provide metabolism

Bactericidal – relating to killing bacterial growth

Bacteriostatic – relating to suppression of bacterial growth by triggering a mechanism that blocks folic acid synthesis, thereby forcing bacteria to synthesize their own folic acid

Broad-spectrum antibiotics – agents that are effective against a wide variety of both gram-positive and gram-negative pathogenic microorganisms

Fungi – microorganisms that grow in single cells or in colonies and are neither plant nor animal

Gram stains – sequential procedures involving crystal violet and iodine solutions followed by alcohol that allow rapid identification of organisms as gram-positive or gram-negative types

Gram-negative – microorganisms that stain red or pink with Gram stain

Gram-positive – microorganisms that stain blue or purple with Gram stain

Infection – the invasion of pathogenic microorganisms that produce tissue damage within the body

Localized infection – involves a specific area of the body such as the skin or internal organs

Mycoplasma – ultramicroscopic organisms that lack rigid cell walls and are considered to be the smallest free-living organisms

Narrow-spectrum antibiotics – antibiotics that are effective against only a few organisms

Porphyria – a group of enzyme disorders that cause skin problems (such as purple discolorations) or neurological complications, or both

Protozoa – single-celled parasitic organisms, many of which are motile (able to move spontaneously)

Rickettsia – intercellular parasites that can only reproduce inside living cells

Red man syndrome – a rash on the upper body caused by vancomycin

Spores – bacteria in a resistant stage that can withstand an unfavorable environment

Systemic infection – impacts the whole body rather than a specific area

Viruses – intracellular parasites that take over the metabolic machinery of host cells and

use it for their own survival and replication; they can live only inside cells. They are minute organisms, and not visible with an ordinary microscope. Viruses are composed only of a single strand of nucleic acid with an enveloping protein sheath

OVERVIEW

Pathogenic microorganisms may cause a wide spectrum of illnesses. They produce infection of different organs or systems of the body, such as upper respiratory tract infections, meningitis, pneumonia, tuberculosis, and urinary tract infections. This chapter focuses on the drugs used to treat a variety of infections.

INFECTIONS

An **infection** is described as the invasion of pathogenic microorganisms that produce tissue damage within the body. Infections may be classified as either local or systemic. A localized infection may involve a specific area of the body, such as the skin or internal organs. A **localized infection** can progress to a systemic infection. A **systemic infection** impacts the whole body rather than a specific area. Infections are also classified as acute or chronic.

Chain of Infection

The chain of infection describes the elements of an infectious process. It is an interactive process that involves the agent, host, and environment. This process must include several essential elements or "links in the chain" for the transmission of microorganisms to occur. Figure 23-1 identifies the six essential links in the chain of infection. Table 23-1 summarizes modes of transmission.

Without the transmission of microorganisms, the infectious process cannot occur. Knowledge about the chain of infection facilitates control or prevention of disease by breaking the links in the chain. This is achieved by altering one or more of the interactive processes of agent, host, or environment.

MICROORGANISMS

Microorganisms are divided into several groups: bacteria, mycoplasma, viruses, fungi, protozoa, and rickettsia. Bacteria are classified according to their shape, such as cocci (spherical), bacilli (rod-shaped), and spirilla (spiral) (Figure 23-2). They are also classified into two groups based upon

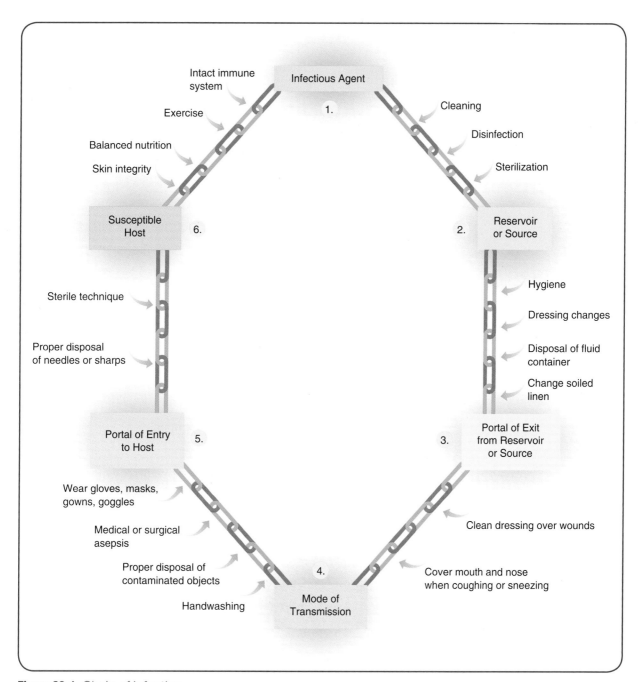

Figure 23-1 Chain of infection.

their capacity to be stained. This staining process is called Gram staining. It involves sequential procedures using crystal violet and iodine solutions followed by alcohol that allow rapid identification of organisms as **gram-positive** or **gram-negative** types. **Gram stains** can identify specific types of bacteria. Gram-negative microorganisms stain red or rose-pink (Figure 23-3). Gram-positive microorganisms stain blue or purple (Figure 23-4). Fungi may also be identified by Gram staining. The culture and sensitivity tests can determine which antibiotics should be prescribed.

TABLE 23-1	Modes of Transmission
Mode	**Examples**
Contact	Direct contact with infected person: • Touching • Bathing • Rubbing • Toileting (urine and feces) • Secretions from client Indirect contact with fomites (inanimate objects capable of carrying pathogens): • Clothing • Bed linens • Dressings • Health care equipment • Instruments used in treatments • Specimen containers used for laboratory analysis • Personal belongings • Personal care equipment • Diagnostic equipment
Airborne	Inhaling microorganisms carried by moisture or dust particles in air: • Coughing • Talking • Sneezing
Vehicle	Contact with contaminated inanimate objects: • Water • Blood • Drugs • Food • Urine
Vector borne	Contact with contaminated animate hosts: • Animals • Insects

Bacteria

Bacteria are small, one-celled microorganisms that lack a true nucleus or mechanism to provide metabolism. Some forms of bacteria produce **spores**, a resistant stage that withstands an unfavorable environment. When proper

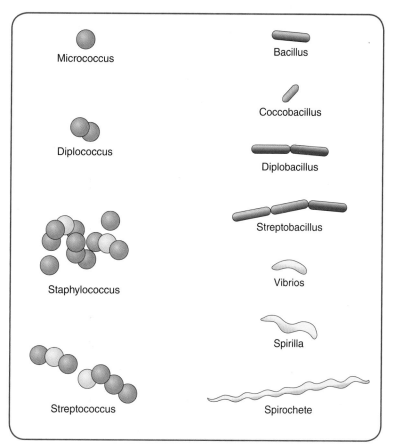

Figure 23-2 Classifications of bacteria.

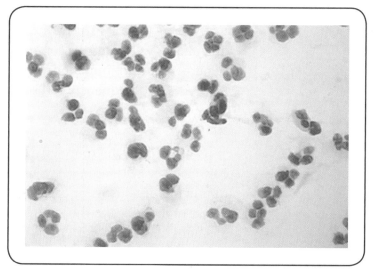

Figure 23-3 Gram-negative.

environmental conditions return, spores germinate and form new cells. Spores are resistant to heat, drying, and disinfectants. Pathogenic bacteria cause a wide range of illnesses, including diarrhea, pneumonia, sinusitis, urinary tract infections, and gonorrhea.

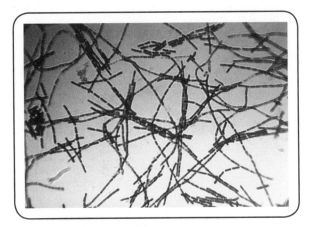

Figure 23-4 Gram-positive.

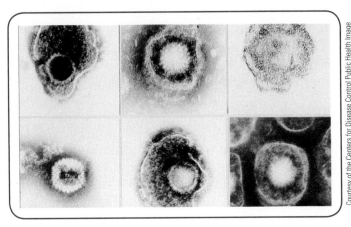

Figure 23-5 Herpes simplex virus.

Courtesy of the Centers for Disease Control Public Health Image Library/Dr. Erskine Palmer

Mycoplasma

Mycoplasma are ultramicroscopic organisms that lack rigid cell walls and are considered to be the smallest free-living organisms. Some are saprophytes (a plant that lives on dead or decaying matter), some are parasites, and many are pathogens. One species is a cause of mycoplasma pneumonia, tracheobronchitis, and pharyngitis.

Viruses

Viruses are organisms that can live only inside cells. They cannot get nourishment or reproduce outside the cell. Viruses contain a core of deoxyribonucleic acid (DNA) or ribonucleic acid (RNA) surrounded by a protein coating. They damage the cell they inhabit by blocking the normal protein synthesis and by using the cell's mechanism for metabolism to reproduce themselves. Viral infections include the common cold, influenza, measles, hepatitis, genital herpes, human immunodeficiency virus (HIV), and the West Nile virus (Figure 23-5). Treatment of viruses will be discussed in Chapter 24.

Fungi

Fungi are unique microorganisms that are neither plant nor animal. They grow in single cells (as in yeast) or in colonies (as in molds) and obtain food from living organisms or organic matter. Diseases caused by fungi occur mainly in individuals who are immunologically impaired. Fungi can cause infections of the hair, skin, nails, and mucous membranes. Athlete's foot is a common example.

Protozoa

Protozoa are single-celled parasitic organisms with the ability to move. Most protozoa obtain their food from dead or decaying organic matter. Infection is spread through ingestion of contaminated food or water, or through insect bites. Common infections are malaria, dysentery, and vaginal infections (Figure 23-6).

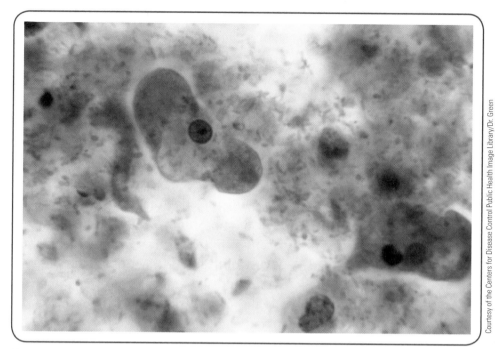

Figure 23-6 Intestinal protozoa *Entamoeba coli*.

Courtesy of the Centers for Disease Control Public Health Image Library/Dr. Green

Rickettsia

Rickettsia are intercellular parasites that need to be in living cells to reproduce. Infection from rickettsia is spread through the bites of fleas, ticks, mites, and lice. Common infections are Lyme disease, Rocky Mountain spotted fever, and typhus.

PRINCIPLES OF ANTI-INFECTIVE THERAPY

Anti-infective agents treat infection by destroying or suppressing the causative microorganisms. The goal is to suppress the causative agent sufficiently so that the body's own defenses can eliminate it. Anti-infective drugs derived from natural substances are called **antibiotics**. Those produced from synthetic substances are called **antimicrobials**. In past years, strong efforts have been made to change antibiotic usage policy rendering prescribing practices clinically stronger, but less costly. There is an emphasis on rapid conversion from parenteral to oral therapy for a variety of infectious processes. Major efforts are being taken to understand the underlying principles associated with the interaction of the antibiotics, host, and pathogens.

Selection of Agents

An anti-infective agent should be chosen on the basis of its pharmacological properties and spectrum of activity, as well as on various patient factors.

1. Pharmacological properties: The drug's ability to reach the infection site and to attain a desired level of concentration in the target tissue.

Key Concept

Probiotics are live microorganisms, usually bacteria, that are similar to the beneficial microorganisms known as "normal flora" in our gastrointestinal tracts. Probiotics are available to consumers primarily in the form of dietary supplements and foods. They are most commonly used to treat irritable bowel syndrome, inflammatory bowel disease, constipation, and chronic diarrhea.

2. Spectrum of activity: To treat an infectious disease effectively, an anti-infective agent must be effective against the causative pathogen. The effectiveness of an anti-infective drug can be confirmed by a sensitivity test. Resistance to an anti-infective agent can arise through mutations in the gene that determines sensitivity or resistance to the agent.

3. Patient factors: There are various patient factors that determine what type of anti-infectives should be administered. These factors include immunity of patients, age, presence of a foreign body, adverse drug reactions, pregnancy and lactation, and underlying disease. Choosing an anti-infective that does not offer enough protection is a common problem. Some commonly used drugs, such as aminoglycosides and vancomycin, are poorly absorbed and can be used to treat gastrointestinal infections without systemic effects. Antimicrobials can be used as prophylactics for people in contact with patients who have meningitis or tuberculosis; in those undergoing surgery to the gastrointestinal, urinary tract, or dental regions; or those with rheumatic fever. Other patient considerations in the use of anti-infective agents include:

- Diminished renal function in the elderly
- Partially developed hepatic function in neonates
- Circulatory problems, such as occur in people with diabetes mellitus

Duration of Anti-Infective Therapy

The most important goal when prescribing anti-infective therapy is to continue it for a sufficient period of time. All antibiotics should be taken for the prescribed treatment period to ensure eradication of the causative organism. Treatment for a chronic infection such as osteomyelitis or endocarditis may require a longer duration, for example, four to six weeks.

Antibiotic Spectrum

Antibiotics may be divided into two groups based on their effectiveness against different organisms. **Broad-spectrum antibiotics** are effective against a wide variety of both gram-positive and gram-negative pathogenic microorganisms. **Narrow-spectrum antibiotics** can be effective on a few gram-positive or gram-negative pathogens.

SUPERINFECTIONS

The normal flora (nonpathogenic microorganisms within the body) may be disrupted by administration of oral antibiotics. This process of destruction of large numbers of normal flora by antibiotics can alter the chemical environment, allowing superinfection (uncontrolled growth of bacteria or fungal microorganisms) to occur. Any antibiotic that is administered for a long time, or a repeated course of therapy, may result in superinfections. A superinfection may develop suddenly and may be serious or life-threatening. Bacterial superinfections involving the large intestine are seen frequently in patients who take oral penicillins. Pseudomembranous colitis is a common bacterial superinfection, and moniliasis is a common type of fungal superinfection.

Methicillin-resistant *Staphylococcus aureus,* commonly known as MRSA, is one of the most prevalent, and deadliest, superinfections in the United States, according to the Centers for Disease Control and Prevention (CDC). The MRSA bacterium is highly resistant to penicillins and other antibiotics that are routinely used today. The superinfection is often transmitted in community areas such as gymnasiums, daycare centers, or health care facilities. Of the 80,000 annual cases in the United States, approximately 11,000 cases are fatal. Prevention of MRSA is essential and requires cleaning, sanitizing, and disinfection with bleach, products such as Lysol® that are described as being able to kill *S. aureus,* hydrogen peroxide disinfectants that are more concentrated than standard formulations, and silver ion products. Treatments for MRSA often begin with sulfamethoxazole/trimethoprim or vancomycin. Other options include clindamycin, minocycline, daptomycin, tigecycline, dalfopristin/quinupristin, and linezolid.

Although MRSA has a higher fatality rate than most other infections, it is actually the sixth most common superinfection in the United States. The top five superinfections are listed below:

- *Streptococcus pneumoniae* (1,200,000 annual cases)
- *Campylobacter* (310,000 annual cases)
- *Clostridium difficile* (250,000 annual cases)
- *Neisseria gonorrhoeae* (246,000 annual cases)
- *Salmonella* (100,000 annual cases)

ANTIBACTERIAL AGENTS

Antibacterial agents are used to treat infections caused by bacteria. The major categories for antibacterial agents include sulfonamides, penicillins, cephalosporins, aminoglycosides, macrolides, tetracyclines, fluoroquinolones, and miscellaneous antibacterial agents.

Sulfonamides

Sulfonamides are the synthetic derivatives of sulfanilamide. These agents were the first drugs to prevent and cure human bacterial infection successfully. They are well absorbed from the gastrointestinal tract and readily

TABLE 23–2	Classification of Sulfonamides		
Generic Name	Trade Name	Route of Administration	Common Dosage Range
Short-Acting (4–8 hours)			
sulfamethizole **(sul-fah-MEH-thih-zohl)**	Thiosulfil Forte®	PO	500 mg–1 g q6-8h
sulfasalazine **(sul-fah-SAH-lah-zeen)**	Azulfidine®	PO	1–2 g/day in 4 divided doses; may increase up to 8 g/day
sulfisoxazole **(sul-fih-SOK-sah-zohl)**	Gantrisin®	PO	2–4 g initially, followed by 1–2 g qid
Intermediate-Acting (7–17 hours)			
sulfadiazine **(sul-fah-DY-ah-zeen)**	Microsulfon®	PO	2–4 g
sulfamethoxazole **(sul-fah-meh-THOK-sah-zohl)**	Gantanol®	PO	2 g initially, followed by 1 g bid
trimethoprim-sulfamethoxazole **(try-MEH-tho-prim sul-fah-MEH-thok-sah-zohl)**	Bactrim®, Septra®	PO	160 mg trimethoprim/800 mg sulfamethoxazole bid
Long-Acting (17+ hours)			
sulfadoxine- pyrimethamine **(sul-fah-DOK-zeen pih-rih-MEH-thah-meen)**	Fansidar®	PO	1 tablet/wk

Key Concept

Sulfonamides were the first antimicrobial agents, but their clinical use has been greatly restricted as a result of the development of resistant bacteria.

Medical Terminology Review

bacteriostatic
bacterio- = bacteria; bacterial
-static = slowing; stoppage
slowing or stopping the growth of bacteria

penetrate the cerebrospinal fluid. Sulfonamides are metabolized to various degrees in the liver, and are eliminated by the kidneys. Although these agents were originally active against a wide range of gram-positive and gram-negative bacteria, the increasing incidence of resistance in bacteria formerly susceptible to sulfonamides has decreased their clinical usefulness. However, sulfonamides remain the drug of choice for certain infections. The major sulfonamides are generally classified as short-acting (e.g., sulfisoxazole), intermediate-acting (e.g., sulfamethoxazole), or long-acting (e.g., sulfadoxine), as shown in Table 23-2. Their rate of action depends on how quickly they are absorbed and eliminated.

Mechanism of Action

Sulfonamides are **bacteriostatic**; that is, they suppress bacterial growth by triggering a mechanism that blocks folic acid synthesis, thereby forcing bacteria to synthesize their own folic acid.

Indications

Sulfonamides are active against gram-positive and gram-negative organisms. They most often are used to treat urinary tract infections caused by

Escherichia coli, including acute and chronic cystitis, and chronic upper urinary tract infections. Prophylactic sulfonamide therapy has been used successfully to prevent streptococcal infections, ulcerative colitis, and rheumatic fever recurrences. Sulfonamides are also used as topical for ocular infections and burn infections.

Adverse Effects

Sulfonamides may cause blood dyscrasias such as hemolytic anemia, aplastic anemia, thrombocytopenia, and agranulocytosis. Hypersensitivity reactions may occur with sulfonamide therapy. Hematuria and crystalluria are two of the major adverse effects of sulfonamide agents. Sulfonamides should be used with caution in patients with renal impairment. Life-threatening hepatitis caused by drugs is a rare adverse effect. Patients who take sulfonamides have increased susceptibility to adverse effects from sun exposure.

Contraindications and Precautions

Sulfonamides must be avoided in patients with a history of hypersensitivity to these drugs. They are contraindicated in the treatment of group A beta-hemolytic streptococcal infections or in infants younger than two months of age (except in the treatment of congenital toxoplasmosis). Sulfonamides must not be used in patients with **porphyria**, advanced kidney or liver disease, intestinal obstruction, or urinary obstruction. They are contraindicated during pregnancy (if near term) and in lactating women. Sulfonamides must be used cautiously in patients with impaired kidney or liver function, severe allergy, bronchial asthma, and blood dyscrasias.

Drug Interactions

Sulfonamides may increase the effects of phenytoin, oral anticoagulants, and sulfonylureas.

Penicillins

Sir Arthur Fleming discovered the antibacterial properties of natural penicillins in 1928 while he was performing research on influenza. In 1938, British scientists realized the effects of natural penicillins on disease-causing microorganisms. In 1941, natural penicillins were used for the treatment of infections.

Natural or semisynthetic antibiotics are produced by or derived from certain species of the fungus *penicillium*. Penicillins are the most widely used anti-infective agents; however, cephalosporin usage has increased in the last decade. Among the most important antibiotics, natural penicillins are the preferred drugs in the treatment of many infectious diseases. The major cause of resistance to penicillin is the production of beta-lactamases (penicillinases). Common organisms that are capable of producing penicillinase include *S. aureus*, *E. coli*, *Pseudomonas aeruginosa*, and species

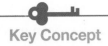

of *Bacillus*, *Proteus*, and *Bactericides*. Penicillins are available as penicillin G, penicillin V, penicillin G procaine, and penicillin G benzathine. Table 23-3 shows common types of penicillins and the route of administration.

Mechanism of Action

Penicillins are **bactericidal**. They inhibit bacterial cell wall synthesis in similar ways to the cephalosporins. Natural penicillins are highly active against gram-positive and some gram-negative cocci. Penicillin G is ten times more active than penicillin V against gram-negative organisms.

TABLE 23-3	Common Penicillins and Routes of Administration		
Generic Name	**Trade Name**	**Route of Administration**	**Common Dosage Range**
Natural Penicillins			
penicillin G potassium **(peh-nih-SIL-lin G poh-TAS-see-um)**	Pentids®	PO	400,000–800,000 units/day
penicillin V potassium **(peh-nih-SIL-lin V poh-TAS-see-um)**	Pen Vee K®, Veetids®	PO	125–250 mg qid
penicillin G procaine **(peh-nih-SIL-lin G PRO-kayn)**	Crysticillin®	IM	600,000–1.2 million units/day
penicillin G benzathine **(peh-nih-SIL-lin G BEN-zah-theen)**	Bicillin L-A®	IM	1.2 million units as a single dose
Penicillinase-Resistant Penicillins			
cloxacillin sodium **(klok-sah-SIL-lin SOH-dee-um)**	Cloxapen®	PO	250–500 mg qid
dicloxacillin sodium **(dy-klok-sah-SIL-lin SOH-dee-um)**	Dycill®, Dynapen®	PO	125–500 mg qid
nafcillin sodium **(naf-SIL-lin SOH-dee-um)**	Nafcil®, Unipen®	PO, IM, IV	500 mg–1 g qid
oxacillin sodium **(ok-sah-SIL-lin)**	Bactocill®	PO, IM, IV	500 mg–1 g qid, IM/IV: 250 mg–1 g q4–6h
Semisynthetic Penicillins			
amoxicillin **(ah-mok-sih-SIL-lin)**	Amoxil®, Trimox®	PO	250–500 mg tid
amoxicillin and clavulanate potassium **(ah-mok-sih-SIL-lin and klah-VYOO-lah-nayt poh-TAS-see-um)**	Augmentin®	PO	250–500 mg q8–12h
ampicillin **(am-pih-SIL-lin)**	Polycillin®, Omnipen®	PO, IM, IV	250–500 mg qid
bacampicillin hydrochloride **(bah-cam-pih-SIL-lin hy-droh-KLOR-ryd)**	Spectrobid®	PO	400–800 mg bid

Indications

Penicillin G is the drug of choice for all *S. pneumoniae* organisms. Penicillins G and V are highly effective against other streptococcal infections, such as bacteremia, pharyngitis, otitis media, and sinusitis. Penicillin G is also the drug of choice against many gonococcal infections, postexposure inhalational anthrax, syphilis, and gas gangrene. Penicillin G procaine is effective against syphilis and uncomplicated gonorrhea. Penicillin G benzathine is very effective against group A beta-hemolytic streptococcal infections. Penicillins G and V may be indicated for prophylactic treatment to prevent streptococcal infection, rheumatic fever, and neonatal gonorrhea ophthalmia.

Adverse Effects

Hypersensitivity occurs in nearly 10% of cases. Reactions from simple rash to anaphylaxis can be observed from two minutes to three days following administration. Anaphylaxis is a life-threatening reaction that most commonly occurs with parenteral administration. Signs and symptoms include severe hypotension, bronchoconstriction, nausea, vomiting, and abdominal pain. Before penicillin therapy begins, the patient's history should be evaluated for allergy to penicillin.

Contraindications and Precautions

Penicillins must be avoided in patients with a history of hypersensitivity to penicillin or cephalosporins. Penicillins should be used cautiously in patients with kidney disease and during pregnancy (category C) and lactation. These drugs are to be used with caution in patients with bleeding disorders, gastrointestinal diseases, and asthma.

Drug Interactions

The most significant drugs that may increase or decrease the effects of penicillin are probenecid, erythromycins, tetracyclines, and chloramphenicol. Probenecid increases blood levels of natural penicillin. On the other hand, chloramphenicol, erythromycins, and tetracyclines are antagonists with penicillin.

Penicillinase-Resistant Penicillins

The penicillin resistance of many gram-positive and gram-negative bacteria derives primarily from penicillin-destroying enzymes called beta-lactamases. The enzymes from staphylococci, enterococci, meningococci, gonococci, and various other bacteria were the first-known beta-lactamases and were called penicillinases.

Resistance of bacteria to penicillin cannot be explained entirely by penicillinase production because many resistant organisms produce little or no penicillinase. Non–penicillinase-mediated resistance, which is referred to as methicillin resistance, may also occur.

> **Key Concept**
>
> Injection of penicillin to a patient may cause anaphylactic reactions within 30 minutes after administration. Therefore, the patient must be monitored for 30 minutes.

Resistant penicillins are used predominantly for penicillinase-producing staphylococcal infections. Most staphylococci are now resistant to benzylpenicillin because they produce a penicillinase. As their name suggests, penicillinase-resistant penicillins are resistant to the action of this enzyme and are therefore indicated in infections caused by penicillin-resistant staphylococcus. Oxacillin, cloxacillin, dicloxacillin, and nafcillin can be given orally. Methicillin is administered parenterally. Nafcillin is used parenterally for more serious infections. Penicillinase-resistant penicillins are used solely in staphylococcal infections resulting from organisms that resist natural penicillins. These agents are less potent than natural penicillins against organisms susceptible to natural penicillins. Penicillinase-resistant penicillins are the preferred choice for skin and soft tissue infections due to staphylococci. Higher doses should be used for severe infections or for infections of the lower respiratory tract. In suspension form, these agents should be taken on an empty stomach, are stable for 14 days after mixing (but refrigeration is required), and are known for having a bitter aftertaste.

Mechanism of Action

Penicillinase-resistant penicillins prevent cell wall synthesis by binding to enzymes called penicillin-binding proteins (PBPs). These enzymes are essential for the synthesis of the bacterial cell wall.

Indications

Indications of penicillinase-resistant penicillins include prevention and treatment of bacterial infections, including streptococcus, enterococcus, and staphylococcus strains.

Adverse Effects

The penicillinase-resistant group can also cause hypersensitivity reactions like natural penicillins. Methicillin may cause nephrotoxicity. Oxacillin can produce hepatotoxicity. They may cause nausea, vomiting, diarrhea, or skin rash.

Contraindications and Precautions

These agents are contraindicated in patients with hypersensitivity to penicillins or cephalosporins. Safe use during pregnancy (category B) is not established.

Penicillinase-resistant penicillins should be used cautiously in patients with a history of, or suspected, allergy (hives, eczema, hay fever, asthma); in premature infants and neonates; and during lactation (which may cause infant diarrhea). They also should be used with great caution in patients with renal or hepatic function impairment.

Medical Terminology Review

nephrotoxicity
nephro- = kidney
-toxicity = the quality or condition of being poisonous
poisoning of the kidney

hepatotoxicity
hepato = liver
toxicity = the quality or condition of being poisonous
poisoning of the liver

Drug Interactions

Penicillinase-resistant penicillins can inactivate aminoglycoside serum samples from patients receiving both drugs.

Semisynthetic Penicillins (Amoxicillin/Clavulanate Potassium)

Streptococcus pneumoniae is the most common cause of acute bacterial sinusitis and community-acquired pneumonia. Amoxicillin/clavulanate potassium is the first FDA-approved antibiotic for both of these infections.

Mechanism of Action

The amoxicillin component of the formulation exerts a bactericidal action against many gram-negative and gram-positive strains. The clavulanate potassium component protects the amoxicillin from degradation by inactivating harmful beta-lactamase enzymes.

Indications

This combination is used in the treatment of respiratory infections caused by susceptible beta-lactamase-producing organisms, including upper respiratory infections such as otitis media, tonsillitis, and sinusitis, and lower respiratory infections such as bronchitis and pneumonia. Urinary tract, skin, and soft tissue infections are also treatable with this combination agent.

Adverse Effects

Amoxicillin/clavulanate potassium should not be used in patients with hepatic dysfunction because of the danger of transient hepatitis and cholestatic jaundice. Serious and occasionally fatal hypersensitivity reactions have been reported in patients receiving penicillin therapy. Diarrhea, nausea, vomiting, urticaria, and candidal vaginitis may occur.

Contraindications and Precautions

This combination should not be used in patients with hypersensitivity to penicillins, infectious mononucleosis, and during pregnancy (category B) and lactation. The combination of amoxicillin and clavulanate potassium shares the toxic potential of ampicillin.

Drug Interactions

Concurrent use of this agent with probenecid may result in increased and prolonged blood levels of amoxicillin. This agent interacts with coumarin or indandione-derivative anticoagulants, heparin, nonsteroidal anti-inflammatory agents (especially aspirin), other platelet aggregation inhibitors or thrombolytic agents, and estrogen-containing oral contraceptives.

Extended-Spectrum Penicillins

This group of penicillins has the widest antibacterial spectrum. Included are the carboxypenicillins and the ureidopenicillins (Table 23-4).

Mechanism of Action

Extended-spectrum penicillins are also bactericidal and inhibit bacterial cell wall synthesis.

Indications

Extended-spectrum penicillins are prescribed mainly to treat serious infections caused by gram-negative organisms. These infections include sepsis, pneumonia, peritonitis, osteomyelitis, and soft tissue infections.

Adverse Effects

As with other penicillins, hypersensitivity reactions may occur. Carbenicillin and ticarcillin may cause hypokalemia. The use of these two drugs may be a danger to patients with congestive heart failure because of the high sodium content of carbenicillin and ticarcillin.

Contraindications and Precautions

These agents are contraindicated in patients with hypersensitivity to penicillins and during pregnancy (category B). Safe use in children is not established.

Extended-spectrum penicillins should be used cautiously in patients with a history of, or suspected, atopy or allergies, or history of allergy to

TABLE 23-4	Extended-Spectrum Penicillins		
Generic Name	Trade Name	Route of Administration	Common Dosage Range
Carboxypenicillins			
carbenicillin (kar-beh-nih-SIL-lin)	Geocillin®	PO	382–764 mg qid
ticarcillin disodium and clavulanate potassium (tih-kar-SIL-lin dy-SOH-dee-um and klah-VYOO-lah-nayt poh-TAS-see-um)	Timentin®	IV	> 60 kg: 3.1 g q4–6h
Ureidopenicillins			
mezlocillin (mez-loh-SIL-lin)	Mezlin®	IM, IV	25–50 mg/kg/day
piperacillin (py-peh-rah-SIL-lin)	Pipracil®	IM, IV	8–16 g/day

cephalosporins; during lactation; in patients with impaired renal and hepatic function; and in patients on sodium-restricted diets.

Drug Interactions

Extended-spectrum penicillins may increase the risk of bleeding if used with anticoagulants. Elimination of ticarcillin is decreased by the use of probenecid.

Cephalosporins

These agents are known as beta-lactam antibiotics. Cephalosporins are semisynthetic antibiotics that are structurally and pharmacologically related to penicillins. Cephalosporins are usually bactericidal in action. The antibacterial activity of the cephalosporin results from inhibition of mucopeptide synthesis in the bacterial cell wall. The cephalosporins are classified into four different "generations." Particular cephalosporins may be differentiated within each group according to the bacteria that are sensitive to them (Table 23-5).

TABLE 23-5	Classification of Cephalosporins		
Generic Name	**Trade Name**	**Route of Administration**	**Common Dosage Range**
First-Generation			
cefadroxil **(sef-ah-DROK-sil)**	Duricef®	PO	1–2 g/day in 1–2 divided doses
cefazolin sodium **(sef-AH-zoh-lin SOH-dee-um)**	Ancef®, Zolicef®, Kefzol®	IM, IV	250 mg–2 g tid
cephalexin **(sef-ah-LEK-sin)**	Keflex®	PO	250–500 mg qid
cephapirin **(sef-ah-PY-rin)**	Cefadyl®	IM, IV	500 mg–1 g q4–6h
cephradine **(SEF-rah-deen)**	Velosef®	PO	250–500 mg q6h
Second-Generation			
cefamandole	Mandol®	IM, IV	500 mg-1g q4-8h
cefoxitin sodium **(sef-OK-sih-tin SOH-dee-um)**	Mefoxin®	IM, IV	1–2 g q6–8h
cefaclor **(SEF-ah-klor)**	Ceclor®	PO	250–500 mg tid

continued on next page

Table 23-5 continued

cefuroxime sodium **(sef-YOO-roh-zeen SOH-dee-um)**	Zinacef®	PO	250–500 mg bid
cefonicid **(sef-ON-ih-sid)**	Monocid®	IM	1–2 g/day
cefprozil **(SEF-pro-zil)**	Cefzil®	PO	250–500 mg, 1–2 times daily
cefmetazole **(sef-MEH-tah-zohl)**	Zefazone®	IV	1–2 g q6–12h
cefotetan **(sef-oh-TEE-tan)**	Cefotan®	IM, IV	1–2 g q12h
Third-Generation			
cefdinir **(SEF-dih-neer)**	Omnicef®	PO	300 mg bid
cefditoren pivoxil **(sef-dih-TOH-ren pih-VOK-zil)**	Spectracef®	PO	200 mg bid
cefpodoxime proxetil **(sef-poh-DOK-zeem PROK-zeh-tihl)**	Vantin®	PO	200 mg bid
ceftazidime **(sef-TAH-zih-deem)**	Fortaz®	IM, IV	1–2 g bid
ceftibuten **(sef-TY-byoo-ten)**	Cedax®	PO	400 mg/day
ceftizoxime sodium **(sef-tih-ZOK-zeem SOH-dee-um)**	Cefizox®	IM, IV	1–2 g bid–tid
cefotaxime sodium **(sef-oh-TAK-zeem SOH-dee-um)**	Claforan®	IM, IV	1–2 g, 12–24 h
cefixime **(sef-IK-zeem)**	Suprax®	PO	400 mg/day in 1–2 divided doses
ceftriaxone sodium **(sef-try-AK-zohn SOH-dee-um)**	Rocephin®	IM, IV	1–2 g, 12–24 h
cefoperazone sodium **(sef-oh-PEH-rah-zohn)**	Cefobid®	IM, IV	.1–2 g, q12h
Fourth-Generation			
cefepime hydrochloride **(SEF-eh-peem hy-droh-KLOR-ryd)**	Maxipime®	IM, IV	500 mg–1 g, q12h

Mechanism of Action

The mechanism of action of cephalosporins lies in preventing cell wall synthesis through binding to PBPs, described earlier. These enzymes are essential for the synthesis of the bacterial cell wall. Cephalosporins are bactericidal against susceptible organisms. Staphylococci that are able to resist methicillin are also resistant to cephalosporins.

Indications

Cephalosporins are the largest, most diverse group of beta-lactam antibiotics. They are used to treat community-acquired and hospital-acquired infections of the skin, soft tissue, urinary tract, and respiratory tract.

- First-generation cephalosporins are effective against most gram-positive organisms and some gram-negative organisms. They are used mainly for *Klebsiella* infections, and in patients who have penicillin- and sulfonamide-resistant urinary tract infections. Indications include uncomplicated skin and soft tissue infections, uncomplicated urinary tract infections, streptococcal pharyngitis, and surgical prophylaxis. Cephapirin and cefazolin are used parenterally; others, such as cephradine, cephalexin, and cefadroxil can be administered orally. First-generation cephalosporins do not penetrate the cerebrospinal fluid, so they are not effective for central nervous system (CNS) infections.

- Second-generation cephalosporins extend the spectrum of the first generation to include *Haemophilus influenzae* and some *Proteus* species. Indications include upper and lower respiratory tract infections, acute sinusitis, otitis media, uncomplicated urinary tract infections, infections of the skin and soft tissues, intra-abdominal infections, gynecological infections, and surgical prophylaxis. Most are administered parenterally except for cefaclor, cefprozil, and cefuroxime, which may be given orally. Other examples of second-generation cephalosporins include cefotetan, cefoxitin, and cefamandole. Second-generation cephalosporins, except for cefuroxime, do not cross the blood-brain barrier, so they are not used for CNS infections.

- Third-generation cephalosporins have even broader gram-negative activity and less gram-positive activity than do second-generation agents. Cefotaxime is an example of these agents, and is potent against *H. influenzae*, *N. gonorrhoeae*, and enterobacteria. Orally administered agents include cefdinir, cefditoren, cefpodoxime, ceftibuten, and cefixime. Parentally administered agents include ceftazidime, ceftizoxime, cefotaxime, ceftriaxone, and cefoperazone. Third-generation agents are used primarily for serious gram-negative infections, alone or in combination with aminoglycosides. Indications include bacillary meningitis, serious *Enterobacteriaceae* infections, upper respiratory tract infections, otitis media, pyelonephritis, skin infections, and soft tissue infections. Ceftriaxone is indicated for Lyme disease and gonorrhea. Many third-generation cephalosporins penetrate the cerebrospinal fluid well, so they can be used for CNS infections.

- Fourth-generation cephalosporins have the greatest action against gram-negative organisms among the four generations and minimal action against gram-positive organisms. Examples of fourth-generation cephalosporins include cefepime, cefluprenam, cefozopran, cefpirome, and cefquinome.

Cefepime and cefpirome are extremely active against hospital-acquired pathogens, and are mostly used for nosocomial infections. Cefepime penetrates the CNS and can be used to treat meningitis. It is the most active fourth-generation cephalosporin, and therefore, is the most commonly used of these agents.

Adverse Effects

The kidneys eliminate all cephalosporins except cefoperazone. Doses must be adjusted for patients with renal impairment. They can cause hypersensitivity reactions similar to those occurring with penicillin. The most common adverse effects include nausea, vomiting, diarrhea, and nephrotoxicity. Adverse effects of cephalosporins include hypoprothrombinemia and bleeding, alcohol intolerance, hypersensitivity reactions, and thrombophlebitis.

Contraindications and Precautions

Cephalosporins are contraindicated if the patient has a history of allergies to these agents or penicillins. Cephalosporins should be avoided in pregnant and lactating women. Cephalosporins are to be used cautiously in patients with renal or hepatic impairment, and in patients with bleeding disorders.

Drug Interactions

Cephalosporins have drug interactions with alcohol, diarrhea medications, birth control pills, anticoagulants, blood viscosity reducing medicines, and antiseizure medicines. Cephalosporins are contraindicated for use with alcohol, alcohol-containing medications, aminoglycosides, anticoagulants, carbenicillin by injection, dipyridamole, divalproex, heparin, pentoxifylline, plicamycin, sulfinpyrazone, ticarcillin, thrombolytic agents, valproic acid, potent diuretics, iron–iron supplements, and probenecid.

Aminoglycosides

Aminoglycosides are broad-spectrum antibiotics. The toxic potential of these drugs limits their use. Since their introduction into clinical use 50 years ago,

Key Concept

Nephrotoxicity may occur with the use of cephalosporins. A decrease in urine output is an early sign of the adverse effect on patients with kidney impairments.

TABLE 23-6 | **Major Aminoglycosides**

Generic Name	Trade Name	Route of Administration	Common Dosage Range
amikacin sulfate (ah-mih-KAY-sin SUL-fayt)	Amikin®	IM, IV	5–7.5 mg/kg/day in 2–3 divided doses
gentamicin sulfate (jen-tah-MY-sin SUL-fayt)	Garamycin®	IM, IV	1.5–2.0 mg/kg/day (standard dose)
kanamycin (kah-nah-MY-sin)	Kantrex®	IM, IV	15 mg/kg q8–12h for serious infections
neomycin sulfate (nee-oh-MY-sin SUL-fayt)	Mycifradin®	PO, IM, Topical	PO: 50 mg/kg in 4 divided doses for 2–3 days; IM: 1.3–2.6 mg/kg qid; Topical: apply 1–3 times daily
netilmicin (neh-til-MY-sin)	Netromycin®	IM	4 mg/kg in 2 divided doses
paromomycin sulfate (pah-roh-moh-MY-sin SUL-fayt)	Humatin®	PO	25–35 mg/kg tid
streptomycin (strep-toh-MY-sin)	(generic only)	IM	15 mg/kg up to 1 g/day as a single dose
tobramycin sulfate (toh-brah-MY-sin SUL-fayt)	Tobrex®	IM, IV	3 mg/kg tid

aminoglycosides have continued to play an important role in the treatment of severe infections. Major aminoglycosides include amikacin, gentamicin, kanamycin, neomycin, netilmicin, streptomycin, and tobramycin. These agents are shown in Table 23-6.

Mechanism of Action

Aminoglycosides are bactericidal; they inhibit bacterial protein synthesis, causing cell death. Their mechanism of action is not fully known.

Indications

Aminoglycosides are prescribed for a variety of disorders and infectious diseases.

- Streptomycin: Used in combination with penicillins, streptomycin is often more effective in enterococcal carditis than regimens that include other aminoglycosides. This combination is also used to treat tularemia, acute brucellosis, bacterial endocarditis, tuberculosis, and plague.

- Amikacin, gentamycin, netilmicin, and tobramycin: These are prescribed for serious gram-negative bacillary infections such as *Enterobacter, Klebsiella,* bacteremia, meningitis, and peritonitis.

- Neomycin: This is used for preoperative bowel sterilization, hepatic coma, and in topical form for burns.
- Spectinomycin: This drug is an aminocyclitol, which is related to the aminoglycosides. Its only use is as a backup drug for the treatment of gonorrhea. Spectinomycin may cause pain at the injection site.

Adverse Effects

Aminoglycosides can cause serious adverse effects such as ototoxicity (including hearing loss) and nephrotoxicity. Neomycin is the most nephrotoxic aminoglycoside, and streptomycin is the least nephrotoxic. Gentamycin and tobramycin are nephrotoxic to the same degree. Aminoglycosides are also potentially neurotoxic, and these adverse effects may cause permanent damage to the organs.

Contraindications and Precautions

Aminoglycosides are contraindicated in those with a history of hypersensitivity or toxic reaction to an aminoglycoside antibiotic. Safety during pregnancy (category C) and lactation, in neonates and infants, or when used for a period exceeding 14 days is not established. Aminoglycosides should be used cautiously in patients with impaired renal function, eighth cranial (auditory) nerve impairment, or in older adults. Other cautions include use in premature infants, neonates, and infants.

Drug Interactions

The risks of nephrotoxicity may increase by using an aminoglycoside with cephalosporins. If an aminoglycoside is used with loop diuretics (furosemide, ethacrynic acid, etc.), there is an increased risk of ototoxicity.

Macrolides

The macrolides include erythromycin, azithromycin, and clarithromycin. Erythromycin is produced by *Streptomyces erythreus*. Macrolides are also used as alternative agents in patients allergic to penicillin. Table 23-7 shows common macrolides.

Mechanism of Action

Macrolides may be bactericidal or bacteriostatic. They inhibit bacterial protein synthesis by binding to cell membranes. Erythromycins generally penetrate the cell wall of gram-positive bacteria more readily than those of gram-negative bacteria.

Indications

Macrolides are effective in the treatment of infections caused by a wide range of gram-negative and gram-positive microorganisms. They are the drug of choice for the treatment of *Mycoplasma pneumoniae, Campylobacter*

TABLE 23-7	Most Commonly Used Macrolides			
Generic Name	Trade Name	Route of Administration	Common Dosage Range	
azithromycin (ah-zith-roh-MY-sin)	Zithromax®, Zmax®	PO	500 mg on day 1, then 250 mg/day	
clarithromycin (klah-rith-roh-MY-sin)	Biaxin®	PO	250–500 mg bid	
dirithromycin (dy-rith-roh-MY-sin)	Dynabac®	PO	500 mg once daily	
erythromycin base (eh-rith-roh-MY-sin BAYS)	Eryc®, Emycin®	PO	250–500 mg qid	
erythromycin estolate (eh-rith-roh-MY-sin eh-STOH-layt)	Ilosone®	PO, IM, IV	250–500 mg	
erythromycin stearate (eh-rith-roh-MY-sin STEER-rayt)	Erythrocin Stearate®	PO	250–500 mg q6–12h	

infections, Legionnaires' disease, chlamydial infections, and pertussis. In patients with penicillin allergy, erythromycins are the best alternatives in the treatment of gonorrhea, syphilis, and pneumococcal pneumonia. Erythromycins may be given prophylactically before dental procedures to prevent bacterial endocarditis.

Adverse Effects

Macrolides rarely cause serious adverse effects. Nausea, vomiting, and diarrhea may occur with all forms of macrolides.

Contraindications and Precautions

Macrolides are contraindicated in patients with hypersensitivity, and in patients with liver diseases. These drugs should be used cautiously during pregnancy and lactation. Erythromycin and azithromycin are contraindicated in pregnancy (category B); and clarithromycin is a pregnancy category C drug. Macrolides must be used with great caution in patients with liver diseases.

Drug Interactions

Macrolides inhibit the hepatic metabolism of theophylline. They may interfere with the metabolism of digoxin, corticosteroids, and cyclosporin. Use of antacids decreases the absorption of most macrolides. Chloramphenicol, clindamycin, and lincomycin are able to decrease the therapeutic activity of the macrolides if they are used concurrently.

TABLE 23-8	Major Tetracyclines and Administration Routes		
Generic Name	Trade Name	Route of Administration	Common Dosage Range
demeclocycline hydrochloride **(deh-mek-loh-SY-kleen hy-droh-KLOR-ryd)**	Declomycin®	PO	150 mg qid or 300 mg bid
doxycycline hyclate **(dok-see-SY-kleen HY-klayt)**	Vibramycin®	PO, IV	100 mg bid on day 1, then 100 mg/day
minocycline hydrochloride **(my-noh-SY-kleen hy-droh-KLOR-ryd)**	Minocin®	PO	4 mg/kg/day–200 mg/day; 200 mg followed by 100 mg bid
oxytetracycline **(ok-see-teh-trah-SY-kleen)**	Terramycin®	PO, IM, IV	PO: 250–500 mg bid–qid; IM: 100 mg tid; IV: 250–500 mg bid
tetracycline hydrochloride **(teh-trah-SY-kleen hy-droh-KLOR-ryd)**	Sumycin®	PO	250–500 mg bid
tigecycline **(ty-geh-SY-kleen)**	Tygacil®	IV	100 mg followed by 50 mg q12h

Tetracyclines

Tetracyclines are broad-spectrum agents that are effective against certain bacterial strains that resist other antibiotics. The major tetracyclines and their administration routes are shown in Table 23-8.

Mechanism of Action

Tetracyclines are bacteriostatic. They inhibit bacterial protein synthesis, which is a process necessary for reproduction of the microorganism.

Indications

Tetracyclines are active against gram-negative and gram-positive organisms, spirochetes, mycoplasmal and chlamydial organisms, rickettsial species, and certain protozoa. They are the drugs of choice in rickettsial infections (e.g., Rocky Mountain spotted fever), chlamydial infections, amebiasis, cholera, brucellosis, and tularemia. Tetracyclines are prescribed as an alternative to penicillin in the treatment of anthrax, syphilis, gonorrhea, Lyme disease, and *H. influenzae* respiratory infections. Oral or topical tetracycline may be used as a treatment for acne. Doxycycline is highly effective in the prophylaxis of "traveler's diarrhea."

Adverse Effects

Abdominal discomfort, nausea, diarrhea, and anorexia are common adverse effects of tetracyclines. Cross-sensitivity within the tetracyclines are also common. Use of the drugs in infants has resulted in retardation of bone growth. Because tetracyclines localize in the dentin and enamel of developing teeth, use of the drugs during tooth development may cause enamel hypoplasia and permanent yellow-gray to brown discoloration of the teeth. Tetracycline can cause fetal toxicity when administered to pregnant women (e.g., retardation of skeletal development). Liver toxicity has occurred following intravenous administration of tetracyclines to pregnant women. Oxytetracycline is the least hepatotoxic. Phototoxicity may occur in patients when they are exposed to strong sunlight (ultraviolet), especially with demeclocycline (Declomycin®). Minocycline can cause vestibular toxicity. Intravenous administration of tetracyclines is irritating and may cause phlebitis.

Contraindications and Precautions

Tetracyclines are contraindicated in patients who are allergic to them, or to any ingredient used in their formulations. Tetracyclines should not be used in children younger than eight years of age unless other appropriate drugs are ineffective or are contraindicated. Tetracyclines should be avoided in patients with severe renal or hepatic impairment. They are also contraindicated in individuals with common bile duct obstruction.

Tetracyclines should be used cautiously in patients with renal function impairment or a history of liver dysfunction. History of allergy, asthma, and undernourished patients are other factors that cause tetracyclines to be used with caution.

Drug Interactions

Certain foods (dairy products) and agents such as iron preparations, laxatives, and antacids that contain aluminum and calcium may lead to reduced tetracycline absorption. Therefore, it is recommended that the drug be taken on an empty stomach. Barbiturates and phenytoin can decrease the effectiveness of tetracyclines.

Fluoroquinolones

Fluoroquinolones (also known as quinolones) are related to nalidixic acid and are bactericidal for growing bacteria. The most commonly used quinolones are shown in Table 23-9.

Mechanism of Action

Fluoroquinolones exert their bactericidal effects by interfering with an enzyme (DNA gyrase) required by bacteria for the synthesis of DNA. This action prevents cell reproduction, resulting in bacterial death.

Indications

Fluoroquinolones are used in the treatment of infections caused by gram-positive and gram-negative microorganisms. Fluoroquinolones are

Key Concept

Tetracyclines should not be used during pregnancy, infancy, and childhood (up to eight years of age), or during lactation, because they cause permanent discoloration of teeth in children.

TABLE 23-9	Fluoroquinolones		
Generic Name	**Trade Name**	**Route of Administration**	**Common Dosage Range**
First-Generation			
nalidixic acid **(nah-lih-DIK-sik AH-sid)**	NegGram®	PO	500 mg–1 g qid
Second-Generation			
ciprofloxacin hydrochloride **(sih-proh-FLOK-sah-sin hy-droh-KLOR-ryd)**	Cipro®, Cipro XR®	PO, IV	PO: 250 mg q12h or 500 mg (Cipro XR®) qd for 3 days; IV: 200 mg q12h, infused over 60 min
lomefloxacin hydrochloride **(loh-meh-FLOK-sah-sin hy-droh-KLOR-ryd)**	Maxaquin®	PO	400 mg qd for 10 days
norfloxacin **(nor-FLOK-sah-sin)**	Noroxin®	PO	400 mg bid
ofloxacin **(oh-FLOK-sah-sin)**	Floxin®	PO	400 mg for 1 dose
Third-Generation			
gatifloxacin **(gah-tih-FLOK-sah-sin)**	Zymar®	PO	400 mg/day
levofloxacin **(leh-voh-FLOK-sah-sin)**	Levaquin®	PO, IV	500 mg/day
Fourth-Generation			
gemifloxacin **(jeh-mih-FLOK-sah-sin)**	Factive®	PO	320 mg/day
moxifloxacin hydrochloride **(mok-see-FLOK-sah-sin hy-droh-KLOR-ryd)**	Avelox®, Vigamox®	PO, IV	400 mg/day

used primarily in the treatment of urinary tract and lower respiratory infections, skin and skin structure infections, and sexually transmitted diseases. Ciprofloxacin, norfloxacin, and ofloxacin are used in ophthalmic forms for eye infections.

Adverse Effects

Fluoroquinolone agents may produce nausea, headache, dizziness, dyspepsia, insomnia, photosensitivity, and hypoglycemia. Crystalluria can occur with high doses at alkaline pH. Therefore, fluoroquinolones should be taken with water and the patient should stay well hydrated. These drugs may cause pain, inflammation, or rupture of a tendon (the most common tendon to be ruptured is the Achilles tendon).

Contraindications and Precautions

Fluoroquinolones are contraindicated in patients with a history of hypersensitivity, during pregnancy (category C) and lactation, and in children younger than 18 years. These agents are also contraindicated in patients who have syphilis, viral infections, tendon inflammation, and tendon pain. Fluoroquinolones should be used cautiously in patients with a history of seizures or renal dysfunction, those undergoing dialysis therapy, or elderly adults.

Drug Interactions

Ciprofloxacin may increase theophylline levels in blood. Fluoroquinolones may increase prothrombin times in patients receiving warfarin. Antacids and iron can decrease the absorption of fluoroquinolones.

Miscellaneous Antibacterial Agents

Some antibiotics are classified as miscellaneous antibacterial agents, such as chloramphenicol, clindamycin, dapsone, spectinomycin, and vancomycin (Table 23-10). A few examples of these drugs are detailed below.

TABLE 23-10 | **Miscellaneous Antibacterial Agents**

Generic Name	Trade Name	Route of Administration	Average Adult Dosage
chloramphenicol (klor-am-FEH-nih-kol)	Chloromycetin®	PO, IV	50 mg/kg qid
clindamycin hydrochloride (klin-dah-MY-sin hy-droh-KLOR-ryd)	Cleocin®	PO, IM, IV	PO: 150–450 mg qid; IM/IV: 600–1200 mg/day in divided doses
dapsone (DAP-sohn)	Aczone®	PO	100 mg/day (with 6 months of rifampin at 600 mg/day for a minimum of 3 years)
ertapenem sodium (er-tah-PEH-nem SOH-dee-um)	Invanz®	IM, IV	1 g/day
lincomycin hydrochloride (lin-koh-MY-sin hy-droh-KLOR-ryd)	Lincocin®	IM, IV	IM: 600 mg q12–24h; IV: 600 mg–1 g bid–tid
methenamine (meh-THEH-nah-meen)	Mandelamine®, Hiprex®	PO	1 g bid (Hiprex®) or qid (Mandelamine®)
nitrofurantoin (ny-troh-FYOO-ran-toh-in)	Furadantin®, Macrobid®	PO	50–100 mg qid
spectinomycin hydrochloride (spek-tih-noh-MY-sin hy-droh-KLOR-ryd)	Trobicin®	IM	2 g as single dose or q12h for 7 days until switched to an oral medication
vancomycin hydrochloride (van-koh-MY-sin hy-droh-KLOR-ryd)	Vancocin®	IV	500 mg qid or 1 g bid

Chloramphenicol

This antibiotic is highly effective against rickettsia as well as many gram-positive and gram-negative organisms.

Mechanism of Action Chloramphenicol is principally bacteriostatic but may be bactericidal against a few bacterial strains (e.g., *H. influenzae*) or when given in higher concentrations. Chloramphenicol inhibits protein synthesis.

Indications Chloramphenicol is used only for specific infections that cannot be treated effectively with other antibiotics. It is particularly effective against typhoid fever, rickettsial infections in pregnant women, and meningococcal infections in cephalosporin-allergic patients. Chloramphenicol is also used for infections in patients who have a history of allergies to tetracycline.

Adverse Effects Chloramphenicol can cause suppression of bone marrow (in high doses) with resulting pancytopenia. This agent can lead to aplastic anemia in rare, non–dose-related cases. Chloramphenicol therapy can also lead to gray baby syndrome in neonates.

Contraindications and Precautions Chloramphenicol is contraindicated in patients with a history of hypersensitivity or toxic reaction to the drug. It should be avoided in the treatment of minor infections, for prophylactic use, in typhoid carrier state, in patients with a past history or family history of drug-induced bone marrow depression, and during pregnancy (category C) and lactation.

Chloramphenicol should be given cautiously to patients with impaired hepatic or renal function. This drug may be used cautiously in premature and full-term infants and children.

Drug Interactions Chloramphenicol may inhibit the metabolism of phenytoin, dicumarol, and tolbutamide, leading to prolonged action and increased effects of these drugs. Phenobarbital can reduce the effect of chloramphenicol therapy. Acetaminophen elevates chloramphenicol levels and may cause toxicity. Penicillins can cause antibiotic antagonism.

Clindamycin

Clindamycin is an antibacterial and antiprotozoal antibiotic that has marked toxicity. It should be prescribed for special infections when it has been determined to be the most effective drug to treat them.

Mechanism of Action Clindamycin is bacteriostatic and inhibits bacterial protein synthesis. This agent is active against most gram-positive and many anaerobic organisms.

Indications Clindamycin is used in serious infections the respiratory tract caused by anaerobes such as those that occur with anaerobic pneumonitis, empyema, and lung abscess that is caused by pneumococci, staphylococci, and streptococci. Clindamycin is also used for serious infections of the

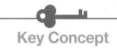

Key Concept

Chloramphenicol may cause non–dose-related and irreversible aplastic anemia and pancytopenia (abnormal reduction in the number of all circulating blood cells).

joints and bones, and intra-abdominal abscess or peritonitis, when less toxic alternatives are inappropriate. Topical applications are used in the treatment of acne vulgaris. Vaginal applications are used in the treatment of bacterial vaginosis in nonpregnant women.

Adverse Effects Clindamycin may cause metallic or unpleasant taste, vomiting, diarrhea, abdominal pain, and pseudomembranous colitis. Leukopenia, neutropenia, and thrombocytopenia may also occur. It also may cause cervicitis, vaginitis, and vulvar irritation.

Contraindications and Precautions Clindamycin is contraindicated in patients with a history of hypersensitivity to clindamycin or lincomycin. This agent also should not be used in patients with a history of regional enteritis, ulcerative colitis, or antibiotic-associated colitis. Clindamycin is contraindicated in pregnancy (category B) and lactation. It must be used cautiously in patients with history of gastrointestinal disease, renal or hepatic disease, eczema, asthma, and hay fever.

Drug Interactions Clindamycin may potentiate the effects of neuromuscular blocking agents, atracurium, tubocurarine, and pancuronium. It is antagonistic to chloramphenicol and erythromycin.

Dapsone

Dapsone is the primary agent in the treatment of all forms of leprosy.

Mechanism of Action Dapsone is bacteriostatic and bactericidal for *Mycobacterium leprae* by blocking folic acid synthesis, thereby forcing microorganisms to synthesize their own folic acid.

Indications Dapsone is the drug of choice for treating leprosy. It is also used prophylactically in contacts of patients with all forms of leprosy except tuberculoid and indeterminate leprosy. Dapsone may be indicated for treatment of dermatitis herpetiformis. The topical (gel) form of dapsone is used for acne vulgaris.

Adverse Effects Nausea, vomiting, and anorexia are common adverse effects of dapsone. This agent may cause skin rash, peripheral neuropathy, blurred vision, hepatitis, hemolysis (destruction of red blood cells), and cholestatic jaundice.

Contraindications and Precautions Dapsone is contraindicated in patients with history of hypersensitivity to sulfones or their derivatives, advanced renal dysfunction, and anemia. Safe use of dapsone during pregnancy (category C) or lactation is not established. Dapsone may be used with caution in patients with hepatic dysfunction, anemia, severe cardiopulmonary disease, and during pregnancy.

Drug Interactions Probenecid can elevate blood levels of dapsone, resulting in toxicity. Otherwise, there are no significant drug-drug interactions associated with the use of dapsone.

Key Concept

Dapsone is excreted in breast milk, and may cause hemolytic reactions in neonates.

Spectinomycin

Spectinomycin is a wide-spectrum antibiotic with moderate activity against both gram-positive and gram-negative bacteria.

Mechanism of Action Its action is usually bacteriostatic, but it has variable activity against a wide variety of gram-negative and gram-positive organisms.

Indications Spectinomycin is used clinically for only one purpose, namely, to treat acute endocervical, rectal, or urethral gonorrhea when the organism is resistant to penicillin, or when the patient is allergic to penicillin. It is not as effective as ceftriaxone.

Adverse Effects Untoward effects include frequent pain at the injection site, an infrequent headache, nausea, vomiting, insomnia, chills, fever, mild pruritus, and urticaria.

Contraindications and Precautions Safety during pregnancy (category B) or lactation, and in infants and children age eight years of age or younger, is not established. Spectinomycin should be used with caution in those with a history of allergies.

Drug Interactions No clinically significant interactions with spectinomycin have been established.

Vancomycin

Vancomycin can destroy most gram-positive organisms.

Mechanism of Action Vancomycin is bactericidal and bacteriostatic. It inhibits bacterial cell wall synthesis and acts against susceptible gram-positive bacteria.

Indications Vancomycin usually is reserved for serious infections, especially those caused by methicillin-resistant staphylococci, or other serious gram-positive infections that do not respond to treatment with other anti-infective agents. It is useful in patients who are allergic to penicillin or cephalosporins. Typical uses include treatment of osteomyelitis, endocarditis, and staphylococcal pneumonia. Vancomycin is used to treat pseudomembranous colitis caused by *Clostridium difficile* and enterocolitis.

Adverse Effects Vancomycin (in higher doses) may cause ototoxicity and nephrotoxicity, which can lead to uremia. It may cause a rash on the upper body, sometimes called **red man syndrome**. This condition may occur along with facial flushing and hypotension in response to rapid infusion of the drug.

Contraindications and Precautions Vancomycin is contraindicated in patients with known hypersensitivity. It is used cautiously in patients with hearing impairment or renal dysfunction and during pregnancy (category C) and lactation.

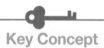

Key Concept

Intravenous administration of vancomycin should occur over a minimum of 60 minutes for a 1-g dose.

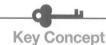

Key Concept

Vancomycin may be used orally only in the treatment of C. difficile colitis.

Drug Interactions Vancomycin may have added toxicity if used with aminoglycosides, cisplatin, polymyxin B, cyclosporine, and amphotericin B. These drugs (with vancomycin) will result in additive effects of ototoxicity and nephrotoxicity.

ANTITUBERCULAR DRUGS

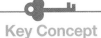

Key Concept

Transmission of tuberculosis (TB) is a serious risk to patients and workers in health care settings such as hospitals. Infection control practices, including the TB test for all patients who have not been tested, can help reduce the risk of transmission.

Tuberculosis is a highly contagious infection caused by *Mycobacterium tuberculosis*. While tuberculosis most commonly affects the lungs, it can also invade any part of the body, including the bone, gastrointestinal tract, and kidneys. Tubercular lesions are characterized by the death of affected tissue, with sloughing of tissue and formation of cavities.

Antitubercular drugs are used to treat tuberculosis by suppressing or killing the slow-growing mycobacteria that causes this disease. Antitubercular agents fall into two main categories: primary (first-line) and retreatment agents (second-line). Because the causative organisms tend to develop resistance to any single drug, combination drug therapy has become standard in the treatment of tuberculosis. Agents chosen for therapy must eradicate mycobacterium. Drugs available include isoniazid, streptomycin, ethambutol, rifampin, pyrazinamide, and rifabutin (Table 23-11). Combination drug therapy is essential. Agents showing the lowest incidence of resistance such as isoniazid, rifampin, and streptomycin are usually used in combination with ethambutol or pyrazinamide. Most patients are started on isoniazid, rifampin, and pyrazinamide. A fourth drug (ethambutol or streptomycin) is added with suspected resistance. Several antitubercular drugs are discussed in detail below.

Primary Antitubercular Drugs

Included in this category are isoniazid, ethambutol, rifampin, pyrazinamide, and streptomycin. These drugs usually offer the greatest effectiveness with the least toxicity. In most cases, the combination of isoniazid, rifampin, and pyrazinamide is most effective. These antibiotics must be administered concurrently during the 6- to 24-month treatment period.

Isoniazid

This agent is the mainstay of antitubercular therapy and is used in all therapeutic regimens.

Mechanism of Action Isoniazid is bacteriostatic and bactericidal, but bacteriostatic for dormant mycobacteria. It is postulated to act by interfering with biosynthesis of bacterial proteins, nucleic acid, and lipids. The mechanism of action is not completely known.

Indications Isoniazid is the most widely prescribed antitubercular drug. It should be used in combination with another antitubercular agent to prevent

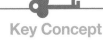

Key Concept

General treatment for any bacterial infection is the administration of a single antibiotic. For tuberculosis, as many as four different drug combinations may be required. These combinations are divided into first- and second-line drugs on the basis of their efficacy, which are also described as "primary" and "retreatment."

TABLE 23-11	Antituberculotics		
Generic Name	**Trade Name**	**Route of Administration**	**Average Adult Dosage**
First-Line Agents			
ethambutol hydrochloride (eh-THAM-byoo-tol hy-droh-KLOR-ryd)	Myambutol®	PO	15–25 mg/kg/day
isoniazid (eye-soh-NY-ah-zihd)	Nydrazid®	PO, IM	5 mg/kg/day
pyrazinamide (py-rah-ZIH-nah-myd)	(generic only)	PO	15–35 mg/kg tid–qid (max: 2 g/day)
rifampin (ry-FAM-pin)	Rifadin®, Rimactane®	PO, IV	600 mg/day as a single dose
rifapentine (rih-fah-PEN-teen)	Priftin®	PO	600 mg twice weekly for 2 mo; then once a week for 4 mo
streptomycin sulfate (strep-toh-MY-sin SUL-fayt)	Streptomycin®	IM	15 mg/kg up to 1 g/day as a single dose
Second-Line Agents			
amikacin sulfate (ah-mih-KAY-sin SUL-fayt)	Amikin®	IM, IV	5–7.5 mg/kg loading dose; then 7.5 mg/kg bid
capreomycin (kah-pree-oh-MY-sin)	Capastat Sulfate®	IM, IV	1 g/day (not to exceed 20 mg/kg/day) for 60–120 days, then 1 g 2–3 times/wk
ciprofloxacin hydrochloride (sih-proh-FLOK-sah-sin hy-droh-KLOR-ryd)	Cipro®	PO	250–750 mg bid
cycloserine (sy-kloh-SEH-reen)	Seromycin®	PO	250 mg q12h for 2 wk; may increase to 500 mg q12h (max: 1 g/day)
ethionamide (eh-thee-OH-nah-myd)	Trecator®	PO	0.5–1.0 g/day divided q8–12h
kanamycin (kah-nah-MY-sin)	Kantrex®	IM, IV	15 mg/kg bid–tid
ofloxacin (oh-FLOK-sah-sin)	Floxin®	PO	400 mg in 1 dose
rifabutin (rih-fah-BYOO-tin)	Mycobutin®	PO	300 mg qid, may give 150 mg bid if nausea is a problem

drug resistance in tuberculosis. In most cases of tuberculosis, isoniazid therapy should be continued for at least six months. However, treatment may require from six months to two years, depending on the severity of the

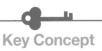

Key Concept

Prophylactic isoniazid may be given alone for up to one year in adults or children who have a positive tuberculin test result, but lack active lesions.

disease. During isoniazid therapy, the patient should be given pyridoxine (vitamin B_6) supplements to prevent neuritis (inflammation of a nerve).

Adverse Effects The most common adverse effects of isoniazid are fever, jaundice, peripheral neuritis, and skin rash. Hepatitis can be severe and fatal. Aplastic or hemolytic anemia and thrombocytopenia may occur. Isoniazid may increase the excretion of pyridoxine, which can lead to peripheral neuritis, particularly in poorly nourished patients.

Contraindications and Precautions Isoniazid is contraindicated in patients with history of isoniazid-associated hypersensitivity reactions, including hepatic injury or acute liver damage (from any cause). Isoniazid should be avoided during pregnancy (category C) unless the risk is warranted.

Isoniazid should be used cautiously in patients with chronic liver disease, renal dysfunction, or chronic alcoholism. This drug must be used cautiously in people older than 35 years, and during lactation.

Drug Interactions Food and antacids that contain aluminum decrease the absorption of isoniazid. Disulfiram may cause coordination difficulties or psychotic reactions. Drinking alcohol with isoniazid may increase the risk of liver damage.

Ethambutol

Ethambutol is a synthetic water-based compound. It is an antituberculosis and anti-infective drug.

Mechanism of Action Ethambutol is bacteriostatic. The actual mechanism of action is unknown, but it appears to inhibit RNA synthesis and thus arrest multiplication of tubercle bacilli. The emergence of resistant strains is delayed by administering ethambutol in combination with other antituberculosis drugs.

Indications Ethambutol is prescribed in the treatment of pulmonary tuberculosis in conjunction with at least one other antituberculosis drug.

Adverse Effects Ethambutol may cause optic neuritis (a decrease in visual acuity and changes in color perception), drug fever, dizziness, confusion, hallucinations, and joint pains.

Contraindications and Precautions Ethambutol is contraindicated in patients with a history of hypersensitivity. The drug should be avoided in children younger than six years of age, and in patients with optic neuritis. Ethambutol should be used with caution in patients with renal and hepatic impairment, and during lactation or pregnancy (category B). Ethambutol is given to patients with diabetic retinopathy because of the danger of optic neuritis.

Drug Interactions Aluminum-containing antacids can decrease absorption of ethambutol.

Rifampin

Rifampin is a complex macrocyclic agent, and an anti-mycobacterial antibiotic. It is a semisynthetic antibiotic derivative of rifamycin.

Mechanism of Action   Rifampin has both bacteriostatic and bactericidal actions. This agent inhibits DNA-dependent RNA polymerase activity in susceptible bacterial cells, thereby suppressing RNA synthesis.

Indications   The combination of rifampin and isoniazid is the most effective drug for treatment of tuberculosis. It should not be given alone because it may cause drug-resistance of organisms. Rifampin may be prescribed in combination with dapsone for the treatment of leprosy. Rifampin is also effective in the prevention of *Neisseria meningitides*, and a wide range of gram-negative and gram-positive organisms.

Adverse Effects   Liver damage can result from rifampin therapy. Liver function tests should be routinely checked. Headache, dizziness, fatigue, confusion, skin rash, nausea, and vomiting may occur.

Contraindications and Precautions   Rifampin is contraindicated in patients with a history of hypersensitivity, hepatic and renal impairment, meningococcal disease, and lactation. Safe use during pregnancy (category C) or in children younger than five years of age is not established. Rifampin should be used cautiously in patients with hepatic disease or history of alcoholism.

Drug Interactions   Rifampin may decrease the effect of many drugs, such as warfarin, oral contraceptives, oral hypoglycemics, digitoxin, and corticosteroids. There is also a decrease in the effects of phenytoin, verapamil, and chloramphenicol. Probenecid may increase blood levels of rifampin.

Streptomycin

Streptomycin is one of the aminoglycosides that is given in combination with other antitubercular agents (see the earlier discussion of aminoglycosides).

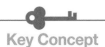

Key Concept

Rifampin may change the colors of urine, tears, saliva, sweat, and feces to orange-red.

Key Concept

Patients who wear soft contact lenses should be instructed that rifampin therapy may permanently stain these lenses.

SUMMARY

The invasion of pathogenic microorganisms may cause either local or systemic infection. The pathogen can be present in the blood circulation, causing bacteremia. Anti-infective drugs, generally called antibiotics, are used to treat infection. Selection of antibiotics depends on various factors such as pharmacological properties and spectrum activity of the drugs, and patient factors such as immunity, age, adverse drugs reactions, and underlying diseases. Pregnancy and lactation also play a major role.

There are broad classifications of anti-infective drugs that may affect specific pathogens such as bacteria, viruses, fungi, protozoa, and mycoplasma. Penicillins are the most widely used anti-infective agents. However, cephalosporin usage has increased in the past decade. There are specific antibiotics that are used predominantly for penicillinase-resistant penicillins. The first drugs used successfully to prevent and treat human bacterial infections were sulfonamides.

EXPLORING THE WEB

Visit any of the following websites to search for information on various types of diseases caused by infectious agents or the drugs used to treat them that were discussed in this chapter.

- **http://www2.caremark.com/**
- **www.cdc.gov**

- **www.mayoclinic.com**
- **www.nfid.org**
- To learn more about the concerns and adverse affects of using antibiotics, review the information found at **www.tufts.edu/med/apua**.

REVIEW QUESTIONS

Multiple Choice

1. Third-generation cephalosporins are potent against all of the following, *except*:

   A. *Neisseria gonorrheae*

   B. *Mycobacterium tuberculosis*

   C. *Haemophilus influenzae*

   D. enterobacteria

2. Which of the following antibiotics should not be used in children younger than age 18 years?

   A. chloramphenicol

   B. penicillins

   C. isoniazid

   D. ciprofloxacin

3. All of the following agents are in the class of macrolide antibiotics *except*:

   A. sulfonamide

   B. erythromycin

   C. azithromycin

   D. clarithromycin

4. Penicillinase may be produced by:

   A. streptococci

   B. *Neisseria gonorrhoeae*

   C. staphylococci

   D. *Haemophilus influenzae*

5. Streptomycin is an aminoglycoside-like antibiotic indicated for the treatment of which of the following:

   A. tuberculosis

   B. gram-negative bacillary septicemia

   C. penicillin-resistant gonococcal infection

   D. syphilis

6. Which of the following antibiotics may cause enamel hypoplasia and permanent yellow-gray color of the teeth in young children?

   A. isoniazid

   B. streptomycin

   C. rifampin

   D. tetracyclines

7. Which of the following antibiotics may lead to gray baby syndrome?

   A. tetracyclines

   B. chloramphenicol

   C. streptomycin

   D. metronidazole

8. A person who lacks resistance to an agent and is vulnerable to a disease is called a:

   A. compromised host

   B. susceptible host

   C. virulent host

   D. parasitic host

9. The presence of viable bacteria in the circulatory system is called:

   A. bacteremia

   B. virimia

   C. anemia

   D. hyperemia

10. The reservoir is a place where:

    A. an infectious agent leaves the body

    B. an organism invades the host

    C. an agent can be spread to others

    D. the agent can survive, colonize, and reproduce

11. Anti-infective drugs derived from natural substances are called:

    A. antivirals

    B. gram stains

    C. antibiotics

    D. antifungals

12. A 42-year-old man has an upper respiratory infection. Four years ago, he experienced an episode of bronchospasm following penicillin V therapy. The culture now reveals gram-positive *Streptococcus pneumoniae* that are sensitive to all of the following drugs. Which of these drugs would be the best choice for this patient?

    A. cefaclor

    B. ampicillin

    C. amoxicillin/clavulanate

    D. erythromycin

13. Isoniazid is a primary antitubercular agent that:

    A. may be nephrotoxic and ototoxic

    B. requires vitamin B_6 (pyridoxine supplementation)

    C. should never be used due to hepatotoxic potential

    D. causes ocular complications that are reversible if the drug is discontinued.

14. All of the following drugs are suitable oral therapy for a lower urinary tract infection due to gram-negative bacteria, *except*:

    A. ciprofloxacin

    B. norfloxacin

    C. sulfadiazine

    D. cefoxitin

15. Which of the following is the drug of choice for chlamydial organisms and rickettsial species?

    A. tetracycline

    B. isoniazid

    C. rifampin

    D. penicillin

Matching

_____ 1. Contraindicated in children younger than eight years of age

_____ 2. Causes aplastic anemia in infants

_____ 3. Changes the color of urine or saliva to orange-red

_____ 4. This agent is used for preoperative bowel sterilization and hepatic coma

_____ 5. The drug of choice for the treatment of Legionnaires' disease and pertussis

_____ 6. The first drug discovered to prevent and cure human bacterial infections

_____ 7. The most widely prescribed antitubercular drug

A. isoniazid

B. erythromycin

C. sulfonamide

D. neomycin

E. rifampin

F. chloramphenicol

G. tetracyclines

Critical Thinking

Christian is a 16-year-old boy who attends a private school. He wanted to work at a local hospital as a volunteer and was required first to have a tuberculin test performed. His physician notes that the TB test is positive with a reading of 16 mm, and orders a chest x-ray. The result of the chest x-ray was negative, so the physician recommends that Christian go to the local health department for tuberculosis evaluation. The staff there determine that he has been exposed to tuberculosis, but does not have the primary form of the disease himself.

1. What drug or drugs would the health department recommend for this patient?

2. How long do you think Christian will need to take the prescribed drug(s)?

3. Since Christian has been exposed to tuberculosis, will his entire family need to receive preventative medications?

CHAPTER 24

Antiviral, Antifungal, and Antiprotozoal Agents

OBJECTIVES

After completing this chapter, the reader should be able to:

1. Describe why antiviral drug treatments are limited compared with other antimicrobial agents.
2. Identify viral diseases that may benefit from drug therapy.
3. Describe the expected outcomes of HIV drug therapy.
4. Define HAART and explain why it is commonly used in the treatment of HIV infection.
5. Explain the mechanisms of action of antiviral, antifungal, and antiprotozoal agents.
6. Explain the four commonly used antifungal agents.
7. Compare the drug therapy of superficial and systemic fungal infections.
8. Name common drugs used for malarial parasites.
9. Explain the important adverse effects of systemic antifungal and antiprotozoal drugs.
10. Name three important amebicides and their mechanisms of action.

GLOSSARY

Acquired immunodeficiency syndrome (AIDS) – a severe immunological disorder caused by the retrovirus HIV, resulting in a defect in cell-mediated immune response

Amebicides and trichomonacides – drugs use to treat amebic and trichomonal infections

Antimalarial agents – drugs used to treat malaria infections

Epidemic – an outbreak of a disease or infection that spreads widely and rapidly

Human immunodeficiency virus (HIV) – a retrovirus that infects helper T cells of the immune system, leading to AIDS

Malaria – a severe, generalized infection caused by the bite of an *Anopheles* mosquito that is infected with a *Plasmodium* protozoon

Mycoses – any disease caused by a fungus

Pro-drug – an inactive or partially active drug that is metabolically changed in the body to an active drug

Replication – the process of reproduction or copying of genetic material

Superficial mycoses – fungal infections involving a surface or a shallow depth of tissue

Systemic mycoses – fungal infections relating to or affecting an entire body or an entire organism

OVERVIEW

Many infections are caused by viruses, fungi, and protozoa. Some of these infections may result in no permanent damage, and usually disappear within seven to ten days if the patient is otherwise healthy. Many of these infections may cause serious viral infections that may be fatal, such as HIV, and may require aggressive drug therapy. Fungal infections are seen commonly in patients with immune deficiency diseases. Fungi and protozoans are more complex than bacteria and there are fewer medications to treat these types of infections.

VIRUSES

Viruses are intracellular parasites that take over the metabolic machinery of host cells and use it for their own survival and replication, often resulting in the destruction of the infected cells. Viral diseases are the most common causes of disease in humans. Viruses result in a wide variety of diseases ranging from the common cold and the "cold sore" of herpes simplex to several types of cancers and AIDS.

Viruses are extremely small, and contain their genetic information in either deoxyribonucleic acid (DNA) or ribonucleic acid (RNA), surrounded by a protein coat (capsid). After infection, viruses usually make multiple copies of their genetic material and produce the necessary viral proteins for replication. Some animal viruses are responsible for diseases such as hemorrhagic fever (Ebola virus), influenza virus, and measles (rubeola virus). In March 2014, an outbreak of the Ebola virus was reported in Western Africa. By March 2015, it had claimed nearly 10,000 lives there. The virus was transmitted to the United States in the fall of 2014 by individuals who had been in Western Africa. This resulted in two deaths.

The Ebola virus is caused by an RNA virus that is spread through direct contact with body fluids of a person who is sick with or had died from Ebola, objects contaminated with the virus, and infected animals. It can only be spread after symptoms begin. Symptoms appear between 2 and 21 days after exposure. They include fever, headache, diarrhea, vomiting, stomach pain, unexplained bleeding or bruising, and muscle pain. It is often fatal, due to internal hemorrhaging from blood vessels and all body organs. However, after 21 days, if an exposed person does not develop symptoms, he or she will not become sick with Ebola. Two new vaccines developed in Canada and Russia are currently in clinical trials.

Antiviral Drugs

Antiviral drugs are used to treat viral infections by influencing viral **replication**. Viruses are not able to independently provide their metabolic activity, and can replicate only within living host cells. Therefore, antiviral

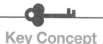

Key Concept

Ebola virus, Dengue virus, and human immunodeficiency virus (HIV) are examples of emerging viruses that threaten the public health and kill thousands of people each year.

agents tend to damage the host as well as viral cells. The majority of antivirals are active against only one virus, either DNA or RNA types. These viruses may include herpes simplex virus (HSV) types 1 and 2, varicella-zoster virus (VZV), cytomegalovirus (CMV), and influenza A. Table 24-1 shows antiviral agents that are currently approved for treatment of some viruses. The following discussion focuses on a few examples of these drugs.

TABLE 24-1 **Antiviral Drugs and Their Therapeutic Uses**

Generic Name	Trade Name	Route of Administration	Common Adult Dosage
Non–HIV Antivirals			
acyclovir (ah-SY-kloh-veer)	Zovirax®	Topical, PO, IV	Topical: Apply 5 times/day for 4 days; PO: 400 mg tid; IV: 5 mg/kg tid
amantadine (ah-MAN-tah-deen)	Symmetrel®	PO	200 mg once daily
cidofovir (sy-DOH-foh-veer)	Vistide®	IV	5 mg/kg once weekly for 2 weeks
famciclovir (fam-SY-kloh-veer)	Famvir®	PO	500 mg tid
ganciclovir (jan-SY-kloh-veer)	Cytovene®	IV	5 mg/kg bid
ribavirin (ry-bah-VY-rin)	Rebetol®, Virazole®	PO	600 mg bid for 24–48 wk
rimantadine (rih-MAN-tah-deen)	Flumadine®	PO	100 mg bid
valacyclovir (vah-lah-SY-kloh-veer)	Valtrex®	PO	1 g tid
HIV Antivirals			
abacavir sulfate (ah-BAH-kah-veer SUL-fayt)	Ziagen®	PO	300 mg bid
didanosine (DDI) (dy-DAN-oh-seen)	Videx®	PO	250 mg once daily
indinavir sulfate (in-DIH-nah-veer SUL-fayt)	Crixivan®	PO	800 mg tid
nevirapine (neh-VY-rah-peen)	Viramune®	PO	200 mg once daily
stavudine (D4T) (STAH-vyoo-deen)	Zerit®	PO	40 mg bid
zidovudine (formerly azidothymidine, AZT) (zy-DOH-vyoo-deen)	Retrovir®	PO, IV	PO: 300 mg bid; IV: 1–2 mg/kg q4h

Acyclovir

Acyclovir is a synthetic acyclic analog of guanosine with activity against various herpes viruses. Herpes viruses can infect neonates, children, and adults, causing a wide spectrum of diseases. Herpes simplex type 1 (HSV-1) virus is responsible for systemic infections involving the liver and other organs, including the central nervous system, and localized infections that may involve the skin, eyes, and mouth. Other medically important herpes viruses include CMV, varicella (chickenpox), and varicella-zoster (shingles). Acyclovir is available in capsules ranging from 200 to 800 mg.

Mechanism of Action Acyclovir is taken up selectively by cells that are infected with herpes viruses. Its activity depends upon conversion to the triphosphate form, which then becomes incorporated into viral DNA and inhibits viral replication.

Indications Acyclovir is most effective against HSV-1 and HSV-2. Intravenous acyclovir is used for HSV encephalitis, neonatal HSV, and life-threatening HSV and VZV infections in immunocompromised patients. Oral acyclovir is indicated for the treatment of primary and recurrent genital herpes. Acyclovir ophthalmic ointment is effective for herpes simplex keratitis.

Adverse Effects Acyclovir may cause nausea, vomiting, and diarrhea. The drug can precipitate in the renal tubules with excessive dosages or when it is given by rapid infusion, which may cause acute renal failure. Other adverse effects of acyclovir include headache, drowsiness, fatigue, uncontrollable rhythmic shaking, confusion, and seizures.

Contraindications and Precautions Acyclovir is contraindicated in patients with hypersensitivity to this agent. It should be used with caution in lactation, pregnancy (category B), dehydration, and renal insufficiency.

Drug Interactions Amphotericin B may raise the plasma and renal concentrations of acyclovir. Probenecid decreases acyclovir elimination. Zidovudine may cause increased drowsiness and lethargy.

Famciclovir

Famciclovir is a **pro-drug** (an inactive or partially active drug that is metabolically changed in the body to an active drug) of the antiviral agent penciclovir.

Mechanism of Action Famciclovir prevents viral replication by inhibition of DNA formation.

Indications Famciclovir is used for the management of acute herpes zoster (shingles) and recurrent genital herpes in immunocompetent patients. It is effective against HSV-1, HSV-2, and VZV.

Adverse Effects Common adverse effects resulting from famciclovir use include fatigue, nausea, diarrhea, vomiting, constipation, and anorexia. Headache is also frequently reported.

Medical Terminology Review

immunocompromised
immune- = relating to the immune system
-compromised = impaired (for example, by disease or treatment)
impairment of the immune system

keratitis
kerat = cornea (of the eye)
the = inflammation
inflammation of the cornea

Key Concept

The patient must be aware that a full therapeutic response to famciclovir may take several weeks.

Medical Terminology Review

immunocompetent
immune- = relating to the immune system
-competent = normal ability to respond
normal functioning of the immune system

Contraindications and Precautions Famciclovir is contraindicated in patients with known hypersensitivity to this agent and during lactation. This drug should be used cautiously in patients with renal or hepatic impairment, or carcinoma; in older adults; and during pregnancy (category B). Safety of this drug in children younger than 18 years is not established.

Drug Interactions Probenecid can increase plasma concentration of penciclovir. Famciclovir may increase digoxin levels.

Amantadine

Amantadine is an antiviral and anticholinergic agent effective for viral respiratory infections such as influenza A virus (it is not effective against influenza B infections), and for Parkinson's disease.

Mechanism of Action The mechanism of the antiviral activity of amantadine is unknown. Its action appears to occur early in the course of viral infection.

Indications Amantadine is indicated for the prophylaxis and treatment of influenza A virus infections, as well as for Parkinson's disease. Individuals who have not received vaccine prophylaxis can benefit from amantadine prophylaxis given for at least 10 days after a known exposure to influenza A.

Adverse Effects Amantadine causes mild adverse effects, including blurred vision, anxiety, insomnia, and dizziness. Urinary retention is another potential adverse effect. Serious adverse effects in patients treated for Parkinson's disease have included congestive heart failure, hypotension, peripheral edema, depression, seizures, psychosis, and leukopenia.

Contraindications and Precautions Amantadine is contraindicated in pregnancy (category C), lactation, and in children younger than one year. Amantadine should be used cautiously in patients with history of epilepsy, congestive heart failure, peripheral edema, postural hypotension (a drop in blood pressure when the patient stands up from a lying or sitting position), psychoses, and hepatic disease.

Drug Interactions Amantadine interacts with anticholinergic drugs to produce atropine-like effects unless the dosage of the anticholinergic drug is reduced. Amantadine prophylaxis or treatment does not interfere with the immune response to influenza vaccination given concurrently.

Ganciclovir

Ganciclovir is an antiviral agent and synthetic purine nucleoside analog that is approved for the treatment of CMV infection.

Mechanism of Action After conversion to ganciclovir triphosphate, ganciclovir is incorporated into viral DNA and inhibits the replication of the virus. By this mechanism, it can terminate viral replication.

Indications Ganciclovir is prescribed for CMV retinitis, as well as prophylaxis and treatment of systemic CMV infections in immunocompromised patients, including HIV-positive and transplant patients.

Adverse Effects Ganciclovir has Black Box Warnings concerning increased potential for dose-limited neutropenia, thrombocytopenia, and anemia. The FDA issues these warnings when a serious problem concerning the use of a drug has been discovered, so that medical practitioners are aware of the problem and its resulting adverse effects. Inflammation of a vein and pain may occur at the site of infusion.

Contraindications and Precautions Ganciclovir is contraindicated in patients with known hypersensitivity, and during lactation. This drug should be used cautiously in patients with renal impairment, in older adults, and during pregnancy (category C). Safety and efficacy in children are not established.

Drug Interactions Probenecid may increase ganciclovir levels and possibly toxicity.

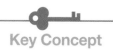

Key Concept

Ganciclovir should not be administered during pregnancy because of its carcinogenic potential.

Antiretroviral Drugs for HIV/AIDS

In 1981, the first cases in what would become an **epidemic** of fatal infections were reported among homosexual men in the United States. The spread of the illness within this group suggested that an infectious agent, transmissible through blood and semen, was causing the symptoms of immunodeficiency that were common to all the patients. The term **acquired immunodeficiency syndrome (AIDS)**, was coined to describe this illness. At the outset of the epidemic, most people with AIDS died within a year of diagnosis. In 1983, researchers isolated the virus that causes AIDS: **human immunodeficiency virus (HIV)**. We have learned much about AIDS since the first case reports. We know its modes of transmission, and who is at risk for HIV infection. We know that HIV kills lymphocytes (cells in the bloodstream necessary to respond to bacteria, fungi, protozoa, and viruses). Antiviral medications for HIV/AIDS slow the growth of HIV in several different ways.

None of the available medications can cure the disease and, due to the rapid mutation of HIV and its resistant strains, new HIV antiviral agents are constantly being developed. The decision of exactly when to begin pharmacotherapy must be made early enough after the diagnosis is established to give each patient the best chance of receiving effective treatment. HIV may remain dormant for either months or years after initial exposure. It is important to begin treatment during the latent stage in order to delay acute symptoms and the onset of full-blown AIDS.

HAART Therapy

Highly active anti-retroviral therapy (HAART) has been shown to reduce viral load and increase CD4 lymphocytes in HIV-infected patients, to delay onset of AIDS, and to prolong survival of those with AIDS. The incidence of and mortality from AIDS have declined substantially since 1996 due to HAART. The benefits of HAART, which involves a combination of three to four drugs with different actions and efficacy against HIV, have been widely publicized. However, HAART presents formidable challenges, including adverse effects and the potential for the rapid spread of drug resistance. Protease inhibitors do not work as well with HIV drugs such as non-nucleoside analogs, and they should not be taken alone. If one of the drugs involved in multiple drug therapy is not well tolerated, or if a patient's HIV infection becomes resistant to it, a whole new set of drugs must be prescribed for the regimen to be effective. Currently, due to the limited number of HAART medications available in the U.S. market, only a few different drug combinations are possible. HAART regimens can also fail because of the lack of viral load response, or poor treatment adherence. Missing a single dose of HAART medication even twice a week can cause the development of drug-resistant HIV—a real danger, because adherence to the drug regimens is difficult. For each group of antiretroviral drugs for HIV/AIDS, only one selected drug will be discussed here. Table 24-2 shows antiretroviral drugs used for HIV/AIDS.

TABLE 24-2   **Antiretroviral Drugs used for HIV/AIDS**

Generic Name	Trade Name	Route of Administration	Adult Dosage
Non-Nucleoside Reverse Transcriptase Inhibitors (NNRTIs)			
delavirdine (deh-lah-VIR-deen)	Rescriptor®	PO	400 mg tid
efavirenz (eh-FAH-vih-renz)	Sustiva®	PO	600 mg/day
nevirapine (neh-VY-rah-peen)	Viramune®	PO	200 mg/day for 14 days, then increase to bid
Nucleoside Reverse Transcriptase Inhibitors (NRTIs)			
abacavir sulfate (ah-BAH-kah-veer SUL-fayt)	Ziagen®	PO	300 mg bid
didanosine (DDI) (dy-DAH-noh-seen)	Videx®	PO	400 mg qd
emtricitabine (em-trih-SIH-tah-been)	Emtriva®	PO	200 mg/day
lamivudine (3TC) (lah-MIH-vyoo-deen)	Epivir®	PO	300 mg/day
stavudine (D4T) (STAH-vyoo-deen)	Zerit®	PO	40 mg bid

Table 24-2 continued

zalcitabine (DDC) **(zal-SIH-tah-been)**	Hivid®	PO	0.75 mg tid
zidovudine (formerly AZT, now ZDV) **(zy-DOH-vyoo-deen)**	Retrovir®	PO, IV	PO: 300 mg bid; IV: 1–2 mg/kg q4h
Protease Inhibitors (PIs)			
amprenavir **(am-PREH-nah-veer)**	Agenerase®	PO	1200 mg bid
atazanavir **(ah-tah-ZAH-nah-veer)**	Reyataz®	PO	400 mg/day
indinavir sulfate **(in-DIH-nah-veer SUL-fayt)**	Crixivan®	PO	800 mg tid
nelfinavir mesylate **(nel-FIH-nah-veer MEH-sih-layt)**	Viracept®	PO	750 mg tid
ritonavir **(ry-TOH-nah-veer)**	Norvir®	PO	600 mg tid with meals
saquinavir mesylate **(sah-KWIH-nah-veer MEH-sih-layt)**	Invirase®	PO	600 mg tid
Miscellaneous Drugs			
enfuvirtide **(en-FYOO-vir-tyd)**	Fuzeon®	SC	90 mg bid
tenofovir disoproxil **(teh-NOH-foh-veer dy-soh-PROK-zil)**	Viread®	PO	300 mg once daily

Delavirdine

Delavirdine is a non-nucleoside reverse transcriptase inhibitor that prevents the replication of the HIV-1 virus.

Mechanism of Actions Delavirdine binds directly to reverse transcriptase of HIV-1 and blocks RNA- and DNA-dependent DNA polymerase activities.

Indications Delavirdine is used in the treatment of HIV infection in combination with other antiretroviral agents.

Adverse Effects Delavirdine may cause headache, fatigue, allergic reaction, chills, edema, and joint pain. Administration of delavirdine may also cause abnormal coordination, amnesia, anxiety, confusion, and dizziness. Common adverse effects of delavirdine include nausea, vomiting, diarrhea, abdominal cramps, and anorexia.

Contraindications and Precautions Delavirdine is contraindicated in patients with hypersensitivity to this agent, and during lactation. Delavirdine must be used cautiously in patients with impaired liver function, and during pregnancy (category C). Safety and efficacy in children younger than 16 years of age have not been established.

Drug Interactions Antacids and H_2-receptor antagonists decrease the absorption of delavirdine. Didanosine and delavirdine should be taken one hour apart to avoid decreased delavirdine levels.

Lamivudine

Lamivudine is one example of a nucleoside reverse transcriptase inhibitor (NRTI). This agent is used in combination with other medications to treat HIV infection in patients with AIDS. It is not a cure, and may not decrease the number of HIV-related illnesses. Lamivudine does not prevent the spread of HIV to other people. It is also used to treat hepatitis B infection. It is often used in combination with zidovudine.

Mechanism of Action NRTIs such as lamivudine work by interfering with viral reproduction. They do so by preventing the creation of new viral RNA. This drug should never be used alone to prevent resistance, which can occur very rapidly.

Indications Lamivudine is used to treat HIV infection in combination with zidovudine. It is also used in the treatment of chronic hepatitis B. The combination of these two drugs may stop the spread of both viruses.

Adverse Effects The most serious adverse effects of lamivudine include rash, stomach pain, vomiting or upset stomach (in children), fever, muscle pain, and a numbness, tingling, or burning sensation in the fingers or toes.

Contraindications and Precautions Lamivudine is contraindicated in patients with hypersensitivity to this agent. Lamivudine should be avoided during lactation. This drug is used with caution in patients with renal impairment, during pregnancy (category C), and in children.

Drug Interactions The use of lamivudine with trimethoprim-sulfamethoxazole can increase the amount of lamivudine in the body. However, it is not necessary to change the dosages of either of these agents. Lamivudine increases the risk of lactic acidosis in combination with other reverse transcriptase inhibitors and antiretroviral agents.

Ritonavir

Ritonavir is an anti-HIV drug that is a protease inhibitor. It is used to treat HIV infection when therapy is warranted.

Mechanism of Action By interfering with the formation of essential proteins and enzymes, ritonavir blocks the maturation of the HIV virus and causes the formation of nonfunctional, immature, noninfectious virions.

Indications Ritonavir is used to treat HIV in adults and children, in combination with other antiretroviral agents. Because it inhibits the metabolism of other protease inhibitors, it is increasingly used for boosting and maintaining plasma concentrations of protease inhibitors.

Adverse Effects One of the more serious effects of ritonavir is potentially fatal pancreatitis. Other serious adverse effects include body fat redistribution and accumulation, increased bleeding in patients with hemophilia type A and B, hyperglycemia, hyperlipidemia, new-onset diabetes mellitus, and the exacerbation of existing diabetes mellitus.

Contraindications and Precautions Ritonavir is contraindicated in patients with hypersensitivity to this drug. Ritonavir should not be given in patients with antimicrobial resistance to protease inhibitors, or those suffering from pancreatitis. Safety and efficacy in children younger than two years of age are not established.

Ritonavir is used with caution in pregnancy (category B), hepatic diseases, advanced HIV disease, diabetes mellitus, hyperlipidemia, and renal insufficiency.

Drug Interactions When ritonavir is given in combination with other protease inhibitors, the dosage of the other protease inhibitors may be reduced. Drug interactions may occur when ritonavir is administered with a wide variety of other drugs, mostly due to pharmacokinetic interactions. Concomitant use of ritonavir with lovastatin or simvastatin is not recommended. Caution should also be taken when ritonavir is used with atorvastatin, cerivastatin, St. John's wort, sildenafil, astemizole, or cisapride.

Tenofovir

Tenofovir is one of the miscellaneous agents for treatment of HIV/AIDS. This agent is an antiviral drug that is approved for the treatment of HIV infection. It is able to reduce the amount of HIV in the blood and, when used in combination with other antiviral drugs, it can help prevent or reverse damage to the immune system and reduce the risk of AIDS-related illnesses. It is also an experimental treatment for hepatitis B.

Mechanism of Action Tenofovir is a potent inhibitor of retroviruses, including HIV-1. It may be active against nucleoside-resistant HIV strains. The active form of tenofovir persists in HIV-infected cells for prolonged periods; thus, it results in sustained inhibition of HIV replication. It reduces the viral load and CD4 counts.

Indications Tenofovir is used in combination with other antiretroviral agents for the treatment of HIV.

Adverse Effects Tenofovir may cause asthenia, anorexia, and neutropenia; as well as increased creatine kinase, liver enzymes (AST, ALT), serum amylase, triglycerides, or serum glucose. Nausea, vomiting, diarrhea, flatulence, abdominal pain, and anorexia are common adverse effects of tenofovir.

Contraindications and Precautions   Tenofovir is contraindicated in patients with hypersensitivity to tenofovir, hepatitis, and lactic acidosis. Tenofovir should be avoided with concurrent administration of nephrotoxic agents, in patients with renal failure, and during lactation. Tenofovir must be used cautiously in patients with hepatic dysfunction, alcoholism, renal impairment, or obesity; during pregnancy (category B); and in children.

Drug Interactions   Tenofovir may increase didanosine toxicity. Use of this agent with acyclovir, amphotericin B, cidofovir, foscarnet, ganciclovir, probenecid, valacyclovir, or valganciclovir may increase tenofovir toxicity by decreasing its renal elimination.

FUNGI

Neither plant nor animal, fungi are a distinct group of organisms that grow in single cells (e.g., yeast) or colonies (e.g., molds) and obtain food from living organisms or organic matter. Fungal diseases are more common in individuals who are immunologically impaired, but may occur in other patients. These infections frequently involve the hair, skin, nails, and mucous membranes. Examples include athlete's foot, histoplasmosis, cryptococcosis, candidal infections, and tinea.

Antifungal Drugs

Antifungal agents are used to treat systemic, local, and topical fungal infections. As fungi are single-celled or multicellular organisms that are more complex than bacteria, most antibacterial agents are ineffective against fungi. The human body is generally resistant to infection by fungi, but patients infected with HIV may frequently exhibit fungal infections, some of which may need intensive drug therapy. Fungal diseases are called **mycoses**.

Fungal infections may be classified into two groups: **superficial mycoses** (of the skin) and **systemic mycoses**, which affect internal organs such as the lungs, digestive organs, and brain. Antifungals are used to treat systemic, local fungal, and topical fungal infections. A table of antifungal drugs can be found in Table 24-3. A selective few agents will be discussed here in detail.

Amphotericin B

Amphotericin B is the most effective agent available for the treatment of most systemic fungal infections.

Mechanism of Action   Amphotericin B is fungistatic, and may be fungicidal at higher concentrations, depending on the sensitivity of the fungus.

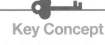

TABLE 24-3	Antifungal Agents		
Generic Name	**Trade Name**	**Route of Administration**	**Common Dosage Range**
amphotericin B (am-foh-TEH-rih-sin B)	Fungizone®, Amphocin®	IV	0.25–0.3 mg/kg/day
butoconazole nitrate (byoo-toh-KOH-nah-zohl NY-trayt)	Femstat 3®, Gynazole-1®	Vaginal	One full applicator hs
caspofungin (KAH-spoh-fun-jin)	Cancidas®	IV	70 mg on day 1; then 50 mg qd thereafter
clotrimazole (kloh-TRY-mah-zohl)	Mycelex®, Lotrimin®	Topical, Vaginal	Topical: 10 mg bid prn; Vaginal: 5–100 mg in applicator hs
econazole nitrate (ee-KOH-nah-zohl NY-trayt)	Spectazole®	Topical	15–85 g prn
fluconazole (floo-KOH-nah-zohl)	Diflucan®	PO, IV	PO: 100–200 mg/day; IV: 200 mg for 14–21 days (max: 400 mg qid)
griseofulvin (GRIH-see-oh-ful-vin)	Grifulvin®, Fulvicin P/G®	PO	500 mg–1 g/day in 1–4 divided doses
itraconazole (eye-trah-KOH-nah-zohl)	Sporanox®	PO	100–400 mg/day
ketoconazole (kee-toh-KOH-nah-zohl)	Nizoral®	PO, Topical	200–400 mg single dose/day
miconazole nitrate (my-KOH-nah-zohl NY-trayt)	Monistat®	Topical, Vaginal	Apply cream or insert suppository into vagina hs
nystatin (ny-STAH-tin)	Mycostatin®	PO, Vaginal, Topical	PO: 500,000–1,000,000 units qid; Vaginal: 1–2 times/day for 2 wk
terbinafine hydrochloride (ter-BIH-nah-feen hy-droh-KLOR-ryd)	Lamisil®	Topical	Apply thin layer to affected area
tioconazole (tee-oh-KOH-nah-zohl)	Vagistat-1®	Vaginal	5 mg (one applicator) once daily
tolnaftate (tol-NAF-tayt)	Tinactin®	Topical	2 oz prn

It has a wide spectrum of activity on most of the fungi pathogenic to humans. Amphotericin B acts by binding to fungal cell membranes, causing them to become permeable.

Indications Amphotericin B is used intravenously for a wide spectrum of potentially fatal systemic fungal (mycotic) infections, including aspergillosis, blastomycosis, coccidiomycosis, cryptococcosis, disseminated candidiasis, and histoplasmosis. Treatment may continue for several months. Unlike antibiotics, resistance to amphotericin B is not common. Topical preparations are used to treat cutaneous and mucocutaneous infections caused by *Candida* (monilia).

Adverse Effects Amphotericin B can cause many serious adverse effects. Therefore, it should be administered in a hospital. Adverse effects include fever, chills, nausea, vomiting, headache, hypotension, muscle pain, dyspnea, and tachypnea. Nephrotoxicity, anaphylactoid reactions, phlebitis, and liver damage may occur. Amphotericin B for parenteral use should only be mixed in 5% dextrose in water (D_5W) and should be protected from light. Sometimes patients may be premedicated with diphenhydramine intravenously or acetaminophen prior to administration.

Contraindications and Precautions Amphotericin B is contraindicated in patients with a known hypersensitivity and during lactation. This agent is used cautiously in patients with severe bone marrow depression or renal function impairment. Amphotericin B should be used during pregnancy (category B) only when there is a life-threatening situation.

Drug Interactions When amphotericin B is given with corticosteroids, severe hypokalemia may occur, and the hypokalemia increases the risk of digitalis toxicity. Aminoglycosides, colistin, furosemide, and vancomycin may interact with amphotericin B, increasing the possibility of nephrotoxicity.

Griseofulvin

Griseofulvin is a drug that is deposited in the skin, and bound to keratin. It is an antifungal, and anti-infective agent.

Mechanism of Action Griseofulvin is fungistatic. It inhibits fungal cell activity. This agent is active against various strains of *Microsporum, Trichophyton,* and *Epidermophyton.* Griseofulvin has no effect on other fungi, including *Candida,* bacteria, and yeast.

Indications Griseofulvin is effective in mycotic infections of the nails, hair, and skin. It is available only in oral form.

Adverse Effects Griseofulvin may produce fatigue, headache, confusion, syncope, and lethargy. It also occasionally causes leukopenia and, in rare cases, serum sickness and hepatotoxicity. Heartburn, nausea, vomiting, diarrhea, flatulence, dry mouth, and unpleasant taste are common adverse effects of griseofulvin.

Contraindications and Precautions Griseofulvin must be avoided in patients with known hypersensitivity and severe liver disease. It is used cautiously during pregnancy (category C) and lactation.

Drug Interactions Griseofulvin may increase the metabolism of antico-agulants and decrease the effects of these agents. Barbiturates can reduce absorption of griseofulvin. A decrease in the effects of an oral contraceptive may occur with the administration of griseofulvin, causing breakthrough bleeding, amenorrhea, or pregnancy. Alcohol consumption can cause flushing and tachycardia when griseofulvin is used.

Nystatin

Nystatin is the common topical treatment for thrush, which can occur in the mouth or on the tongue, gums, or skin. Its chemical structure is similar to that of amphotericin B. It is not considered a systemic antifungal, but acts locally. Nystatin is available in tablets or a liquid suspension, as well as a cream, ointment, and topical powder; and therapy is usually continued for two weeks to be effective.

Mechanism of Action Nystatin is fungicidal and fungistatic. It is effective against a variety of yeasts and fungi (candidal infections).

Indications Nystatin is prescribed primarily in the treatment of local infections of the skin and mucous membranes caused by *Candida albicans* (e.g., vulvovaginal, orpharyngeal, and intestinal candidiasis). It is also used for candidal diaper rashes. It is often used prophylactically on the diaper area when an oral *Candida* infection is present.

Adverse Effects Nystatin can temporarily affect the sense of taste, and thus decrease appetite. Other adverse effects include nausea, vomiting, diarrhea, and stomach pain. If used to treat vaginal infections, the patient should avoid using sanitary napkins and refrain from sexual contact until the infection subsides.

Contraindications and Precautions Vaginal tablets of nystatin are contraindicated during pregnancy (category C), and with vaginal infections caused by *Trichomonas* species. Nystatin should be used cautiously during lactation.

Drug Interactions There are no listed drug interactions with nystatin.

Itraconazole

Itraconazole is an antifungal agent indicated in the treatment of histoplasmosis, aspergillosis, and blastomycosis. Liver function should be monitored during treatment with itraconazole.

Mechanism of Action Itraconazole is fungistatic, and may also be fungicidal depending on the concentration. The drug interferes with the formation of ergosterol, the principal sterol in the fungal cell membrane that, when depleted, interrupts membrane functions.

Indications Itraconazole is used in the treatment of systemic fungal infections caused by blastomycosis, histoplasmosis, and aspergillosis due to dermatophytes of the toenail with or without fingernail involvement, or mouth and throat candidiasis.

Adverse Effects Itraconazole may cause heart failure. With high doses, hypertension may occur. Other adverse effects include headache, dizziness, fatigue, euphoria, drowsiness, gynecomastia, hypokalemia (low potassium level), hypertriglyceridemia, impotence, rash, pruritus, and adrenal insufficiency.

Contraindications and Precautions Itraconazole is contraindicated in patients with a known hypersensitivity or renal failure, and during pregnancy (category C) and lactation.

Itraconazole should be used cautiously in patients with hypochlorhydria, hepatitis, and HIV. Itraconazole also must be used with great caution in patients with pulmonary, renal, and valvular heart diseases.

Drug Interactions Itraconazole may increase levels and toxicity of oral hypoglycemic agents. Combination with oral midazolam, pimozide, levomethadyl, or quinidine may cause severe cardiac events, including cardiac arrest or sudden death. Itraconazole levels are decreased by carbamazepine, phenytoin, phenobarbital, isoniazid, and rifampin.

Fluconazole

Fluconazole is an antifungal agent used in the treatment of both systemic and superficial mycoses.

Mechanism of Action Fluconazole interferes with the formation of ergosterol, resulting in decreased cell wall integrity and leakage of essential cellular components. Fluconazole is fungistatic and it may also be fungicidal, depending on the concentration used.

Indications Fluconazole has been shown to be effective against meningitis, as well as oropharyngeal and systemic candidiasis, both of which are commonly seen in AIDS patients. Fluconazole is also used for vaginal candidiasis.

Adverse Effects The most common adverse effects of fluconazole include elevated liver enzymes, gastrointestinal complaints, headache, and skin rash.

Contraindications and Precautions Fluconazole is contraindicated in patients with known hypersensitivity and during pregnancy (category C) and lactation. Fluconazole is used cautiously in patients with renal impairment. This agent may be given during pregnancy if the benefit of the drug outweighs any possible risk to the fetus.

Drug Interactions Fluconazole administration may increase the effect of oral hypoglycemics and decreases the metabolism of phenytoin and warfarin.

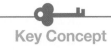

Key Concept

Herbal supplements such as St. John's wort and garlic may affect itraconazole levels.

Key Concept

When fluconazole is used in the treatment of elderly patients or those who have renal impairments, a creatinine clearance test should be performed before administration of the drug.

Ketoconazole

Ketoconazole is an antifungal agent effective in the treatment of candidiasis, histoplasmosis, blastomycosis, and aspergillosis.

Mechanism of Action Ketoconazole is fungistatic and may also be fungicidal depending on the concentration used. The drug interferes with the formation of ergosterol, the principal sterol in the fungal cell wall, interrupting membrane function.

Indications Ketoconazole is used for severe systemic fungal infections, including candidiasis (e.g., oral thrush, candiduria), and chronic mucocutaneous and pulmonary candidiasis. Topical forms are available for superficial mycoses.

Adverse Effects Ketoconazole is usually well-tolerated. In some cases, nausea, vomiting, dizziness, headache, abdominal pain, and pruritus have been reported. Most adverse effects are mild and transient. In rare cases, fatal hepatic necrosis may occur. Periodic liver function tests should be used to monitor for hepatotoxicity.

Contraindications and Precautions Ketoconazole is contraindicated in patients with known hypersensitivity to ketoconazole or to any component in its formulation, as well as those with chronic alcoholism. Safe administration of ketoconazole during pregnancy (category C) and lactation, or in children younger than two years of age is not established.

Drug Interactions Ketoconazole increases the anticoagulant effects of warfarin and causes hepatotoxicity when administered with alcohol. The absorption of ketoconazole is decreased when this agent is given with histamine antagonists and antacids.

> **Key Concept**
>
> Postexposure prophylaxis for various types of fungi includes either local or systemic medications as soon as possible after exposure. Since the structure and chemical makeup of fungi make them difficult to kill, antifungal medications may need to be administered for several months.

PROTOZOA

Protozoa are single-celled parasitic organisms, many of which are motile. They generally obtain their food from dead or decaying organic matter. Some protozoa are agents of disease, transmitting infection through contamination of food or water, or through insect bites. These organisms cause infections that are among the most serious known to humanity. Common protozoal infections include amebiasis, malaria, toxoplasmosis, trypanosomiasis, trichomoniasis, and giardiasis. Although many of these diseases are rare in the United States, travelers to Africa, South America, and Asia may acquire them overseas and return home with the infection. Table 24-4 shows the characteristics of each group.

Antiprotozoal Drugs

Antiprotozoal drugs fall into two main categories: **amebicides and trichomonacides**, which are prescribed to treat amebic and trichomonal infections, and **antimalarial agents** used to treat malaria infections.

TABLE 24-4	Protozoa That Cause Major Diseases and Preferred Site of Infection		
Protozoan Group	Genus	Preferred Site of Infection	Disease
Amoebae	*Entamoeba*	Intestine	Amebiasis
Sporozca	*Plasmodium*	Bloodstream, liver	Malaria
	Toxoplasma	Intestine	Toxoplasmosis
Flagellates	*Trypanosoma*	Blood	Trypanosomiasis
	Trichomonas	Genital tract	Trichomoniasis
	Giardia	Intestine	Giardiasis

Amebicides and Trichomonacides

These drugs are very important in the treatment of amebiasis, giardiasis, and trichomoniasis. They include metronidazole, iodoquinol, and paromomycin (Table 24-5).

Metronidazole

Metronidazole is an antitrichomonal, amebicide, and antibiotic.

Mechanism of Action Metronidazole is a synthetic compound with direct trichomonacidal and amebicidal activity as well as antibacterial activity against anaerobic bacteria and some gram-negative bacteria.

Indications Metronidazole is the drug of choice in amebic dysentery, giardiasis, and trichomoniasis. It is used in asymptomatic and symptomatic dysentery, which is a gastrointestinal disorder resulting from ulcerative inflammation of the colon caused chiefly by infection with *Entamoeba histolytica*. Entamoeba, giardia, toxoplasma, and trypanosomal infections are commonly found in Africa, Asia, and Latin America. These infections are rare in the United States. *Trichomonas vaginalis* is usually transmitted through sexual contact and is frequently seen in men and women in the United States. Metronidazole is also used in the treatment of amebic liver abscess, and for preoperative prophylaxis in colorectal surgery, elective hysterectomy, or vaginal repair. Intravenous metronidazole is used for the treatment of serious infections caused by susceptible anaerobic bacteria in intra-abdominal infections, skin infections, and septicemia.

Adverse Effects Metronidazole causes nausea, vomiting, diarrhea, metallic taste or bitter taste, and, occasionally, neurological reactions. This agent may also cause polyuria, dysuria, pyuria, incontinence, cystitis, decreased libido, and vaginal dryness.

Contraindications and Precautions Metronidazole is contraindicated in patients with known hypersensitivity, blood dyscrasias, and active central

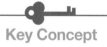

Key Concept

Alcohol must be avoided while a patient is taking metronidazole to prevent profound vomiting.

TABLE 24-5	Drug Effects on Protozoal Infections		
Generic Name	**Trade Name**	**Route of Administration**	**Common Adult Dosage**
Antiprotozoals (nonmalarial)			
metronidazole (meh-troh-NIH-dah-zohl)	Flagyl®	PO, IV	PO: 250–500 mg tid; IV loading dose: 15 mg/kg; Maint dose: 7.5 mg/kg q6h
pentamidine isoethionate (pen-TAH-mih-deen eye-soh-eh-THY-oh-nayt)	Nebupent®	IM, IV	4 mg/kg daily for 14–21 days; infuse over 60 min
trimetrexate (try-meh-TREK-sayt)	Neutrexin®	IV	45 mg/m² daily
Antimalarials			
atovaquone (ah-TOH-vah-kwohn)	Mepron®	PO	750 mg bid for 21 days
chloroquine phosphate (KLOH-roh-kween FOS-fayt)	Aralen®	PO	600 mg initial dose, then 300 mg weekly
hydroxychloroquine (hy-drok-see-KLOH-roh-kween)	Plaquenil®	PO	620 mg initial dose, then 310 mg weekly
mefloquine hydrochloride (MEF-loh-kween hy-droh-KLOR-ryd)	Lariam®	PO	Prevention: begin with 250 mg weekly for 4 weeks, then 250 mg every other week; Treatment: 1250 mg as a single dose
primaquine phosphate (PRY-mah-kween FOS-fayt)	Primaquine®	PO	30 mg/day
pyrimethamine (pih-rih-MEH-thah-meen)	Daraprim®	PO	25 mg weekly for 10 weeks
quinine (KWY-nyn)	Quinamm®	PO	260–650 mg tid for 3 days
Amebicides			
doxycycline (dok-see-SY-kleen)	Vibramycin®	PO	100 mg/day
iodoquinol (eye-oh-doh-KWIH-nol)	Yodoxin®	PO	650 mg t.i.d. × 20 days (max: 2 g/day)
paromomycin sulfate (pah-roh-moh-MY-sin SUL-fayt)	Humatin®	PO	25–35 mg/kg in 3 doses (with meals) for 5–10 days

nervous system disease. Metronidazole cannot be used in the first trimester of pregnancy (category B), or during lactation. This drug should be cautiously used in patients with coexistent candidiasis, alcoholism, and liver disease, and during the second and third trimesters of pregnancy.

Drug Interactions In patients taking metronidazole, alcohol may elicit disulfiram reaction, which consists of flushing, a throbbing headache, nausea, vomiting, arrhythmias, and many other unpleasant effects. Trimethoprim and nitroglycerin, if used with metronidazole, also may elicit disulfiram reaction due to the alcohol content of the dosage form. Metronidazole interacts with many drugs, including oral solutions of citalopram ritonavir and intravenous formulations of sulfamethoxazole. Phenobarbital increases metronidazole metabolism.

Antimalarial Agents

Malaria is a severe, generalized infection caused by the bite of an *Anopheles* mosquito that is infected with *Plasmodium* protozoa. *Plasmodium* is the most important human parasite among the sporozoa. There are four species, which cause different types of malaria: *Plasmodium falciparum*, *Plasmodium malariae*, *Plasmodium vivax*, and *Plasmodium ovale*. According to **Integrated** Regional Information Networks (www.irinnews.org), it is estimated that more than 100 million people are infected with malaria, and about one million die annually in Africa alone. Antimalarial agents are selectively active during different phases of the protozoan life cycle and include chloroquine, primaquine, quinine, and hydroxychloroquine. Agents that are employed in the prevention of malaria include mefloquine, quinacrine, and folic acid antagonists. Mefloquine is chemically related to quinine. It is used both in the prevention of malaria and in the treatment of acute malarial infections. Quinacrine was once the most popular drug for malaria prophylaxis, but its use has declined sharply with the development of safer and more effective agents. Folic acid antagonists such as pyrimethamine and sulfa drugs interfere with the synthesis of folic acid. They may be used alone or in combination to suppress and prevent malaria caused by susceptible strains of *Plasmodium*.

Mechanism of Action Chloroquine and hydroxychloroquine bind to and alter the properties of *Plasmodium*. The mechanism of action of primaquine and quinine is unknown.

Indications Chloroquine is the drug of choice to suppress malaria symptoms and treat acute attacks resulting from *P. falciparum* and *P. malariae* infections. Chloroquine is the most useful antimalarial agent. Hydroxychloroquine is prescribed as an alternative to chloroquine in patients who cannot tolerate chloroquine or when chloroquine is unavailable. Primaquine is used to cure relapses of *P. vivax* and *P. ovale* malaria, to prevent malaria in exposed persons, and in the prevention and treatment of chloroquine-resistant strains of *P. falciparum*. Quinine is prescribed for acute malaria caused

Key Concept

Chloroquine may cause irreversible retinal damage in patients who receive this drug for long-term therapy.

Key Concept

Patients must stop taking quinine if they experience itching, rash, fever, difficulty breathing, or vision problems.

Key Concept

In the United States, most protozoal infections are linked to dirty living conditions in poorer communities. Health care workers who are most at risk are those who work with the homeless. Health care workers who travel to impoverished countries are also at higher risk, and if conditions such as traveler's diarrhea are contracted, treatment involves loperamide (in the absence of dysentery) and a fluoroquinolone such as ciprofloxacin.

by chloroquine-resistant strains. Quinine is always given in combination with another antimalarial agent.

Adverse Effects Chloroquine and hydroxychloroquine can concentrate in the liver and must be used carefully in patients with liver diseases. They may cause visual disturbances, headache, and skin rash.

Primaquine may cause anemia, granulocytopenia, nausea, vomiting, and abdominal cramps.

Quinine overdose or hypersensitivity reactions may be fatal. Toxicity of quinine produces visual and hearing disturbances, headache, fever, syncope, and cardiovascular collapse.

Contraindications and Precautions Chloroquine is contraindicated in patients with hypersensitivity to this agent, renal disease, or psoriasis. It should be avoided for long-term therapy in children and during pregnancy (category C) and lactation. Safe use in women of childbearing potential has not been established.

Chloroquine should be used with caution in patients with impaired hepatic function, alcoholism, or eczema, and in infants and children.

Primaquine is contraindicated in patients with rheumatoid arthritis and lupus erythematosus. Primaquine is also contraindicated in patients with recent or concomitant use of agents capable of bone marrow depression (e.g., quinacrine). This drug is not used during pregnancy (category C) or lactation.

Quinine is contraindicated in patients with myasthenia gravis, tinnitus, and optic neuritis, and during pregnancy (category X). This drug should be avoided during lactation. Quinine is used cautiously in patients with cardiac arrhythmias.

Since millions of U.S. residents travel to countries where malaria is present every year, and about 1500 cases of malaria are diagnosed in this country annually, travelers should be individually assessed as to needed precautions. The Centers for Disease Control and Prevention (CDC) publish malaria information, by country, at this web location: http://www.cdc.gov/malaria/travelers/country_table/a.html. This website also lists the recommended medications for each country. Based on the risk assessment, specific malaria prevention interventions will be indicated. These may include antimalarial medications, mosquito repellants, and the use of insecticide-treated bed nets. The CDC also publishes the "Yellow Book," which details infectious diseases related to travel, at this web location: http://wwwnc.cdc.gov/travel/yellowbook/2014/chapter-3-infectious-diseases-related-to-travel/malaria.

Drug Interactions Antacids containing aluminum and magnesium decrease chloroquine absorption. Toxicity of both primaquine and quinacrine are increased. Quinine may increase digoxin levels. Anticonvulsants, barbiturates, and rifampin increase the metabolism of quinine.

SUMMARY

Most antiviral drugs act by inhibiting viral DNA or RNA replication in the virus, causing viral death. These agents have limited use because they are effective against only a small number of specific viral infections. However, the arsenal of antiretroviral drugs is constantly changing as new products are added to the market. This area is of intense research interest, and new information is being discovered every day that will influence the treatment of patients with immunodeficiency problems.

Superficial mycotic (fungal) infections occur on the surface of, or just below, the skin or nails. Deep mycotic infections develop inside the body, such as the lungs. Treatment for deep mycotic infections is often difficult and prolonged. Antiprotozoal drugs include antimalarial, antiamebia, antitrichomoniasis, and others. Diseases caused by protozoa are rare in the United States. They are seen commonly in Africa, Asia, and Latin America.

EXPLORING THE WEB

Look for additional information on HIV and AIDS and the treatments used to combat the diseases on the following sites:

- **www.aids.gov**

- **www.thebodypro.com**

- **www.unicef.com**

- **http://www.cdc.gov/malaria/travelers/country_table/a.html**

- **http://wwwnc.cdc.gov/travel/yellowbook/2014/chapter-3-infectious-diseases-related-to-travel/malaria**

REVIEW QUESTIONS

Multiple Choice

1. Amantadine is prescribed for the prophylaxis and treatment of:

   A. malaria

   B. candidal infections

   C. HIV

   D. influenza A

2. Which of the following antimicrobial agents is similar in chemical structure to amphotericin B?

   A. ribavirin

   B. streptomycin

   C. amantadine

   D. nystatin

3. Which of the following are parasitic, minute organisms that may invade normal cells and cause disease?

   A. fungi

   B. protozoa

   C. viruses

   D. bacteria

4. Herpes simplex virus type 2 (HSV-2) causes which of the following conditions or diseases?

   A. cold sores

   B. AIDS

   C. fever blisters

   D. genital herpes

5. Ketoconazole is contraindicated in children younger than what age?

   A. 2 years

   B. 6 years

   C. 12 years

   D. 18 years

6. All of the following parasitic organisms include the classification of protozoa, *except:*

   A. flagellates

   B. spirochetes

   C. sporozoa

   D. amoebae

7. Intravenous metronidazole is used in the treatment of which of the following serious infections?

   A. susceptible anaerobic bacteria

   B. trichomoniasis

   C. giardiasis

   D. amebic dysentery

8. Which of the following explains the sharp decline in the use of quinacrine in the treatment of malaria?

   A. less safe and less effective

   B. more expensive

   C. product discontinued

   D. none of the above

9. Which of the following agents is indicated to treat cytomegalovirus?

   A. zidovudine

   B. abacavir

   C. ganciclovir

   D. nelfinavir

10. The trade names of enfuvirtide (miscellaneous drug for treatment of HIV/AIDS) include which of the following?

    A. Fuzeon®

    B. Viread®

    C. Hivid®

    D. Norvir®

11. Which of the following antiviral drugs may be indicated for treatment of Parkinson's disease?

    A. famciclovir

    B. ritonavir

    C. acyclovir

    D. amantadine

12. All of the following diseases may be caused by protozoa, *except:*

    A. giardiasis

    B. aspergillosis

    C. trichomoniasis

    D. malaria

13. HAART therapy in HIV/AIDS patients has been shown to:

    A. increase CD4 lymphocytes

    B. increase viral lode

    C. decrease CD4 lymphocytes

    D. have only limited effect upon survival

14. The first cases of AIDS in the United States were reported in which of the following years?

    A. 1969

    B. 1975

    C. 1981

    D. 1996

15. Chloroquine is the drug of choice to suppress symptoms of

    A. systemic mycoses

    B. genital herpes

    C. malaria

    D. superficial mycoses

Matching

Generic Names

_____ 1. tioconazole

_____ 2. fluconazole

_____ 3. nystatin

_____ 4. ketoconazole

_____ 5. miconazole

_____ 6. griseofulvin

_____ 7. amphotericin B

_____ 8. itraconazole

Trade Names

A. Fulvicin P/G®

B. Monistat®

C. Nizoral®

D. Sporanox®

E. Fungizone®

F. Diflucan®

G. Mycostatin®

H. Vagistat-1®

Critical Thinking

A young female client who was recently diagnosed with insulin-dependent diabetes has been given a prescription for metronidazole (Flagyl®) to treat a vaginal infection.

1. What should the physician tell this patient about the potential adverse effects of metronidazole?

2. What foods or beverages must be avoided with this medication?

Pharmacology for Specific Populations

CHAPTER 25

Drug Therapy During Pregnancy and Lactation

OUTLINE

OBJECTIVES

After completing this chapter, the reader should be able to:

1. Identify normal physiological changes with pregnancy that alter the pharmacokinetics of drug therapy.

2. Define "teratogenic effect" and its relevance in managing drug therapy in pregnant patients.

3. Differentiate the classifications of drugs for use in pregnancy.

4. Describe why adverse effects of drug therapy may be overlooked in pregnant patients.

5. Identify how drug therapy in pregnant or breastfeeding patients may vary from drugs in other groups.

6. Discuss FDA pregnancy categories.

7. Identify potential drugs that cause problems during breastfeeding.

8. Explain pharmacodynamics of drugs during pregnancy.

9. Describe the common conditions affecting pregnant patients.

10. Define preeclampsia and eclampsia.

GLOSSARY

Affinity – the measure of the binding strength of two drugs

Eclampsia – the gravest form of pregnancy-induced hypertension. It is characterized by grand mal seizures, coma, hypertension, proteinuria, and edema

Floppy infant syndrome – a condition of abnormally low muscle tone, often with reduced muscle strength; also called infantile hypotonia

Hemodynamic – related to the physical aspects of blood circulation, including cardiac function and peripheral vascular physiologic characteristics

Hyperemesis gravidarum – pernicious vomiting during pregnancy

Organogenesis – the period from implantation to about 60 days thereafter; the time when major fetal organs form

Preeclampsia – an abnormal condition of pregnancy characterized by elevated blood pressure and protein in the urine occurring after the 24th week of pregnancy; it may also cause swelling of the face and hands

Teratogenic – the ability of any substance, agent, or process to interfere with normal prenatal development, causing the formation of one or more developmental abnormalities in the fetus

OVERVIEW

Medical Terminology
Review

preeclampsia
pre- = before
-eclampsia = a serious
complication of pregnancy
involving convulsions
a condition that exists prior
to a more serious condition
of pregnancy

A developing fetus must always be carefully considered when drugs are administered to a pregnant woman. Each drug prescribed for a woman during pregnancy must be evaluated for its utmost effectiveness while weighing this against its potential adverse effects. Practitioners must always consider the dangers these drugs may present to the fetus. There are many conditions that occur secondary to pregnancy, including preeclampsia (high blood pressure, weight gain, and protein in the urine), eclampsia (a seizure disorder that may follow preeclampsia), and gestational diabetes. Sometimes, fetal conditions are treated by administering drugs to the mother, who passes them to the fetus through the placenta. An example of this is digoxin, used to treat fetal congestive heart failure or tachycardia.

PHARMACOKINETICS DURING PREGNANCY

During pregnancy, physiological and anatomical changes occur that can alter drug pharmacokinetics. These changes involve the endocrine, cardio-vascular, circulatory, gastrointestinal, and renal systems.

Absorption

The function of the gastrointestinal tract may be greatly altered by hormonal action during pregnancy. Peristalsis and gastric emptying may be slowed to such a degree as to affect the amount of drug absorbed from the gut. Gastric acid secretion is also more erratic, which can affect the degree of absorption of acidic agents. However, because of individual differences in the effects of pregnancy, the observed effects on absorption can vary greatly and are difficult to predict. Nevertheless, an awareness of the kinds of pharmacokinetic effects that can be expected during pregnancy is valuable, even if these effects do not occur every time.

Distribution

Because of **hemodynamic** changes involving the mechanics of blood circulation, many alterations occur in a pregnant woman's body. The heart rate increases by about 10 to 15 beats per minute. The blood volume increases by 40%. Plasma volume increases by 50% throughout pregnancy. These changes alter drug transportation and distribution. Other factors that determine distribution during pregnancy include plasma protein concentration and **affinity** for the drug, body fluid levels, drug solubility, body fat content, and the blood flow to tissues, all of which can undergo changes. Therefore, distribution of drugs in pregnant women can be altered.

The fetus receives drugs from the mother's circulatory system, which passes them through the placenta. Drugs are affected by pregnancy hormones; this can result in a larger than normal amount of free drugs in circulation, which can easily cross the placental membrane. Fat-soluble drugs, in particular, pass through the placenta's lipid membrane with ease.

Drugs can be distributed in a mother's breast milk, usually in low concentrations. It is important to note that drugs with increased lipid solubility and low protein binding (such as central nervous system agents), may be present in high concentrations in breast milk. Since breast milk contains a high percentage of fats, lipophilic (fat-soluble) drugs pass easily through breast milk. Other drugs that easily diffuse in breast milk include those with lower molecular weights or organic bases.

Drug levels in breast milk are not the same as drug levels in the mother's blood, because of the influence of factors that were discussed earlier. If bioavailability of the drug is poor, high concentrations are usually not achieved in a neonate's circulation. Consequently, less than 2% of the mother's total dose of these drugs is usually ingested by a nursing infant.

Metabolism

Drug metabolism may be altered by liver disease, hepatic blood flow, conditions that affect hepatic enzyme levels, or diet in general, but drug metabolism is not altered by breastfeeding or pregnancy.

Excretion

During pregnancy, increases in renal plasma flow (usually 40% to 50%), glomerular filtration rates, and tubular reabsorption cause changes in renal function. Increased renal plasma flow causes greater capillary pressure and increased glomerular filtration (by approximately 50%). Drug excretion rates are therefore increased during pregnancy.

PHARMACODYNAMICS

The mechanism of action of any drug that is used in pregnant women has important clinical applications. By the 32nd week of pregnancy, a woman's cardiac output has increased by 50%. Her arterial blood pressure increases, beginning in the second trimester. Because of these changes, a drug's pharmacodynamics must be carefully evaluated before administration. Knowledge of therapeutic indexes, dose-response relationships, and drug receptor interactions will help pharmacy technicians provide cautious, safe, and effective treatment during pregnancy.

PREGNANCY DRUG CATEGORIES

Pregnancy drug categories were developed in 1980 by the Food and Drug Administration (FDA) to help classify drugs according to the risks they pose to a developing fetus. See Table 25-1 for a listing of these categories.

TABLE 25-1	Pregnancy Drug Categories
Category	**Explanation**
A	Controlled studies in pregnant women show no risk to the fetus (examples: doxylamine, magnesium sulfate, levothyroxine sodium)
B	Animal studies fail to show fetal risk, but no controlled human studies were conducted; or animal studies show fetal risk that is not confirmed in human studies (examples: nitrofurantoin, low-molecular-weight heparins, metformin)
C	Animal studies show fetal risk, but no controlled human studies were conducted; or there are no animal or human studies—these drugs are given if their benefit justifies their risks (examples: chloramphenicol, fluoroquinolones, trimethoprim)
D	Controlled human studies show fetal risk; the benefit of these drugs may be acceptable, despite risks, in life-threatening situations (examples: aminoglycosides, streptomycin, tetracycline)
X	Controlled human studies show fetal risk that outweighs any possible benefit; these drugs are contraindicated for use in pregnant or potentially pregnant women (examples: warfarin, methotrexate, isotretinoin)

Drug manufacturers are required to state these pregnancy categories in all printed drug reference materials and package inserts. There are many stated concerns about these categories and how accurate they are in describing the dangers of various drugs. Category C, in particular, is being revised because it contains drugs that have undergone no human studies, but animal studies have indicated fetal harm. Animal studies do not always accurately predict human responses to the studied drug. The FDA is working to clarify the categorization of drugs with more focus on their actual fetal risks.

Adverse Effects

There are two major considerations when evaluating the adverse effects of drug therapy in pregnant women:

1. Common side effects of pregnancy

2. Adverse effects that maternal drug therapy can have upon the fetus

Many of the side effects of pregnancy can mask the adverse effects of drug therapy in pregnant patients. These signs and symptoms include:

- Light-headedness or hypotension
- Constipation
- Heartburn
- Nausea and vomiting
- Heart palpitations

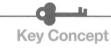

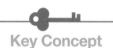

- Fatigue

- Frequent urination

The dose and duration of drug therapy, the type of adverse effects that may occur, and the stage of pregnancy must all be considered in determining drug administration and potential fetal risks. Before a fertilized ovum is implanted in the uterus, certain drugs such as alcohol can produce a hostile environment capable of preventing implantation or causing a spontaneous abortion.

Some drugs that are not normally **teratogenic** (causing developmental malformations) can have effects that impede a neonate's ability to adapt to life outside the uterus (Table 25-2). Benzodiazepines can cause **floppy infant syndrome**, while nonsteroidal anti-inflammatory drugs such as aspirin or indomethacin can cause premature closure of the neonate's ductus arteriosus.

Contraindications and Precautions

Some drugs are contraindicated for use during the first trimester of pregnancy. Caution is advised for others because certain drugs may pass through the placenta to the fetus, causing teratogenic effects. Some others should not

TABLE 25-2	Common Nonteratogenic Drugs with Adverse Fetal Effects
Nonteratogenic Agents	**Adverse Fetal Effects**
acetaminophen (ah-see-tah-MIH-noh-fen)	Renal failure
adrenocortical hormones (ah-dree-noh-KOR-tih-kal HOR-mohns)	Adrenocortical suppression, electrolyte imbalance
amphetamines (am-FEH-tah-meens)	Withdrawal
cocaine (koh-KAYN)	Vascular disruption, withdrawal, intrauterine growth retardation
meperidine (meh-PEH-rih-deen)	Neonatal depression
phenobarbital (if excessively used) (fee-noh-BAR-bih-tahl)	Neonatal bleeding, death
smoking tobacco products (cigarettes, etc.)	Premature births, intrauterine growth retardation
thiazide diuretics (THY-ah-zyd dy-yoo-REH-tiks)	Thrombocytopenia, salt and water depletion, possible neonatal death

be used at all during pregnancy and lactation. As the preceding categories of drugs show, the prescription or administration of medications during pregnancy must be done cautiously.

During the period of **organogenesis** (from implantation to about 60 days thereafter; the time when major fetal organs form), teratogenic drugs may cause serious malformations, or even spontaneous abortion, to occur (Table 25-3). Drug therapy should be delayed until after this time if possible.

TABLE 25-3	Common Teratogenic Drugs
Drug or Drug Class	**Indications**
aminopterin (ah-mih-NOP-teh-rin), busulfan (byoo-SUL-fan), cyclophosphamide (sy-kloh-FOS-fah-myd), methylaminopter (meh-thil-ah-mih-NOP-ter), thalidomide (thah-LIH-doh-myd)	Antineoplastic
androgenic hormones (an-droh-JEE-nik HOR-mohns), diethylstilbestrol (dy-eh-thil-stil-BES-trol)	Hormone replacement
coumarin (KOO-mah-rin)	Anticoagulant
etretinate (eh-TREH-tih-nayt)	Psoriasis
isotretinoin (eye-soh-TREH-tih-noyn)	Recalcitrant cystic acne
lithium (LITH-ee-um)	Antimanic
methimazole (meh-THIH-mah-zohl)	Antithyroid
penicillamine (peh-nih-SIL-lah-meen)	Cystinuria and rheumatoid arthritis
phenytoin (FEH-nih-toh-in), trimethadione (try-meh-THAH-dee-ohn), valproic acid (val-PROH-ik AH-sid)	Anticonvulsant
tetracycline (teh-trah-SY-kleen)	Antibiotic

The embryonic phase is completed at about 60 days, when the fetal phase begins. Effects that may occur during this latter phase include:

- Damage to structures or organs that were normally formed during organogenesis
- Damage to systems currently undergoing tissue development
- Retardation of growth
- Fetal death or stillbirth

Combinations of drug effects may occur, with growth retardation being the most common fetal effect. For example, coumarin derivatives that are used as anticoagulants can produce eye and brain defects as a result of hemorrhagic accidents in the developing fetus.

> ### Key Concept
> The minimum therapeutic dose should be used for as short a time as possible during pregnancy. If possible, drug therapy should be delayed until after the first trimester of pregnancy.

LACTATION DRUG CATEGORIES

The American Academy of Pediatrics published a report in 2001 that identified several categories of drugs that may cause problems during breastfeeding. These categories are listed below:

- Cytotoxic drugs that can interfere with a nursing infant's cellular metabolism
- Abused drugs with reported adverse effects on nursing infants
- Radioactive agents that require the stopping of breastfeeding
- Drugs that have unknown but possibly dangerous effects on nursing infants
- Drugs that have caused harm to some nursing infants and should be given to nursing mothers only with caution
- Maternal medications that are usually compatible with breastfeeding
- Food and environmental agents that affect nursing infants

It is recommended that all drugs of abuse be avoided by lactating women, regardless of documented effects on nursing infants. Women should not breastfeed while they are taking active radioactive agents. Drugs that have unknown neonatal effects include antianxiety drugs, antidepressants, and neuroleptics and must be used with caution. Nursing mothers should be informed that these drugs may be passed to their infant, and can affect the development of the central nervous system with long-term effects. Other drugs that may have adverse effects on neonates include anti-infectives, aspirin, phenobarbital, and sulfasalazine. While most drugs that are administered to nursing mothers are safe for use, with only minimal effects, many drugs are not part of large research studies and realistically need to be further tested in order to ensure safety.

> ### Key Concept
>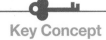
> Drugs may be excreted into breast milk, although the total amount received by the infant is a small percentage of the maternal dose.

COMMON CONDITIONS AFFECTING THE PREGNANT PATIENT

Pregnant patients who have preexisting conditions requiring drug therapy have special needs. Physicians must consider how drug therapy will affect the developing fetus. Also, any adverse effects caused by pregnancy must be identified so that drug therapy may be changed if needed. If the pregnancy causes health changes that require new drug therapy, adverse effects of these new drugs upon the fetus must also be considered.

During pregnancy, special attention should be given to cardiovascular problems that may develop. The cardiovascular system changes and experiences more stress during pregnancy, possibly requiring changes in drug selection or dosage. The use of over-the-counter drugs, which can pose additional risks to the fetus, must also be assessed.

Seizure Disorders

A woman with a seizure disorder who is planning to become pregnant must first discuss her condition with her physician and seriously consider how anticonvulsant drug therapy might affect her fetus. Physicians, in turn, must carefully assess how pregnant women with seizure disorders should be treated to avoid possible teratogenic effects to the fetus. It is believed by many experts that seizures in a pregnant woman can cause fetal hypoxia, which leads to central nervous system damage. But anticonvulsant drug therapy may also adversely affect a developing fetus. The anticonvulsants trimethadione and valproic acid should be avoided in pregnant women. However, only drugs of pregnancy category X are strictly contraindicated. The decision whether to maintain therapy with category D or even category C drugs must be made based on the ratio of risks to benefits.

Depression

Though little accurate information exists, the use of antidepressants by pregnant women must be carefully controlled. Drugs such as selective serotonin reuptake inhibitors (SSRIs) do not appear to cause increased risk for fetal complications. However, high doses of fluoxetine (Prozac®) have been shown to cause low birth weight.

Diabetes

According to the FDA, approximately 9% of all women in the United States have diabetes mellitus and about one-third of these women do not know they have the disorder. Furthermore, gestational diabetes may develop in 2% to 5% of all pregnancies. During pregnancy, production of hormones increases; thus, insulin demands also increase. This can cause insulin resistance in the pregnant patient. Insulin therapy may be required to prevent hyperglycemia, which can cause congenital anomalies that can harm the fetus. Insulin is preferred over oral hypoglycemic drugs during pregnancy because it does not cross the placenta. After the baby is delivered, insulin therapy is usually no longer required for women who have developed gestational diabetes, because their blood glucose levels return to normal.

Women with diabetes or who acquire diabetes during their pregnancies are at risk for having babies with higher birth weights, leading to an increased incidence of cesarean deliveries. These women are also at an increased risk of developing toxemia.

Hyperemesis During Pregnancy

Hyperemesis gravidarum (pernicious vomiting during pregnancy) may require antiemetic drug therapy. This currently consists of piperazines and phenothiazines. Of these classes of antiemetic drugs, piperazines are not known to be teratogenic, while the phenothiazines are generally considered safe in low, infrequent doses.

Preeclampsia

Preeclampsia is a hypertensive condition developing usually after the 24th gestational week. It is characterized by hypertension, cerebral edema, and proteinuria. Preeclampsia may lead to eclampsia, and the primary goal of preeclampsia treatment is to prevent this condition from developing. Treatment is aimed at decreasing central nervous system irritability and reducing maternal blood pressure. The drugs of choice for preeclampsia are magnesium sulfate (to prevent convulsions) and hydralazine (to treat hypertension). Other medications used in the treatment of hypertension in preeclampsia include diazoxide, nifedipine, and labetalol (see Chapter 13).

Eclampsia

Eclampsia is a more serious condition in which the blood pressure is higher, and kidney dysfunction is indicated by proteinuria, weight gain, and generalized edema (of the face, hands, feet, and legs). In some patients, the blood pressure becomes extremely high, and generalized seizures (grand mal) or coma develops. Immediate hospitalization is required for adequate treatment of eclampsia.

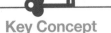

Key Concept

When using antiemetics, especially during the first trimester, the risk for adverse fetal effects must be considered.

SUMMARY

Drug therapy may be required to manage preexisting or newly developed conditions in pregnant or lactating women. However, drug therapy can adversely affect the fetus or infant. Since physiological changes related to pregnancy can alter drug absorption, distribution, and elimination, potential risks must always be considered before administering any drug. Also, potential fetal risks must be compared with maternal benefits when drug therapy is needed. Drugs may be excreted into breast milk in varying amounts. Limiting drug use during pregnancy and lactation decreases adverse effects to both the mother and infant.

EXPLORING THE WEB

Visit **www.aafp.org**

- Search for and read the article "Medications in the Breast-Feeding Mother."

Visit the following websites and search for "pregnancy"; read additional articles relevant to the discussion presented in this chapter.

- **http://drugtopics.modernmedicine.com**
- **http://emedicine.medscape.com**
- **www.fda.gov**
- **www.perinatology.com**
- **www.uspharmacist.com**

REVIEW QUESTIONS

Multiple Choice

1. Which of the following is a result of pharmacokinetics of orally administered drugs that may be altered by progesterone during pregnancy?

   A. increased opening of the center of the iris of each eye

   B. decreased volume of the respiratory system to absorb more inhaled medications

   C. decreased gastric tone and motility

   D. increased time required for the urinary bladder to empty

2. Which of the following is a true statement?

   A. drug levels in breast milk are more than the drug levels in the mother's blood.

   B. drug levels in breast milk are not the same as the drug levels in the mother's blood.

   C. drugs with increased lipid solubility and low protein binding may be present in low concentrations in breast milk.

   D. fat-soluble drugs are not able to pass easily through breast milk.

3. By the eighth month of pregnancy, a woman's cardiac output has:

   A. increased by 50%

   B. increased by 80%

   C. decreased by 50%

   D. decreased by 80%

4. Which of the following pregnancy drug categories is absolutely contraindicated for use in pregnant women?

   A. category B

   B. category C

   C. category D

   D. category X

5. Women should not breastfeed while they are taking:

   A. tetracycline

   B. aspirin

   C. acetaminophen

   D. radioactive agents

6. Which of the following drugs is nonteratogenic and may be used during pregnancy?

   A. cocaine

   B. magnesium sulfate

   C. meperidine

   D. thiazide diuretics

7. Methimazole is a teratogenic drug that is indicated for:

   A. congestive heart failure

   B. hypertension

   C. thyroid conditions

   D. diabetes mellitus

8. Which of the following conditions during pregnancy may be accompanied by convulsions?

   A. depression

   B. diabetes

   C. preeclampsia

   D. eclampsia

9. Seizures in pregnant women can cause fetal:

   A. hypertension

   B. hypoxia

   C. pernicious vomiting

   D. all of the above

10. Administration of high doses of fluoxetine (Prozac®) during pregnancy may cause which of the following effects in newborns?

    A. low birth weight

    B. high birth weight

    C. low blood glucose

    D. high blood glucose

11. Which of the following drugs may be required to prevent hyperglycemia during pregnancy?

    A. oral hypoglycemics

    B. insulin

    C. vitamin B_6

    D. none of the above

12. Which of the following medications may be used for pernicious vomiting during pregnancy?

    A. vitamin C

    B. vitamin B_{12}

    C. piperazine

    D. minocycline

13. Drug excretion rates during pregnancy are:

    A. increased

    B. decreased

    C. not changed

    D. changed only in depressed women

14. Which of the following classes of drugs are safer during pregnancy in women with severe depression?

    A. monoamine oxidase inhibitors

    B. tricyclic antidepressants

    C. selective serotonin reuptake inhibitors

    D. A and B

15. Which of the following is an adverse fetal effect of acetaminophen during pregnancy?

    A. renal failure

    B. heart failure

    C. liver failure

    D. low birth weight

Critical Thinking

A 37-year-old woman had a root canal procedure at her local dentist's office. The dentist ordered ibuprofen to be taken every four hours for pain. The woman had another painkiller at home, so she did not get her dentist's prescription filled. Every four hours, she took this painkiller, which was Tylenol No. 3®. Unknowingly, she continued to breastfeed her 4-month-old baby while taking the drug. After several sessions of breastfeeding, the baby went into a deep sleep, from which it could not be awakened. The baby was rushed to the emergency department, where it died.

1. What was the likely cause of the baby's death?

2. What drugs are combined in Tylenol No. 3®?

3. If this woman had filled her dentist's prescription and used it as instructed, would there have been any danger to her baby?

Drug Therapy for Pediatric Patients

OBJECTIVES

After completing this chapter, the reader should be able to:

1. Understand the factors affecting pharmacokinetics and pharmacodynamics in children.

2. Recognize common childhood respiratory diseases.

3. Identify treatment of asthma in children.

4. Describe otitis media in children.

5. Describe diabetes mellitus in pediatrics.

6. Identify cardiovascular and blood disorders.

7. Describe factors that place infants at risk for iron deficiency anemia.

8. Define sickle cell anemia.

9. List five common examples of infectious diseases in pediatrics.

10. Explain acute bacterial meningitis.

GLOSSARY

Apnea – the cessation of respiration for more than 20 seconds with or without cyanosis, hypotonia, or bradycardia

Bacteremia – a condition in which bacteria are recovered from blood cultures of a patient and may or may not be associated with the disease

Croup – a viral infection that affects the larynx and the trachea

Epiglottitis – an acute bacterial infection of the epiglottis (an appendage that closes the glottis while food or drink is passing through the pharynx) and the surrounding areas, causing airway obstruction

Eustachian tubes – tubes within the ear by which fluids drain

Gestational age – the time from the first day of the mother's last menstrual cycle to the current date of the pregnancy

Insulin-dependent diabetes mellitus (IDDM) – a disorder caused by failure of the pancreas to secrete sufficient insulin

Iron deficiency anemia – anemia characterized by low serum iron, increased serum iron-binding capacity, decreased serum ferritin, and decreased marrow iron stores

Kernicterus – yellow staining and degenerative lesions in basal ganglia associated with high levels of unconjugated bilirubin in infants; also known as *bilirubin encephalopathy*

Neonatal period – the time from birth to approximately 28 days of age

Otitis media – an inflammation of the middle ear

Patent ductus arteriosus – a condition in which the normal channel between the pulmonary artery and the aorta fails to close at birth

Pediatric period – the period from birth to approximately age 18 years

Pneumonia – an inflammation or infection of the pulmonary parenchyma; caused by viruses, bacteria, mycoplasma, and aspiration of foreign substances

Pneumonitis – inflammation of the lungs

Respiratory distress syndrome (RDS) – a condition that results from absence, deficiency, or alteration of the components of pulmonary surfactant

Respiratory syncytial virus (RSV) – the major cause of bronchiolitis and pneumonia in infants younger than one year of age; caused by a virus and produces mild cold-like symptoms

Septicemia – bacteremia associated with active disease, whether localized or systemic

Sickle cell anemia – an inherited disorder characterized by the presence of crescent-shaped red blood cells containing abnormal hemoglobin, termed hemoglobin S (HbS)

OVERVIEW

Pediatric drug therapy is a special consideration in medicine. It is problematic even for practitioners with extensive experience. To put it simply, a child's age, weight, and developmental status, combined with incomplete clinical information about how specific agents affect pediatric patients, can complicate drug therapy. Although a drug undergoes the same processes in a child as it does in an adult, a child's body is distinctive and constantly changing, which affects how it responds to the drug.

Drug administration, usage, and research in pediatric patients continue to pose challenges. Children are not merely miniature adults, and knowledge about pediatric medications cannot simply be extrapolated from the adult research, literature, and clinical trials. As a general rule, if a label does not contain a pediatric dosage, it should not be assumed that the drug is safe for anyone younger than 12 years of age. In these cases, the pharmacy technician should be sure that a drug is safe for children by asking the doctor or pharmacist. Effective and safe drug therapy in newborns, infants, and children requires an understanding of maturational changes that affect drug action, metabolism, and disposition. Pediatric drug dosages must be adjusted for the characteristics of individual drugs, and for the patient's age, disease states, sex, and individual needs, to prevent ineffective treatment or toxicity.

DEFINING THE NEONATAL AND PEDIATRIC POPULATION

The **neonatal period** generally covers the time from birth to approximately 28 days of age. This general category also includes premature infants of varying gestational ages. **Gestational age** (the time from the first day of the mother's last menstrual cycle to the current date of the pregnancy) will factor in dosing for various medications and may even preclude the use of some. The **pediatric period** covers a wide range of ages, from birth to approximately age 18 years (Table 26-1).

TABLE 26-1	Stages of Childhood Growth and Development
Age	**Description**
Newborn	Birth to one month
Infancy	One month to one year
Toddlerhood	One to three years
Preschool age	Three to six years
School age	Six to 12 years
Adolescence	12 to 18 years

UNIQUE CHARACTERISTICS IN PEDIATRIC MEDICATION ADMINISTRATION

Key Concept

Children younger than two years of age should not be given any over-the-counter OTC drug without a physician's approval. Children will respond differently to some drugs than adults. For example, certain barbiturates that make adults feel sluggish will make a child hyperactive. Conversely, amphetamines, which stimulate adults, can calm children.

Key Concept

Body surface area (BSA) is the measured or calculated surface area of a human body. It is a better indicator of metabolic mass than body weight because it is less affected by abnormal amounts of adipose tissue. Body surface area varies, based on age. Newborns have an average BSA of 0.25 square meters (m²); a 9-year-old child has a BSA of 1.07 m²; a 12-year-old child has a BSA of 1.33 m²; and an average adult has a BSA of 1.73 m².

A child's body surface area, metabolism, development, and tolerance are quite different from those of an adult. Childhood rates of absorption, distribution, and excretion are also different, since their development is ongoing. For many drugs, safe and effective use in children requires additional pharmacokinetic and pharmacodynamic data. According to the American Academy of Pediatrics, 20% of all medications marketed today do not have U.S. Food and Drug Administration (FDA) approved labeling for use in neonates, infants, children, and adolescents, and only 5 of the 80 drugs most often used in newborns and infants are labeled for pediatric use. The FDA has recently made regulatory changes to facilitate labeling of drugs for pediatric use.

To complicate matters further, most drugs are not tested on children. In many instances, no one knows for sure if a given drug is safe or effective in children, or what dosage is appropriate. Only about 30% of FDA-approved drugs have been approved for specific pediatric indications, and few approved drugs come in child-appropriate dosage forms, which means that health care professionals must formulate pediatric doses.

It is essential that pharmacy technicians be familiar with most common diseases and conditions of neonatal and young children, the principles of pharmacology, and the required drug therapy. The technician should also consider the four processes involved in pharmacokinetics: absorption, distribution, metabolism, and excretion.

Pharmacokinetics

Pharmacokinetics focuses on how drugs move throughout the body. This includes the processes of absorption, distribution, biotransformation, and excretion. Pharmacokinetics deals with how drugs enter the body, reach their site of action (in what concentration), and how the body eliminates them. The body's effects on drugs, or how the body handles drugs, can be described as pharmacokinetics.

Neonates, infants, and children have different pharmacokinetic processes than adults. It is important to understand the developmental differences of children in order to understand how drugs are concentrated at the site of action, how intense their effects will be, and how long their action will last.

Absorption

Absorption involves the movement of drugs from their site of administration into the bloodstream. Two factors that influence oral drug absorption are gastric emptying time and pH. In neonates and infants, gastric emptying time is slower than in adults, reaching adult values at around six months of age. Delayed gastric emptying delays drug absorption of drugs designed to be absorbed from the intestine. More complete absorption may occur for drugs that are absorbed mostly from the stomach.

In newborns, gastric pH is more alkaline that in later childhood, becoming more acidic at around two to three years of age. Acidic drugs are better absorbed from an acidic environment while basic (alkaline) drugs are better absorbed from an alkaline environment. Thus, during infancy, basic drugs are more easily absorbed from the stomach, while acidic drugs are less well absorbed. This difference in comparison to older children and adults is important when treating infants and young children.

Topical medications are absorbed more rapidly by infants and children. On reason for this is because they have a greater ratio of body surface area (BSA) to weight. Also, their skin is thinner, and thus more permeable.

Distribution

The movement or transport of drugs throughout the body is known as distribution. In this process, drugs are made available to body tissues and fluids. Body composition, fluid distribution, blood flow to the tissues, special membrane barriers, and protein binding all influence drug distribution in the body.

Neonates, infants, and young children have more body water than adults. Premature neonates have 85% body water, neonates have 70% to 75%, and adults have 50% to 60%. The percentage of body fat differs, too, based on age and gender, as well as individual variation. A neonate's body is composed of 15% to 16% fat; however, premature infants may have as little as 1% fat. Body fat percentage peaks at about nine months of age, decreasing (between one and five years) to between 8% and 12%, and increasing again around adolescence. Girls have a higher percentage of body fat than boys.

Lipid-soluble drugs can be stored in body fat, and have a high affinity for adipose (fat) tissue. As a result, lower levels of drug may remain in circulation, decreasing availability at the site of action. Children and adolescents with higher percentages of body fat need a higher milligram-per-kilogram dose of lipid-soluble drugs than do those who have a lower percentage of body fat.

Children younger than two years of age have an immature blood-brain barrier that allows relatively easy access to the central nervous system (CNS). Therefore, they are more sensitive to drugs that affect the brain, with increased risk of CNS toxicity. To protect young children from undesired drug effects, lower doses of certain drugs may be required.

Metabolism

Metabolism (biotransformation) involves the alteration or transformation of chemicals from their original form, aiding in the eventual excretion of the substance by the renal system. Most biotransformation of drugs

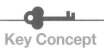

Key Concept

Sulfonamide antimicrobials compete with serum bilirubin for binding to albumin. Drugs given to a neonate with jaundice can displace bilirubin from albumin. Because of the greater permeability of the neonatal blood-brain barrier, substantial amounts of bilirubin may enter the brain and cause **kernicterus** (yellow staining and degenerative lesions in basal ganglia associated with high levels of unconjugated bilirubin in infants; also known as bilirubin encephalopathy).

happens in the liver. In infants and neonates, liver immaturity influences drug-metabolizing capacity. Hepatic enzyme activity does not mature until one to two years of age. Thus, during infancy drugs metabolized by the liver have a longer half-life (the time needed for 50% of the administered dose to be eliminated) and there is more chance for toxicity. As a result, reduction of some drug dosages and less frequent drug administration may be required for this age group.

Young children have higher metabolic rates and metabolize drugs more rapidly than other age groups. Between two and six years of age, this physiological state is more pronounced. Consequently, higher doses or more frequent administration of medications is required for this age group, and this need can persist until 10 to 12 years of age.

Excretion

The process of removing drugs, active metabolites, and inactive metabolites from the body is known as excretion. Most drugs are excreted by the kidneys. Renal function increases rapidly during infancy, reaching adult levels by 6 to 12 months of age. During infancy, reduced renal excretion results in longer drug half-lives and the increased possibility of toxicity for drugs that are primarily excreted through the renal system. Especially during the neonatal period, reduced dosages are required. By three years of age, drugs are eliminated more rapidly because the glomerular filtration rate surpasses the adult rate. Consequently, in toddlers, a drug's half-life may be shorter than in older children and adults.

Pharmacodynamics

How drugs affect the body and the way in which they accomplish is referred to as pharmacodynamics. This process involves the biochemical and physical effects of drugs (drug effects and the responses resulting from drug action) and the mechanisms of drug action. Most drugs are believed to act at the cellular level. They do this by attaching to cellular receptors, where they block or mimic the action of endogenous molecules that regulate cell action.

A drug's mechanism of action is the same in all individuals. However, drug effects may differ in infants and children because of immaturity of target organs and the sensitivity of receptors. As a result, an infant or child may need either a lower or higher dose of a drug than might be expected in an adult, and usually has a heightened sensitivity to drugs.

> **Key Concept**
>
> The kidneys of infants younger than six months of age are not well developed. These infants should not be given water to drink because it will remove sodium ions and cause an increase in potassium ions in their blood. Breast milk and formula supply all of their needed fluids.

FEVER

Fever is a common reason why parents seek medical attention for their children, and approximately 30% of visits to pediatricians are fever related. Parents often think of fever as a disease rather than a symptom. In fact, fever is part of the febrile response, which includes the activation of numerous physiological, endocrinological, and immunological responses. Microbes, toxins, or products of microbial origin, antigen-antibody complexes, complement (a group of proteins in the blood that assist the function of antibodies in the immune system), and other chemical agents are pyrogens that cause fever.

This evidence indicates that fever is an important defense mechanism and that treating the fever may have detrimental effects. For example, in children infected with varicella virus (chickenpox), acetaminophen prolongs the time of crusting of skin lesions. Nevertheless, many clinicians and caregivers believe that fever is harmful. A small percentage of children younger than five years of age may develop a seizure when they have a fever.

Acetaminophen is one of the most widely used antipyretics. Like aspirin and other nonsteroidal anti-inflammatory drugs, acetaminophen blocks the conversion of arachidonic acid to prostaglandin (see Chapter 22). Current evidence continues to suggest that acetaminophen is the drug of choice for antipyresis in children.

Ibuprofen (Motrin®) is another option as an antipyretic. It was shown to provide a greater temperature reduction in febrile children and a longer duration of antipyresis than occurred with acetaminophen when these drugs were administered in equal doses (10 mg/kg). Physical methods to reduce temperature are ineffective if shivering is not prevented, and such methods do not alter the hypothalamic set point.

CHILDHOOD RESPIRATORY DISEASES

The patterns of respiratory tract diseases in childhood are modified by age, sex, race, season, geography, and environmental and socioeconomic conditions. Immediately after birth, tuberculosis can be transmitted to the newborn, presenting after several weeks of life as a severe **pneumonitis**. Lung immaturity and other events related to the perinatal period predispose to hyaline membrane disease. The incidence of respiratory tract infections also peaks during the first two to three years of school. Respiratory diseases affect many children each year. Respiratory syncytial virus (RSV) and asthma are two specific problems quite often treated in the pediatric/neonatal patient population. Apnea is seen in the neonatal age group, especially in premature infants.

Apnea

Apnea is the cessation of respiration for more than 20 seconds with or without cyanosis, hypotonia, or bradycardia. Apnea may be a symptom of another disorder that resolves upon treatment of the disorder. Examples include infection, gastroesophageal reflux, hypoglycemia, metabolic disorders, drug

Medical Terminology
Review

pneumonitis
pneumo(n)- = breathing; the lungs
-itis = inflammation; condition
inflammation of the lungs impairing breathing

toxicity, hydrocephalus, or thermal instability in newborns. Immaturity of the CNS often accounts for apnea of the newborn, which occurs most commonly during active sleep and in premature infants.

Treatment for Apnea

The treatment of central apnea that is most commonly used for premature infants includes minimizing potential causes such as temperature variances and feeding intolerance. The use of xanthine medications such as caffeine and theophylline (see Chapter 16) provide CNS stimulation. Pulmonary function support may include the use of supplemental oxygen and continuous positive airway pressure at low pressures. Apnea monitors are used in many situations.

Sudden Infant Death Syndrome (SIDS)

Sudden infant death syndrome is the leading cause of death in infants between one month and one year of age. Approximately 2500 infants die from SIDS every year in the United States. Although the mechanism underlying SIDS was initially believed to be linked to apnea, recent studies have refuted this. By definition, SIDS is the sudden, unexplained death of an infant. It occurs without warning in babies who are otherwise healthy, usually during sleep. Most deaths occur between the ages of two and four months, with increased incidence in cold weather. Native American infants are three times as likely to die from SIDS as Caucasian infants, and African-American infants are twice as likely. There is also a distinct gender difference; more male infants die from SIDS than female infants.

Treatment for Sudden Infant Death Syndrome

Although SIDS remains poorly understood and clearcut treatment measures are lacking, the risk of its occurrence can be greatly reduced by placing infants on their backs to sleep. Additional risk factors include smoking, drinking, or drug use during pregnancy; prematurity or low birth weight; mothers younger than age 20; poor prenatal care; tobacco smoke exposure after birth; and overheating due to excessive sleepwear or bedding.

Respiratory Syncytial Virus (RSV)

Respiratory syncytial virus (RSV) is the major cause of bronchiolitis and pneumonia in infants younger than one year. It is the most important respiratory tract pathogen of early childhood. It causes mild cold-like symptoms in infants and most children. However, RSV can cause a more serious respiratory disease in premature infants that sometimes requires hospitalization. The at-risk group includes infants born before 36 weeks of gestation or those with chronic lung disease. The respiratory disease occurs because of the immaturity of the infants' lungs and because these infants have not received sufficient antiviral substances from their mothers. In most parts of the

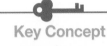

Key Concept

As a preventive measure against SIDS, infants should never be placed face down on their stomachs to sleep.

United States, RSV infection occurs seasonally, generally from fall through spring (October through March). At-risk infants are now treated before discharge from the hospital to provide some immunoprophylaxis.

Treatment for Respiratory Syncytial Virus

Palivizumab (Synagis®) is used for immunoprophylaxis against severe lower respiratory tract RSV infections. In infants with uncomplicated bronchiolitis, treatment is symptomatic. Humidified oxygen is usually indicated for hospitalized infants because most have hypoxia. Fluids should be carefully administered. Often, intravenous or tube feeding is helpful when sucking is difficult. Bronchodilators should not be routinely used. However, a course of epinephrine should be used in children with wheezing who are older than one year, and bronchodilators should be administered if found to be beneficial. The use of corticosteroids is not indicated except as a last resort in patients whose condition is critical. Sedatives are rarely necessary. The antiviral drug ribavirin, delivered by small-particle aerosol and breathed along with the required concentration of oxygen for 20 to 24 hours per day for three to five days, has a beneficial effect on the course of pneumonia caused by RSV.

Asthma

Asthma is a leading cause of chronic illness in childhood, and is responsible for a significant proportion of school days missed because of chronic illness. As discussed in Chapter 16, asthma is a chronic, reversible obstruction of the bronchial airways. The airways become overreactive because of this inflammation and increased mucous secretion; mucosal swelling and muscle contraction then occur. This leads to airway obstruction, chest tightness, coughing, wheezing, and, if asthma is severe, shortness of breath and low blood oxygen levels. Most children experience their first symptoms by four to five years of age. Allergies, viral respiratory infections, and airborne irritants produce the inflammation that can lead to asthma. Childhood asthma is a disease with a strong allergic component and a genetic predisposition. Approximately 75% to 80% of children with asthma have allergies.

Treatment for Asthma

Treatment for asthma generally involves two types of medications: quick-relief medications (also called bronchodilators), and controller medications. Controller medications get their name because they help control inflammation to make breathing easier. These medications must be taken daily to be effective. Medications in the bronchodilators and controller group are listed in Table 26-2.

Respiratory Distress Syndrome

Respiratory distress syndrome (RDS), or hyaline membrane disease, is the result of the absence, deficiency, or alteration of the components of

TABLE 26-2	Bronchodilators and Controller Groups for Asthma	
Generic Name	Trade Name	Route of Administration
Bronchodilators		
albuterol (al-BYOO-teh-rol)	Proventil®, Ventolin®	PO
epinephrine (eh-pih-NEH-frin)	Adrenalin®	SC, IM, IV, Nasal spray
isoproterenol hydrochloride (eye-soh-proh-TEH-reh-nol hy-droh-KLOR-ryd)	Isuprel®	IV
metaproterenol sulfate (meh-tah-proh-TEH-reh-nol SUL-fayt)	Alupent®, Metaprel®	PO, Inhalation
pirbuterol acetate (pir-BYOO-teh-rol AH-seh-tayt)	Maxair®	Inhalation
salmeterol xinafoate (sal-MEH-teh-rol zih-NAH-foh-ayt)	Serevent Diskus®	Inhalation
terbutaline sulfate (ter-BYOO-tah-leen SUL-fayt)	Terbutaline Sulfate Tablets®, Terbutaline Sulfate Injection®	PO, SC
Xanthine Derivatives		
aminophylline (ah-mih-NAW-fil-leen)	Truphylline®	PO, IV
theophylline (thee-AW-fil-leen)	Elixophyllin®	PO, IV
Leukotriene Inhibitors		
montelukast (mon-TEL-yoo-kast)	Singulair®	PO
zafirlukast (zah-FIRL-yoo-kast)	Accolate®	PO
Corticosteroids		
beclomethasone sodium phosphate (bek-loh-MEH-thah-zone SOH-dee-um)	Beconase AQ®	Intranasal
budesonide nasal (byoo-DEH-soh-nyd NAY-zal)	Rhinocort Aqua®	Intranasal
dexamethasone (dek-sah-MEH-thah-zohn)	Decadron®	PO, IM, IV

Table 26-2 continued

fluticasone propionate (floo-TIH-kah-zohn)	Flovent®, Flonase®	Oral inhalation (Flovent®), Nasal spray (Flonase®)
hydrocortisone sodium (hy-droh-KOR-tih-zohn SOH-dee-um)	Solu-Cortef®	PO
prednisolone (pred-NIH-zoh-lohn)	Prelone®	PO
Mast Cell Stabilizers		
cromolyn sodium (KROH-moh-lin SOH-dee-um)	Intal®	Oral inhalation
nedocromil sodium (neh-DOH-kroh-mil SOH-dee-um)	Tilade®	Oral inhalation

Medical Terminology
Review

lipoprotein
lipo = fats; triglycerides
protein = amino acid complex
amino acid complex with fatty substance

pulmonary surfactant. Surfactant, a lipoprotein complex, is an ingredient of the film-like surface of each alveolus that prevents alveolar collapse. When the amount of surfactant is inadequate, alveolar collapse and hypoxia result. The younger an infant is, the greater is the incidence of RDS. However, the occurrence of RDS appears to be more dependent on lung maturity than on actual gestational age. The severity of RDS is decreased in infants whose mothers received corticosteroids 24 to 48 hours before delivery.

Corticosteroids are most effective when the fetus is less than 34 weeks' gestational age, and they are administered to the mother for at least 24 hours, but no longer than seven days before delivery.

Treatment for Respiratory Distress Syndrome

Infants at risk for RDS, as well as infants with respiratory failure due to meconium aspiration syndrome, persistent pulmonary hypertension, or pneumonia, are treated with natural, animal-derived, or synthetic surfactant. Continuous positive airway pressure using nasal prongs is required to prevent volume loss during expiration, or mechanical ventilation using an endotracheal tube for severe hypoxemia or hypercapnia. Aerosol administration of bronchodilators is also prescribed.

Croup

Croup, or acute laryngo-tracheobronchitis, is a viral infection that affects the larynx and the trachea, resulting in subglottic edema and upper respiratory tract obstruction accompanied by thick secretions. Children are susceptible to airway obstruction because the diameter of the subglottic area at this stage is narrow. Croup can be caused by any virus associated with upper respiratory tract infection. Spasmodic croup is a sudden attack of croup, which usually occurs during the night and can be associated with an upper respiratory tract infection, fever, or allergies. The incidence of croup is higher in the late fall and early winter. Children between six months and six years of age are usually affected. The peak age of onset is two years.

Treatment for Croup

When a child with suspected croup is seen at the hospital, supplemental humidified oxygen is given as indicated by the child's appearance, results of pulse oximetry, and vital signs. The child can be treated with bronchodilators, usually administered with epinephrine if humidification alone is ineffective. The use of corticosteroids is controversial. Children who receive corticosteroids need endotracheal intubation less often, and their stridor is more quickly resolved. Antibiotics are administered if secondary bacterial infection is suspected.

Epiglottitis

Epiglottitis is an acute bacterial infection of the epiglottis (an appendage that closes the glottis while food or drink is passing through the pharynx) and the surrounding areas, causing airway obstruction. The infection is caused by *Haemophilus influenzae* type b or, on rare occasions, streptococci and pneumococci. The use of *H. influenzae* type b (Hib) vaccine in infants has resulted in a dramatic reduction in the incidence of epiglottitis. Onset is sudden and infection progresses rapidly, causing acute respiratory difficulty. This condition requires emergency airway stabilization and medical measures because a fatal outcome can occur. Boys between the ages of two and seven years are most often affected. The incidence of epiglottitis is highest in the winter.

> **Medical Terminology Review**
>
> **epiglottitis**
> epi = above
> glott = the tongue
> itis = inflammation; condition
> inflammation of the tissue above the tongue in the airway

Treatment for Epiglottitis

Visual examination of the throat is contraindicated until a tracheostomy is performed. The child is observed in the intensive care area until swelling of the epiglottis decreases (usually by the third day). Antibiotics are given for a total of 7 to 10 days.

Pneumonia

Pneumonia is an inflammation or infection of the pulmonary parenchyma. Pneumonia is caused by viruses, bacteria, mycoplasma organisms, and aspiration of foreign substances. Viral pneumonia occurs more often than bacterial pneumonia.

Treatment for Pneumonia

Medical treatment is primarily supportive and includes oxygen and respiratory treatments to improve oxygenation. Antibiotics are used to treat bacterial pneumonia based on culture and sensitivity testing. Hospitalization depends on the severity of illness, the child's age, and the suspected organism.

COMMON CHILDHOOD ILLNESSES

It is beyond the scope of this text to discuss the full range of pediatric disorders and illnesses, or their varied treatments. However, selected examples of the most common childhood illnesses will be discussed to highlight drug-related therapies that pharmacy technicians should understand.

Otitis Media

Otitis media is an inflammation of the middle ear. Children six years of age and younger are at particular risk for otitis media because their **eustachian tubes** are shorter and more horizontal than those in adults. Otitis media is the most commonly encountered diagnosis in office visits for children younger than 15 years of age in the United States. It occurs most often in children between three months and three years of age, with peak incidences occurring between 5 to 24 months and 4 to 6 years. Boys have more ear infections than girls. Rupture of the tympanic membrane (eardrum) with discharge and short-term conductive hearing loss are common complications of otitis media.

Treatment for Otitis Media

The efficacy of steroid therapy, decongestants, and antihistamines for the resolution of otitis media has not been proven, and their use should not be encouraged. Surgical removal of tonsils or adenoids is not recommended for the treatment of otitis media with effusion in the absence of specific pathological conditions of the tonsils or adenoids. The first-line antibiotic medication most often prescribed is amoxicillin or ampicillin. The second-line medication regimen (to be used when an amoxicillin-resistant organism is suspected) includes amoxicillin with clavulanate, cefaclor, cotrimoxazole, erythromycin, or sulfisoxazole. In the penicillin-allergic child, erythromycin with a sulfonamide or trimethoprim-sulfamethoxazole may be used. Generic names, trades names, and routes of administration of these agents were discussed in Chapter 23. Myringotomy is the surgical procedure of inserting pressure-equalizing tubes into the tympanic membrane. This allows ventilation of the middle ear, relieves the negative pressure, and permits drainage of fluid. The tubes usually fall out after 6 to 12 months.

Diabetes Mellitus

Insulin-dependent diabetes mellitus (IDDM), or type 1 (juvenile-onset) diabetes, occurs when the pancreas fails to secrete sufficient insulin in response to increases in blood glucose. Insulin is necessary for many physiological functions of the body. Insulin deficiency results in unrestricted glucose production without appropriate use, leading to hyperglycemia and increased production of ketones in the blood. Age ranges of peak incidence are five to seven years and puberty. Among children 5 to 10 years of age, the disease is more commonly diagnosed in girls. Type 1 diabetes usually starts with polyphagia, weight loss, polydipsia, and polyuria. Long-term effects of IDDM include failure to grow at a normal rate, neuropathy (the impairment of sensory and motor nerve functions), recurrent infection, renal microvascular disease, and ischemic heart disease.

Treatment for Insulin-Dependent Diabetes Mellitus (IDDM)

As soon as hyperglycemia or glucosuria is detected, immediate medical attention is needed because of the potential for rapid deterioration of the child's condition. The initial therapy will depend on how early the diagnosis is made, and on the state of the child. Medical management includes the regulation of serum glucose, fluid, and electrolyte levels. Once glucose levels are stabilized, the child's insulin dose is typically dictated by a sliding scale based on the serum glucose level. Regulation of nutrition and exercise is also a key factor in managing diabetes. For older children, or children who are in the midst of the adolescent growth spurt, a regimen of twice-daily injections of a mixture of preferably NPH and regular insulin before breakfast and before supper may be started immediately. Table 26-3 shows types and action of insulins (see also Chapter 18).

Treatment of Hyperglycemia in Infants

Symptomatic hyperglycemia can occur in newborn infants. These babies usually suffer from severe intrauterine malnutrition and, therefore, are small for their gestational age. They are hypoinsulinemic and their pancreas fails to release insulin in response to any of the standard body demands. They must be treated with divided doses of exogenous insulin of up to 1–2 units/kg/24 h. Insulin requirements are best established by starting a continuous intravenous insulin infusion at rates that provide at least 0.5 units/kg/24 h. Insulin treatment is simplified by using diluted insulin so that inadvertent overdoses do not occur. In most cases, pancreas function develops sometime between the age of 6 and 12 weeks. The children do well after the newborn period and do not appear to be at increased risk of developing type 1 diabetes at a later age, though it is possible. See Chapter 18 for more information on the endocrine system, hormones, and related subjects.

Seizure Disorders

A seizure is a sudden, transient alteration in brain function as a result of abnormal neuronal activity and excessive cerebral electric discharge. The causes of seizure are varied and include perinatal factors, infectious disease (encephalitis and meningitis), febrile illness, metabolic disorders, trauma,

TABLE 26-3	Types and Action of Insulin		
		Action	
Type and Onset of Action		Peak	Duration
Fast			
Insulin (regular) (Novolin®; Humulin R®)	30–60 minutes; 15 minutes	2–4 hours	6–8 hours
Prompt insulin zinc suspension (Semilente®)	60–90 minutes	2–8 hours	12–16 hours
Intermediate			
Isophane insulin (NPH) (Novolin N®; Humulin N®)	2 hours	8–12 hours	18–24 hours
Insulin zinc suspension (lente) (Humulin L®; Novolin L)	60–150 minutes	8–12 hours	18–24 hours
Slow			
Extended insulin zinc suspension (Ultralente®; Humulin U®)	4–8 hours	16–18 hours	36 hours
Protamine zinc insulin suspension (PZI®)	4–8 hours	16–20 hours	36 hours

neoplasms, toxins, circulatory disturbances, and degenerative diseases of the nervous system. Epilepsy is a disorder characterized by recurrent, unprovoked seizures, in which seizures are of primary cerebral origin, indicating underlying brain dysfunction. Epilepsy is not a disease in itself.

Treatment for Epilepsy

Antiepileptic drug therapy is the mainstay of medical management. Single-drug therapy is the most desirable, with the goal of establishing a balance between seizure control and adverse side effects. The drug of choice is based on seizure type, epileptic syndrome, and patient variables. Drug combinations may be needed to achieve seizure control. Complete control is achieved in only 50% to 75% of children with epilepsy. The most commonly used anticonvulsants were discussed in Chapter 9.

CARDIOVASCULAR AND BLOOD DISORDERS

Medications to support cardiovascular functions in the pediatric/neonatal patient population differ little from those used with adults. Digoxin, diuretics, and, occasionally, antihypertensives are utilized. Discussion in this section focuses on patent ductus arteriosus and congestive heart failure, well as iron deficiency anemia and sickle cell anemia. The pharmacy technician needs to recognize the medications used for these conditions and how to prepare them for proper use.

Patent Ductus Arteriosus

During fetal life, most of the pulmonary arterial blood is shunted through the ductus arteriosus into the aorta. Functional closure of the ductus normally occurs soon after birth, but if the ductus remains patent when pulmonary vascular resistance falls, aortic blood is shunted into the pulmonary artery. **Patent ductus arteriosus** (PDA) is one of the most common congenital cardiovascular anomalies associated with maternal rubella (German measles) infection during early pregnancy. The entire phenomenon of transition is not completely understood, and the transition period of infants is a particularly important time. In uncomplicated PDA, the ductus closes spontaneously within the first weeks or months of life.

Treatment for Patent Ductus Arteriosus

When a large symptomatic PDA is present, general treatment may include fluid restriction, correction of anemia, digitalization, and diuretic therapy. Ductus arteriosus patency is mediated through the prostaglandins, and the ductus arteriosus in the preterm infant with RDS can be constricted and closed by the administration of inhibitors of prostaglandin synthesis such as indomethacin. Early administration of indomethacin in the course of RDS associated with large ductal left-to-right shunts is approximately 80% effective in closing the ductus. Surgical closure is a safe and effective backup technique for management when indomethacin is contraindicated or indomethacin treatment has not been successful. Administration is by intravenous infusion over at least 30 minutes to minimize adverse effects on cerebral, renal, and gastrointestinal blood flow. Usually, three doses per course are given, with a maximum of two courses. Urine output must be closely monitored and if anuria (no urine output) or oliguria occurs, subsequent doses should be delayed.

Congestive Heart Failure

Congestive heart failure (CHF) occurs when the heart cannot pump the blood returning to the right side of the heart or provide adequate circulation to meet the needs of organs and tissues in the body. There are two main causes of CHF:

1. High output state, usually related to congenital heart diseases in which there is increased pulmonary blood flow returning to the right side of the heart

2. Low output state, related to (a) congenital heart diseases in which there are left-side heart obstructions causing the heart to pump harder to

bypass the restrictive area (e.g., coarctation of the aorta or aortic valve stenosis), (b) a primary heart muscle disease (e.g., cardiomyopathy), or (c) rhythm disturbances (e.g., tachycardia or bradycardia).

Ninety percent of infants with congenital heart defects develop CHF within the first year of life. The majority of affected infants manifest symptoms within the first few months of life.

Treatment for Congestive Heart Failure

The initial management of CHF involves pharmacological agents that act to improve the function of the heart muscle and reduce the workload on the heart. Digitalis is given to increase cardiac output by slowing conduction through the atrioventricular node to make each contraction stronger. Diuretics decrease preload volume because their actions result in decreased extracellular fluid volume. Fluids are usually restricted to two-thirds of maintenance levels, and attention is given to nutrition and rest. Medical management continues with the plan for interventional cardiac catheterization or surgical intervention if indicated. See Chapter 12 for more information about the cardiovascular system and related subjects.

Iron Deficiency Anemia

Iron deficiency anemia is the most common form of anemia affecting children in North America. The full-term infant born of a well-nourished, non-anemic mother has sufficient iron stores until the birth weight is doubled, generally at four to six months of age. After that period, iron must be available from the diet to meet the child's nutritional needs. If dietary iron intake is insufficient, iron deficiency anemia results, generally after nine months of age.

Preterm infants, those with significant perinatal blood loss, or infants born to a poorly nourished mother with iron deficiency, may have inadequate iron stores. These infants have a significantly higher risk for iron deficiency anemia before the age of six months. Iron deficiency anemia may also result from chronic blood loss. In infants, such blood loss may be due to chronic intestinal bleeding caused by the heat-labile protein in cow's milk. Other causes of iron deficiency anemia include nutritional deficiencies such as folate (vitamin B_{12}) deficiency, sickle cell anemia, infections, and chronic inflammation.

Treatment for Iron Deficiency Anemia

Treatment efforts are focused on prevention and intervention. Prevention includes encouraging mothers to begin supplement breastfeeding with other foods after the infant reaches the age of four to six months. Mothers must also eat foods that are rich in iron during pregnancy and while breastfeeding, and take iron-fortified prenatal vitamins (approximately 1 mg/kg of iron supplement per day) to ensure sufficient fetal stores of iron before birth.

Therapy to treat iron deficiency anemia consists of a medication regimen. Iron is administered to the infant or child by mouth in doses of 2 to 3 mg/kg of elemental iron. All forms of iron (ferrous sulfate, ferrous fumarate, ferrous succinate, and ferrous gluconate) are equally effective. Vitamin C must be administered simultaneously with iron (ascorbic acid increases iron absorption). Iron is best absorbed when it is taken one hour before a meal. Iron therapy should continue for a minimum of six weeks after the anemia is corrected to replenish iron stores. Injectable iron is seldom used unless small bowel malabsorption disease is present.

Sickle Cell Anemia

Sickle cell anemia is an inherited disorder. Children with sickle cell anemia have abnormal hemoglobin, termed hemoglobin S (HbS). Sickled red blood cells are crescent-shaped, have decreased oxygen-carrying capacity, and are destroyed at a higher rate than that for normal red blood cells. Sickling results in clumping of red blood cells in the vessels, decreased oxygen transport, and increased destruction of red blood cells. Ischemia and tissue death result from the obstruction of vessels and decreased blood flow. Sickle cell trait occurs in 8% to 10% of African Americans. Most commonly, death occurs in children at one to three years of age from organ failure or thrombosis of major organs, usually the lungs and brain. With new treatments, 85% of affected individuals survive to the age of 20 years.

Treatment of Sickle Cell Anemia

Medical management focuses on pain control, oxygenation, hydration, and careful monitoring for other complications of vasoocclusion. Administration of prophylactic penicillin to prevent septicemia should be initiated at two to three months of age and continued through five years of life. Additional immunizations required are:

- Pneumococcal vaccine at two years of age with a booster at four to five years

- Influenza vaccine

Analgesics are used to control pain during a crisis period. The only cure is thought to be bone marrow transplantation, which also involves risks. This may be a promising treatment modality in the near future.

INFECTIOUS DISEASES

Various types of infectious agents have effects on different body systems in newborns and children, which can cause infectious diseases. Discussion of the many infectious diseases that affect children is beyond the scope of this text, but the following sections present symptoms or complications resulting from infectious diseases that are of particular concern when seen in children.

Diarrhea

Diarrhea is one of the most common problems encountered by pediatricians. Diarrhea is defined as an increase in frequency, fluidity, and volume of feces. During the first three years of life, it is estimated that a child will experience an acute, severe episode of diarrhea one to three times. It may be caused by a variety of infectious agents such as bacteria, viruses, protozoans, and parasites. Hospitalization is usually necessary for severe diarrhea because of the possibility of bacterial disease, which should be treated there, and because hydration often requires fluid therapy.

Treatment for Diarrhea

Treatment for diarrhea is symptomatic. Antipyretic drugs are recommended for fever. Codeine, morphine, and the phenothiazine derivatives, often used for pain and vomiting but rarely needed for children, should be avoided because they may induce misleading signs and symptoms.

Bacteremia and Septicemia

The terms bacteremia and septicemia describe the presence of bacteria in the blood. In **bacteremia**, bacteria are recovered from blood cultures of a patient and may or may not be associated with the disease. **Septicemia** is bacteremia associated with active disease, whether localized or systemic. In some patients, bacteremia or septicemia may be associated with focal infection (e.g., pneumonia, osteomyelitis, endocarditis, or meningitis). Primary bacteremia, however, also occurs in normal infants and children.

Treatment for Bacteremia and Septicemia

Treatment may be initiated with ampicillin and a semisynthetic penicillinase-resistant penicillin (methicillin, oxacillin, nafcillin) administered intravenously. In some patients, the use of chloramphenicol may also be indicated.

Acute Bacterial Meningitis

The incidence of bacterial meningitis (especially that caused by *H. influenzae* type b and group B beta-hemolytic streptococci) is increasing. Mortality and morbidity are significant, but the reported number of deaths has decreased over time. Acute bacterial meningitis may be caused by several types of bacteria; the most common pathogens vary depending on the age of the child. Table 26-4 shows the most common causative agents in different age groups.

Treatment for Meningitis

Initial therapy includes immediate administration of multiple antibiotics including a third-generation cephalosporin (e.g., ceftriaxone or cefotaxime) after an intravenous line has been placed and blood has been drawn for cultures. Vancomycin, with or without rifampin, is usually added,

Medical Terminology Review

bacteremia
bacter = bacteria; bacterial
emia = blood
bacteria in the blood
septicemia
septic = presence of pathogens or toxins
emia = blood
pathogens in the blood

TABLE 26-4	Most Common Infectious Agents Causing Meningitis in Different Age Groups
Age Group	Infectious Causes
Neonates	Group B streptococci, *Escherichia coli*
Infants	*Haemophilus influenzae* type b, *Streptococcus pneumoniae*
Young children	*S. pneumoniae* or *Neisseria meningitidis*

Key Concept

For an intramuscular injection in a young child, the vastus lateralis is the preferred site. Because of underdevelopment of the gluteal muscles, they are not recommended for use in children younger than three years of age.

as is ampicillin or gentamycin. Heparin therapy should be considered for patients with the syndrome of disseminated intravascular coagulation. Corticosteroids have been suggested as a therapeutic adjunct that may reduce cerebral edema and inflammation.

Streptococcal Infections

Streptococci are among the most common causes of bacterial infections in infancy and childhood. Group A streptococci are the most common bacteria causing acute pharyngitis.

Treatment for Streptococcal Infections

Penicillin is the drug of choice for the treatment of streptococcal infections. The goal of therapy is to maintain, for at least 10 days, blood and tissue levels of penicillin sufficient to kill streptococci. Various subjects related to antimicrobial infections and the agents used to treat them were covered in Chapter 23.

Human Immunodeficiency Virus and Acquired Immunodeficiency Syndrome

The cause of acquired immunodeficiency syndrome (AIDS) is the human immunodeficiency virus (HIV). This virus attaches to lymphocytes and other immunological cells, which results in a gradual destruction of T-helper lymphocytes. Therefore, HIV is able to reduce and damage immune functions of the body. The virus is transmitted only through direct contact with infected blood or blood products and body fluids through intravenous drug use, sexual contact, perinatal transmission from mother to infant, and breastfeeding. There is no evidence that HIV infection is acquired through casual contact.

Zidovudine is given to pregnant HIV-infected women, which significantly reduces the probability of transmission from mother to child. Infants infected through perinatal transmission from infected mothers accounts for more than 85% of children with AIDS who are younger than 13 years. This may occur during pregnancy, labor, delivery, or breastfeeding. Most children who are HIV-positive live in sub-Saharan Africa. Throughout the world, there are more than 3.2 million children living with HIV. However, there has been a 43% drop in new childhood HIV infections since 2009. It is vital that HIV-positive children receive treatment, and preventing mother-to-child transmission is very successful today, with proper funding, training, and resources.

Treatment for AIDS

There is currently no cure for HIV infection and AIDS. Management begins with a staging evaluation to determine disease progression and the appropriate course of treatment. Drugs such as zidovudine (formerly AZT, now ZDV), didanosine (DDI), zalcitabine (DDC), and lamivudine (3TC) slow down multiplication of the virus. Combination drug treatment is used, and many children are enrolled in research drug protocols. Trimethoprim-sulfamethoxazole (Septra®, Bactrim®) and pentamidine are used for treatment and prophylaxis of *Pneumocystis carinii* pneumonia. Monthly administration of intravenous immunoglobulin has been useful in preventing serious bacterial infections in children, as well as hypogammaglobulinemia. Immunizations are recommended for children with HIV infection, but instead of the oral poliovirus vaccine, the inactivated poliovirus vaccine is given. See Chapter 24 for more information about immunological agents and related subjects.

SUMMARY

The administration of drugs to a growing and developing infant or child may present a unique problem to the physician, who must be constantly aware of the changes in drug dosages that are required because of altered pharmacokinetics at different ages. Underlying this approach is the concept that there are complex changes in anatomy, physiology, biochemistry, and behavior from one stage of development to another from conception to adulthood. Drugs are double-edged swords. Although they can save lives, they can also endanger lives. Effective and safe drug therapy in neonates, infants, and children requires an understanding of the differences in drug action, metabolism, and disposition that are apparent during growth and development. Virtually all pharmacokinetic parameters change with age. Therefore, pediatric drug dosage regimens must be adjusted for age, disease state, sex, and individual needs. Failure to make such adjustments may lead to ineffective treatment or even to toxicity. Pharmacy technicians must be educated so that they have the required knowledge about, and can pay proper attention to, this important matter. It is impossible to cover each topic or aspect of pediatric diseases, conditions, and pharmacology in this chapter. Therefore, special consideration was given to highlighting selected diseases and their therapies for discussion in this chapter.

EXPLORING THE WEB

Visit **www.aap.org**

- Look for information on the disorders covered in this chapter. You may also find information on disorders that are not covered in this chapter. Create flashcards of the diseases and disorders and their treatments to use for preparation of exams.

- Visit the following websites to research articles related to pediatric illnesses and treatments:

- **http://emedicine.medscape.com**

- **www.medscape.com**

- **Visit www.nichd.nih.gov** and search for the information related to the Pediatric Pharmacology Research Units (PPRU) Network. What are the goals of this network? What research is being conducted? What are the results of some of the research to date?

REVIEW QUESTIONS

Multiple Choice

1. Which of the following factors may cause slower drug excretion and increase the risk of drug toxicity in an infant?

    A. kidney stones

    B. pyelonephritis

    C. urethritis

    D. renal immaturity

2. Which of the following is not a risk factor for sudden infant death syndrome?

    A. sleep apnea

    B. Native American ancestry

    C. drug use during pregnancy

    D. premature birth

3. Palivizumab (Synagis®) is used for immuno-prophylaxis against which of the following infections?

   A. epiglottitis

   B. pneumonia

   C. respiratory syncytial virus

   D. asthma

4. At which of the following ages do children exhibit the peak onset for croup?

   A. 1

   B. 2

   C. 4

   D. 6

5. Which of the following is the most commonly encountered diagnosis of respiratory disorders in office visits for children younger than the age of 15 in the United States?

   A. pneumonia

   B. flu

   C. epiglottitis

   D. otitis media

6. Patent ductus arteriosus is one of the most common congenital cardiovascular anomalies associated with which of the following maternal infections?

   A. hepatitis B

   B. rubella

   C. AIDS

   D. pneumonia

7. Ninety percent of infants with congenital heart defects develop which of the following complications within the first year of life?

   A. iron deficiency anemia

   B. cystic fibrosis

   C. sickle cell anemia

   D. congestive heart failure

8. The most common cause of death in children between 1 and 3 years who are suffering from sickle cell anemia is:

   A. thrombosis of major organs

   B. encephalitis

   C. kidney failure

   D. meningitis

9. The first-line antibiotic medication most often prescribed for otitis media is:

   A. tetracycline

   B. gentamycin

   C. tobramycin

   D. amoxicillin

10. Which of the following infectious diseases may be related to bacteremia?

   A. hepatitis B

   B. cystitis

   C. osteomyelitis

   D. epiglottitis

11. The goal of therapy for treatment of streptococcal infections is to:

   A. maintain for at least 10 days blood and tissue levels of penicillin sufficient to kill streptococci

   B. prevent myocarditis by using corticosteroids

   C. maintain for at least 3 days blood and tissue levels of corticosteroids to deal with stress

   D. prevent nephritic syndrome by using antineoplastic agents

12. Which of the following infectious diseases probably requires monthly administration of intravenous immunoglobulin to prevent serious bacterial infections in children?

   A. epiglottitis

   B. croup

   C. asthma

   D. AIDS

13. Which of the following types of insulins is classified as intermediate action?

   A. NPH

   B. regular

   C. ultralente

   D. protamine zinc

14. The drug of choice for epilepsy is based on which of the following factors?

    A. types of seizure

    B. pregnancy

    C. maturation of patients

    D. race and age of patients

15. Treatment for patent ductus arteriosus includes which of the following agents?

    A. oxygen

    B. morphine

    C. indomethacin

    D. acetaminophen

Fill in the Blank

1. In children, bacteremia may be associated with infections such as:

    a. _____

    b. _____

    c. _____or _____

2. The two mainstays of treatment for congestive heart failure are _____ and _____ .

3. The most common congenital cardiovascular anomaly is _____, which may indicate the need for indomethacin therapy.

4. Ninety-seven percent of all juvenile patients with newly diagnosed diabetes have type _____, also known as _____ .

5. Epiglottitis is commonly caused by _____, type b.

6. Respiratory distress syndrome or hyaline membrane disease is the result of the absence of _____.

7. The most widely used antipyretic in children is _____.

Critical Thinking

A 15-month-old girl who has been breastfed since birth without receiving formula or other foods is brought to the pediatrician's office. He examines her and orders blood tests, which reveal that she has severe anemia.

1. With this history of the infant, what type of anemia do you think she has?

2. What would be the way to prevent an infant from developing this type of anemia?

3. What other types of anemia can be seen in children of this age?

CHAPTER 27 Drug Therapy for Geriatrics Patients

OUTLINE

OBJECTIVES

After completing this chapter, the reader should be able to:

1. Identify the most popular types of drugs that elderly patients need.

2. Discuss clinical concerns of drug therapy and the way elderly patients react to certain drugs differently than younger patients.

3. Compare the way aging affects drug interaction, absorption, and distribution.

4. Understand how drug metabolism changes with age.

5. Discuss differences in renal function in elderly patients.

6. List some of the adverse effects that certain drugs have upon older patients.

7. Review some of the ways aging can be slowed with a healthy diet and exercise.

8. Identify age-related changes to the integumentary system.

9. Discuss common disorders in the elderly.

10. Describe the use of cold remedies in elderly people, and potential related consequences.

GLOSSARY

Collagen – a strong fibrous protein found in connective tissue

Dermis – a thick layer of loose connective tissue that is well supplied with blood vessels, lymphatic vessels, nerves, and accessory organs

Elastin – an extracellular connective tissue protein

Pharmacodynamic interactions – differences in effects produced by a given plasma level of a drug

Pharmacokinetic interactions – differences in the plasma levels of a drug achieved with a given dose of that drug

Polypharmacy – the practice of prescribing multiple medicines to a single patient simultaneously

OVERVIEW

The phenomenon of aging is unavoidable because aging is a universal process. The difference between aging and disease is that the aging process is intrinsic and depends on genetic factors, whereas disease is intrinsic and extrinsic, depending on both genetic and environmental factors. Aging is always progressive, whereas disease may be discontinuous, and may progress, regress, or be arrested entirely. Aging is irreversible, whereas disease may be treatable and often has a known cause. Elderly patients often have organs that are not functioning as well as those of younger adults. The average life expectancy in the United States has increased largely because of improvements in sanitation, food and water supplies, and the advent of antibiotics and vaccinations.

AGING PATIENTS

The impact of age on medical care is substantial, and thus a significantly altered approach to treatment is needed for the older patient. As individuals age, they are more likely to be affected by many chronic disorders and disabilities. Consequently, they use more drugs than any other age group. Combined with a decrease in physiological reserve and organs that may not be functioning fully, these added burdens (if present) make the older person more vulnerable to environmental, pathological, or pharmacological illnesses. Understanding these facts is essential for optimal care of older patients. Aging alters pharmacodynamics and pharmacokinetics, with implications for the choice, dose, and rate of administration of many drugs. Rates of absorption, distribution, metabolism, and excretion are usually less than those in younger adults. In addition, pharmacotherapy may be complicated by an elderly patient's inability to purchase or obtain drugs, or to comply with drug regimens.

Many drugs benefit elderly people. Some can save lives, such as antibiotics and thrombolytic therapy in acute illness. Oral hypoglycemic drugs can improve independence and quality of life while controlling chronic disease. Antihypertensive drugs and influenza vaccines can help prevent or decrease morbidity. Analgesics and antidepressants can control debilitating symptoms. Therefore, the appropriateness of the potential benefits in outweighing the potential risks should guide therapy. The health problems and medical management of elderly patients differ from those of younger ones in important ways, which explains the development of training in geriatrics as a medical specialty. Prescribing medications for elderly patients is always a challenge for physicians. Body functions decline dramatically in elderly patients. Therefore, the normal aging process can lead to altered drug effects and the need for altered doses. Safe, effective pharmacotherapy remains one of the greatest challenges in the practice of clinical geriatrics.

PHYSIOLOGICAL AGING

Not all functions in the human body show age-related changes. For example, the hematocrit does not change with age. However, levels of testosterone, cortisol, thyroxine, and insulin do show age-related declines.

It is extremely difficult to differentiate among primary (physiological), secondary (pathophysiological), and tertiary (sociogenic and behavioral) changes associated with aging. Age-related changes may be responsible for the atypical presentation of diseases in elderly people, which can be observed in hyperthyroidism, depression, uncontrolled diabetes mellitus, and rheumatoid arthritis. Although age-related changes may lessen the severity of some diseases, they may also be responsible for more severe presentations. For example, normal human aging is associated with a progressive reduction in dopamine concentrations in the brain, which may influence the onset or severity of Parkinson's disease. Menopause clearly is related to an increase in osteoporosis and atherosclerosis. Arteriosclerosis accounts for the age-related increase in diastolic blood pressure, a major risk factor for cerebrovascular disease (stroke).

Blood and Lymphatic Systems

The effect of the aging process on the blood results mainly from a reduced capacity to make new blood cells quickly when disease has occurred. After age 70 (approximately), the amount of bone marrow space occupied by tissue that produces blood cells declines progressively. This decrease in the ability to produce new blood cells when disease has occurred is a serious problem for elderly patients.

In the lymphatic system, age-related changes affect immune responses. Specific antibody responses to foreign antigens are impaired by the aging process. Elderly individuals may be more susceptible to infections and malignancies due to decreased immunity. In the elderly, infections are a leading cause of morbidity and mortality (Table 27-1).

Cardiovascular System

With advancing age, the heart weight increases significantly. In the myocardium (the heart muscle) fat, **collagen** (a strong fibrous protein found in

TABLE 27-1	Common Infections in the Elderly	
Disorder	**Causes**	**Prevention or Treatment**
Pneumonia	Bacterial	Vaccine and antibiotics
Influenza	Viral	Vaccine
Urinary Tract	Bacterial	Antibiotics
Herpes zoster (shingles)	Viral	Vaccine

connective tissue), and **elastin** (an extracellular connective tissue protein) increase. Arterial compliance in the internal and external carotid pathways significantly decrease. Fibrous plaques are present in many individuals' arteries by the age of 15 to 24 years. Within another decade of life, 85% of blood vessels have these plaques. More than 60% of hearts at ages 55 to 64 years show vascular calcification. Narrowing heart vessels are also more prevalent with age, and occlusion may occur in at least one of the three major coronary arteries. See Chapter 12 for more information on the cardiovascular system.

Urinary System

Age-associated kidney changes can be categorized as anatomical or functional. Anatomical changes include loss of glomeruli, decreased kidney size, renal tubular changes, and renal vascular changes. Anatomical changes involving the lower urinary tract make men more susceptible to prostatic hypertrophy. Women become prone to pelvic relaxation, urinary incontinence, urinary tract infections, and the development of uterine and cervical cancers. Renal function declines progressively starting in the fifth decade, so that by age 70 normal renal function is greatly reduced in comparison to that at age 30. Glomerular filtration rate declines by about 1 mL/min/year. Even in the absence of cardiovascular, renal, or acute illness, the decline is more rapid in men than in women. Renal blood flow and plasma flow also decrease with age. Drug metabolism is often impaired in the elderly because of a decrease in the glomerular filtration rate, as well as reduced hepatic clearance. See Chapter 14 for more information on the urinary system.

Endocrine System

Specific age-related disturbances in extrahepatic hormonal regulatory mechanisms have been proposed. The reduced availability of hormones results in diminished endocrine regulatory mechanisms, deficiencies in hormonal feedback mechanisms, and decreased binding affinities and receptors. Altered pancreatic and adrenal hormone concentrations decrease glucose tolerance with age. Insulin release is impaired in some older individuals, whereas others have fewer insulin receptors or exhibit postreceptor abnormalities. The peripheral glucose disposal rate is significantly lower in older than in younger people. Production of sex hormones also decreases with age. In postmenopausal women, reduced estrogen concentrations have been linked to increased incidences of osteoporosis and cardiovascular disease. See Chapter 18 for more information on the endocrine system.

Skeletal System

Normal age-related changes of the musculoskeletal system affect the mobility of most elderly people. The musculoskeletal system gradually loses bone mass after age 50 because bone formation and resorption becomes unstable.

The skeletal system of elderly people also is affected by a decrease in total body mass. Bone mass, density, and strength all decrease, and at the same time, bone fragility increases. In the elderly, skeletal system diseases and disorders are influenced by these factors. See Chapter 11 for more information on the musculoskeletal system.

Respiratory System

The respiratory system changes as we age. The diameters of the trachea and central airways increase, enlarging anatomical dead space. The volume of the alveolar ducts increases, whereas the membranous bronchioles narrow. Lung weight decreases dramatically, and chest wall compliance also decreases. These and other changes result in less elastic recoil in the lung, increased closing volume, and decreased maximal expiratory flow.

Thus, elderly people have an increased risk for respiratory failure. Aspiration or inhalation of foreign material into the tracheobronchial tree can produce major respiratory illness, which is more likely to occur in older than younger people. Finally, asthma in the elderly must be differentiated from other causes of airflow obstruction, such as acute bronchitis or congestive heart failure. See Chapter 16 for more information on the respiratory system.

Gastrointestinal System

The gastrointestinal system also changes with age. The gastrointestinal system starts with the oral cavity, where age-related changes reflect perturbation in oral health resulting from poor hygiene, disease, or disease treatment, rather than from dysfunction directly related to age. Nevertheless, oral disorders are common among elderly people. As many as 50% of older people experience traumatic lesions of the oral cavity, which may be ulcerative, atrophic, or hyperplastic. These changes make the oral mucosa more susceptible to disease, a problem that can be exacerbated by corticosteroids, antibiotics, cytotoxic agents, and immunosuppressive therapy. Elderly people may have an increased risk of local adverse drug reactions such as fixed eruptions (round or oval patches of reddened blisters on the skin), swelling, glossitis (inflammation of the tongue), and stomatitis (inflammation of the mouth).

Gastric secretion declines with age. Gastric cell function decreases and gastric pH rises. Gastric emptying is about 2.5 times faster in younger than in older people, perhaps because it is under the control of the central nervous system (CNS), which may lose efficiency with advancing age. Slowing of gastric emptying also follows a reduction in gastric acid secretion. Gastric emptying is reduced by stress, lack of ambulation, gastric ulcer, intestinal obstruction, myocardial infarction, and diabetes mellitus. Emptying is delayed by fatty meals in the elderly more so than in younger people. Bleeding is a fairly common complication of ulcers in elderly people. The normal aging process leads to a reduction in vitamin D absorption and a profound decline in the intestinal absorption of calcium. There is little existing evidence that the motility of the small intestine is altered by the aging process. Constipation is common because of alteration of motility in the large intestine.

The liver is the organ least affected by primary changes of aging. It continues to function in those individuals not affected by disease. In general, just a small part can perform the tasks of the entire liver. Liver weight correlates with body weight, and both decrease starting in the fifth or sixth decade.

Primary aging may be responsible for decreased hepatic blood flow, which in turn probably affects the metabolic clearance of certain drugs. These functional changes are thought to be most relevant with drugs that have a high first-pass extraction ratio. Clearance is limited by the capacity of the organ, and hepatic clearance cannot exceed hepatic blood flow, which is approximately 1.5 L/min. Thus, reduced blood flow can alter drug action in the elderly. For at least some drugs, hepatic metabolism in the elderly apparently is altered.

The reduction in hepatic clearance is due to the decreased activity of microsomal enzymes and reduced hepatic perfusion with aging. The distribution of drugs is also affected. In addition, serum albumin levels decrease, especially in sick patients, so that protein binding of some drugs (such as warfarin and phenytoin) is reduced. This leaves more free (active) drugs available. Also, older individuals often have altered responses to a given serum drug level. See Chapter 17 for more information on the gastrointestinal system.

Nervous System

With age, cellular brain mass and cerebral blood flow decrease. Sensory conduction takes longer, and the blood-brain barrier may become more permeable. These changes may decrease coordination, prolong reaction time, and impair short-term memory. Manifestations include more falls (particularly among elderly women), urinary incontinence, and confusion. Homeostatic response (the balance of the internal body systems) also declines.

In short, the brain shrinks with advancing age and loses nerve cells. The brain weighs less at 70 years of age than it weighs at age 30. Various areas of the brain lose substantial amounts of their nerve cells, although the nerve cells that control eye movement are not affected. The greatest loss of cells appears to take place in the temporal area, but the functional effect is surprisingly small. Cerebral blood flow is controlled by autoregulation, metabolic regulation, and chemical factors. Its regulation is influenced by the disease processes prevailing in old age, such as dementia, atherosclerosis, diabetes mellitus, stroke, and hypertension.

Short-term memory is significantly affected by aging, a loss that can be minimized by teaching methods of memorization to older adults. The declines in both learning facility and information retrieval, and perhaps also the loss in processing speed, appear to contribute to failing short-term memory.

The neurotransmitter serotonin is widely distributed throughout the CNS. It is implicated in a variety of neural functions, such as pain, feeding, sleep, sexual behavior, cardiac regulation, and cognition. Changes in the serotonin system occur in association with healthy aging. See Chapter 5 for more information on the nervous system.

Special Senses (Eye and Ear)

Vision impairment is one of the three most common medical problems among the elderly. Significant visual difficulties are caused by the aging process. Visual changes result in difficulty reading, and progressive changes can eventually make it difficult to conduct daily activities independently. With aging, the size of the pupil decreases, necessitating brighter lighting in order to see. Sensitivity to glare also increases because of age-related changes in the opacity of the lens. As we age, color discrimination decreases and depth perception becomes altered.

Hearing impairment is the second-most common health problem seen in elderly patients. High frequencies may become inaudible by the age of 50, with a marked decline occurring after age 65. The term "hard of hearing" may relate more to high-frequency hearing loss than an overall decline in hearing perception. Therefore, it is usually easier for an elderly adult to hear male voices, telephones, doorbells, and horns since they have lower tones and are of high intensity.

Integumentary System

Cells in the epidermis that contain melanocytes (which produce the pigment melanin), must be continuously replaced with new cells that divide, by mitosis, in the lower layers. The rate of production of these new cells decreases between the ages of 20 and 70 years. It is clear that during long periods of time, individual epidermal cells are exposed to carcinogens (cancer-causing agents), such as ultraviolet light from the sun. Furthermore, the number of melanocytes and the amount of protective melanin pigment decrease with age, making ultraviolet light more dangerous.

The **dermis** is a thick layer of loose connective tissue that is well supplied with blood vessels, lymphatic vessels, nerves, and accessory organs. The predominant cells found in the dermis are fibroblasts, mast cells, and macrophages. Fibroblasts produce and release collagen and elastin into the extracellular matrix, giving the skin its strength and elasticity, respectively.

The amount of collagen and elastin in the dermis decrease as people age, accounting for thinning and wrinkling of the skin in the elderly. Loss of collagen makes the skin more susceptible to wear and tear, whereas loss of elastin causes skin to lose its resiliency over time.

Perhaps the most striking age-related changes in the integumentary system are the graying, thinning, and loss of the hair. Hair color depends on varying amounts of melanin pigment within the specialized cells.

Reproductive System

As men age, testosterone levels decrease, sperm production slows, the scrotum loses muscle tone, and the testicles lose size and firmness. With age, the prostate gland enlarges considerably. Sexual activity is still normal and possible in elderly patients if they have no major health problems.

In women, physical changes occur after menopause. The ovaries cease producing ova (eggs), and lowered estrogen levels may cause physiological symptoms. Women experience a general atrophy of the genitalia that is related to hormonal changes, including less fat, the loss of external hair, and flattening of the labia. An elderly female's uterus is about one-half the size of the uterus in a young adult female. With age, the vagina also becomes drier and narrower.

After menopause, women experience changes in breast tissue resulting in less glandular tissue, reduced elasticity, more connective tissue, and more fat. As a result, the breasts experience sagging, though the size of the breasts may not change. Many of the physiological changes in body systems are summarized in Table 27-2.

PRINCIPLES OF DRUG THERAPY IN ELDERLY PATIENTS

The principal clinical concerns of drug therapy include efficacy and safety, dosage, complexity of regimen, number of drugs, cost, and patient compliance. There are several reasons for the greater incidence of adverse reactions of drugs in the elderly population. The elderly are more sensitive to some drugs, (e.g., opioids), and less sensitive to others (e.g., beta-blocking agents). The older patient with multiple chronic conditions is likely to be receiving many drugs, including nonprescribed agents. Drug doses in elderly patients must often be reduced, although dose requirements may vary considerably from person to person. In general, starting doses of about one-third to one-half the usual adult dose are indicated for drugs with a low therapeutic index.

THE PHYSIOPATHOLOGY OF AGING

Many of the physiological changes associated with aging can be slowed to some extent with a healthy diet and consistent regimen of moderate exercise. Many of the chronic diseases prevalent in elderly persons are either preventable or modifiable with healthy lifestyle habits. Reduction of dietary fat (especially saturated fats and cholesterol) is widely believed to lower the risk of coronary artery disease and stroke, as well as breast and colon cancer.

TABLE 27-2	Physiological Changes Due to Aging
System or Process	**Changes**
Cardiovascular system	The heart becomes less efficient, working harder to pump blood
Blood lipids	Level of good (HDL) cholesterol falls while bad (LDL) cholesterol rises
Urinary system	Kidney function declines; muscles of the bladder weaken, causing loss of urine control; in men, the prostate enlarges, also causing loss of urine control
Endocrine system	Ability to use glucose declines, increasing the risk of developing diabetes
Skeletal system	Bones lose calcium, weakening them
Muscular system	Strength and flexibility decline
Gastrointestinal system	Peristaltic motions decrease, altering digestion; gastric secretions decrease, altering defecation; mouth secretions decrease, causing greater tooth decay; speech, swallowing, and taste may be affected
Nervous system	Motor nerves deteriorate, slowing reaction time
Brain processes	Memory becomes less efficient; reflexes become slower; coordination decreases
Special senses	Degeneration of eye structures causes poor vision; tear production declines; hearing ability decreases
Integumentary system	Skin thins and dries, becoming wrinkled; nail growth slows
Reproductive system	The vagina narrows and becomes drier; the penis becomes less able to achieve or maintain erections
Metabolism	Slows, generally causing weight gain
Body temperature	Ability to maintain normal temperature declines

It is clear that our health and well being depend on the degree to which our organ systems can successfully work together to maintain homeostasis (internal stability) in the body. Diminished function in one organ system is lessened by appropriate compensatory mechanisms in other systems. The aging process affects all body systems physiologically.

COMMON DISORDERS IN THE ELDERLY

Some disorders occur almost exclusively in elderly persons, and some occur in persons of all ages but are far more common in elderly persons than in other age groups. For example, multiple disorders, accidental hypothermia, and urinary incontinence are almost exclusively found in elderly persons. Some other examples include lymphoma, chronic lymphocytic leukemia, prostate cancer, degenerative osteoarthritis, dementia, falls, hip fracture, osteoporosis, parkinsonism, hypertension, heart failure, stroke, and herpes zoster. These disorders are available for study and review in many medical textbooks. In this chapter, the most common disorders in elderly persons will be discussed selectively.

Multiple Disorders

Normal and abnormal effects of the aging process on different systems of the body in elderly persons may cause multiple disorders after middle age. A patient may suffer from several disorders, such as peptic ulcer, hypertension, and diabetes mellitus. Therefore, some patients are receiving several different medications that may cause drug interactions and side effects.

Cardiovascular Disorders

The incidence and prevalence of most cardiovascular disorders increases markedly with advancing age. Significant fat accumulations and calcifications in blood vessels of the heart (coronary arteries), brain, or peripheral arterial system are found in the majority of men and women older than 70 years of age. The combined effects of the pathological and physiological changes contribute to a high prevalence of problems, such as heart failure and cardiac arrhythmias in the elderly. There is good evidence that risk factors such as hypertension and hyperlipidemia can be successfully modified in older people, reducing the risk of ischemic vascular events. Multiple disorders are common in old age and coexistent diseases often can influence the choice of drugs for a cardiovascular condition. In addition, both pharmacokinetic and pharmacodynamic drug profiles may be altered in older subjects. These can influence both choice of drug and dosing regimen.

Ischemic Heart Disease

Aging is associated with a progressive rise in morbidity and mortality due to heart disease, which is the most common cause of death in the United States. The three main groups of drugs used to treat angina pectoris are beta-adrenergic receptor blocking agents, calcium channel blockers, and nitrates, which are discussed in Chapter 12.

Acute Myocardial Infarction

Acute myocardial infarction (AMI) is painless in many persons older than 70 years of age. The mortality from AMI is greater in older subjects than in young and middle-aged subjects. This is due to a number of factors, including increased severity of underlying coronary artery disease, a greater prevalence of previous myocardial infarction, and an associated increase in the incidence of cardiac failure. The aims of treatment are to relieve symptoms, reduce mortality, and prevent late cardiovascular disability. Pain relief is usually attempted by the use of intravenous opiates such as diamorphine.

Intravenous nitrates are sometimes used to reduce opiate requirements, and may also be helpful in the treatment of associated cardiac failure; however, adverse effects, including hypotension and bradycardia, are more common in elderly subjects. When used in elderly persons, the dosage should be reduced.

Aspirin has been shown to significantly reduce mortality, reinfarction, and stroke rate after AMI in older patients. Treatment with the combination of thrombolytic agents and oral aspirin confers additional benefit.

Cardiac Failure

The incidence and prevalence of cardiac failure increase sharply with increasing age. In postmortem examinations of elderly persons, the most common underlying pathological conditions are ischemia and hypertensive heart disease. The appropriate treatment of cardiac failure depends on accurate diagnosis, including the underlying cardiac pathological conditions. Treatments for cardiac failure are discussed in Chapter 12.

Hypertension

The major causes of death and morbidity associated with hypertension are myocardial infarction and stroke. In addition, congestive heart failure is more common in elderly hypertensive patients than in their younger counterparts. Blood pressure rises with age up to about 75 years. Hypertension is perhaps best defined as the blood pressure level at which treatment is likely to be beneficial.

The best choice of antihypertensive treatment for elderly patients remains highly controversial. Drugs that are effective in younger patients also will lower blood pressure in those who are elderly. In the absence of specific contraindications, different agents seem to be tolerated equally well in elderly patients, though some may develop adverse reactions requiring a change of drug. Treatment of hypertension is discussed in Chapter 13.

Cerebrovascular Disease

Stroke continues to be a significant public health problem in the United States. According to the American Heart Association, it is estimated that every four minutes, one person in the United States suffers a stroke, making it the third leading cause of death and the major cause of long-term disability in adults. Because two thirds of all patients affected by stroke are older than 65 years, this disease mostly affects the elderly population.

The most significant nonmodifiable risk factor for stroke is advanced age. The risk for stroke in African Americans is much higher than in Caucasians, even after controlling for the effects of age, hypertension, and diabetes. Cigarette smoking and excessive alcohol consumption are important independent risk factors for stroke. Hypertension is by far the most important modifiable risk factor. It is a contributing factor in more than two-thirds of strokes, and lowering diastolic blood pressure significantly reduces stroke risk by 40%.

General therapeutic measures for stroke patients include maintaining an open airway, hydration with intravenous fluids, and judicious treatment of hypertension and hypoglycemia.

Cancer

The management of cancer with aging is an increasingly common problem as the number of elderly patients with cancer grows. Elderly persons currently comprise approximately 12% of the U.S. population and by 2030 are projected to comprise nearly 20%. After heart disease, cancer is the second leading cause of death in the United States.

Malignant tumor incidence increases progressively with age, although the increase is not uniform for each type of cancer. The reason for the increased incidence of cancer with age is not fully understood. The duration of carcinogenesis (agents that cause cancers), and the prolonged exposure to chemical, physical, or biological carcinogens may explain the association.

Cancer in older persons should be considered differently because of the physiological effects of aging. There are two important pharmacokinetic factors that occur with aging: a change in the volume of distribution, and a decrease in the concentration of serum albumin. The treatment of different cancers was discussed in Chapter 21.

Arthritis

Arthritis is the most common chronic ailment in elderly persons. Most people aged 70 years or older report having arthritis, occasionally resulting in physical limitations. After age 65, the prevalence is approximately 50%, and it increases every decade thereafter. The two most common forms of arthritis in elderly persons are rheumatoid arthritis (RA) and osteoarthritis (OA).

Rheumatoid Arthritis

The clinical manifestations of RA in elderly people may differ from those of the typical younger adult patient with this disease. The abrupt appearance of symptoms is more common in elderly-onset disease, whereas bone erosions and nodules are less common. A multidisciplinary treatment approach is required for elderly patients with RA. It includes physical therapy, occupational therapy, pharmacotherapy, and, occasionally, surgical intervention. The goals of therapy for elderly patients are the same as those for younger patients: to relieve symptoms, reduce inflammation, avoid joint destruction, prevent deformities, maintain functional capacity, and preserve quality of life.

The pharmacotherapy of RA is similar in young and old patients. Age alone does not contraindicate the use of the first- or second-line antirheumatic drugs. However, the adverse effects of some drugs are more pronounced in elderly patients. Nonsteroidal anti-inflammatory drugs (NSAIDs), including aspirin and nonacetylated salicylates, are useful in treating arthritic symptoms in elderly subjects. Drug therapy must be monitored vigilantly in elderly patients because of the increased risk of complications. NSAIDs in elderly patients may result in include cardiovascular (congestive heart failure and hypertension), CNS (confusion, dizziness, headaches, and hearing loss), gastrointestinal (gastritis, ulcers, and epigastric pain), and renal (electrolyte imbalances, fluid retention, and renal insufficiency) complications. Chapter 11 provides details of antirheumatic pharmacotherapy.

Osteoarthritis

Osteoarthritis (OA) is characterized by degeneration of cartilage, bone remodeling, and overgrowth of bone. This form of arthritis, also referred to as degenerative joint disease, is the most common form in elderly people. Radiographic evidence of OA is present in the majority of those older than age 65, yet many are asymptomatic. Pain is the primary complaint of patients with OA but can be absent despite severe joint damage. Joint stiffness, pain at night, pain at rest, and crepitus (a feeling of crackling as the joint is moved) also are common symptoms. Commonly affected joints include the interphalangeal joints of the hands, knees, hips, first metatarsophalangeal joint, and the lumbar and cervical spine.

The primary goals in treating OA are to minimize joint pain, maintain functional mobility, and allow use of the affected joints. A combination of pharmacotherapy and nonpharmacological therapeutic interventions is often necessary. Resting the joints sometimes relieves pain. Joint replacement may be the treatment of choice in patients with severe OA that cannot be adequately managed with other modalities. For more information for pharmacotherapy, refer to Chapter 11.

Osteoporosis

Osteoporosis is a metabolic bone disorder in which the rate of bone reabsorption accelerates while the rate of bone formation slows down, causing a loss of bone mass. Bones affected by this disease lose calcium and phosphate salts, and thus become porous, brittle, and abnormally vulnerable to fractures. Osteoporosis may be primary or secondary to an underlying disease. Primary osteoporosis is often called postmenopausal osteoporosis because it develops more commonly in postmenopausal women.

Osteoporosis is a major risk factor for vertebral compression fractures and hip fractures in the elderly. It can develop insidiously with increasing deformity, kyphosis, and loss of height. As bones weaken, spontaneous wedge fractures, pathological fractures of the neck or femur and hip, become increasingly common. The condition is often discovered when an elderly person bends to lift something, hears a snapping sound, and then feels a sudden pain in the lower back.

The aims of treatment are to prevent additional fractures and control pain. A physical therapy program, emphasizing gentle exercise and activity, is an important part of the treatment. Hormone replacement therapy (HRT) with estrogen and progesterone may retard bone loss and prevent the occurrence of fractures. HRT decreases bone reabsorption and increases bone mass. Other medications may include alendronate (Fosamax®) and calcitonin; however, adequate calcium and vitamin D intakes are needed for maximum effect. Drug therapy merely arrests osteoporosis; it does not cure it. Surgery can correct pathological fractures.

Ophthalmic Disorders

One of the consequences of aging is a gradual impairment of vision. Like other tissues and organs in the body, the eye is constantly undergoing changes, both physical and functional. Changes may be a consequence of the aging process, diet, environment, or disease. Conditions that are commonly associated with age-related deterioration of ocular function include reduction in precorneal tear production; changes affecting the clarity and flexibility of the crystalline lens; an elevation in intraocular pressure, and changes in vessels supplying blood to regions in the eye.

Dry Eye Syndrome

Dry eye syndrome (xerosis) in elderly persons may be caused by a number of conditions, including trachoma, vitamin A deficiency, chemical burn, radiation, and chemotherapy. Dry eye is a common disorder affecting the elderly population, especially individuals older than 40 years. In elderly persons, a thinned conjunctiva and diminished corneal sensation add to the problem of dry eyes.

The primary treatment for dry eyes is replacement of deficient tear production with artificial tear preparations. Sterile isotonic saline preparations have been used to replace aqueous tear deficiencies, but the duration of relief is extremely short, requiring frequent dosing. Relief can be prolonged by the addition of water-soluble polymers, which increase the viscosity of the solution and provide an aqueous film over the corneal surface for an extended period.

Presbyopia

In the normal resting state, the eye can focus on an image of a distant object. However, to focus on a near object, the refractive power of the lens must increase. This is accomplished by contraction of the ciliary muscles, which causes the lens to become more spherical. This process is referred to as accommodation. The closest distance that the eye is able to accommodate (near point) is extremely short in infancy, and it progressively increases with age. When a person reaches the mid-40s, presbyopia, a condition in which the near point of accommodation moves beyond a comfortable reading distance, gradually develops. Presbyopia is presently treated using corrective eyeglasses. Bifocal or trifocal contact lenses are also available, but they have had limited acceptance.

Cataract

A cataract is defined as any opacity or loss in transparency in the crystalline lens of the eye. When a cataract interferes with transmission of light to the retina, some loss in visual acuity, and possibly complete loss of vision, may result. Cataracts are a leading cause of blindness and visual impairment worldwide.

Cataracts may be congenital or acquired (secondary). Most cataracts have no known cause, and they usually occur in individuals older than 50 years of age. There is significant correlation between age and the occurrence of lens opacities, which are found to some degree in most people older than 60.

At present, no medical treatment will restore an opaque lens to its transparent state. Surgery remains the only effective method of treatment.

Glaucoma

Glaucoma includes a group of ocular diseases that are characterized by increased intraocular pressure, which may produce compression of the optic disk, resulting in damage to the optic nerve that leads to loss of the peripheral visual field and visual acuity.

Glaucoma is the second leading cause of blindness in the world. According to the Glaucoma Foundation, it is estimated that 67 million people worldwide have primary glaucoma. It is also a common cause of blindness in the United States.

The treatment of glaucoma centers on the reduction of the elevated intraocular pressure. Currently, this is accomplished with medical, laser, or surgical treatment.

DRUG INTERACTIONS

A drug interaction occurs whenever the pharmacological action of a drug is altered by a second substance. This change may be related to **pharmacokinetic interactions** (differences in the plasma levels of a drug achieved with a given dose of that drug), and **pharmacodynamic interactions** (differences in effects produced by a given plasma level of a drug). The duration and intensity of the action of a drug are a function of the plasma level of the drug, which is related directly to the absorption, distribution, metabolism, and excretion of that drug. These rates may be altered by previous drug therapy, dietary factors, and exposure to environmental chemicals (chemicals not used for therapeutic purposes). Physical factors such as ambient temperature and effects of disease (e.g., fever) may also have an impact.

Pharmacokinetics

As discussed in Chapter 3, pharmacokinetics is the study of the activities of drugs occurring within the body after a drug is administered, including absorption, distribution, excretion, and metabolism. It also involves the amount of time that each of these processes requires. Pharmacokinetics is also the study of the onset of action, duration of effect, biotransformation, and routes of excretion of the metabolites of the drug. It is difficult to determine the amount of drug reaching its site of action as a function of time after administration. In most cases, this is not feasible; therefore, it is the plasma concentration of the drug that is measured. This provides useful information, since the amount of drug in the tissues is related to plasma concentration. Pharmacokinetics are also greatly affected by the aging process.

Drug Absorption

Physiological changes with aging, such as changes in gastric pH, slowed gastric emptying rate, reduced cardiac output (blood flow), reductions of absorptive surfaces, and slowed gastrointestinal tract motility, are factors that affect not only drug absorption but also drug distribution and metabolism. Different diseases and conditions of the gastrointestinal tract are also obvious factors that affect drug absorption. Examples are peptic ulcer, diarrhea, and constipation.

Drug Distribution

Alterations in drug distribution noted in elderly patients are linked to many factors, such as reduced total body water content, decreased plasma albumin concentration, reduced lean body mass, and increased body fat. Many drugs, especially acidic ones, bind to plasma proteins. Drugs can compete for plasma protein-binding sites. Plasma protein-binding sites are especially significant when a high percentage of the drug (more than 90%) is normally protein bound, as with coumarin anticoagulants, sulfonamides, salicylates, indomethacin, and most other NSAIDs. Lipid-soluble drugs such as lidocaine and diazepam have a large volume of distribution in elderly persons, whereas water-soluble drugs such as ethanol and acetaminophen have a smaller volume of distribution. Digoxin also has a lower volume of distribution in elderly persons; therefore, doses must be reduced.

Drug Metabolism

The most common and most important cause for differences in the plasma levels of a drug is a change in the rate of biotransformation of the drug. Variations in a person's plasma drug levels are more common with drugs that undergo extensive gastrointestinal metabolism or first-pass hepatic metabolism. The total liver blood flow declines significantly with aging because of a reduction of cardiac output. Therefore, if severe and progressive liver damage is present in an elderly person, drug metabolism would be affected. Otherwise, the decline in the ability of elderly persons to metabolize most drugs is relatively small and difficult to predict. In older persons, presystemic (first-pass) metabolism of some drugs given orally is decreased and their serum concentration and bioavailability are increased. Examples of these drugs include labetalol, propranolol, and verapamil. Consequently, initial doses of these drugs should be reduced as required. However, presystemic metabolism of other metabolized drugs such as imipramine, amitriptyline, morphine, and meperidine is not decreased. The effects of cigarette smoking, diet, and alcohol consumption may be more important than the physiological changes in the liver.

Drug Elimination

Drugs may be eliminated from the body by many routes, including urine, feces (e.g., unabsorbed drugs or those secreted in bile), saliva, sweat, tears, breast milk, and lungs (e.g., alcohols and anesthetics). Any route may be important for a given drug, but the kidney is the most important route for the elimination of the majority of drugs. Some drugs are excreted unchanged in the urine, whereas other drugs are so extensively metabolized that only a small fraction of the original chemical substance is excreted unchanged. Different responses to drug therapy may be seen in elderly individuals because of a decline in hepatic and renal function, which is often accompanied by a concurrent disease process. The rate of elimination of any drug by the kidney is reduced in elderly persons. Renal blood flow, mainly in the renal cortex, decreases significantly with aging. This physiological change causes a decrease in renal drug elimination.

Because renal function is dynamic, maintenance doses of drugs should be adjusted when a patient becomes acutely ill or dehydrated or has recently recovered from dehydration. In addition, because renal function continues to decline, the dose of drugs given long-term should be reviewed periodically. Examples of these drugs are the aminoglycosides, chlorpropamide, digoxin, and lithium carbonate. To prevent drug toxicity, renal function must be estimated, and the dosage of the drug should be adjusted. Most elderly patients do not have normal renal function, and the majority require adjustments in the dosages of drugs that are eliminated primarily by the kidneys. See Chapter 3 for more information on drug elimination and the renal system.

Pharmacodynamics

Drug action is defined as physiological changes in the body caused by a drug, or responses to the pharmacological effects of a drug. Pharmacodynamics refers to the chemical reaction of drugs in the body, a topic that was previously introduced in Chapter 3. This can be different in elderly persons because of physiological changes that occur with aging. Drugs can modify the way the body acts, but they do not give body organs and tissues new functions. They usually either slow down or speed up ordinary cell processes.

The most common way in which drugs display their action is by forming a chemical bond with specific receptors within the body. This binding may occur if the drug and its receptors have a compatible chemical shape. Figure 27-1 illustrates a drug-receptor interaction.

The effects of similar concentrations of drugs at the site of action may be greater or lesser in elderly persons than they are in younger persons. The difference may be due to changes in drug-receptor interactions. The increased sensitivity that occurs with aging must be considered when drugs that can have serious adverse effects are used. These drugs include morphine, pentazocine, warfarin, angiotensin-converting enzyme inhibitors, diazepam (especially when it is given parenterally), and levodopa. Some drugs whose effects are reduced in elderly persons include tolbutamide, glyburide, and beta-blockers, which should also be used with caution because serious dose-related toxicity can still occur, and signs of toxicity may be delayed.

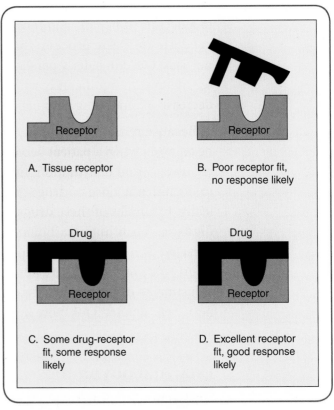

Figure 27-1 Drug-receptor interaction.

POLYPHARMACY

Polypharmacy is the practice of prescribing multiple medicines simultaneously to a single patient. It increases costs for treatment as well as the chances for drug interactions and multiple adverse effects. Polypharmacy is more common in elderly patients because they often need several medical specialists and also may be using over-the-counter (OTC) drugs and herbal supplements. Herbal supplements must be considered to be drugs because of their potential to interact adversely with prescribed and OTC drugs. Approximately two-thirds of people over the age of 65 use prescription and OTC drugs.

Liver dysfunction, confusion, falls, and malnutrition may all be caused by polypharmacy. Liver dysfunction contributes to confused mental states and delirium, with perception disturbances and misinterpretations of information commonly seen.

SPECIFIC DRUG CONSIDERATIONS FOR THE ELDERLY

Several classes of drugs that are commonly prescribed for elderly persons will be selectively discussed here. They include cardiovascular drugs, CNS drugs, anti-inflammatory drugs, and gastrointestinal drugs. However, there are many different types of drugs that are potentially inappropriate for use by the elderly. These are listed in the *Beers Criteria for Potentially Inappropriate Medication Use in Older Adults*, which is commonly referred to as the *Beers List*. It is a guideline for health care professionals to help improve the safety of prescribing medications for older adults. Drugs that are dangerous if used by people older than 65 years of age are listed in Table 27-3.

Cardiovascular Drugs

Almost one-third of all deaths in Western countries can be attributed to heart disease. Many cardiovascular drugs must be used cautiously in the elderly for the treatment of hypertension, congestive heart failure, myocardial infarction, and stroke, among other disorders and conditions.

Blood pressure increases with age, leading to serious health problems. Treatment of hypertension is effective in older patients. Antihypertensive drugs include thiazides, which are the most commonly prescribed class of diuretics. In the elderly, because of potential adverse effects, these agents should be used in lowered doses. Unfortunately, thiazides can worsen gout, which is a common elderly condition. Beta-blockers and angiotensin-converting enzyme inhibitors are prescribed less often than thiazides because they may conflict with certain disorders in the elderly. Alpha$_1$ blockers are infrequently used for elderly patients because of their adverse effects.

Key Concept

The Beers List of potentially inappropriate medications for older adults is now under the management of the American Geriatrics Society (AGS). These medications include a variety of anticholinergics, antiparkinson agents, antispasmodics, alpha$_1$ blockers, antiarrhythmic drugs, antipsychotics, barbiturates, and many others. The complete list is located at: http://www .americangeriatrics.org/ files/documents/beers/ PrintableBeersPocket-Card.pdf.

TABLE 27-3	Dangerous Medications for Adults Older Than 65 Years of Age	
Classification	**Generic Name**	**Trade Name**
Analgesics	meperidine hydrochloride **(meh-PEH-rih-deen hy-droh-KLOR-ryd)**	Demerol®
	pentazocine **(pen-TAH-zoh-seen)**	Talwin®
Antiarrhythmics	disopyramide **(dy-soh-PIH-rah-myd)**	Norpace®
Antidepressants	amitriptyline hydrochloride **(ah-mih-TRIP-tih-leen hy-droh-KLOR-ryd)**	(generic only)
	doxepin hydrochloride **(DOK-zeh-pin hy-droh-KLOR-ryd)**	Sinequan®
	fluoxetine hydrochloride **(floo-OK-zeh-teen hy-droh-KLOR-ryd)**	Prozac®
Antiemetics	trimethobenzamide hydrochloride **(try-meh-thoh-BEN-zah-myd hy-droh-KLOR-ryd)**	Tigan®
Antihistamines	chlorpheniramine maleate **(klor-feh-NIH-rah-meen MAH-lee-ayt)**	Chlor-Trimeton®
	diphenhydramine hydrochloride **(dy-fen-HY-drah-meen hy-droh-KLOR-ryd)**	Benadryl®, Tylenol PM®
	hydroxyzine pamoate **(hy-DROK-sih-zeen PAH-moh-ayt)**	Vistaril®, Atarax®
	promethazine hydrochloride **(proh-MEH-thah-zeen hy-droh-KLOR-ryd)**	Phenergan®
Antihypertensives	clonidine hydrochloride **(KLAW-nih-deen hy-droh-KLOR-ryd)**	Catapres®
	hydrochlorothiazide **(hy-droh-klor-oh-THY-ah-zyd)**	Esidrix®, HydroDIURIL®
	methyldopa **(meh-thil-DOH-pah)**	Aldomet®
	propranolol **(proh-PRAN-oh-lol)**	Inderal®
	reserpine **(REH-zer-peen)**	(generic only)

Table 27-3 continued

Anti-infectives	nitrofurantoin **(ny-troh-fyoo-RAN-toh-in)**	Macrodantin®
Antipsychotics	haloperidol **(hah-loh-PEH-rih-dol)**	Haldol®
	thioridazine hydrochloride **(thy-oh-RIH-dah-zeen hy-droh-KLOR-ryd)**	Mellaril®
Antispasmodics	belladonna alkaloids **(bel-lah-DON-nah AL-kah-loydz)**	Donnatal®
	dicyclomine hydrochloride **(dy-CY-kloh-meen hy-droh-KLOR-ryd)**	Bentyl®
	hyoscyamine sulfate **(hy-oh-SY-ah-meen SUL-fayt)**	Levsin®
	oxybutynin chloride **(ok-see-BYOO-tih-nin KLOR-ryd)**	Ditropan®
	tolterodine tartrate **(tol-TEH-roh-deen TAR-trayt)**	Detrol®
Decongestants	oxymetazoline **(ok-see-MEH-tah-zoh-leen)**	Afrin®, Dristan®
	phenylephrine hydrochloride **(feh-nil-EH-freen hy-droh-KLOR-ryd)**	Neo-Synephrine®
	pseudoephedrine hydrochloride **(soo-doh-eh-FEH-dreen hy-droh-KLOR-ryd)**	Sudafed®
Histamine H$_2$ blockers	cimetidine **(sih-MEH-tih-deen)**	Tagamet®
Iron	ferrous sulfate **(FER-rus SUL-fayt)**	Feosol®, Feratab®
Muscle relaxants	carisoprodol **(kah-rih-soh-PROH-dol)**	Soma®
	cyclobenzaprine hydrochloride **(sy-kloh-BEN-zah-preen hy-droh-KLOR-ryd)**	Flexeril®
	methocarbamol **(meh-thoh-KAR-bah-mol)**	Robaxin®
	orphenadrine **(or-FEN-ah-dreen)**	Norflex®
NSAIDs	indomethacin **(in-doh-MEH-thah-sin)**	Indocin®

continued on next page

Table 27-3 continued

	ketorolac tromethamine **(keh-TOH-roh-lak tro-MEH-thah-meen)**	Toradol®
	phenylbutazone **(feh-nil-BYOO-tah-zohn)**	Butazolidin®
Oral hypoglycemics	chlorpropamide **(klor-PRO-pah-myd)**	Diabinese®
Platelet inhibitors	dipyridamole **(dy-pih-RIH-dah-mol)**	Persantine®
Sedative-hypnotics	alprazolam **(al-PRAH-zoh-lam)**	Xanax®
	chlordiazepoxide **(klor-dy-ah-zeh-POK-zyd)**	Librium®, Limbitrol®
	diazepam **(dy-AH-zeh-pam)**	Valium®
	flurazepam **(floo-RAH-zeh-pam)**	Dalmane®
	lorazepam **(loh-RAH-zeh-pam)**	Ativan®
	meprobamate **(meh-PROH-bah-mayt)**	Miltown®
	oxazepam **(ok-ZAH-zeh-pam)**	Serax®
	temazepam **(teh-MAH-zeh-pam)**	Restoril®
	triazolam **(try-AH-zoh-lam)**	Halcion®

The toxic effects of cardiac glycosides are particularly dangerous in elderly patients because of their increased susceptibility to arrhythmias. Renal function should be considered when dosing regimens are being contemplated. Digoxin is considered safe for older adults if there is close monitoring of serum digoxin levels, creatinine clearance tests, and monitoring of vital signs.

Because older people exhibit changes in hemodynamic reserve, treating patients in this age group who have arrhythmias (dysrhythmias) is challenging. Disopyramide should be avoided because of its major toxicities. Patients with arrhythmias should receive therapy that is designed to control their ventricular rate without conversion to normal sinus rhythm.

The prevention of possible thromboembolism in chronic atrial fibrillation is an important goal.

Anticoagulants

Many elderly patients with atrial fibrillation are not given anticoagulants because physicians fear injuries and secondary bleeding due to falls. Head injuries from falling are usually of greatest concern. Given that anticoagulation can result in an annual absolute reduction in the risk of stroke, the benefits of anticoagulation outweigh the risks of falling in most instances (see Chapter 15).

Central Nervous System Drugs

Many central nervous system drugs act by blocking receptors and preventing transmitters from binding them. Among the CNS drugs used in the treatment of geriatric patients are sedative-hypnotics, narcotic analgesics, antidepressants, antipsychotics, and drugs used for Alzheimer's disease.

The second most common group of drugs prescribed for (or taken OTC) by the elderly are sedatives and hypnotics. The half-lives of many of these drugs show the greatest age-related increase in people who are 60 to 70 years of age. Reduced renal function or liver disease affects the rate at which these drugs can be eliminated. Ataxia and other motor impairments should be closely watched for in older patients when they are taking these drugs, which include barbiturates and benzodiazepines.

Narcotic analgesics may cause dose-related adverse effects in the elderly. Because of the way respiratory function changes as we age, geriatric patients are often more sensitive to the respiratory effects of these drugs. Use of narcotics may cause hypotension in the elderly. Opioids are often underutilized in the elderly, though good pain management plans are easily obtained for this age group.

Antidepressants and antipsychotics have sometimes been overused in the elderly for the treatment of such disorders as schizophrenia, dementia, aggressiveness, delirium, and paranoia. Older drugs of this type, such as chlorpromazine, should be avoided in the elderly because they induce orthostatic hypotension. According to the patient's tolerance, drug doses should be gradually increased to achieve the desired therapeutic effect, with close monitoring for adverse effects.

Some phenothiazines should be started at just a fraction of the amounts used for young adults when they are being used for the elderly. Due to its clearance by the kidneys, lithium must be dosage-adjusted, and it should never be used concurrently with thiazide diuretics. Antidepressants often cause more toxicity in older adults, and those with reduced antimuscarinic effects (such as nortriptyline and desipramine) should be used. Major depression and senile dementia must be carefully differentiated because they can sometimes resemble each other.

Alzheimer's disease is characterized by progressive impairment of memory and cognitive function. Cholinomimetic drugs are usually used for this condition, to decrease the release of gamma-aminobutyric acid (GABA), and increase the release of norepinephrine, dopamine, and serotonin from nerve endings. Some agents, such as donepezil, rivastigmine, and galantamine have been shown to improve cognitive activity in some Alzheimer's patients and may even reduce morbidity from other diseases. This is important in prolonging the life of the patient. However, these agents should be used with caution in patients receiving other cytochrome P450 enzyme inhibitors.

Anti-Inflammatory Drugs

About one-half of patients with cancer who are dying have severe pain. Patients perceive pain differently, depending on factors such as fatigue, insomnia, anxiety, depression, and nausea. Addressing these factors together with a supportive environment can help control pain.

The choice of analgesic depends largely on pain intensity, which can be determined only by talking with and observing the patient. All pain can be relieved by an appropriately potent drug at the right dosage, which may also produce sedation or confusion. Commonly used drugs are aspirin, acetaminophen, or NSAIDs for mild pain; codeine or oxycodone for moderate pain; and hydromorphone or morphine for severe pain. For a detailed discussion of analgesic use, see Chapter 22.

Cold Remedies

Over-the-counter cold remedies often cause adverse effects in elderly people. The anticholinergic properties of many of these drugs create confusion, impair bladder emptying, or cause constipation, and decongestants may cause urinary hesitance or retention in men.

Gastrointestinal Drugs

Many seriously ill patients experience nausea, often without vomiting. Contributors to nausea include gastrointestinal problems such as constipation and gastritis, metabolic abnormalities such as hypercalcemia and uremia (elevation of urea in blood), drug side effects, and increased intracranial pressure due to brain cancer. Treatment should be guided by the probable etiology, such as discontinuation of NSAIDs and administration of H_2-receptor blockers such as ranitidine (Zantac®), famotidine (Pepcid®), and cimetidine (Tagamet®) in a patient with gastritis. In contrast, a patient with known or suspected brain metastasis may have nausea due to increased intracranial pressure and would best be treated with a course of corticosteroids. Metoclopramide, orally or by injection, is useful for nausea caused by

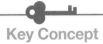

Key Concept

For the administration of drugs in elderly patients, neurological status and parameters relating to renal, liver, cardiac, and respiratory function should be noted.

gastric distension. If a reason for mild nausea is not identifiable, nonspecific treatment with phenothiazines such as promethazine or prochlorperazine before meals may be given. Anticholinergic drugs such as scopolamine and the antihistamine meclizine prevent recurrent nausea in many patients. Second-line drugs for intractable nausea include haloperidol and granisetron. Constipation is common in elderly people because of inactivity, use of opioid and anticholinergic drugs, and decreased fluid and dietary fiber intake. Laxatives help prevent fecal impaction, especially for those receiving opioids. Laxative drugs are discussed in Chapter 17.

Antimicrobial Drugs

Due to alterations in their T-lymphocyte function, many elderly patients appear to have reduced host defenses and are more susceptible to serious infections and diseases such as cancer. It is important to remember that decreased renal function greatly affects the use of certain antimicrobial drugs, such as aminoglycosides, in the elderly. Antimicrobial drugs that are considered safe for the elderly include penicillins, cephalosporins, sulfonamides, and tetracyclines. Drug doses should be decreased if the patient has decreased renal drug clearance or the drug has a prolonged half-life.

SUMMARY

Throughout the aging process, individuals are more likely to be affected by many chronic disorders and disabilities. Consequently, elderly persons use more drugs than any other age group. The normal function of each system and organ of the body changes during the aging process. However, some functions in the human body do not show age-related changes. There are three factors that are associated with the aging process: physiological, pathophysiological, and sociogenic or behavioral. The principles of drug therapy in elderly patients are based on efficacy and safety, dosage, complexity of regimen,

number of drugs, cost, and patient compliance. Many disorders and conditions are more common in elderly men, women, or both. The most common diseases seen in elderly persons in the United States have been selectively discussed. Several classes of drugs that are commonly prescribed for elderly patients should be given special consideration because of their side effects, drug interactions, and dosages. They include anticoagulants, glaucoma medications, analgesics, antihypertensives, cold remedies, antiemetics, and benzodiazepines.

EXPLORING THE WEB

Visit the following websites and search for articles and information related to the body as it ages and the effects of pharmacotherapy in the elderly:

- **www.nlm.nih.gov/medlineplus**
- **https://postgradmed.org**
- **http://healthlibrary.stanford.edu**
- **www.adaa.org**
- **www.americangeriatrics.org**
- **http://www.americangeriatrics.org/files/ documents/beers/PrintableBeersPocketCard .pdf**

REVIEW QUESTIONS

Multiple Choice

1. Which of the following disorders is the most common cause of death in the United States?

    A. cancer

    B. AIDS

    C. rheumatoid arthritis

    D. heart disease

2. The goal of treatment for osteoporosis includes:

    A. stopping the aging process

    B. preventing additional fractures and controlling pain

    C. preventing surgery for pathologic fractures and controlling pain

    D. stopping the use of hormone replacement

3. In postmenopausal women, reduced estrogen blood levels have been linked to increased incidence of which of the following conditions or diseases?

    A. upper respiratory tract infections

    B. rheumatoid arthritis

    C. breast cancer

    D. cardiovascular disease

4. Which of the following drugs requires a lower dosage in elderly persons because of reduction of renal function?

    A. warfarin

    B. gentamicin

    C. digoxin

    D. ranitidine

5. Which of the following medications in elderly patients may cause falls and hip fractures?

    A. thiazides

    B. diazepam

    C. vitamin B$_{12}$

    D. cimetidine

6. Which of the following is not linked to the physiological changes that occur with aging?

    A. reduction of cardiac output

    B. reduction of absorptive surfaces

    C. increased gastric emptying rate

    D. changes in gastric pH

7. All of the following are reasons for the greater incidence of adverse reactions of drugs in elderly individuals, *except*:

    A. increased total body fluid

    B. impaired drug metabolism

    C. decreased serum albumin levels

    D. medication errors are more likely to occur

8. Which of the following drugs has a large volume of distribution?

    A. diazepam

    B. acetaminophen

    C. digoxin

    D. ethanol

9. Which of the following body systems is the most important for elimination of the majority of drugs?

    A. digestive

    B. respiratory

    C. reproductive

    D. urinary

10. Which of the following agents can cause adverse effects such as gastritis, hypertension, and congestive heart failure?

    A. benzodiazepines

    B. antihistamines

    C. anticoagulants

    D. NSAIDs

11. The number of melanocytes and the amount of protective melanin in elderly people:

    A. increases

    B. decreases

    C. does not change

    D. depends on what types of medications are being taken

12. The most important route for the elimination of the majority of drugs includes which of the following?

    A. sweat

    B. saliva

    C. lungs

    D. kidneys

13. The effects of similar drug concentrations at the site of action are called:

    A. pharmacology

    B. pharmacokinetics

    C. pharmacodynamics

    D. pharmacogenetics

14. In the United States, how many people older than 65 years of age take prescription and non-prescription (over-the-counter) drugs?

    A. one half

    B. one fourth

    C. two thirds

    D. three fifths

15. Primary changes of aging are also known as:

    A. physiological aging changes

    B. pathophysiological aging changes

    C. sociogenic aging changes

    D. tertiary aging changes

Fill in the Blank

1. Anticholinergic properties of many over-the-counter cold remedies often cause adverse effects in elderly people. These effects include:

   a. _____

   b. _____

   c. _____

   d. _____

2. Scopolamine and the antihistamine meclizine prevent recurrent _____ in many elderly patients.

3. Longer-acting benzodiazepines should be avoided in elderly people because _____.

4. Many elderly patients with atrial fibrillation are not given anticoagulants because physicians fear _____ and secondary bleeding due to _____.

5. The most significant unmodifiable risk factor for stroke is _____.

6. Digoxin has a lower volume of distribution in elderly patients; therefore, doses _____.

7. Topical beta-blockers can cause systemic side effects in elderly patients, such as _____, _____, and _____.

Critical Thinking

A 65-year-old man has had a history of alcoholism for the past 20 years. He has been taking warfarin for the past 10 days. It is known that with cirrhosis of the liver, serum albumin decreases, as does hepatic blood flow.

1. What would be the consequences of taking warfarin in his condition?

2. Explain the hepatic clearance in elderly people who are suffering from liver diseases.

3. If this patient also takes phenytoin, what would be the potential outcome?

OUTLINE

OBJECTIVES

After completing this chapter, the reader should be able to:

1. Describe the terms *drug abuse* and *drug misuse*.
2. Explain tolerance, withdrawal, and addiction.
3. Identify the difference between physical and psychological dependence.
4. Discuss the most commonly abused drugs.
5. Explain the metabolism of alcohol.
6. Describe the symptoms of withdrawal from alcohol.
7. Identify the effects of nicotine on the brain.
8. Discuss the pharmacology of marijuana.
9. Describe the withdrawal symptoms of opioids.
10. Explain "club drugs."

GLOSSARY

Addiction – the condition of persistently and compulsively needing a substance or behavior; it may involve physical dependence, psychological dependence, or both

Cross-tolerance – extension of the tolerance for a substance to other substances of the same class, such as between alcohol and barbiturates

Delirium tremens – an acute, sometimes fatal episode of delirium usually caused by withdrawal or abstinence from alcohol following habitual excessive drinking; characterized by sweating, trembling, anxiety, confusion, and hallucinations

Ethanol – ethyl alcohol; a transparent, colorless, volatile, flammable liquid that is the primary ingredient of alcoholic beverages

Hallucinogens – agents capable of producing hallucinations, distortions of sensory perceptions, and disturbed emotions, judgments, and memories

Nucleus accumbens – a structure forming the floor of the caudal anterior area of the lateral brain ventricle; it is the area of the brain affected by most substances of abuse

Physical dependence – a form of dependence in which there is evidence of tolerance to a substance, withdrawal, or both

Psychological dependence – a form of dependence in which there is a need to use a substance in order to achieve a pleasurable mental experience

Rebound effects – emergence or reemergence of symptoms that were absent or controlled while taking a substance, but appear when that same substance is discontinued or reduced in dosage

Schedule drugs – drugs that have strict prescribing and availability criteria because of their potential for addiction or abuse

Sedatives – tranquilizers; substances that induce sedation by reducing irritability or excitement

Substance abuse – patterned use of a substance, often a drug, in which users consumes it in amounts or with methods that are harmful to themselves or to others

Tachyphylaxis – an acute, sudden decrease in response to a drug after it is administered

Withdrawal syndrome – a set of symptoms occurring in discontinuation or dosage reduction of various substances; it is more likely to occur in relation to higher dosages and longer periods of use

OVERVIEW

There are many drugs that are regularly misused and abused, as well as highly addictive. When a person self-administers a drug in a way that is not the intended, beneficial use, the term **substance abuse** is used to describe this situation. This term is preferred over the term *drug abuse* since many abused substances are not thought to be "drugs" by the people who use them. Today, substance abuse affects people from every socioeconomic class, often with devastating consequences. A controlled substance is one that has restricted usage by the Comprehensive Drug Abuse Prevention and Control Act of 1970, and its later revisions, including the Controlled Substances Act. Five drug schedules were created by this act to classify drugs of abuse. Therefore, **schedule drugs** are classified based on their potential for abuse as well as toxicity, with Schedule I drugs having the most serious effects, and Schedule V having the least.

The National Institute on Drug Abuse (NIDA) estimates that 10% of adults in the United States have abused drugs during their lifetimes. Trends show that more and more Americans accept that substance abuse is a *relatively normal* component of life. Though millions of dollars have been spent attempting to educate people and eradicate substance abuse, the results have not been outstanding. Pre-teenage children are now trying various substances, often becoming dependent upon them, at higher rates than ever before.

DRUG MISUSE AND ABUSE

> ## Medical Terminology Review
>
> **hallucination**
> hallucin- = to wander in mind
> -ation = action or process
> a sensory experience of something that does not exist outside the mind

The misuse and abuse of drugs often lead to **addiction**, which is the overwhelming desire to repeat use of the drug, even with serious consequences to health and lifestyle. Substance misuse is the improper use of substances that have been prescribed or acquired for legitimate therapeutic purposes. Continued abuse of substances is extremely individualized. Regardless of whether the desired effects are euphoria, sedation, pleasure, satisfaction, or even hallucinations, users often say that they enjoy the drug-taking experience and therefore continue these behaviors. Habituation defines repeated substance use in which the user feels better taking the substance than when not taking it.

So many factors have an influence on drug misuse and abuse that it is difficult to list them all. Substances that are abused differ in their costs and availability, speeds at which their effects occur, lengths that effects last, and types of administration—most commonly being smoked, swallowed, inhaled, or injected. People with more extreme risk-taking behaviors are often drawn into substance abuse. Often, a person with chronic pain becomes a substance abuser simply because of the desire to remove painful sensations. Users often state that they were pressured by their peers, or the conventions of their social groups or communities. In lower amounts, certain individuals begin using substances to expand their minds or consciousness.

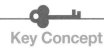

Key Concept

According to the National Institute on Drug Abuse, the abuse of alcohol, illicit drugs, and tobacco costs over $600 billion every year in relation to crimes, health care, and lost productivity. Of these, the overall cost of alcohol abuse is most expensive, totaling about $235 billion annually.

Long-term use of a legally prescribed drug such as a narcotic analgesic, used to relieve pain, often results in addiction. A patient with chronic pain may find that he or she is able to sleep or live without pain, or with significantly reduced pain, and becomes comfortable with these changes, desiring them to continue for life. Often, patients increase the dosages of these pain-relieving drugs over time, leading to a state of serious addiction. Significantly, use of prescription medications according to accepted medical standards *rarely* results in addiction. Risks of addiction from prescription medications are related to the doses taken and the length of continuance of the medication. Therefore, potentially addicting prescription medications are prescribed at the lowest effective doses, for the shortest time necessary.

INFLUENCE OF BEHAVIOR UPON DRUG ABUSE

Friends, family members, or casual acquaintances that abuse substances are often extremely influential upon another person's decision to do so. Substance abuse is often associated with specific surroundings and environments. Often, a person who has stopped abusing a substance returns to the behavior once he or she reenters a certain social situation in which abuse previously occurred.

The criterion for substance dependence, which may involve either physical and psychological dependence, or both, involves a maladaptive pattern of use that leads to clinically significant distress or impairment. This is manifested by three or more of the following factors, occurring at any time within a 12-month period:

- **Tolerance** – the individual requires highly increased amounts of the substance in order to achieve the desired effect or intoxication, and continued use of the same amount results in a greatly decreased effect. Tolerance is defined as a biological condition, in which the body adapts to a substance after continued administration. Development of tolerance is common for drugs that affect the nervous system. Tolerance is a natural result of continued use of a substance, but does not mean that an individual is addicted to or abusing the substance. Tolerance to various effects of a substance differs among these effects. Examples of slowly developing tolerance include drugs that reduce pain, and examples of quickly developing tolerance include drugs that cause nausea. With illicit drugs, tolerance is more dangerous, since increased dosages to achieve the same effect are more likely to result in an overdose. After discontinuing an abused drug, tolerance fades, often within 10 days to 2 weeks. However, if the individual returns to taking the drug at the same high dosage, it may be fatal. Rapid development of tolerance is known as tachyphylaxis, such as with amphetamines or cocaine, but also with prescribed medications

Medical Terminology
Review

tachyphylaxis
tachy- = swift or rapid
-phylaxis =protection
against an agent
a rapidly diminishing
response (tolerance) to
successive doses of a
drug.

Key Concept

It should be understood that "tolerance" is different from "resistance" or "immunity." Both resistance and immunity refer to the immune system, and not to the development of tolerance to a substance. Although a patient may become tolerant to morphine, he or she does not become resistant to its effects.

---

such as nitroglycerin. Tachyphylaxis can occur to adverse as well as therapeutic drug effects. Between two closely related or pharmacologically similar drugs, **cross-tolerance** may develop.

- **Withdrawal** – there is a characteristic withdrawal syndrome for the substance, and the same—or a closely related—substance is taken to avoid or relieve symptoms of withdrawal

- **Overdosage** – larger amounts of the substance are taken than were intended, or the substance is taken over a longer period of time than intended

- **Addiction** – the individual desires to control or reduce usage of the substance, but is unsuccessful in being able to do so

- **Time loss** – the individual spends much of his or her time trying to obtain the substance, use the substance, or recover from its effects

- **Activity loss** – use of the substance results in the individual giving up important recreational, occupational, or social activities

- **Awareness** – though the individual understands that he or she is physically or psychologically addicted, use of the substance continues; this may be true even when serious health problems begin to occur

Physical Dependence

When an individual's body adapts to repeated use of a substance and normal physiology becomes altered, **physical dependence** occurs. The cells of the body actually begin to treat the substance as "normal." Physical dependence is reversible by discontinuing use, but often results in uncomfortable, and sometimes severe, withdrawal symptoms. Extremely fast physical dependence often occurs with the use of *opioids* such as heroin or morphine, especially when they are injected intravenously. With extended use over time, physical dependence can easily occur from the use of alcohol, nicotine, central nervous system (CNS) depressants, and certain stimulants.

Physical dependence is not the same as addiction, and may occur during normal courses of therapy with prescription medications. A good example is physical dependence upon narcotic analgesics while a person is being treated for chronic pain. Withdrawal symptoms may occur when the substance is discontinued, but the person is not considered to be *addicted*. Rather, the term **addiction** is considered to mean compulsive and destructive substance use. In addicted patients, physical dependence is certainly a component of their addiction. Physical dependence is often overcome within a few days or weeks after the substance is discontinued.

Psychological Dependence

In **psychological dependence**, the individual has an overwhelming desire to continue use of the substance even though obvious negative physical, social, or economic consequences are occurring. This type of dependence produces no physical discomfort. Sometimes, psychological dependence is related to the individual's social contacts or a living situation that is not supportive. Psychological dependence often causes return to drug-seeking behaviors or relapses while the individual is in substance abuse therapy. With drugs such as antianxiety medications or marijuana, psychological dependence usually results from relatively high doses taken over a long period of time. However, an example of a substance that may cause psychological dependence after only one or a few uses is *crack cocaine*. Unlike physical dependence, psychological dependence on a substance may require months, years, or the individual's entire lifetime to overcome after the substance is discontinued.

COMMONLY ABUSED DRUGS

Though abused substances belong to many different classifications, the major factor that they share is that they affect the brain, often causing euphoria by enhancing dopamine secretion. This occurs in the area of the brain called the **nucleus accumbens**. One primary exception is the abuse of *anabolic steroids*, which affect the muscular system instead of the brain. Though federally listed illegal drugs such as heroin are routinely abused, many abused substances are prescription medications, such as alprazolam (Xanax®), methamphetamine (Desoxyn®), hydrocodone (Vicodin®), and oxycodone (OxyContin®). Tobacco products and alcohol are also among the most commonly abused substances. Illegal substances that are among the most abused include club drugs such as *ecstasy* and hallucinogens such as *lysergic acid diethylamide (LSD)*. Although cocaine is listed as a Schedule II drug, it is popular among illegal users, and is regularly abused.

Alcohol (Ethanol)

Ethanol is the most commonly abused substance in the United States. It is actually a CNS depressant, and is a form of alcohol that is also known as *ethyl alcohol*. Although small quantities of alcohol consumed on a daily basis have been shown to reduce the risk of stroke and heart attack, abuse may have devastating effects. According to the National Institute on Alcohol Abuse and Alcoholism, more than 15 million Americans have an alcohol use disorder, and according to the Centers for Disease Control and Prevention (CDC), more than half of Americans aged 12 and older have used alcohol at least once in the last month.

Alcohols are easily absorbed across the gastrointestinal tract, mostly from the small intestine, though foods slow absorption rates. Once alcohol enters the bloodstream, it is distributed to the tissues immediately and crosses the blood-brain barrier easily (Figure 28-1). Therefore, its effects on the brain may be seen in as little as 5 to 30 minutes after being consumed.

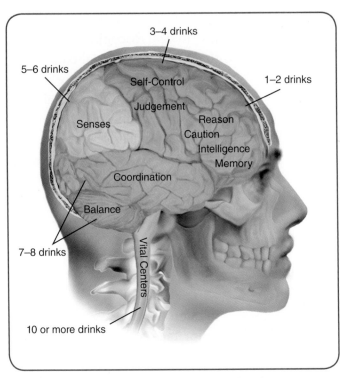

Figure 28-1 Alcohol and the blood-brain barrier.

Its metabolism and excretion is at a constant rate through the activity of the liver enzymes alcohol dehydrogenase and aldehyde dehydrogenase. Metabolism first yields acetaldehyde, and then acetic acid, which is also known as acetate (Figure 28-2). Differences in enzymatic activity between various groups of people mean that alcohol metabolism rates also differ. Those who drink alcohol more regularly have higher amounts of the metabolizing enzymes, meaning they can drink larger quantities without becoming intoxicated.

Elimination of blood alcohol declines at approximately 15 milligrams (mg) per hour, which is an unchangeable rate by any other substance. The average rate of metabolism is approximately one serving of alcohol per hour.

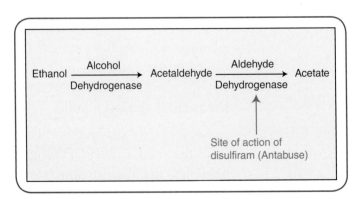

Figure 28-2 The metabolism of alcohol.

Breath testing to determine the amount of alcohol in the bloodstream is effective since it is vaporized and excreted by the lungs. Alcohol is classified as a CNS depressant because it reduces the ability of the brain to remain alert and wakeful. Symptoms of alcohol intoxication include relaxation, sedation, incoordination, decreased inhibition, and reduced judgment. It may also cause various degrees of amnesia, increased blood flow to the face, and in large amounts, severe hypotension, vomiting, respiratory failure, coma, and death.

When consumption of alcohol is chronic, the individual becomes both physically and psychologically dependent. The liver is the organ most damaged by alcohol abuse, with up to 90% of heavy drinkers developing hepatitis, or inflammation of the liver. Alcoholism often results in cirrhosis, which is a condition in which the liver cannot perform its normal, vital functions. Cirrhosis often results in the death of the alcoholic individual. When the liver is impaired, there may be abnormal blood clotting, nutritional deficiencies, and heightened sensitivity to other drugs. The brain is also damaged by chronic alcohol abuse, with memory and cognitive abilities becoming impaired.

Chronic alcoholism and its related malnutrition causes a deficiency of thiamine (vitamin B_1), which may result in Wernicke's encephalopathy. This condition is signified by mental status disorders, oculomotor abnormalities, and ataxia. Thiamine deficiency can cause cerebellar degeneration as well as neuropathy, which may involve cerebral hemorrhages. If treatment is delayed, a type of amnesia known as Korsakoff's amnestic syndrome may develop, or the patient may die from Wernicke's encephalopathy. It is essential to administer high doses of intravenous thiamine, as well as treat magnesium deficiency, as soon as possible.

For persons with alcoholism, doses of other drugs should be decreased in order to avoid toxicity, adverse drug effects, and drug interactions. Alcohol should never be combined with nonsteroidal anti-inflammatory agents (NSAIDs) such as aspirin because of the risk of gastrointestinal hemorrhage. When alcohol is combined with acetaminophen (Tylenol®), fatal liver damage can occur. Alcohol should also not be combined with other CNS depressants due to possible cumulative effects resulting in profound sedation, coma, and death. Combination with opioids, barbiturates, and benzodiazepines is often fatal. Pregnant women must avoid alcohol completely because of the risk of fetal alcohol syndrome, which causes birth defects and serious risks to normal health.

Withdrawal from alcohol is severe and possibly life threatening. Between 5% and 10% of withdrawal cases cause **delirium tremens**. Symptoms of this condition include confusion, intense agitation, paranoia, panic attacks, terrifying hallucinations, and uncontrollable tremors. One-third of patients with delirium tremens will die if untreated. This condition, as well as

Medical Terminology Review

cirrhosis
cirrh- = yellow/brown color (in reference to the liver)
-osis =process or disease condition
liver condition in which normal cells are replaced by scar tissue.

alcohol-related seizures *must* be prevented, which involves use of a benzodiazepine such as diazepam (Valium®) or lorazepam (Ativan®). If the patient is hallucinating, an antipsychotic agent such as haloperidol (Haldol®) may also be needed.

Alcohol dependence often requires long-term therapy with behavioral counseling and self-help groups such as Alcoholics Anonymous. Medications include disulfiram (Antabuse®) and naltrexone (Revia®). Disulfiram stops continued alcohol abuse by making the patient vomit, along with other unpleasant symptoms. It does this by causing the toxic substance acetaldehyde to build up in the patient's system. This agent is also the chemical responsible for causing a hangover after a night of binge drinking. However, disulfiram should not be used in patients who are at high risk of returning to their abuse of alcohol because reactions to the drug can be fatal.

To reduce the psychological craving for alcohol, naltrexone (Revia®) is indicated. It appears to act by blocking the "pleasant" effects of alcohol when it is first consumed. Without being able to enjoy its effects, the alcoholic therefore loses the craving. This drug is also used for opiate dependence and has been used to treat nicotine withdrawal. However, due to the potential severe opioid withdrawal, this drug should not be given to a patient who has taken opioids within five to seven days of administration.

The drug acamprosate calcium is used as an oral anti-alcoholic drug. It interacts with glutamate and gamma-aminobutyric acid (GABA) neurotransmitter systems, restoring the balance between neuronal excitation and inhibition that is altered by alcohol use. It is not metabolized by the liver, so patients with impairment of liver function can receive acamprosate calcium in the same dosages as those with normal liver function. This drug is not effective in patients who are still consuming alcohol, but has promising results in those who have stopped drinking and wish to remain alcohol-free. It does not affect withdrawal symptoms, and patients must be monitored for suicidal ideation and behaviors. It is used along with counseling and psychosocial support programs.

Nicotine

Nicotine stimulates the cardiovascular and central nervous systems, and is a significantly addictive drug. It is classified differently from the CNS stimulants, however. Nicotine is a legal drug, found in all tobacco products. Though the tar and chemicals found in tobacco products are carcinogenic, nicotine itself has not been proven to have cancer-causing properties. It is the single most heavily used legal and addictive drug in the United States, with more than 29% of the population affected. Through education, use of tobacco products is decreasing, but more than half of all teenagers admit to having tried cigarettes. This is important for everyone, since even nonsmokers are prone to lung cancer from inhaling second-hand smoke.

Nicotine is most commonly inhaled by smoking cigarettes, pipes, or cigars. There are several thousand chemicals in tobacco smoke, many of which are carcinogenic. Nicotine reaches the brain in 15 seconds, and its effects last between 30 minutes and several hours. Its half-life is only two to three hours, but the drug accumulates and is only released slowly from body tissues. Most body systems are affected by nicotine, and it works by stimulating release of epinephrine to directly stimulate the reticular activating system of the brain.

Symptoms caused by nicotine use include increased alertness and focus, relaxation, light-headedness, general overall pleasure, accelerated heart rate, and increased blood pressure. The cardiovascular effects of nicotine are significant, but more serious in smokers who also take oral contraceptives. These people have a risk of fatal myocardial infarction that is five times higher than nonsmokers who take oral contraceptives. Nicotine produces muscle tremor in moderate doses, and convulsions in high doses. In general, body weight is reduced since metabolism is increased and appetite is decreased. Chronic smoking leads to emphysema, heart disease, and lung cancer. Smoking also leads to infertility, birth defects, and low birth weight of infants.

Nicotine causes quick psychological and physical dependence. Users usually continue to use tobacco products for many years, finding themselves unable to quit even though they are aware of the negative aspects of the habit. Of those people who try to quit smoking, only one out of four remain tobacco-free within one year. The withdrawal symptoms when quitting the use of tobacco products include agitation, problems concentrating, anxiety, weight gain, headache, and severe cravings for the drug. Withdrawal syndrome peaks at 24 to 48 hours after the final dose, but may continue over several weeks. Each individual has a different experience trying to quit, and symptoms are not consistent compared with duration of use or doses that were usually taken. About 90% of individuals quit smoking without any form of treatment.

Drugs for smoking cessation were discussed in detail in Chapter 16. Nicotine replacement therapy (NRT) is based on proven results of falling blood nicotine levels, which prompt cravings for nicotine. This form of therapy may be administered by chewing gum, transdermal patches, or nasal sprays (see Table 16-8). They work by raising serum nicotine levels to reduce unpleasant withdrawal symptoms. This is not effective on its own for many patients. The drug bupropion, sold as Zyban®, helps to reduce cravings and doubles the chance that the individual will remain tobacco-free if it is continued for three to six months. Bupropion was originally designated only as an antidepressant, but helps nearly half of all former smokers to quit successfully. It is often given along with NRT.

The newest drug used to manage nicotine withdrawal is varenicline (Chantix®), which is administered in increased dosages over an eight-day period, and then at a maintenance level for 12 to 24 weeks. It activates nicotine receptors in the brain, reducing withdrawal symptoms and cravings. Varenicline also blocks nicotine from reaching its receptors, so that those who relapse and restart smoking can derive no pleasure from the habit. The drug often causes nausea and vomiting, and carries an alert warning patients to watch for agitation, behavior changes, depression, and suicidal ideation. Some patients have attempted suicide while taking the drug, and unfortunately, some have succeeded.

Marijuana and Other Cannabinoids

Marijuana is classified as a cannabinoid, and is the most frequently abused illicit substance. Cannabinoids are naturally derived products from the hemp plant (*Cannabis sativa*), which is most prevalent in tropical regions. Other cannabinoids include hashish and hash oil. Hashish is a solid and dry resin of the plant that has high potency, while hash oil is made by dissolving either hashish or marijuana in alcohol or another solvent, and allowing the liquid to evaporate. This forms a thick and oily concentrated form of cannabis.

There are over 70 natural cannabinoid substances, with the primary psychoactive properties provided by *tetrahydrocannabinol (THC)*. This agent increases pulse rate, has differing effects on blood pressure, creates a feeling of euphoria, and reddens the conjunctiva. It also affects the senses, memory, and cognition while decreasing motor coordination and increasing appetite. Through selective cultivation and plant breeding, varieties of *Cannabis* today have much higher THC concentrations than in previous times. Hash oil contains the most THC, between 30% and 80% of its content, followed by hashish with 20% to 60% and marijuana with 5% to 25%.

Humans, as well as many other animals, produce natural *endocannabinoids* that allow for intercellular communication. Endocannabinoids have similar characteristics as neurotransmitters and are able to modulate neuronal function. They are structurally similar to THC, and bind to the same cannabinoid receptors (CB1 and CB2). Both agonists and antagonists to these receptors are being researched to develop new pharmacological agents.

Marijuana is commonly known as pot, weed, dope, grass, or reefer. More than 40% of the population over the age of 12 years in the United States has tried marijuana. It is most commonly smoked as cigarettes called joints, but is also used in pipes, teas, or mixed into foods such as brownies and other desserts. However, marijuana that is consumed orally results in a lower serum blood level than when it is inhaled. When marijuana is inhaled, effects begin within a few minutes and last from one to three hours. Motor activities and coordination decrease and thoughts become disconnected as euphoria develops. The use of marijuana is usually pleasant, causing laughter and increased perception of colors, sounds, and thoughts. When the drug is taken with other people, the experience is usually more pleasant than when taken alone. Perception of time is altered, and the user is hungrier and thirstier than usual, most commonly craving sweets such as chocolate. The eyes become red because of dilation of optic blood vessels.

However, after the euphoria of cannabinoids subsides, the user may become depressed, sleepy, or paranoid. Driving is partially impaired when cannabinoids are used alone, but since these drugs are often combined with alcohol, can become particularly dangerous. Most significant is the fact that marijuana or hashish smoke introduces *four times* as many particulates such as tar into the lungs as tobacco smoking. This is because cannabinoids are inhaled much more deeply and held in the lungs for a longer period of time. Therefore, daily smoking of cannabinoids greatly increases the risk of lung cancer and respiratory disorders. Chronic use results in apathy and lack of motivation. Extremely high doses cause hallucinations. Since THC accumulates in reproductive tissues, cases of decreased spermatogenesis and amenorrhea have been reported.

Marijuana produces very little physical dependence or tolerance in its usual doses. Withdrawal symptoms are generally mild or nonexistent. Chronic abuse of high doses, however, causes irritability, insomnia, and restless when the drug is discontinued, and psychological dependence also occurs. It is easy to determine if a person has used THC since its metabolites remain in the body for months to years. It can also be detected in the urine if used within three to five days prior to the test, even if only a single dose was taken.

Today, marijuana is legal in certain states, but this remains controversial. Clinically, THC reduces eyeball pressure in patients with glaucoma, and reduces nausea and vomiting in patients on chemotherapy. It also reduces muscle spasticity in patients with multiple sclerosis and similar disorders. However, the current drugs used for these same conditions have been proven to be more effective and safer to use. The medical value of marijuana has not been proven, and federally, it remains a Schedule I drug, with no FDA-approved uses.

Cocaine

Cocaine is a CNS stimulant that is naturally derived from the coca plant of South America. In the Andes mountain regions, the coca plant is chewed for its effects, or tea is made from its leaves. The majority of cocaine that enters the United States comes from Columbia, followed by other South American countries. Cocaine was formerly used as a legal anesthetic. It is a Schedule II drug with psychoactive and physiological actions that are similar to amphetamines, but with faster, more intense actions. The drug is usually diluted with various powders before it is sold, so that by the time a user purchases it, it is only about 40% as pure as its initial form.

Cocaine is the second-most commonly used illicit drug in the United States. It is most commonly inhaled, but also is smoked and injected. Inhalation or injection causes instant euphoria that lasts for 10 to 20 seconds. Small doses of cocaine produce intense euphoria, illusions of strength, decreased hunger and pain, and increased sensory perception. In large doses, these effects increase, but less pleasurable effects also occur, including dysrhythmias, rapid heartbeat, pupil dilation, elevated body temperature, and sweating. Cocaine users often appear hyperexcited, very talkative, and impulsive in their actions.

Cocaine has a short half-life of between 60 and 90 minutes when injected, and tolerance quickly develops. The short half-life results in addicts taking the drug at intervals of 10 to 45 minutes, often over several days in a row. Cardiovascular damage from the drug is slowly progressive. After the last dose, cocaine remains in the user's hair cells for between two and six months.

If cocaine is taken when a woman is pregnant, the fetus experiences prolonged drug effects, since the immature liver cannot metabolize it. This results in preterm labor, increased risk of miscarriage, low birth weight, and sometimes, birth defects. The newborn has difficulties in feeding, is easily startled, and experiences increased irritability.

Adverse effects of cocaine are similar to those of amphetamines. The metabolite formed by the liver is more toxic than the drug itself. Once the user loses the sense of euphoria, he or she usually experiences exhaustion, irritability, depression, insomnia, and extreme distrust. The skin may "crawl," as if covered with insects. Those who inhale the drug develop a chronically runny nose, crusting and redness around the nostrils, and deterioration of nasal cartilage. Cocaine overdose often causes dysrhythmias, seizures, stroke, or death from respiratory arrest. Psychological dependence often leads to intense cravings for cocaine.

Amphetamines and Methylphenidate

Amphetamines and methylphenidate, like cocaine, are also CNS stimulants, which increase the activity of the central nervous system. Although CNS stimulants are legally prescribed to treat attention deficit/hyperactivity disorder (ADHD), as well as narcolepsy, they are commonly abused. Many of these agents are used as club drugs, though they are not hallucinogens.

Amphetamines increase the effects of norepinephrine, dopamine, and serotonin. The activity of norepinephrine on the brain's reticular formation results in heightened awareness, wakefulness, self-confidence, euphoria, elevated mood, and empowerment. The appetite is suppressed, and the individual can perform without fatigue for an extended period of time. Many of the physiological actions of various amphetamines are similar to actions of the sympathetic nervous system. They also increase heart rate, breathing rate, and blood pressure. Additional symptoms include sweating, dilated pupils, and tremors. However, certain stimulants, when taken excessively, cause dysrhythmias, seizures, stroke, and cardiac arrest.

Long-term use of amphetamines results in anxiety, restlessness, defensiveness, and often when "coming down" from lengthy periods of use, extreme rage. When used chronically, amphetamines can cause psychosis that is similar to paranoid schizophrenia, though this usually subsides after a few days following discontinuation of the drugs. Tolerance to amphetamines occurs very quickly, especially if they are injected.

Though previously prescribed for various medical conditions up to the 1970s, amphetamines and dextroamphetamines now have only limited therapeutic uses because of their adverse effects and abuse potential. They are now usually obtained from illegal laboratories. Interestingly, physical dependence is unusual, and the only significant withdrawal symptom is depression. Dextroamphetamine, under the trade name Dexedrine®, is used for short-term weight loss when all other attempts have failed, and also for narcolepsy.

Methamphetamine, commonly known as ice, meth, or speed, is used recreationally because of its intense euphoria. This drug is one of the most popular and dangerous of all amphetamines. It is usually taken in powder or crystal form, with this latter form being known as crystal meth, though the drug can also be smoked. Methamphetamine is a Schedule II drug, legally marketed under the trade name Desoxyn®. Illegally, it can be easily synthesized from the over-the-counter (OTC) decongestant pseudoephedrine. Therefore, most states require pharmacies to keep pseudoephedrine behind the counter and require purchasers to register when they buy it. The quantities that can be purchased are limited by law. Manufacturers are now replacing pseudoephedrine in their cold and flu remedies with other drugs. Similar in structure to methamphetamine, a drug known as methcathinone or Cat, is a Schedule I agent that is made illegally. It is administered by inhalation, orally, or by intravenous injection.

Methylphenidate (Ritalin®) is a CNS stimulant used for children with attention deficit/hyperactivity disorder because it calms inattentive or hyperactive symptoms. It stimulates alertness and the ability to focus. This Schedule II drug acts in similar ways to cocaine and amphetamines. Therefore, it is often abused by teenagers and adults to experience euphoria, increased alertness, or to suppress the appetite. Commonly, tablets are crushed so that they can be inhaled or dissolved in liquid for intravenous injection. Ritalin® is occasionally mixed with heroin in a combination referred to as a speedball. It is usually obtained illegally by diverting legal prescriptions, by patients selling or sharing it with others, and by theft.

Caffeine

Caffeine is a CNS stimulant found naturally in more than 63 species of plants. It is commonly found in coffee, chocolate, tea, ice cream, and soft drinks.

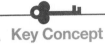

Key Concept

Recent studies have shown that caffeine, in recommended amounts, has antioxidant activity that fights the free radicals that are linked to heart disease and Alzheimer's disease. Therefore, drinking two to three cups of coffee per day, but no more, may have significant antioxidant benefits.

Caffeine is added to certain OTC stimulants and analgesics to increase their effects. The drug is quickly distributed throughout the body, and requires several hours to be completely metabolized and eliminated. It causes significant diuresis. Caffeine produces increased alertness, nervousness, restlessness, insomnia, and irritability. The blood pressure increases, respiratory passages dilate, stomach acid production increases, and blood glucose levels are altered. When use of caffeine is repeated, there may be physical dependence and tolerance. Withdrawal from caffeine causes fatigue, severe headache, depression, and impaired ability to perform daily activities.

Opioids

Opioids are CNS depressants and are also known as opiates or narcotic analgesics. Like all of these depressants, they cause relaxation or sedation. Most CNS depressants are legal substances, but their high abuse potential causes them to be strictly controlled. Opioids are prescribed for anesthesia, severe pain, persistent pain, and diarrhea that may be life threatening. This class of drugs include natural substances that come from the seeds of the poppy plant *Papaver somniferum*, including opium, codeine, and morphine. Also included are synthetic drugs such as fentanyl (Duragesic®), meperidine (Demerol®), methadone (Dolophine®), oxycodone (OxyContin®), and the illegal drug heroin.

Effects of opioids begin in 30 minutes and can last longer than 24 hours. If opium is smoked or injected, the rush of euphoria is immediate. Effects include extreme pleasure, profound sedation, slowed body activities, constricted pupils (miosis), slurred speech, increased pain threshold, and respiratory depression. Tolerance usually develops quickly, with addicts often needing 10 times higher doses to achieve desired effects. Dependence also occurs rapidly. Though these substances often cause initial sweating, itching, nausea, and vomiting, these symptoms are transitory and usually cease soon after use becomes regular. Over time, the pleasant effects far exceed the unpleasant effects.

Withdrawal causes intense, unpleasant symptoms within only a few hours after parenteral agents are discontinued, and within three to five days after oral opiates are discontinued. Withdrawal symptoms include diaphoresis, dysphoria, lacrimation, violent yawning, pupil dilation (mydriasis), rhinorrhea, diarrhea, fever, goose bumps, muscle cramping, and tremor. However, withdrawal is usually not life threatening, and there is no delirium. Withdrawal peaks within 36 to 72 hours after discontinuation of parenteral opioids. For withdrawal from low to moderate doses, withdrawal symptoms resemble those of influenza, and are relatively mild. An infant born to a mother using opioids will experience withdrawal symptoms after birth.

Although methadone is also addictive, it is a narcotic that has been the conventional treatment of choice for opioid addiction, such as from heroin.

Methadone acts as an antagonist to heroin. In some cases, methadone treatment is maintained over the life of the patient to combat recurrent heroin addiction. Otherwise, methadone is gradually reduced over approximately six months, with less intense symptoms but more prolonged withdrawal. Additional treatments for opioid dependence include buprenorphine (Subutex®) and buprenorphine/naloxone (Suboxone®). Outpatient management is preferred. A significant problem with buprenorphine is that abusers may crush the pills, dissolve the powder, and inject it intravenously. This is the reason why naloxone is added, since it is an opioid antagonist that blocks the euphoric effects of buprenorphine and also induces withdrawal symptoms if the combination drug is injected.

The use of oxycodone (OxyContin®) as an abused drug has become extremely prevalent in recent years. It contains 10 to 160 mg of active drug per tablet, in comparison to the 2.5 to 10 mg of active drug found in earlier formulations known as Percodan® or Percocet®. When Oxycontin® tablets are crushed, dissolved, and injected, the rush of euphoria resembles those of heroin or morphine. Usually, this drug is obtained by being diverted from medical sources through fake prescriptions, selling of prescriptions to other individuals, and theft from pharmacies or other patients.

Heroin has continued to be in the news because it is widely trafficked, especially in urban areas. Users often commit criminal acts in order to support their addiction, and the drug has claimed the lives of many people, including successful and wealthy celebrities. Death from heroin abuse is most prevalent in urban males between 15 and 35 years of age. Unlike many other abused substances, heroin use is increasing in the United States.

For all opioids, there are now many programs that are based on total abstinence from using all types of drugs. Many of these programs are run by formal drug users, who offer firsthand experience and support. They aim at helping addicts develop a more positive self-image and to learn how to be a valuable member of society without the use of substances.

Sedatives and Antianxiety Drugs

Sedatives are also known as tranquilizers and sedative-hypnotics. They are CNS depressants mostly prescribed for sleep disorders and certain types of epilepsy. The primary classes of sedatives are barbiturates and nonbarbiturate sedative-hypnotics, which have similar actions, uses, addiction potentials, and safety profiles. Over time, high levels of barbiturates cause both physical and psychological dependence. Barbiturates are often dangerously combined with alcohol or CNS stimulants. Once addicted, individuals often use barbiturates to sleep and amphetamines to stay awake—a severe and damaging cycle of abuse.

Signs and symptoms of sedative abuse include slurred speech, incoordination, and an apathetic attitude toward life. Commonly abused barbiturates include amobarbital (Amytal®), pentobarbital (Nembutal®), phenobarbital (Luminal®), and secobarbital (Seconal®). Today, safer alternatives to barbiturates and nonbarbiturate sedative-hypnotics are prescribed more frequently. Still, overdoses of both of these types of sedatives are very dangerous because they suppress the brain's respiratory centers. Extremely high doses often cause coma, cessation of breathing, and death. Withdrawal syndrome from these drugs is similar to that of alcohol, and may be fatal.

Benzodiazepines began to replace barbiturates in the 1970s due to their relative safeness for use. They are classified as antianxiety agents rather than sedatives. Benzodiazepines are prescribed frequently, which has recently resulted in a significant rise in their abuse by younger adults and teenagers. As well as treating anxiety, they are prescribed for seizures, muscle spasms, and sleep disorders. Common benzodiazepines include alprazolam (Xanax®), clonazepam (Klonopin®), diazepam (Valium®), midazolam (Versed®), temazepam (Restoril®), and triazolam (Halcion®).

One of the most common benzodiazepines reported as an abused drug is flunitrazepam (Rohypnol®) because it causes anterograde amnesia, in which the user cannot remember anything that happened while under its influence. Its effects begin within 30 minutes and last for eight hours or more, leaving the user conscious but unaware of the actions of themselves or others. This has resulted in it being called the date-rape drug, because it has been used by sexual predators who have "dosed" others with flunitrazepam in order to commit physical assaults. This benzodiazepine is not approved by the FDA for specific medical conditions, but has been used for patients with insomnia who do not respond to conventional medications. It is listed as a Schedule IV drug.

Abusers of benzodiazepines often mix them with alcohol, cocaine, or heroin, often with lethal results. High doses of benzodiazepines cause disorientation, sleepiness, and a "detached" or worry-free attitude toward life. Serious respiratory depression does not occur, and death from overdose is rare when these drugs are used on their own. Withdrawal symptoms are not as severe as those of barbiturates. However, abrupt discontinuance of these agents results in anxiety, restlessness, shaking, and weakness within 12 hours. Additional symptoms may include nausea, vomiting, orthostatic hypotension, tremors, and seizures. Withdrawal symptoms are worse at two to three days after discontinuance, but then gradually subside over the next three to five days.

A naturally occurring substance known as *gamma-hydroxybutyric acid (GHB)* is another commonly abused CNS depressant. Under the trade name Xyrem®, GHB is used for narcoleptics who have excessive sleepiness during the daytime, or weak or paralyzed muscles, which are known as cataplexy. Confusingly, the FDA classifies GHB as a Schedule I drug, but its inclusion as part of the formula of Xyrem® is classified as Schedule III. It is abused in order to produce euphoria, even at low doses. The active ingredient *GHB* has the same properties as flunitrazepam, and it has also been used as a date-rape drug. It is often slipped into a beverage without any indication of it being present, and consumed by the intended victim. Overdose may result in severe respiratory depression, seizures, vomiting, coma, and death. There is no known antidote.

Anabolic Steroids

Anabolic steroids are commonly abused in an attempt to increase muscle strength and physical performance. They do not affect the nervous system like the other drugs of abuse. The effects of anabolic steroids are slow, requiring months in order to be seen. The term *anabolic* means growth, and anabolic steroids are similar to testosterone, which is the primary androgen or male sex hormone. They add to skeletal muscle mass and increase the user's strength; hence their abuse most commonly occurs in athletes. Anabolic steroids have been proven to greatly improve physical performance. They are now banned by most sports organizations, and athletes are regularly tested for the presence of steroids. When these agents are found in user's systems, they are usually disqualified and eliminated from competition. Other users take anabolic steroids to enhance their physical appearance.

Medically, anabolic steroids are administered as replacement therapy for men who secrete inadequate amounts of testosterone, as well as being sometimes used to treat certain types of cancer. Therapeutic doses are 10 to 100 times lower than the amounts used by abusers of anabolic steroids. They are usually obtained by diversion from prescription medications, or from illegal laboratories. Anabolic steroids are administered as intramuscular injections, tablets, ointments, or through transdermal patches. Often, the abuser takes two or more types of steroids at the same time, often in different routes of administration, which is a process called *stacking*. An abuser may also take steroids in a cyclical pattern known as *pyramiding*, with doses progressively increased over 6 to 12 weeks, then slowly decreased until they are no longer taken. It is commonly believed that stacking and pyramiding are safe methods of using anabolic steroids, but this has not been proven.

Eventually, anabolic steroids produce opposite effects to those that they initially caused. Although masculinity is enhanced at first, eventually these substances cause impotence, infertility, gynecomastia, and testicular atrophy. When women take these drugs, they develop masculine characteristics such as hirsutism, menstrual irregularities, deepening of the voice, and shrinkage of breast tissue. In both sexes, the most serious adverse effects include elevated cholesterol, hepatic cysts, myocardial infarction, and stroke. The personality may change, with users becoming aggressive, violent, depressed, anorexic, and experiencing decreased libido and insomnia.

Anabolic steroids are Schedule II drugs because of their abuse potential. The U.S. Congress passed the Anabolic Steroid Control Act in 2004 to control androstenedione (Andro®), as well as 25 other steroid precursors. These precursor agents had been sold as dietary supplements legally, but were found to metabolize to steroids once inside the body, with the same health risks. One strange fact is that the popular supplement *dehydroepiandrosterone (DHEA)* was intentionally omitted from the list of banned precursors and is still legally sold OTC. This agent is a natural steroid precursor that is secreted by the adrenal glands, and many people believe it has performance-enhancing and anti-aging properties. Its exclusion from the banned list of precursors may be because it is considered safer than the other precursors, or because of political lobbying by the dietary supplement manufacturers.

LSD, Club Drugs, and Other Hallucinogens

Hallucinogens produce a state of consciousness that can be described as "dream-like." Many users experience a feeling of being more connected with other people, as well as a higher "plane" of consciousness that seems spiritual. Commonly called *psychedelics,* hallucinogens first came to significant public awareness in the 1960s with the drug known as lysergic acid diethylamide (LSD). Other hallucinogens have been more recently termed *club drugs* because they are used in nightclubs to intensify the social and musical experiences that exist there. The effects of hallucinogens differ widely, based on the drugs used and individual expectations. These drugs are seldom taken on a continual basis, but are used for special events and occasions.

Lysergic acid diethylamide was a legal agent until it began to be popularly used in the 1960s. Common names for LSD include acid, blotter acid, California sunshine, and the beast. It is derived from a fungus that grows on grains such as rye, and is usually administered orally in liquid, capsule, or tablet forms. Often, LSD liquid is placed onto papers that are printed with images of the drug culture or cartoon characters. Once dried, the paper is cut into small squares, with each square representing one dose. The squares are consumed so that the drug can take effect. Even as little as 25 micrograms (mcg) of LSD can produce an effect. The drug is distributed throughout the body quickly, with effects beginning within one hour, and lasting from 6 to 12 hours. The drug affects the central and autonomic nervous systems. The user experiences increased blood pressure and body temperature, dry mouth, dilated pupils, piloerection or erection of the hair, and increased heart rate.

Hallucinogens such as LSD are used for their psychoactive effects, and not their physical effects. The user often experiences deep personal insights, religious revelations, and laughter, with many people reporting hallucinations and afterimages projected onto others whenever they move. Bright lights and vivid colors are common. Some people report hearing voices that are not actually there, or reverse sensibilities known as *synesthesia,* such as "hearing colors" or "seeing sounds." The sense of time is altered, and the user is able to focus thoughts with more intensity.

Serious adverse effects of LSD include acute anxiety, terrifying perceptions, confusion, panic attacks, paranoia, and severe depression. If use is repeated, the individual may lack reasoning abilities and experience impaired memory. Flashbacks, which may occur with no warning, are common. They involve experiencing the effects of the drug weeks, months, or years after it was taken. Though LSD is a recreational drug that rarely causes dependence, tolerance occurs very quickly, often within two to three days. There are no withdrawal symptoms.

Drugs that are similar to LSD include psilocybin, mescaline, and dimethyltryptamine (DMT). In general, these agents are not as potent, and they are less commonly abused. Psilocybin is the main psychoactive ingredient in over 100 species of mushrooms that grow mostly in Mexico and Central America. Commonly known as magic mushrooms or shrooms, psilocybin is metabolized to an active form known as psilocin. Possession of mushrooms containing psilocybin is illegal, and both psilocybin and psilocin are listed as Schedule I drugs. Users cultivate the mushrooms indoors and the drug is taken by either eating the fresh mushrooms or ingesting dried extracts.

Mescaline comes from the peyote cactus and similar species in Mexico and Central America. In most cases, the drug is packaged into capsules that contain dried forms of the cactus. These plants grow very slowly in their natural states, and are rare because of overharvesting. Peyote is an illegal drug in the United States, except for members of the Native American Church, where it is part of religious ceremonies.

Dimethyltryptamine is a natural substance that actually exists in humans in tiny amounts, but is also found in many plants growing in the Caribbean islands, Central America, and South America. This hallucinogen was also used to induce visions by native cultures during spiritual ceremonies. DMT is usually smoked, but is also taken by inhalation, injection, or in oral forms. It is closely related to the hallucinogen known as *5-MeO-DMT*, which is a powerful psychedelic tryptamine used by South American shamans for centuries.

Club drugs include a large variety of hallucinogens preferred by younger people to enhance nightclub and party environments. Many people combine club drugs with large amounts of alcohol. Also, there are other club drugs that are not classified as hallucinogens. Of the hallucinogenic club drugs, perhaps the most popular is *MDMA* or *3,4-methylenedioxymethamphetamine,* which is commonly called ecstasy or XTC, and more recently, Molly. It is a synthetic amphetamine with both hallucinogenic and stimulant effects that lasts for three to six hours when taken orally. The user's emotions and general awareness are enhanced, and he or she is able to remain awake and active for a long time, often becoming socially extroverted in behaviors. The drug has a narrow therapeutic index, and may be fatal if overdosage occurs. Chronic users experience anxiety, depression, hostility, and insomnia.

Because of the common belief that it enhances sexual desire, *MDA or 3,4-methylenedioxyamphetamine* is called the love drug. It is sometimes a component of ecstasy. Also used in "rave parties," the drug commonly known as *STP* has effects similar to those of LSD, but which last longer. Its actual name is *2,5 dimethoxy-4-methylamphetamine (DOM).*

A drug that originated as a prescribed anesthetic, but which was removed from the market in 1965, *phencyclidine* is used to produce a trance-like state, with no loss of consciousness, for several days. Commonly known as PCP, angel dust, or crystal, this drug is taken by inhalation, tablet forms, or by sprinkling on marijuana and smoking the mixture. Phencyclidine is responsible for many deaths because of its effects, which include detachment from reality, slurred speech, a sense of "floating," time distortion, violent panic attacks, seizures, and coma. Tolerance develops with continuous use, and hallucinations are not produced.

A similar drug to phencyclidine, ketamine was formerly used as an anesthetic. It is commonly known as special K, kitkat, or K. It is often stolen from veterinary offices so that its liquid form may be mixed into drinks or injected. It also may be evaporated to a solid form that can be inhaled or taken in pills. Ketamine is now more popular than phencyclidine as a club drug, with similar effects, though these last for only 35 to 40 minutes. High doses may cause amnesia and loss of consciousness. With continued use, psychoses can develop.

One of the only substances used as a club drug that is legally sold is known as *dextromethorphan, DXM, or robo.* Dextromethorphan is an ingredient in OTC cold remedies, in which it acts as a cough suppressant. People abusing this drug will use the extra-strength cold remedies, but take them in large quantities to experience effects that are similar to phencyclidine and ketamine. These include dizziness, slurred speech, drowsiness, euphoria, and lack of coordination. If overdose occurs, the individual may experience brain damage, seizures, stroke, and hypothermia. Death may result. The combination of dextromethorphan with antihistamines, aspirin, or acetaminophen in various OTC cold remedies can result in toxicity when these remedies are consumed in larger than recommended quantities. Pure dextromethorphan is also available illegally compounded into high-dosage tablets.

Inhalants

Inhalants are vaporized substances that are breathed to achieve a high, a process known on the street as huffing. Some inhalants are in gaseous form while others are in liquid form, and they may be inhaled at room temperature, or heated. Many inhalants are soaked into a cloth or placed in a plastic or paper bag prior to being inhaled. Nearly any chemical that can be vaporized can be used. Commonly abused products include glues, adhesives, aerosols, cleaning agents, fuels, and solvents. These are easily obtained from office supply or hardware stores, and the majority of users are teenagers and older children. Other inhalants include legal anesthetics such as nitrous oxide, which are sometimes used by people with access to them in the medical workplace. A recreational inhalant that is often used in party environments is *amyl nitrite*, commonly referred to as "poppers."

Inhaled substances act very quickly, with the majority able to enter the brain since they are lipid-soluble. General effects of inhalants include drowsiness, light-headedness, euphoria, and exhilaration. Many people report experiencing hallucinations. Many parents are unaware of exactly what their child or teenager is doing since the effects resemble alcohol intoxication. Most of the psychoactive effects disappear within a few minutes, causing users to continue huffing many times over a few hours. This is extremely dangerous, since high doses and repeated exposures are linked to coma and even death.

Dangerous chemicals found in various inhalants are quite diverse. Gasoline, rubber cement, and spray paints contain *toluene*, which has claimed the lives of not only abusers but people who worked in manufacturing facilities that used the substance. Other inhaled substances found in workplaces and various industries, with serious potential dangers, include chlorinated hydrocarbons, hexane, benzene, methylene chloride, and butane.

Physical dependence is usually not seen since inhalants commonly are used only on occasion. Tolerance has not been documented. Some users experience a hangover-like syndrome after psychoactive effects have disappeared. Chronic abuse of inhalants is most common in adult males, resulting in serious and permanent effects, mostly upon the nervous system. Symptoms of chronic inhalant use include cognitive impairment, incoordination, tremors, hallucinations, dementia, and psychosis. Certain inhalants cause nephrotoxicity. Users may have reduced breathing reflexes. There are documented cases of users placing plastic bags over their heads and suffocating. Treatment for inhalant abuse is based on symptoms, often requiring long-term behavioral therapy to help the user understand that continued and chronic abuse results in permanent damage.

TREATING ADDICTION

When a person has been determined to be physically dependant upon a substance, treatment begins with discontinuance of the substance. In cases where abrupt discontinuance occurs, the patient experiences a **withdrawal syndrome**. This may range between extremely severe and prolonged symptoms, or only minor symptoms, based on characteristics of the substance itself. In nearly all cases, withdrawal should be managed in a substance abuse treatment facility. Abrupt dosage reduction is avoided for specific medications due to health risks. Often, antagonist drugs are administered to assist in lessening withdrawal symptoms. Table 28-1 lists the treatments and withdrawal symptoms for commonly abused substances.

TABLE 28-1	Treatments and Withdrawal Symptoms for Commonly Abused Substances	
Substance	**Treatment**	**Withdrawal Symptoms**
Alcohol	Antiseizure agents, benzodiazepines; after withdrawal is over, disulfiram (Antabuse®) and naltrexone (Revia®) are used	Fatigue, tremors, abdominal cramping, anxiety, confusion, hallucinations, delirium, seizures
Nicotine	Bupropion (Wellbutrin®) or nicotine replacement therapy	Anxiety, irritability, headaches, restlessness, increased appetite, insomnia, decreased heart rate and blood pressure, inability to concentrate
Marijuana	No treatment required	Irritability, insomnia, restlessness, chills, tremor, weight loss
Cocaine and amphetamines	Behavioral therapy; no specific pharmacological treatment is available	Anxiety, mental depression, agitation, extreme fatigue, irritability, disturbed sleep, hunger, psychological craving
Opioids	Buprenorphine (Suboxone®)/methadone (Methadose®) therapy; clonidine (Catapres®; to reduce agitation, anxiety, cramping, and sweating); oxazepam (Serax®; to reduce insomnia and muscle spasms); antiemetics; detoxification usually completed in 2–3 days; withdrawal may be sped up with naltrexone along with propofol (Diprivan®), ondansetron (Zofran®), or octreotide (Sandostatin®); for other symptoms, clonidine and benzodiazepines may be used	Excessive sweating, dilated pupils, restlessness, agitation, goose bumps, tremor, increased heart rate and blood pressure, violent yawning, nausea, vomiting, abdominal cramps and pain, muscle spasms with kicking movement, weight loss
Barbiturates and other sedative-hypnotics	Same as alcohol: Antiseizure agents, benzodiazepines; after withdrawal is over, disulfiram (Antabuse®) and naltrexone (Revia®) are used	Anxiety, insomnia, abdominal cramps, weakness, anorexia, tremor, hallucinations, seizures, delirium
Benzodiazepines	Dosage must be gradually tapered over weeks or months; if there is acute intoxication, flumazenil (generic) is given by rapid IV infusion over 15–20 seconds	Insomnia, abdominal pain, irritability, nausea, headache, sensitivity to light and sound, fatigue, tremors
Anabolic steroids	Behavioral therapy; symptomatic treatment may require antidepressants	Fatigue, mood swings, anorexia, restlessness, insomnia, depression, reduced sex drive, psychological craving
Hallucinogens	Treatment not usually required; symptoms will resolve in approximately 12 hours; if PCP is involved, excretion is based on pH, with urine acidification increasing the clearance rate by about 100 times	Varied symptoms based on the type of hallucinogen; may include anxiety, insomnia, mental depression, panic attacks, paranoid delusions, lethargy

Key Concept

For all forms of addiction, effective treatment takes time as the former addict's brain slowly readjusts to normal, and new behaviors replace bad behaviors. The needs of the individual must be addressed, and treatment methods are often changed as therapy continues. While all treatments for substance addiction begin with detoxification, the patient's psychiatric and emotional balance must also be addressed in order for therapy to remain effective.

Some prescription drugs cause significant withdrawal symptoms when discontinued but are still not considered drugs of abuse. These include antidepressants, beta-blockers, anticonvulsants, and corticosteroids, which all cause physical dependence but not actual addiction. Patients do not realistically administer these drugs for any reason other than prescribed treatment regimens. These medications should be tapered off, and not stopped abruptly.

Commonly, withdrawal symptoms are generally opposite to the effects of the substance. A drug used to reduce anxiety usually causes anxiety when withdrawn, and a drug used to stay awake usually causes drowsiness when withdrawn. These are known as **rebound effects**. When they become severe, the individual often takes higher doses of the substance in order to counteract them. Often, addicted people say that they continue drug use in order to avoid withdrawal symptoms. This results in a cycle of continued substance abuse.

To break the cycle of substance abuse, counselors and therapists often encourage recovering individuals to avoid people who shared their behaviors. They are instructed about forming new social contacts and joining self-help groups, such as Alcoholics Anonymous or Narcotics Anonymous.

SUMMARY

Addiction is a serious consequence of substance misuse and abuse. People abuse substances for a variety of reasons, with the list of abused substances ranging from those that are legal, such as alcohol, to those that have no medical use, such as heroin. Many substance abusers are influenced to do so by friends, family members, and casual acquaintances that have similar behaviors. Many drugs result in the development of tolerance, causing the user to require increasing amounts in order to achieve the same effects. Dependence upon a substance may be physical, psychological, or both. The most commonly abused drugs are alcohol, nicotine, cannabinoids such as marijuana, cocaine and other CNS stimulants, opioids and other CNS depressants, anabolic steroids, hallucinogens, and inhalants. Treatment for substance abuse and addiction usually requires discontinuance, withdrawal, antagonist drugs, counseling, and self-help groups.

EXPLORING THE WEB

Visit the following websites and search for articles and information related to misused, abused, and addictive drugs:

- http://www.streetdrugs.org
- http://whyquit.com
- www.aa.org (Alcoholics Anonymous)
- www.ca.org (Cocaine Anonymous)
- www.drugabuse.gov
- www.drugfree.org
- www.drugs.com
- www.marijuana.com
- www.na.org (Narcotics Anonymous)
- www.preventteendruguse.org
- www.stopcocaineaddiction.com

REVIEW QUESTIONS

Multiple Choice

1. Rapid development of tolerance to a drug is called:

   A. intoxication

   B. anaphylactic shock

   C. tachyphylaxis

   D. tachyarrhythmia

2. Which of the following abused substances may cause psychological dependence after only one or a few uses?

   A. crack cocaine

   B. alcohol

   C. marijuana

   D. alprazolam

3. To reduce the psychological craving for alcohol, which of the following drugs may be used?

   A. methyl alcohol

   B. alprazolam

   C. oxycodone

   D. naltrexone

4. All of the following are synthetic opioid drugs, *except*:

   A. fentanyl

   B. cocaine

   C. methadone

   D. heroin

5. Which of the following drugs is used in patients for alcohol withdrawal delirium tremens?

   A. disulfiram (Antabuse®)

   B. lorazepam (Ativan®)

   C. methadone (Dolophine®)

   D. naloxone (Narcan®)

6. The effects of tetrahydrocannabinol include all of the following, *except*:

   A. reddened conjunctiva

   B. euphoria

   C. decreased appetite

   D. increased pulse rate

7. All of the following are major withdrawal symptoms from alcohol, *except*:

   A. seizures

   B. tremors

   C. nausea

   D. hypotension

8. Which of the following is an antagonist to heroin?

   A. pentobarbital

   B. methadone

   C. amobarbital

   D. alprazolam

9. Which of the following benzodiazepines is not approved by the FDA for any specific medical condition?

   A. flunitrazepam (Rohypnol®)

   B. alprazolam (Xanax®)

   C. temazepam (Restoril®)

   D. clonazepam (Klonopin®)

10. Withdrawal symptoms of anabolic steroids include all of the following, *except*:

    A. insomnia

    B. reduced sex drive

    C. increased energy

    D. restlessness

11. Which of the following is the drug of choice to treat Wernicke's encephalopathy?

    A. IV potassium chloride

    B. IV glucose

    C. IV thiamine

    D. IV lorazepam

12. Which of the following are clinical manifestations of cocaine toxicity?

    A. diaphoresis and dilated pupils

    B. tachycardia and hypotension

    C. pinpoint pupils and insomnia

    D. tremors and constriction of the pupils

13. Nicotine replacement therapy forms include all of the following, *except*:

    A. transdermal patches

    B. subcutaneous injections

    C. chewing gum

    D. nasal sprays

14. All of the following may cause hallucinations, *except*:

    A. LSD

    B. methadone

    C. ecstasy

    D. alcohol

15. Which of the following drugs is used for overdose of morphine?

    A. naloxone

    B. heroin

    C. varenicline

    D. potassium chloride

Fill in the Blank

1. The condition of persistently needing a substance, which may involve physical or psychological dependence is called _____.

2. Extension of tolerance for a substance to others of the same class is known as _____.

3. Another name for a tranquilizer is a _____.

4. The cardiovascular effects of nicotine are more serious in smokers who also take oral _____.

5. Anabolic steroids cause impotence, infertility, gynecomastia, and _____.

Critical Thinking

A 19-year-old woman was brought to the emergency department by the police, who picked her up outside of a college sorority. She had been acting abnormally, excited and odd, and would not stop talking even inside the police car. The officers had found a white powdered substance in a small bag in her purse. Her pupils were dilated, she was sweating, and upon examination, her heart was racing.

1. Which drug most likely fits this scenario?

2. If this patient was pregnant, how would this drug affect the fetus?

1. A 4-year-old boy presents with the following symptoms. He is experiencing a fever of 101.9°F, chills, sore throat, and rash. The best recommendation for treating this child's fever is:

   A. choline salicylate, because it is in the liquid form, and therefore more easily swallowed
   B. acetaminophen, since the specific disease condition is not known
   C. pediatric aspirin, because it is flavored and will ensure patient compliance
   D. any of the above recommendations are acceptable

Questions 2–4

A 60-year-old hypertensive woman brings three prescriptions to your pharmacy. They include furosemide, enalapril, and irbesartan.

2. Which of the following is an example of an ACE inhibitor?

   A. furosemide
   B. enalapril
   C. digoxin
   D. irbesartan

3. Which of the following is the trade name of furosemide?

   A. Midamor®
   B. Hygroton®
   C. Aldactone®
   D. Lasix®

4. Irbesartan is classified as which of the following types of antihypertensive drugs?

   A. peripheral vasodilator
   B. angiotensin II receptor antagonist
   C. adrenergic blocker
   D. angiotensin-converting enzyme inhibitor

5. A 31-year-old woman presents with a 2-month history of depressed mood, absence of pleasure from the performance of any act, increased appetite, weight gain, and suicidal ideation. This is the patient's first episode of major depression. Which of

the following agents would be most appropriate in the treatment of this patient?

   A. sertraline (Zoloft®)
   B. chlorpromazine (Thorazine®)
   C. thioridazine (Mellaril®)
   D. ritodrine (Yutopar®)

Questions 6–7

A 56-year-old man has been diagnosed with acute gouty arthritis of the right large toe.

6. Which of the following is the drug of choice for relieving pain and inflammation, and for ending the acute gout attack?

   A. mivacurium
   B. gold sodium thiomalate
   C. aspirin
   D. colchicine

7. If the traditional drug of choice is not an analgesic, which of the following agents may be used in combination in the management of pain for acute gout?

   A. succinylcholine
   B. allopurinol
   C. acetaminophen
   D. oxycodone

Questions 8–9

A 72-year-old man with advanced inoperable throat cancer is hospitalized for pain management. He is given a morphine solution (40 mg orally) every 3 hours for pain. He complains of difficulty swallowing and about the frequency with which he must take the morphine.

8. An appropriate analgesic alternative for this patient would be:

   A. intramuscular methadone
   B. controlled-release oral morphine
   C. transdermal fentanyl
   D. not another medication; simply increase the dose of the oral morphine solution

9. If there is no other analgesic alternative and the attending physician increases the oral dosage of morphine, which of the following might be the consequence?

   A. excellent pain relief
   B. worsening renal function
   C. excessive appetite
   D. overdose

Questions 10–12

A 21-year-old, previously healthy man is brought to the emergency department with a 2-week history of excessive elimination of urine, excessive thirst, and an unintentional weight loss of 25 pounds. No retinopathy is present. Laboratory values reveal high blood glucose and high glucose in the urine.

10. What is the most likely diagnosis for this patient?

    A. type 1 diabetes mellitus
    B. type 2 diabetes mellitus
    C. type 3 diabetes mellitus
    D. diabetes insipidus

11. Which of the following is the appropriate initial therapy?

    A. intravenous fluids and a sulfonylurea agent
    B. intravenous fluids and intravenous regular insulin
    C. intravenous fluids and 10 units of subcutaneous regular insulin
    D. intravenous fluids alone

12. The patient is at risk for developing which of the following complications?

    A. coronary artery disease
    B. retinopathy
    C. hypoglycemia
    D. all of the above

Questions 13–15

A 75-year-old man with a history of cigarette smoking for 50 years is brought to the emergency department with a fever of 103°F (which he has had for 4 days), cough, chills, and chest pain. Chest x-ray reveals pneumonia with confirmation via blood tests.

13. If this patient was diagnosed with bacterial pneumonia, which of the following antibiotics is the most appropriate to administer intravenously?

    A. chloramphenicol
    B. cephradine
    C. amphotericin B
    D. rifampin

14. If the patient has an allergy to the drug of choice (which is one of the four choices in Question 13), which of the following would be the best alternate drug of choice?

    A. chloramphenicol
    B. cephradine
    C. amphotericin B
    D. rifampin

15. The physician orders chloramphenicol 50 mg/kg/day in divided doses (every 6 hours). Which of the following is the most serious adverse effect of this drug?

    A. ototoxicity
    B. nephrotoxicity
    C. phlebitis at injection site
    D. bone marrow suppression

Questions 16–17

A 25-year-old man has burns on over 75% of his body. He has been admitted for two weeks at a local hospital, where he developed Zollinger-Ellison syndrome (a hypersecretion condition of the stomach with gastric ulcers).

16. Which of the following prototypes of H_2-receptor antagonists is used in the treatment of this condition?

    A. cimetidine
    B. famotidine
    C. nizatidine
    D. ranitidine

17. Which of the following prototype H_2-receptor antagonists is the most potent?

    A. ranitidine
    B. cimetidine
    C. famotidine
    D. nizatidine

18. Erythromycin 500 mg bid for 8 days is prescribed. The pharmacy technician has only the 250 mg dose in stock. How many capsules will the technician dispense for this patient?

   A. 16
   B. 24
   C. 32
   D. 48

Questions 19–21

A 62-year-old woman has been diagnosed with congestive heart failure and pulmonary edema. Her physician orders digitalis, a diuretic, ACE inhibitors, and beta-blockers.

19. Which of the following diuretics are preferred?

   A. loop diuretics
   B. thiazide and thiazide-like diuretics
   C. potassium-sparing diuretics
   D. carbonic anhydrase inhibitors

20. If the order is for thiazide or loop diuretics, which of the following is the most dangerous adverse effect?

   A. hypertension
   B. hyperkalemia
   C. hypokalemia
   D. loss of appetite

21. If the physician orders spironolactone, which of the following adverse effects may occur?

   A. hyperkalemia
   B. gynecomastia
   C. hyponatremia
   D. all of the above

22. A pediatrician orders penicillin for an 11-year-old patient without closely checking the patient's chart. While the pharmacy technician is dispensing the prescription, he notices that the computer chart indicates that the patient has an allergy to penicillin. Which of the following would be the best drug of choice in this case?

   A. ciprofloxacin
   B. clarithromycin
   C. amikacin
   D. vancomycin

23. A 75-year-old patient with advanced metastatic prostate cancer and a long history of renal failure presents with severe bone pain. He is given meperidine. Two days later, he develops a generalized seizure condition. What is the likely mechanism of this complication?

   A. worsening renal failure
   B. buildup of meperidine metabolite levels
   C. hypercalcemia
   D. brain metastasis

24. A 55-year-old patient with a history of hypertension and recent edema in her legs is treated with a thiazide diuretic. She should be monitored regularly for altered plasma levels of:

   A. uric acid
   B. calcium
   C. glucose
   D. potassium

25. A 27-year-old woman who breastfeeds her 7-month-old infant presents with chronic panic disorder. Her physician prescribes a benzodiazepine for her. All of the following properties of this drug are desirable for breastfeeding, *except*:

   A. hepatic metabolism to inactive metabolites
   B. a tendency to bind to milk proteins
   C. a rapid onset of action
   D. a short half-life

Answer Key

1. B	2. B	3. D	4. B	5. A	6. D
7. B	8. C	9. D	10. A	11. B	12. D
13. B	14. A	15. D	16. A	17. C	18. C
19. A	20. C	21. D	22. B	23. B	24. D
25. B					

Brand Name	Generic Name	Drug Class
Vicodin®	hydrocodone/APAP	Analgesic
Levothroid®, Levoxyl®, Synthroid®	levothyroxine sodium	Thyroid product
Prinivil®, Zestril®	lisinopril	Antihypertensive, angiotensin-converting enzyme (ACE) inhibitor
Zocor®	simvastatin	Antihyperlipidemic, HMG-CoA reductase inhibitor
Zithromax®	azithromycin	Antibiotic, macrolide
ProAir HFA®	albuterol (salbutamol)	Sympathomimetic
Crestor®	rosuvastatin calcium	Antihyperlipidemic, HMG-CoA reductase inhibitor
Nexium®	esomeprazole magnesium	Proton pump inhibitor
Lipitor®	atorvastatin calcium	Antihyperlipidemic, HMG-CoA reductase inhibitor
Motrin®	ibuprofen (Rx)	Nonsteroidal anti-inflammatory
Oleptro®	trazodone HCl	Antidepressant
Lopressor®	metoprolol tartrate	Beta-adrenergic blocker
Coumadin Tabs®	warfarin sodium	Anticoagulant, coumarin derivative
Cymbalta®	duloxetine hydrochloride	Antidepressant, selective serotonin and norepinephrine reuptake inhibitor
Flovent HFA®	fluticasone propionate	Glucocorticoid
Singulair®	montelukast sodium	Antiasthmatic, leukotriene receptor antagonist
Dyazide®	hydrochlorothiazide	Diuretic, thiazide
Ventolin HFA®	albuterol sulfate	Sympathomimetic

Brand Name	Generic Name	Drug Class
Advair Diskus®	fluticasone propionate and salmeterol xinafoate	Anti-asthmatic combination drug
Pravachol®	pravastatin sodium	Antihyperlipidemic, HMG-CoA reductase inhibitor
Amoxil®	amoxicillin	Antibiotic, penicillin
Norvasc®	amlodipine besylate	Calcium channel blocker
Prilosec®	omeprazole (Rx)	Proton pump inhibitor
Prinzide®, Zestoretic®	lisinopril/hydrochlorothiazide	Antihypertensive (combination ACE inhibitor and thiazide diuretic)
Lopressor®	metoprolol succinate	Beta-adrenergic blocker
Percocet®	oxycodone/APAP	Analgesic
Zoloft®	sertraline hydrochloride	Antidepressant, selective serotonin reuptake inhibitor
Diovan®	valsartan	Antihypertensive, angiotensin II receptor blocker
Xanax®	alprazolam	Antianxiety, benzodiazepine
Fortamet®	metformin HCl	Antidiabetic
Diflucan®	fluconazole	Antifungal
Bactrim®	sulfamethoxazole/trimethoprim	Antibacterial
Ativan®	lorazepam	Antianxiety, benzodiazepine
Mobic®	meloxicam	Nonsteroidal anti-inflammatory
Deltasone®	prednisone	Glucocorticoid
Klonopin®	clonazepam	Anticonvulsant
Ultram®	tramadol HCl	Analgesic
Lasix®	furosemide	Diuretic
Plavix®	clopidogrel bisulfate	Antiplatelet drug
Diovan HCT®	valsartan/hydrochlorothiazide	Antihypertensive
Drisdol®	ergocalciferol (vitamin D2) (Rx)	Provitamin/Organic compound

Brand Name	Generic Name	Drug Class
Flovent, Flonase®	fluticasone propionate	Glucocorticoid
Celexa®	citalopram HBr	Antidepressant, selective serotonin reuptake inhibitor
Lantus®, Lantus Solostar®	insulin glargine	Insulin
Augmentin®	amoxicillin trihydrate/clavulanate potassium	Antibiotic, penicillin
Vyvanse®	lisdexamfetamine dimesylate	Central nervous system (CNS) stimulant
Cipro®, Proquin XR®	ciprofloxacin HCl	Antibiotic, fluoroquinolone
Lexapro®	escitalopram oxalate	Antidepressant, selective serotonin reuptake inhibitor
Spiriva®	tiotropium bromide	Anticholinergic
Celebrex®	celecoxib	Nonsteroidal anti-inflammatory drug, cyclooxygenase-2 (COX-2) inhibitor
Ambien®	zolpidem tartrate	Sedative-hypnotic, nonbenzodiazepine
Lyrica®	pregabalin	Anticonvulsant, miscellaneous
Tenormin®	atenolol	Beta-adrenergic blocker
Nasonex®	mometasone furoate monohydrate	Glucocorticoid
Coreg®, Coreg CR®	carvedilol	Alpha/Beta-adrenergic blocker
Keflex®	cephalexin	Cephalosporin, first generation
Effexor XR®	venlafaxine HCl ER	Antidepressant
Flexeril®, Amrix®	cyclobenzaprine HCl	Skeletal muscle relaxant, centrally acting
Abilify®	aripiprazole	Antipsychotic
Januvia®	sitagliptin phosphate	Antidiabetic

Brand Name	Generic Name	Drug Class
Naprosyn®	naproxen	Nonsteroidal anti-inflammatory
Concerta®, Ritalin-SR®	methylphenidate ER	CNS stimulant
Viagra®	sildenafil citrate	Erectile dysfunction, pulmonary arterial hypertension
Toprol XL®	metoprolol succinate	Beta-adrenergic blocker
Micro-K 10 Extencaps®	potassium chloride	Electrolyte
Zetia®	ezetimibe	Antihyperlipidemic
Suboxone®	buprenorphine and naloxone	Opioid and opioid antagonist
Namenda®	memantine hydrochloride	Anti-Alzheimer's disease
Klonopin®	clonazepam	Anticonvulsant
Ativan®	lorazepam	Antianxiety
Cialis®	tadalafil	Erectile dysfunction
Adderall®	amphetamine salts	CNS stimulant
Medrol®	methylprednisolone	Glucocorticoid
Protonix®	pantoprazole sodium	Proton pump inhibitor
Valium®, Diastat®	diazepam	Antianxiety, benzodiazepine
Aloprim®, Zyloprim®	allopurinol	Antigout
Gabarone®, Neurontin®	gabapentin	Anticonvulsant
Zantac®	ranitidine HCl	Histamine H_2 receptor blocker
Digoxin®	digoxin	Cardiac glycoside
Bystolic®	nebivolol	Beta-adrenergic blocker
Elavil®	amitriptyline HCl	Antidepressant, tricyclic
Loestrin 24 Fe®	ethinyl estradiol	Oral contraceptive
Risperdal®	risperidone	Antipsychotic
Pitocin®	oxytocin	Oxytocic
Paxil®	paroxetine HCl	Antidepressant, selective serotonin reuptake inhibitor
Dyazide®, Mazide®	triamterene/hydrochlorothiazide	Antihypertensive

Brand Name	Generic Name	Drug Class
Atridox®, Vibramycin®	doxycycline hyclate	Antibiotic, tetracycline
Wellbutrin®	bupropion HCl XL	Antidepressant
Mevacor®	lovastatin	Antihyperlipidemic, HMG-CoA reductase inhibitor
Tylenol w/ Codeine®	acetaminophen/ codeine (APAP/ CD)	Non-narcotic analgesic
Klor-Con M20®	potassium salts	Electrolyte
Tricor®	fenofibrate	Antihyperlipidemic
Restoril®	temazepam	Sedative-hypnotic
Pepcid®	famotidine	Histamine H_2 receptor blocker
Nasocort®	triamcinolone acetonide	Glucocorticoid
Fosamax®	alendronate sodium	Bone growth regulator
Cleocin®	clindamycin HCl	Antibiotic
Flomax®	tamsulosin hydrochloride	Alpha-adrenergic blocker
Benicar HCT®	olmesartan medoxomil	Antihypertensive
Symbicort®	budesonide/ formoterol fumarate dihydrate	Corticosteroid

Brand Name	Generic Name	Drug Class
Bactroban Nasal®	mupirocin	Antibiotic
Niaspan®	niacin (nicotinic acid)	Vitamin B complex
Lovaza®	omega-3-acid ethyl esters	Lipid-regulating agent
Premarin®	estrogens	Estrogen
NuvaRing®	etonogestrel/ethinyl estradiol vaginal ring	Contraceptive
Dexilant®	dexlansoprazole	Proton pump inhibitor
Cheratussin AC®	codeine phosphate	Analgesic
Penicillin VK®	penicillin V potassium	Antibiotic, penicillin
Flagyl®	metronidazole	Trichomonacide, amebicide
Actos®	pioglitazone hydrochloride	Antidiabetic
Cozaar®	losartan potassium	Antihypertensive, angiotensin II receptor blocker
Lidoderm®	lidocaine	Analgesic

Source: Rx List—www.rxlist.com

Common Look-alike and Sound-alike Drugs

Generic Names	Trade Names	Possible Dangers
celecoxib citalopram hydrobromide fosphenytoin	Celebrex® Celexa® Cerebyx®	Mix-ups may cause decreased mental ability, lack of pain or seizure control, and other serious adverse events
cisplatin carboplatin	Platinol® Paraplatin®	Though the generic names are similar, safe doses of carboplatin usually exceed the maximum safe dose of cisplatin, potentially causing toxicity and death
clonidine clonazepam	Catapres® Klonopin®	Easily confused generic or trade names
concentrated liquid morphines versus conventional liquid morphine concentrations	Concentrated: Roxanol®, MSIR® Conventional: morphine oral liquid	Concentrated forms can be confused with standard concentrations, which can lead to fatal errors due to differences in labeling or prescribing by volume versus milligrams, e.g., 10 mg versus 10 mL
ephedrine epinephrine	Ephedrine® Adrenalin®	Similar names and clinical uses can cause these drugs to be stored close to each other; also, they are packaged in similar amber-colored vials and ampules
fentanyl sufentanil	Sublimaze® Sufenta®	These non interchangeable drugs have very different potencies, and can cause respiratory arrest if misused
hydromorphone injection morphine injection	Dilaudid® Astramorph®, Duramorph®, Infumorph®	Hydromorphone is not the generic equivalent of morphine and they are not interchangeable; due to close storage and similar concentrations, they may be easily misused, causing death because of potency differences influencing respiratory arrest
insulin glargine insulin zinc suspension human insulin insulin lispro human insulin aspart 70% isophane insulin NPH/ 30% insulin regular 70% insulin aspart protamine suspension and 30% insulin aspart	Lantus® Lente® Humulin®, Novolin® Humalog® Novolog® Novolin 70/30® Novolog Mix 70/30®	Similar names, strengths, and concentrations can cause medication errors; also mix-ups between 100 units/mL and 500 units/mL can occur

lipid-based:
   doxorubicin liposomal
   daunorubicin citrate liposomal
conventional:
   daunorubicin
   doxorubicin
	Doxil®
	Daunoxome®
	
	Cerubidine®
	Adriamycin®, Rubex®
		Confusion between liposomal and conventional formulations can occur easily, but these products are not interchangeable; accidental use of liposomal forms instead of conventional forms has resulted in severe side effects and death

nefazodone quetiapine	Serzone® Seroquel®	Similar names and available dosages, as well as use in similar clinical settings, can cause many adverse events and potentially dangerous drug interactions with other agents that may be used concurrently

Drug	U.S. Drug Schedule	Canadian Drug Schedule
alfentanil	II	I
alprazolam	IV	IV
amobarbital	II	IV
amphetamine	II	III
aprobarbital	III	IV
benzphetamine	III	III
buprenorphine	III	I
butabarbital	III	IV
butorphanol	IV	IV
chloral hydrate	IV	Not controlled, but pharmaceutical forms require a prescription
chlordiazepoxide	IV	IV
clonazepam	IV	IV
clorazepate	IV	IV
cocaine	II	I
codeine	II	I
dexmethylphenidate	II	III
dextroamphetamine	II	III
dextropropoxyphene (bulk)	II	I
dextropropoxyphene (dosage forms)	IV	I
diazepam	IV	IV
diethylpropion	IV	IV
difenoxin products	V	I
diphenoxylate products	V	I
dronabinol	III	Not available
estazolam	IV	IV
ethchlorvynol	IV	IV
fentanyl	II	I
fluoxymesterone	III	IV
flurazepam	IV	IV
glutethimide	II	IV
halazepam	IV	IV

Drug	U.S. Drug Schedule	Canadian Drug Schedule
hydrocodone	Only available in C-II combination drugs	I
hydromorphone	II	I
ketamine	III	I
levorphanol	II	I
lorazepam	IV	IV
mazindol	IV	IV
meperidine (called *pethidine* in Canada)	II	I
mephobarbital	IV	IV
meprobamate	IV	IV
methadone	II	I
methamphetamine	II	III
methandrostenolone (called *metandienone* in Canada)	III	IV
methylphenidate	II	III
methyltestosterone	III	IV
midazolam	IV	IV
modafinil	IV	Not controlled, but requires a prescription
morphine	II	I
nandrolone	III	IV
opium	II	I
opium products	V	I
oxandrolone	III	IV
oxazepam	IV	IV
oxycodone	II	I
oxymetholone	III	IV
oxymorphone	II	I
paraldehyde	IV	Not available
paregoric	III	Not available
pemoline	IV	IV
pentazocine	IV	I

Drug	U.S. Drug Schedule	Canadian Drug Schedule
pentobarbital sodium (PO)	II	IV
pentobarbital sodium (rectal)	III	IV
phencyclidine	II	I
phendimetrazine	III	IV
phenobarbital	IV	IV
phentermine	IV	IV
prazepam	IV	IV
quazepam	IV	IV
remifentanil	II	I
secobarbital	II	IV
sibutramine	IV	Not available
stanolone (called *androstanolone* in Canada)	III	IV
stanozolol	III	IV
sufentanil	II	I
temazepam	IV	IV
testosterone	III	IV
thiopental	III	IV
triazolam	IV	IV
zaleplon	IV	Not available
zolpidem	IV	IV

Drug Dosage Calculations

Using Ratios and Proportions to Calculate Dosages

1. Ratios may be written as follows: 3 : 4, which means 3 parts of drug #1 to 4 parts of solution or solvent. Ratios are used to express the relationship between two or more quantities. Ratios are usually expressed as fractions in drug calculations, as follows:

$$\frac{3 \text{ parts of drug #1}}{4 \text{ parts of a solution}} = \frac{3}{4}$$

Proportions show the relationship between two ratios, as follows:

$$\frac{\text{Dose on hand}}{\text{Quantity on hand}} = \frac{\text{Desired dose}}{\text{Desired quantity (X)}}$$

The same formula can be written as follows by using cross multiplication:

$$\text{Desired quantity (X)} = \frac{\text{Desired dose}}{\text{Dose on hand} \times \text{quantity on hand}}$$

If the dose on hand is 200 mg, the desired dose is 400 mg, and the quantity on hand is 10 mL, what is the desired quantity (X)?

$$\frac{\text{Dose on hand (200 mg)}}{\text{Quantity on hand (10 mL)}} = \frac{\text{Desired dose (400 mg)}}{\text{Desired quantity (X)}}$$

When cross-multiplying, we find:

$$200 \times X = 10 \text{ mL} \times 400$$

$$200X = 4000 \text{ mL}$$

$$X = 20 \text{ mL}$$

The dose to be administered is 20 mL.

2. The same proportion method can solve solid dosage calculations, as follows:

If the dose on hand is available as 5 mg tablets, and the desired dose is 25 mg/day, how many tablets should be administered each day?

$$\frac{\text{Dose on hand (5 mg)}}{1 \text{ tablet}} = \frac{\text{Desired dose (25 mg)}}{\text{Desired quantity (X)}}$$

By cross-multiplying, it is found that:

$$5 \text{ mg} \times X = 25 \text{ mg} \times 1 \text{ tablet}$$

$$5X = 25 \text{ mg}$$

$$X = 5 \text{ tablets/day}$$

Therefore, 5 tablets should be administered daily.

Dosage Calculations by Weight

Drug dosages are often expressed as milligrams per unit of body weight (usually kilograms rather than pounds), and are commonly used in depicting pediatric dosages. An example of a recommended dosage of a drug might be 1 mg/kg/24 hours. This information can be used to calculate the dose for a specific patient, or to check that prescribed dosages are correct and not significantly under or over the required dosages for that patient.

Caution must always be used in converting between pounds and kilograms. The formula that should be understood is as follows:

Body weight × (dose in mg/kg) = X mg of drug

Example: Chewable tablets for a 110-pound child are to be administered at the rate of 20 mg/kg/dose. How many tablets, if they are 500 mg each, should be administered to this patient for each dose?

First, convert the patient's weight to kilograms as follows:

$$1 \text{ kg} = 2.2 \text{ lbs}$$

$$\frac{1 \text{ kg}}{2.2 \text{ lbs}} = \frac{X \text{ mg}}{110 \text{ lbs}}$$

$$X = 50 \text{ mg}$$

Next, calculate the total daily dose as follows. For each kilogram of body weight, you should give 20 mg of the drug.

$$\frac{20 \text{ mg}}{1 \text{ kg}} = \frac{X \text{ kg}}{50 \text{ kg}}$$

$$X = 1000 \text{ kg}$$

Finally, calculate the number of tablets needed to supply 1000 mg per dose. Remember that the concentration of the tablets on hand is 500 mg per tablet.

$$\frac{500 \text{ mg}}{1 \text{ tablet}} = \frac{1000 \text{ mg}}{X \text{ tablets}}$$

$$X = 2 \text{ tablets per dose}$$

Calculating Dosage by Body Surface Area

Using body surface area to calculate pediatric dosages is a very accurate method. Nomograms are charts that use patient weight and height to determine body surface area in square meters (m²). This body surface area (BSA) is then placed into a ratio with the average adult's body surface area (1.73 m²). The following formula is then used:

$$\text{Child's dose} = \frac{\text{Child's BSA in m}^2}{1.73 \text{ m}^2} \times \text{Adult dose}$$

Nomogram scales contain metric and avoirdupois values for height and weight, enabling BSA to be determined in pounds and inches or kilograms and centimeters without needing to make conversions. See the figure of the nomogram scale at the end of this Appendix.

WEST NOMOGRAM

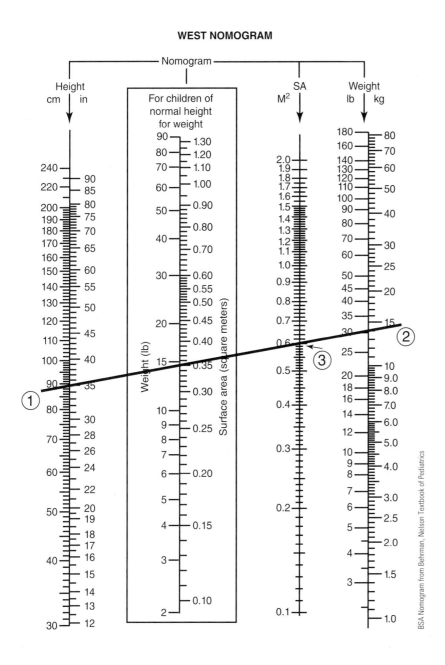

BSA Nomogram from Behrman, Nelson Textbook of Pediatrics

To determine BSA, a ruler or straightedge is recommended. After determining the patient's height and weight, place the ruler or straightedge on the nomogram and connect the two points on the height and weight scales that represent the patient's values. Where the ruler or straightedge crosses the center column (BSA), the corresponding reading is the value of the BSA in square meters. Substitute the BSA value in the formula to calculate the dosage for this patient. If this child's BSA is 0.52 m², and the adult dosage of the required drug is 500 mg, use the following formula to determine the child's dose:

$$\text{Child's dose} = \frac{0.52 \text{ m}^2}{1.73 \text{ m}^2} \times \text{Adult dose (500 mg)}$$

$$= 0.3 \times 500 \text{ mg}$$

$$= 150 \text{ mg (child's dose)}$$

Calculating IV Infusion Rates

To calculate the flow rate using the ratio and proportion method, follow these steps:

1. Determine the number of milliliters the patient will receive per hour.

2. Determine the number of milliliters the patient will receive per minute.

3. Determine the number of drops per minute that will equal the number of milliliters calculated above. The IV set's drop rate must be considered. This is expressed as a ratio of drops per milliliter (gtt/mL).

Example: The prescriber orders 3000 mL of dextrose 5% in water (D_5W) IV over 24 hours. If the IV set delivers 15 drops per milliliter, how many drops must be administered per minute?

First, calculate mL/h

$$\frac{3000 \text{ mL}}{24 \text{ h}} = \frac{X \text{ mL}}{1 \text{ h}}$$

$$X = 125 \text{ mL/h or}$$

$$125 \text{ mL/60 min}$$

Next, calculate mL/min.

$$\frac{125 \text{ mL}}{60 \text{ min}} = \frac{X \text{ mL}}{1 \text{ min}}$$

$$X = 2 \text{ mL/min}$$

Finally, calculate gtt/min using the drop rate per minute of the IV set. (IV set drop rate = 15 drops/mL)

$$\frac{15 \text{ gtt}}{1 \text{ mL}} = \frac{X \text{ gtt}}{2 \text{ mL (amount needed/min)}}$$

$$X = 30 \text{ gtt/min}$$

Recommended Immunization Schedules for Persons Aged 0 Through 18 Years
UNITED STATES, 2015

This schedule includes recommendations in effect as of January 1, 2015. Any dose not administered at the recommended age should be administered at a subsequent visit, when indicated and feasible. The use of a combination vaccine generally is preferred over separate injections of its equivalent component vaccines. Vaccination providers should consult the relevant Advisory Committee on Immunization Practices (ACIP) statement for detailed recommendations, available online at http://www.cdc.gov/vaccines/hcp/acip-recs/index.html. Clinically significant adverse events that follow vaccination should be reported to the Vaccine Adverse Event Reporting System (VAERS) online (http://www.vaers.hhs.gov) or by telephone (800-822-7967).

The Recommended Immunization Schedules for
Persons Aged 0 Through 18 Years are approved by the

Advisory Committee on Immunization Practices
(http://www.cdc.gov/vaccines/acip)

American Academy of Pediatrics
(http://www.aap.org)

American Academy of Family Physicians
(http://www.aafp.org)

American College of Obstetricians and Gynecologists
(http://www.acog.org)

 U.S. Department of Health and Human Services
Centers for Disease Control and Prevention

Figure 1. Recommended immunization schedule for persons aged 0 through 18 years – United States, 2015.
(FOR THOSE WHO FALL BEHIND OR START LATE, SEE THE CATCH-UP SCHEDULE [FIGURE 2]).

These recommendations must be read with the footnotes that follow. For those who fall behind or start late, provide catch-up vaccination at the earliest opportunity as indicated by the green bars in Figure 1. To determine minimum intervals between doses, see the catch-up schedule (Figure 2). School entry and adolescent vaccine age groups are shaded.

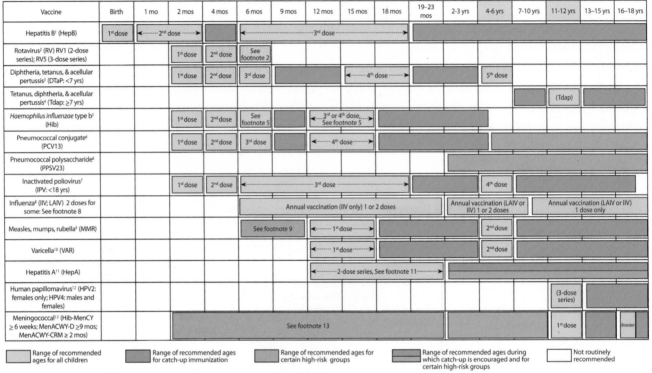

This schedule includes recommendations in effect as of January 1, 2015. Any dose not administered at the recommended age should be administered at a subsequent visit, when indicated and feasible. The use of a combination vaccine generally is preferred over separate injections of its equivalent component vaccines. Vaccination providers should consult the relevant Advisory Committee on Immunization Practices (ACIP) statement for detailed recommendations, available online at http://www.cdc.gov/vaccines/hcp/acip-recs/index.html. Clinically significant adverse events that follow vaccination should be reported to the Vaccine Adverse Event Reporting System (VAERS) online (http://www.vaers.hhs.gov) or by telephone (800-822-7967). Suspected cases of vaccine-preventable diseases should be reported to the state or local health department. Additional information, including precautions and contraindications for vaccination, is available from CDC online (http://www.cdc.gov/vaccines/recs/vac-admin/contraindications.htm) or by telephone (800-CDC-INFO [800-232-4636]).

This schedule is approved by the Advisory Committee on Immunization Practices (http://www.cdc.gov/vaccines/acip), the American Academy of Pediatrics (http://www.aap.org), the American Academy of Family Physicians (http://www.aafp.org), and the American College of Obstetricians and Gynecologists (http://www.acog.org).

NOTE: The above recommendations must be read along with the footnotes of this schedule.

FIGURE 2. Catch-up immunization schedule for persons aged 4 months through 18 years who start late or who are more than 1 month behind —United States, 2015.

The figure below provides catch-up schedules and minimum intervals between doses for children whose vaccinations have been delayed. A vaccine series does not need to be restarted, regardless of the time that has elapsed between doses. Use the section appropriate for the child's age. Always use this table in conjunction with Figure 1 and the footnotes that follow.

Vaccine	Minimum Age for Dose 1	Minimum Interval Between Doses			
		Dose 1 to Dose 2	Dose 2 to Dose 3	Dose 3 to Dose 4	Dose 4 to Dose 5
Children age 4 months through 6 years					
Hepatitis B[1]	Birth	4 weeks	8 weeks *and* at least 16 weeks after first dose. Minimum age for the final dose is 24 weeks.		
Rotavirus[2]	6 weeks	4 weeks	4 weeks[2]		
Diphtheria, tetanus, and acellular pertussis[3]	6 weeks	4 weeks	4 weeks	6 months	6 months[3]
Haemophilus influenzae type b[5]	6 weeks	4 weeks if first dose was administered before the 1st birthday. 8 weeks (as final dose) if first dose was administered at age 12 through 14 months. No further doses needed if first dose was administered at age 15 months or older.	4 weeks[5] if current age is younger than 12 months **and** first dose was administered at younger than age 7 months, **and** at least 1 previous dose was PRP-T (ActHib, Pentacel) or unknown. 8 weeks *and* age 12 through 59 months (as final dose)[5] • if current age is younger than 12 months **and** first dose was administered at age 7 through 11 months; OR • if current age is 12 through 59 months **and** first dose was administered before the 1st birthday, **and** second dose administered at younger than 15 months; OR • if both doses were PRP-OMP (PedvaxHIB; Comvax) **and** were administered before the 1st birthday. No further doses needed if previous dose was administered at age 15 months or older.	8 weeks (as final dose) This dose only necessary for children 12 through 59 months who received 3 doses before the 1st birthday.	
Pneumococcal[6]	6 weeks	4 weeks if first dose administered before the 1st birthday. 8 weeks (as final dose for healthy children) if first dose was administered at the 1st birthday or after. No further doses needed for healthy children if first dose administered at age 24 months or older.	4 weeks if current age is younger than 12 months and previous dose given at <7months old. 8 weeks (as final dose for healthy children) if previous dose given between 7-11 months (wait until at least 12 months old); OR if current age is 12 months or older and at least 1 dose was given before age 12 months. No further doses needed for healthy children if previous dose administered at age 24 months or older.	8 weeks (as final dose) This dose only necessary for children aged 12 through 59 months who received 3 doses before age 12 months or for children at high risk who received 3 doses at any age.	
Inactivated poliovirus[7]	6 weeks	4 weeks[7]	4 weeks[7]	6 months[7] (minimum age 4 years for final dose).	
Meningococcal[13]	6 weeks	8 weeks[13]	See footnote 13	See footnote 13	
Measles, mumps, rubella[8]	12 months	4 weeks			
Varicella[10]	12 months	3 months			
Hepatitis A[11]	12 months	6 months			
Children and adolescents age 7 through 18 years					
Tetanus, diphtheria; tetanus, diphtheria, and acellular pertussis[4]	7 years[4]	4 weeks	4 weeks if first dose of DTaP/DT was administered before the 1st birthday. 6 months (as final dose) if first dose of DTaP/DT was administered at or after the 1st birthday.	6 months if first dose of DTaP/DT was administered before the 1st birthday.	
Human papillomavirus[12]	9 years	Routine dosing intervals are recommended.[12]			
Hepatitis A[11]	Not applicable (N/A)	6 months			
Hepatitis B[1]	N/A	4 weeks	8 weeks **and** at least 16 weeks after first dose.		
Inactivated poliovirus[7]	N/A	4 weeks	4 weeks[7]	6 months[7]	
Meningococcal[13]	N/A	8 weeks[13]			
Measles, mumps, rubella[8]	N/A	4 weeks			
Varicella[10]	N/A	3 months if younger than age 13 years. 4 weeks if age 13 years or older.			

NOTE: The above recommendations must be read along with the footnotes of this schedule.

U.S. Department of Health and Human Services, Centers for Disease Control and Prevention

Footnotes — Recommended immunization schedule for persons aged 0 through 18 years—United States, 2015

For further guidance on the use of the vaccines mentioned below, see: http://www.cdc.gov/vaccines/hcp/acip-recs/index.html.
For vaccine recommendations for persons 19 years of age and older, see the Adult Immunization Schedule.

Additional information

- For contraindications and precautions to use of a vaccine and for additional information regarding that vaccine, vaccination providers should consult the relevant ACIP statement available online at http://www.cdc.gov/vaccines/hcp/acip-recs/index.html.
- For purposes of calculating intervals between doses, 4 weeks = 28 days. Intervals of 4 months or greater are determined by calendar months.
- Vaccine doses administered 4 days or less before the minimum interval are considered valid. Doses of any vaccine administered ≥5 days earlier than the minimum interval or minimum age should not be counted as valid doses and should be repeated as age-appropriate. The repeat dose should be spaced after the invalid dose by the recommended minimum interval. For further details, see *MMWR, General Recommendations on Immunization and Reports / Vol. 60 / No. 2; Table 1. Recommended and minimum ages and intervals between vaccine doses* available online at http://www.cdc.gov/mmwr/pdf/rr/rr6002.pdf.
- Information on travel vaccine requirements and recommendations is available at http://wwwnc.cdc.gov/travel/destinations/list.
- For vaccination of persons with primary and secondary immunodeficiencies, see Table 13, *"Vaccination of persons with primary and secondary immunodeficiencies,"* in *General Recommendations on Immunization (ACIP),* available at http://www.cdc.gov/mmwr/pdf/rr/rr6002.pdf.; and American Academy of Pediatrics. "Immunization in Special Clinical Circumstances," in Pickering LK, Baker CJ, Kimberlin DW, Long SS eds. *Red Book: 2012 report of the Committee on Infectious Diseases. 29th ed.* Elk Grove Village, IL: American Academy of Pediatrics.

1. Hepatitis B (HepB) vaccine. (Minimum age: birth)

Routine vaccination:

At birth:

- Administer monovalent HepB vaccine to all newborns before hospital discharge.
- For infants born to hepatitis B surface antigen (HBsAg)-positive mothers, administer HepB vaccine and 0.5 mL of hepatitis B immune globulin (HBIG) within 12 hours of birth. These infants should be tested for HBsAg and antibody to HBsAg (anti-HBs) 1 to 2 months after completion of the HepB series at age 9 through 18 months (preferably at the next well-child visit).
- If mother's HBsAg status is unknown, within 12 hours of birth administer HepB vaccine regardless of birth weight. For infants weighing less than 2,000 grams, administer HBIG in addition to HepB vaccine within 12 hours of birth. Determine mother's HBsAg status as soon as possible and, if mother is HBsAg-positive, also administer HBIG for infants weighing 2,000 grams or more as soon as possible, but no later than age 7 days.

Doses following the birth dose:

- The second dose should be administered at age 1 or 2 months. Monovalent HepB vaccine should be used for doses administered before age 6 weeks.
- Infants who did not receive a birth dose should receive 3 doses of a HepB-containing vaccine on a schedule of 0, 1 to 2 months, and 6 months starting as soon as feasible. See Figure 2.
- Administer the second dose 1 to 2 months after the first dose (minimum interval of 4 weeks), administer the third dose at least 8 weeks after the second dose AND at least 16 weeks after the **first** dose. The final (third or fourth) dose in the HepB vaccine series should be administered **no earlier than age 24 weeks**.
- Administration of a total of 4 doses of HepB vaccine is permitted when a combination vaccine containing HepB is administered after the birth dose.

Catch-up vaccination:

- Unvaccinated persons should complete a 3-dose series.
- A 2-dose series (doses separated by at least 4 months) of adult formulation Recombivax HB is licensed for use in children aged 11 through 15 years.
- For other catch-up guidance, see Figure 2.

2. Rotavirus (RV) vaccines. (Minimum age: 6 weeks for both RV1 [Rotarix] and RV5 [RotaTeq])

Routine vaccination:

Administer a series of RV vaccine to all infants as follows:
1. If Rotarix is used, administer a 2-dose series at 2 and 4 months of age.
2. If RotaTeq is used, administer a 3-dose series at ages 2, 4, and 6 months.
3. If any dose in the series was RotaTeq or vaccine product is unknown for any dose in the series, a total of 3 doses of RV vaccine should be administered.

Catch-up vaccination:

- The maximum age for the first dose in the series is 14 weeks, 6 days; vaccination should not be initiated for infants aged 15 weeks, 0 days or older.
- The maximum age for the final dose in the series is 8 months, 0 days.
- For other catch-up guidance, see Figure 2.

3. Diphtheria and tetanus toxoids and acellular pertussis (DTaP) vaccine. (Minimum age: 6 weeks. Exception: DTaP-IPV [Kinrix]: 4 years)

Routine vaccination:

- Administer a 5-dose series of DTaP vaccine at ages 2, 4, 6, 15 through 18 months, and 4 through 6 years. The fourth dose may be administered as early as age 12 months, provided at least 6 months have elapsed since the third dose. However, the fourth dose of DTaP need not be repeated if it was administered at least 4 months after the third dose of DTaP.

3. Diphtheria and tetanus toxoids and acellular pertussis (DTaP) vaccine (cont'd)

Catch-up vaccination:

- The fifth dose of DTaP vaccine is not necessary if the fourth dose was administered at age 4 years or older.
- For other catch-up guidance, see Figure 2.

4. Tetanus and diphtheria toxoids and acellular pertussis (Tdap) vaccine. (Minimum age: 10 years for both Boostrix and Adacel)

Routine vaccination:

- Administer 1 dose of Tdap vaccine to all adolescents aged 11 through 12 years.
- Tdap may be administered regardless of the interval since the last tetanus and diphtheria toxoid-containing vaccine.
- Administer 1 dose of Tdap vaccine to pregnant adolescents during each pregnancy (preferred during 27 through 36 weeks' gestation) regardless of time since prior Td or Tdap vaccination.

Catch-up vaccination:

- Persons aged 7 years and older who are not fully immunized with DTaP vaccine should receive Tdap vaccine as 1 dose (preferably the first) in the catch-up series; if additional doses are needed, use Td vaccine. For children 7 through 10 years who receive a dose of Tdap as part of the catch-up series, an adolescent Tdap vaccine dose at age 11 through 12 years should NOT be administered. Td should be administered instead 10 years after the Tdap dose.
- Persons aged 11 through 18 years who have not received Tdap vaccine should receive a dose followed by tetanus and diphtheria toxoid (Td) booster doses every 10 years thereafter.
- Inadvertent doses of DTaP vaccine:
  - If administered inadvertently to a child aged 7 through 10 years may count as part of the catch-up series. This dose may count as the adolescent Tdap dose, or the child can later receive a Tdap booster dose at age 11 through 12 years.
  - If administered inadvertently to an adolescent aged 11 through 18 years, the dose should be counted as the adolescent Tdap booster.
- For other catch-up guidance, see Figure 2.

5. *Haemophilus influenzae* type b (Hib) conjugate vaccine. (Minimum age: 6 weeks for PRP-T [ACTHIB, DTaP-IPV/Hib (Pentacel) and Hib-MenCY (MenHibrix)], PRP-OMP [PedvaxHIB or COMVAX], 12 months for PRP-T [Hiberix])

Routine vaccination:

- Administer a 2- or 3-dose Hib vaccine primary series and a booster dose (dose 3 or 4 depending on vaccine used in primary series) at age 12 through 15 months to complete a full Hib vaccine series.
- The primary series with ActHIB, MenHibrix, or Pentacel consists of 3 doses and should be administered at 2, 4, and 6 months of age. The primary series with PedvaxHib or COMVAX consists of 2 doses and should be administered at 2 and 4 months of age; a dose at age 6 months is not indicated.
- One booster dose (dose 3 or 4 depending on vaccine used in primary series) of any Hib vaccine should be administered at age 12 through 15 months. An exception is Hiberix vaccine. Hiberix should only be used for the booster (final) dose in children aged 12 months through 4 years who have received at least 1 prior dose of Hib-containing vaccine.
- For recommendations on the use of MenHibrix in patients at increased risk for meningococcal disease, please refer to the meningococcal vaccine footnotes and also to *MMWR* February 28, 2014 / 63(RR01):1-13, available at http://www.cdc.gov/mmwr/PDF/rr/rr6301.pdf.

U.S. Department of Health and Human Services, Centers for Disease Control and Prevention

For further guidance on the use of the vaccines mentioned below, see: http://www.cdc.gov/vaccines/hcp/acip-recs/index.html.

5. **Haemophilus influenzae type b (Hib) conjugate vaccine (cont'd)**

Catch-up vaccination:
- If dose 1 was administered at ages 12 through 14 months, administer a second (final) dose at least 8 weeks after dose 1, regardless of Hib vaccine used in the primary series.
- If both doses were PRP-OMP (PedvaxHIB or COMVAX), and were administered before the first birthday, the third (and final) dose should be administered at age 12 through 59 months and at least 8 weeks after the second dose.
- If the first dose was administered at age 7 through 11 months, administer the second dose at least 4 weeks later and a third (and final) dose at age 12 through 15 months or 8 weeks after second dose, whichever is later.
- If first dose is administered before the first birthday and second dose administered at younger than 15 months, a third (and final) dose should be given 8 weeks later.
- For unvaccinated children aged 15 months or older, administer only 1 dose.
- For other catch-up guidance, see Figure 2. For catch-up guidance related to MenHibrix, please see the meningococcal vaccine footnotes and also *MMWR* February 28, 2014 / 63(RR01);1-13, available at http://www.cdc.gov/mmwr/PDF/rr/rr6301.pdf.

Vaccination of persons with high-risk conditions:
- Children aged 12 through 59 months who are at increased risk for Hib disease, including chemotherapy recipients and those with anatomic or functional asplenia (including sickle cell disease), human immunodeficiency virus (HIV) infection, immunoglobulin deficiency, or early component complement deficiency, who have received either no doses or only 1 dose of Hib vaccine before 12 months of age, should receive 2 additional doses of Hib vaccine 8 weeks apart; children who received 2 or more doses of Hib vaccine before 12 months of age should receive 1 additional dose.
- For patients younger than 5 years of age undergoing chemotherapy or radiation treatment who received a Hib vaccine dose(s) within 14 days of starting therapy or during therapy, repeat the dose(s) at least 3 months following therapy completion.
- Recipients of hematopoietic stem cell transplant (HSCT) should be revaccinated with a 3-dose regimen of Hib vaccine starting 6 to 12 months after successful transplant, regardless of vaccination history; doses should be administered at least 4 weeks apart.
- A single dose of any Hib-containing vaccine should be administered to unimmunized* children and adolescents 15 months of age and older undergoing an elective splenectomy; if possible, vaccine should be administered at least 14 days before procedure.
- Hib vaccine is not routinely recommended for patients 5 years or older. However, 1 dose of Hib vaccine should be administered to unimmunized* persons aged 5 years or older who have anatomic or functional asplenia (including sickle cell disease) and unvaccinated persons 5 through 18 years of age with human immunodeficiency virus (HIV) infection.

    Patients who have not received a primary series and booster dose or at least 1 dose of Hib vaccine after 14 months of age are considered unimmunized.

6. **Pneumococcal vaccines. (Minimum age: 6 weeks for PCV13, 2 years for PPSV23)**

Routine vaccination with PCV13:
- Administer a 4-dose series of PCV13 vaccine at ages 2, 4, and 6 months and at age 12 through 15 months.
- For children 14 through 59 months who have received an age-appropriate series of 7-valent PCV (PCV7), administer a single supplemental dose of 13-valent PCV (PCV13).

Catch-up vaccination with PCV13:
- Administer 1 dose of PCV13 to all healthy children aged 24 through 59 months who are not completely vaccinated for their age.
- For other catch-up guidance, see Figure 2.

Vaccination of persons with high-risk conditions with PCV13 and PPSV23:
- All recommended PCV13 doses should be administered prior to PPSV23 vaccination if possible.
- For children 2 through 5 years of age with any of the following conditions: chronic heart disease (particularly cyanotic congenital heart disease and cardiac failure); chronic lung disease (including asthma if treated with high-dose oral corticosteroid therapy); diabetes mellitus; cerebrospinal fluid leak; cochlear implant; sickle cell disease and other hemoglobinopathies; anatomic or functional asplenia; HIV infection; chronic renal failure; nephrotic syndrome; diseases associated with treatment with immunosuppressive drugs or radiation therapy, including malignant neoplasms, leukemias, lymphomas, and Hodgkin's disease; solid organ transplantation; or congenital immunodeficiency:
    1. Administer 1 dose of PCV13 if any incomplete schedule of 3 doses of PCV (PCV7 and/or PCV13) were received previously.
    2. Administer 2 doses of PCV13 at least 8 weeks apart if unvaccinated or any incomplete schedule of fewer than 3 doses of PCV (PCV7 and/or PCV13) were received previously.
    3. Administer 1 supplemental dose of PCV13 if 4 doses of PCV7 or other age-appropriate complete PCV7 series was received previously.
    4. The minimum interval between doses of PCV (PCV7 or PCV13) is 8 weeks.
    5. For children with no history of PPSV23 vaccination, administer PPSV23 at least 8 weeks after the most recent dose of PCV13.

6. **Pneumococcal vaccines (cont'd)**
- For children aged 6 through 18 years who have cerebrospinal fluid leak; cochlear implant; sickle cell disease and other hemoglobinopathies; anatomic or functional asplenia; congenital or acquired immunodeficiencies; HIV infection; chronic renal failure; nephrotic syndrome; diseases associated with treatment with immunosuppressive drugs or radiation therapy, including malignant neoplasms, leukemias, lymphomas, and Hodgkin's disease; generalized malignancy; solid organ transplantation; or multiple myeloma:
    1. If neither PCV13 nor PPSV23 has been received previously, administer 1 dose of PCV13 now and 1 dose of PPSV23 at least 8 weeks later.
    2. If PCV13 has been received previously but PPSV23 has not, administer 1 dose of PPSV23 at least 8 weeks after the most recent dose of PCV13.
    3. If PPSV23 has been received but PCV13 has not, administer 1 dose of PCV13 at least 8 weeks after the most recent dose of PPSV23.
- For children aged 6 through 18 years with chronic heart disease (particularly cyanotic congenital heart disease and cardiac failure), chronic lung disease (including asthma if treated with high-dose oral corticosteroid therapy), diabetes mellitus, alcoholism, or chronic liver disease, who have not received PPSV23, administer 1 dose of PPSV23. If PCV13 has been received previously, then PPSV23 should be administered at least 8 weeks after any prior PCV13 dose.
- A single revaccination with PPSV23 should be administered 5 years after the first dose to children with sickle cell disease or other hemoglobinopathies; anatomic or functional asplenia; congenital or acquired immunodeficiencies; HIV infection; chronic renal failure; nephrotic syndrome; diseases associated with treatment with immunosuppressive drugs or radiation therapy, including malignant neoplasms, leukemias, lymphomas, and Hodgkin's disease; generalized malignancy; solid organ transplantation; or multiple myeloma.

7. **Inactivated poliovirus vaccine (IPV). (Minimum age: 6 weeks)**

Routine vaccination:
- Administer a 4-dose series of IPV at ages 2, 4, 6 through 18 months, and 4 through 6 years. The final dose in the series should be administered on or after the fourth birthday and at least 6 months after the previous dose.

Catch-up vaccination:
- In the first 6 months of life, minimum age and minimum intervals are only recommended if the person is at risk of imminent exposure to circulating poliovirus (i.e., travel to a polio-endemic region or during an outbreak).
- If 4 or more doses are administered before age 4 years, an additional dose should be administered at age 4 through 6 years and at least 6 months after the previous dose.
- A fourth dose is not necessary if the third dose was administered at age 4 years or older and at least 6 months after the previous dose.
- If both OPV and IPV were administered as part of a series, a total of 4 doses should be administered, regardless of the child's current age. IPV is not routinely recommended for U.S. residents aged 18 years or older.
- For other catch-up guidance, see Figure 2.

8. **Influenza vaccines. (Minimum age: 6 months for inactivated influenza vaccine [IIV], 2 years for live, attenuated influenza vaccine [LAIV])**

Routine vaccination:
- Administer influenza vaccine annually to all children beginning at age 6 months. For most healthy, nonpregnant persons aged 2 through 49 years, either LAIV or IIV may be used. However, LAIV should NOT be administered to some persons, including 1) persons who have experienced severe allergic reactions to LAIV, any of its components, or to a previous dose of any other influenza vaccine; 2) children 2 through 17 years receiving aspirin or aspirin-containing products; 3) persons who are allergic to eggs; 4) pregnant women; 5) immunosuppressed persons; 6) children 2 through 4 years of age with asthma or who had wheezing in the past 12 months; or 7) persons who have taken influenza antiviral medications in the previous 48 hours. For all other contraindications and precautions to use of LAIV, see *MMWR* August 15, 2014 / 63(32);691-697 [40 pages] available at http://www.cdc.gov/mmwr/pdf/wk/mm6332.pdf.

For children aged 6 months through 8 years:
- For the 2014-15 season, administer 2 doses (separated by at least 4 weeks) to children who are receiving influenza vaccine for the first time. Some children in this age group who have been vaccinated previously will also need 2 doses. For additional guidance, follow dosing guidelines in the 2014-15 ACIP influenza vaccine recommendations, *MMWR* August 15, 2014 / 63(32);691-697 [40 pages] available at http://www.cdc.gov/mmwr/pdf/wk/mm6332.pdf.
- For the 2015–16 season, follow dosing guidelines in the 2015 ACIP influenza vaccine recommendations.

For persons aged 9 years and older:
- Administer 1 dose.

U.S. Department of Health and Human Services, Centers for Disease Control and Prevention

For further guidance on the use of the vaccines mentioned below, see: http://www.cdc.gov/vaccines/hcp/acip-recs/index.html.

9. **Measles, mumps, and rubella (MMR) vaccine. (Minimum age: 12 months for routine vaccination)**
   Routine vaccination:
   - Administer a 2-dose series of MMR vaccine at ages 12 through 15 months and 4 through 6 years. The second dose may be administered before age 4 years, provided at least 4 weeks have elapsed since the first dose.
   - Administer 1 dose of MMR vaccine to infants aged 6 through 11 months before departure from the United States for international travel. These children should be revaccinated with 2 doses of MMR vaccine, the first at age 12 through 15 months (12 months if the child remains in an area where disease risk is high), and the second dose at least 4 weeks later.
   - Administer 2 doses of MMR vaccine to children aged 12 months and older before departure from the United States for international travel. The first dose should be administered on or after age 12 months and the second dose at least 4 weeks later.
   Catch-up vaccination:
   - Ensure that all school-aged children and adolescents have had 2 doses of MMR vaccine; the minimum interval between the 2 doses is 4 weeks.

10. **Varicella (VAR) vaccine. (Minimum age: 12 months)**
    Routine vaccination:
    - Administer a 2-dose series of VAR vaccine at ages 12 through 15 months and 4 through 6 years. The second dose may be administered before age 4 years, provided at least 3 months have elapsed since the first dose. If the second dose was administered at least 4 weeks after the first dose, it can be accepted as valid.
    Catch-up vaccination:
    - Ensure that all persons aged 7 through 18 years without evidence of immunity (see *MMWR* 2007 / 56 [No. RR-4], available at http://www.cdc.gov/mmwr/pdf/rr/rr5604.pdf) have 2 doses of varicella vaccine. For children aged 7 through 12 years, the recommended minimum interval between doses is 3 months (if the second dose was administered at least 4 weeks after the first dose, it can be accepted as valid); for persons aged 13 years and older, the minimum interval between doses is 4 weeks.

11. **Hepatitis A (HepA) vaccine. (Minimum age: 12 months)**
    Routine vaccination:
    - Initiate the 2-dose HepA vaccine series at 12 through 23 months; separate the 2 doses by 6 to 18 months.
    - Children who have received 1 dose of HepA vaccine before age 24 months should receive a second dose 6 to 18 months after the first dose.
    - For any person aged 2 years and older who has not already received the HepA vaccine series, 2 doses of HepA vaccine separated by 6 to 18 months may be administered if immunity against hepatitis A virus infection is desired.
    Catch-up vaccination:
    - The minimum interval between the two doses is 6 months.
    Special populations:
    - Administer 2 doses of HepA vaccine at least 6 months apart to previously unvaccinated persons who live in areas where vaccination programs target older children, or who are at increased risk for infection. This includes persons traveling to or working in countries that have high or intermediate endemicity of infection; men having sex with men; users of injection and non-injection illicit drugs; persons who work with HAV-infected primates or with HAV in a research laboratory; persons with clotting-factor disorders; persons with chronic liver disease; and persons who anticipate close personal contact (e.g., household or regular babysitting) with an international adoptee during the first 60 days after arrival in the United States from a country with high or intermediate endemicity. The first dose should be administered as soon as the adoption is planned, ideally 2 or more weeks before the arrival of the adoptee.

12. **Human papillomavirus (HPV) vaccines. (Minimum age: 9 years for HPV2 [Cervarix] and HPV4 [Gardasil])**
    Routine vaccination:
    - Administer a 3-dose series of HPV vaccine on a schedule of 0, 1-2, and 6 months to all adolescents aged 11 through 12 years. Either HPV4 or HPV2 may be used for females, and only HPV4 may be used for males.
    - The vaccine series may be started at age 9 years.
    - Administer the second dose 1 to 2 months after the first dose (minimum interval of 4 weeks); administer the third dose 24 weeks after the first dose and 16 weeks after the second dose (minimum interval of 12 weeks).
    Catch-up vaccination:
    - Administer the vaccine series to females (either HPV2 or HPV4) and males (HPV4) at age 13 through 18 years if not previously vaccinated.
    - Use recommended routine dosing intervals (see Routine vaccination above) for vaccine series catch-up.

13. **Meningococcal conjugate vaccines. (Minimum age: 6 weeks for Hib-MenCY [MenHibrix], 9 months for MenACWY-D [Menactra], 2 months for MenACWY-CRM [Menveo])**
    Routine vaccination:
    - Administer a single dose of Menactra or Menveo vaccine at age 11 through 12 years, with a booster dose at age 16 years.
    - Adolescents aged 11 through 18 years with human immunodeficiency virus (HIV) infection should receive a 2-dose primary series of Menactra or Menveo with at least 8 weeks between doses.
    - For children aged 2 months through 18 years with high-risk conditions, see below.
    Catch-up vaccination:
    - Administer Menactra or Menveo vaccine at age 13 through 18 years if not previously vaccinated.
    - If the first dose is administered at age 13 through 15 years, a booster dose should be administered at age 16 through 18 years with a minimum interval of at least 8 weeks between doses.
    - If the first dose is administered at age 16 years or older, a booster dose is not needed.
    - For other catch-up guidance, see Figure 2.
    Vaccination of persons with high-risk conditions and other persons at increased risk of disease:
    - Children with anatomic or functional asplenia (including sickle cell disease):
      1. Menveo
         o *Children who initiate vaccination at 8 weeks through 6 months:* Administer doses at 2, 4, 6, and 12 months of age.
         o *Unvaccinated children 7 through 23 months:* Administer 2 doses, with the second dose at least 12 weeks after the first dose and after the first birthday.
         o *Children 24 months and older who have not received a complete series:* Administer 2 primary doses at least 8 weeks apart.
      2. MenHibrix
         o *Children 6 weeks through 18 months:* Administer doses at 2, 4, 6, and 12 through 15 months of age.
         o If the first dose is given at or after 12 months of age, a total of 2 doses should be given at least 8 weeks apart to ensure protection against serogroups C and Y meningococcal disease.
      3. Menactra
         o *Children 24 months and older who have not received a complete series:* Administer 2 primary doses at least 8 weeks apart. If Menactra is administered to a child with asplenia (including sickle cell disease), do not administer Menactra until 2 years of age and at least 4 weeks after the completion of all PCV13 doses.
    - Children with persistent complement component deficiency:
      1. Menveo
         o *Children who initiate vaccination at 8 weeks through 6 months:* Administer doses at 2, 4, 6, and 12 months of age.
         o *Unvaccinated children 7 through 23 months:* Administer 2 doses, with the second dose at least 12 weeks after the first dose AND after the first birthday.
         o *Children 24 months and older who have not received a complete series:* Administer 2 primary doses at least 8 weeks apart.
      2. MenHibrix
         o *Children 6 weeks through 18 months:* Administer doses at 2, 4, 6, and 12 through 15 months of age.
         o If the first dose of MenHibrix is given at or after 12 months of age, a total of 2 doses should be given at least 8 weeks apart to ensure protection against serogroups C and Y meningococcal disease.
      3. Menactra
         o *Children 9 through 23 months:* Administer 2 primary doses at least 12 weeks apart.
         o *Children 24 months and older who have not received a complete series:* Administer 2 primary doses at least 8 weeks apart.
    - For children who travel to or reside in countries in which meningococcal disease is hyperendemic or epidemic, including countries in the African meningitis belt or the Hajj, administer an age-appropriate formulation and series of Menactra or Menveo for protection against serogroups A and W meningococcal disease. Prior receipt of MenHibrix is not sufficient for children traveling to the meningitis belt or the Hajj because it does not contain serogroups A or W.
    - For children at risk during a community outbreak attributable to a vaccine serogroup, administer or complete an age- and formulation-appropriate series of MenHibrix, Menactra, or Menveo.
    - For booster doses among persons with high-risk conditions, refer to *MMWR* 2013 / 62(RR02);1-22, available at http://www.cdc.gov/mmwr/preview/mmwrhtml/rr6202a1.htm.

    For other catch-up recommendations for these persons, and complete information on use of meningococcal vaccines, including guidance related to vaccination of persons at increased risk of infection, see MMWR March 22, 2013 / 62(RR02);1-22, available at http://www.cdc.gov/mmwr/pdf/rr/rr6202.pdf.

U.S. Department of Health and Human Services, Centers for Disease Control and Prevention

Specific Antidotes

Poisonings account for approximately 5 million injuries per year in the United States. Of these, 5000 people die annually. Poisonings are responsible for 9% of all ambulance transports, 10% of all hospital emergency visits, and 5% of all hospital inpatient admissions. In children, many poisonings result from failure to store hazardous household substances and medications in a safe place. Poisons are often classified according to the body organ they primarily affect. The following table lists the specific antidotes for toxic substances.

Toxin	Antidote (s)
Acetaminophen	acetylcysteine (Mucomyst®)
Anticholinergic agents (e.g., tricyclic antidepressants)	physostigmine salicylate (Antilirium®)
Anticholinesterase agents (e.g., organophosphate insecticides)	pralidoxime chloride, PAM (Protopam Chloride®)
Arsenic	dimercaprol (BAL in Oil®)
Benzodiazepines	flumazenil (Romazicon®)
Calcium and digitalis	edetate disodium (Endrate®, Sodium Versenate®)
Cholinergic agents	atropine
Cyanide	amyl nitrite, sodium thiosulfate
Digoxin	digoxin immune FAB (Digibind®)
Folic acid antagonists (e.g., methotrexate)	leucovorin calcium
Gold	dimercaprol
Heparin	protamine sulfate
Ifosfamide	mesna (Mesnex®)
Insulin	glucagon
Iron	deferoxamine mesylate (Desferal Mesylate®)
Lead	edetate calcium disodium (Calcium Disodium Versenate®), succimer (Chemet®), dimercaprol, penicillamine (Cuprimine®)
Mercury	dimercaprol
Narcotics (opiates)	naloxone HCl (Narcan®), nalmefene HCl (Revex®)
Warfarin	vitamin K

Medical errors can potentially cause great harm to patients. Hundreds of thousands of people die each year as a result of medical errors or accidents. Some studies have shown that medication errors account for 10% to 25% of all medical errors. The following form is used by the U.S. Food and Drug Administration (FDA) to document adverse events related to medications, medical devices, and other medical products.

DEPARTMENT OF HEALTH AND HUMAN SERVICES Food and Drug Administration	Form Approved: OMB No. 0910-0291 Expiration Date: 6/30/2015 *(See PRA Statement below)*

MedWatch Consumer Voluntary Reporting
(FORM FDA 3500B)

When do I use this form?

- You were hurt or had a bad side effect (including new or worsening symptoms) after taking a drug or using a medical device or product.

- You used a drug, product, or medical device incorrectly which could have or led to unsafe use.

- You noticed a problem with the quality of the drug, product, or medical device.

- You had problems with how a drug worked after switching from one maker to another maker.

Don't use this form to report:

- Vaccines – report problems to the Vaccine Adverse Event Reporting System (VAERS)

- Investigational drugs or medical devices (those being studied, not yet approved) – report problems to your doctor or to the contact person listed in the clinical trial

Will the information I report be kept private?

The FDA recognizes that privacy is an important concern, so you should know:

- We ask only for the name and contact information of the person filling out the form in case we need more information. This information will not be given out to the public.

- Information about the problem may be shared with the company that makes the product to help them better understand the problem you are reporting, unless you request otherwise (see Section E).

What types of products should I use this form for?

- Drugs, including prescription or over-the-counter medicines, and biologics, such as human cells and tissues used for transplantation (for example, tendons, ligaments, and bone) and gene therapies

- Medical devices, including any health-related kit, test, tool, or piece of equipment (such as breast implants, pacemakers, diabetes glucose-test kits, hearing aids, breast pumps, and many others)

- Nutrition products, including vitamins and minerals, herbal remedies, infant formulas, and medical foods, such as those labeled for people with a specific disease or condition

- Cosmetics or make-up products

- Foods (including beverages and ingredients added to foods)

Are there specific instructions for filling out the form?

- Fill in as much information as possible and send in the report even if you do not have all the information.

- You can fill out this form yourself or have someone fill it out for you. If you need help, you may want to talk with your health professional.

- Feel free to include or attach an image. Please do not send the products to the FDA.

How will I know the FDA has received my form?

- You will receive a reply from the FDA after we receive your report. We will personally contact you only if we need additional information.

- Your report will become part of a database so that it can be reviewed and compared to other reports by an FDA safety evaluator who will determine what steps to take.

How can I contact the FDA if I have questions?

Toll-free line: 1-800-332-1088
www.fda.gov/reportinghelp
To report online: www.fda.gov/medwatch/report.htm

The information below applies only to requirements of the Paperwork Reduction Act of 1995.

The burden time for this collection of information is estimated to average 25 minutes per response, including the time to review instructions, search existing data sources, gather and maintain the data needed and complete and review the collection of information. Send comments regarding this burden estimate or any other aspect of this information collection, including suggestions for reducing this burden, to the address to the right:

OMB Statement: "An agency may not conduct or sponsor, and a person is not required to respond to, a collection of information unless it displays a currently valid OMB number."

Department of Health and Human Services
Food and Drug Administration
Office of Chief Information Officer
Paperwork Reduction Act (PRA) Staff
PRAStaff@fda.hhs.gov

DO NOT SEND YOUR COMPLETED FORM TO THIS PRA STAFF EMAIL ADDRESS.

FORM FDA 3500B (4/13)   **MedWatch** Consumer Voluntary Reporting   **General Information Page**

DEPARTMENT OF HEALTH AND HUMAN SERVICES
Food and Drug Administration

Form Approved: OMB No. 0910-0291
Expiration Date: 6/30/2015
(See PRA Statement on preceding general information page)

MedWatch Consumer Voluntary Reporting
(FORM FDA 3500B)

Section A – About the Problem

What kind of problem was it? *(Check all that apply)*

☐ Were hurt or had a bad side effect *(including new or worsening symptoms)*

☐ Used a product incorrectly which could have or led to a problem

☐ Noticed a problem with the quality of the product

☐ Had problems after switching from one product maker to another maker

Did any of the following happen? *(Check all that apply)*

☐ Hospitalization – admitted or stayed longer

☐ Required help to prevent permanent harm *(for medical devices only)*

☐ Disability or health problem

☐ Birth defect

☐ Life-threatening

☐ Death *(Include date)*: _____

☐ Other serious/important medical incident *(Please describe below)*

_____

Date the problem occurred *(mm/dd/yyyy)*

_____

_____

Tell us what happened and how it happened. *(Include as many details as possible)*

_____

_____

_____   Continuation Page

List any relevant tests or laboratory data if you know them. *(Include dates)*

_____

_____

_____   Continuation Page

For a problem with a product, including

- prescription or over-the-counter medicine
- biologics, such as human cells and tissues used for transplantation (for example, tendons, ligaments, and bone) and gene therapies
- nutrition products, such as vitamins and minerals, herbal remedies, infant formulas, and medical foods
- cosmetics or make-up products
- foods (including beverages and ingredients added to foods)

⇨ **Go to Section B**

For a problem with a medical device, including

- any health-related test, tool, or piece of equipment
- health-related kits, such as glucose monitoring kits or blood pressure cuffs
- implants, such as breast implants, pacemakers, or catheters
- other consumer health products, such as contact lenses, hearing aids, and breast pumps

⇨ **Go to Section C
(Skip Section B)**

For more information, visit *http://www.fda.gov/MedWatch*

Submission of a report does not constitute an admission that medical personnel or the product caused or contributed to the event.

FORM FDA 3500B (4/13)   **MedWatch** Consumer Voluntary Reporting   Page 1 of 3

U.S. Department of Health and Human Services

Section B – About the Products

Name of the product as it appears on the box, bottle, or package *(Include as many names as you see)*

Name of the company that makes the product

Expiration date *(mm/dd/yyyy)*	Lot number	NDC number

Strength *(for example, 250 mg per 500 mL or 1 g)*	Quantity *(for example, 2 pills, 2 puffs, or 1 teaspoon, etc.)*	Frequency *(for example, twice daily or at bedtime)*	How was it taken or used *(for example, by mouth, by injection, or on the skin)?*

Date the person first started taking or using the product *(mm/dd/yyyy)*: _____

Date the person stopped taking or using the product *(mm/dd/yyyy)*: _____

Why was the person using the product *(such as, what condition was it supposed to treat?)*

_____

_____

_____

Did the problem stop after the person reduced the dose or stopped taking or using the product? ☐ Yes ☐ No

Did the problem return if the person started taking or using the product again?

☐ Yes ☐ No ☐ Didn't restart

Do you still have the product in case we need to evaluate it? *(Do not send the product to FDA. We will contact you directly if we need it.)*

☐ Yes ☐ No

⬛➡ **Go to Section D (Skip Section C)**

Section C – About the Medical Device

Name of medical device

Name of the company that makes the medical device

Other identifying information *(The model, catalog, lot, serial, or UDI number, and the expiration date, if you can locate them)*

_____

_____

_____

Was someone operating the medical device when the problem occurred?

☐ Yes

☐ No

If yes, who was using it?

☐ The person who had the problem

☐ A health professional *(such as a doctor, nurse, or aide)*

☐ Someone else *(Please explain who)*

_____

For implanted medical devices ONLY *(such as pacemakers, breast implants, etc.)*

Date the implant was put in *(mm/dd/yyyy)*	Date the implant was taken out *(If relevant) (mm/dd/yyyy)*

⬛➡ **Go to Section D**

For more information, visit *http://www.fda.gov/MedWatch*

Submission of a report does not constitute an admission that medical personnel or the product caused or contributed to the event.

FORM FDA 3500B (4/13)   **MedWatch** Consumer Voluntary Reporting   Page 2 of 3

U.S. Department of Health and Human Services

608   APPENDIX H • Reporting of Medical Errors

Section D – About the Person Who Had the Problem

Person's Initials	Sex	Age (at time the problem occurred) or Birth Date	Weight (Specify lbs or kg)	Race
	☐ Female ☐ Male			

List known medical conditions (such as diabetes, high blood pressure, cancer, heart disease, or others)

_____

_____

Please list all allergies (such as to drugs, foods, pollen, or others).

List any other important information about the person (such as smoking, pregnancy, alcohol use, etc.)

List all current prescription medications and medical devices being used.

_____

_____ | Continuation Page |

List all over-the-counter medications and any vitamins, minerals, supplements, and herbal remedies being used.

| Continuation Page |

▭▷ **Go to Section E**

Section E – About the Person Filling Out This Form

We will contact you only if we need additional information. Your name will not be given out to the public.

Last name	First name
Number/Street	City and State/Province
Country	ZIP or Postal code

Telephone number	Email address	Today's date (mm/dd/yyyy)

Did you report this problem to the company that makes the product (the manufacturer)? ☐ Yes ☐ No	May we give your name and contact information to the company that makes the product (manufacturer) to help them evaluate the product? ☐ Yes ☐ No

Send This Report by Mail or Fax

Keep the product in case the FDA wants to contact you for more information. Please do not send products to the FDA. Mail or fax the form to:

Mail: MedWatch Food and Drug Administration 5600 Fishers Lane Rockville, MD 20857	**Fax:** 1-800-332-0178 (toll-free)

Thank you for helping us protect the public health.

For more information, visit http://www.fda.gov/MedWatch	Submission of a report does not constitute an admission that medical personnel or the product caused or contributed to the event.

FORM FDA 3500B (4/13)   **MedWatch** Consumer Voluntary Reporting   Page 3 of 3

U.S. Department of Health and Human Services

Continued Entries

CONTINUED ENTRY FOR: Tell us what happened and how it happened. *(Include as many details as possible)*

Back to Form

CONTINUED ENTRY FOR: List any relevant tests or laboratory data if you know them. *(Include dates)*

Back to Form

CONTINUED ENTRY FOR: List all current prescription medications and medical devices being used.

Back to Form

CONTINUED ENTRY FOR: List all over-the-counter medications and any vitamins, minerals, and herbal remedies being used.

Back to Form

FORM FDA 3500B (4/13)   **MedWatch** – Consumer Voluntary Reporting   **Continuation Page**

U.S. Department of Health and Human Services

APPENDIX I

Drug/Food Interactions

A. DRUGS THAT SHOULD BE TAKEN WHILE FASTING

Alendronate

Ampicillin

Bethanechol (may experience nausea and vomiting)

Bisacodyl

Captopril (take 1 hour before meals)

Ceftibuten (Cedax®)

Cetirizine (Zyrtec®)

Chloramphenicol

Cilostazol (Pletal®)

Cyclosporine gel caps only (avoid fatty meals)

Demeclocycline (avoid high calcium foods/dairy products)

Dicloxacillin

Didanosine (Videx®)

Digitalis preparations (not with high-fiber foods)

Digoxin (avoid high-fiber cereals and oatmeal)

Erythromycin base/estolate

Etidronate (Didronel®)

Felodipine (Plendil®)

Ferrous salts (not with tea, coffee, egg, cereals, fiber, or milk)

Fexofenadine

Flavoxate

Indinavir (Crixivan®)

Ketoprofen (if gastrointestinal [GI] distress occurs, may take with food)

Lansoprazole

Levodopa (not with high-protein foods; meals delay absorption and peak plasma concentration; avoid caffeine)

Levothyroxine

Lomustine (empty stomach will reduce nausea)

Loracarbef (Lorabid®)

Loratadine (Claritin®)

Methotrexate (milk, cream, or yogurt may decrease absorption)

Methyldopa (not with high-protein foods; meals delay absorption and peak plasma concentration; avoid caffeine)

Nafcillin (inactivated by stomach acid; absorption variable with/without food)

Norfloxacin (milk, cream, or yogurt may decrease absorption)

Omeprazole

Oxacillin

Oxytetracycline (avoid dairy products and foods high in calcium)

Penicillamine (antacids, iron, and food decrease absorption)

Perindopril (Aceon®)

Phenytoin (if GI distress occurs, may take with food; food effect depends on preparation)

Propantheline

Repaglinide (Prandin®)

Rifabutin (Mycobutin®)

Rifampin

Riluzole (Rilutek®)

Roxithromycin (take at least 15 min before or after meal)

Sotalol

Sucralfate

Sulfadiazine

Sulfamethoxazole-Trimethoprim (Bactrim®)

Terbutaline sulfate

Tetracycline (avoid dairy products and foods high in calcium)

Theophylline (absorption of controlled release varies by preparation)

Thyroid hormone preparations (limit foods containing goitrogens)

Tolcapone (Tasmar®)

Trientine (antacids, iron, and food reduce absorption)

Zafirlukast (Accolate®)

Zalcitabine (Hivid®)

B. DRUGS THAT SHOULD BE TAKEN WITH FOOD

Allopurinol (after meal)

Amiodarone (Cordarone®)

Aspirin

Atovaquone (Mepron®)

Augmentin

Baclofen (Lioresal®)

Bromocriptine (Parlodel®)

Buspirone

Carbamazepine (erratic absorption; Tegretol®)

Carvedilol (Coreg®)

Cefpodoxime (Vantin®)

Chloroquine

Chlorothiazide

Cimetidine (Tagamet®)

Clofazimine

Diclofenac (Voltaren®)

Divalproex (Depakote®)

Doxycycline

Felbamate (Felbatol®)

Fenofibrate (TriCor®)

Fenoprofen

Fiorinal

Fludrocortisone

Gemfibrozil

Glyburide (take with breakfast)

Griseofulvin (high-fat meals)

Hydrocortisone

Hydroxychloroquine (Plaquenil®)

Indomethacin

Iron products (take between meals, unless GI upset)

Isotretinoin

Itraconazole capsules

Ketorolac

Lithium

Mebendazole

Methenamine
Methylprednisolone
Metronidazole
Misoprostol (Cytotec®)
Naltrexone
Naproxen
Nelfinavir (Viracept®)
Niacin
Nifedipine (grapefruit juice
  increases bioavailability)
Nitrofurantoin
Olsalazine
Oxcarbazepine
Pentoxifylline
Pergolide
Perphenazine
Piroxicam
Potassium salts
Prednisone
Probucol (high-fat meals)
Procainamide
Ritonavir (Norvir®)
Salsalate
Saquinavir
Sevelamer (Renagel®)
Spironolactone
Sulfasalazine
Sulfinpyrazone
Sulindac
Ticlopidine
Tolmetin
Trazodone
Troglitazone
Valproic acid
Verapamil SR (absorption varies
  by manufacturer; too-rapid
  absorption may cause heart block)

C. CONSTIPATING AGENTS

Antacids (aluminum and calcium
  containing)
Anticholinergic drugs
Anticonvulsants
Antidepressants

Antihistamines
Antiparkinsonian drugs
Antipsychotic drugs
Antispasmodics
Bisphosphonates
Blood pressure drugs (calcium
  channel blockers)
Calcium supplements
Clonidine
Diuretics
Ganglionic blocking agents
Iron supplements
Monamine oxidase (MAO)
  inhibitors
Muscle relaxants
Narcotics
Nonsteroidal anti-inflammatory
  drugs (NSAIDs)
Octreotide
Opioids
Phenothiazines
Prostaglandin synthesis inhibitors
Tranquilizers
Tricyclic antidepressants

D. DIARRHEAL AGENTS

Adrenergic neuron blockers:
  reserpine, guanethidine
Antacids (Mg^{2+} containing)
  H_2 receptor antagonists (e.g.,
  ranitidine) proton pump inhibitors
  (e.g., omeprazole)
Antiarrhythmics (e.g., quinidine)
Antibiotics (especially broad-
  spectrum agents)
Antidepressants (fluoxetine,
  sertraline)
Antihypertensives (beta-blockers,
  angiotensin-converting enzyme
  [ACE] inhibitors)
Anti-inflammatory drugs (NSAIDs,
  colchicine)
Antivirals
Chemotherapy agents

Cholinergic agonists and
  cholinesterase inhibitors
Colchicine
Corticosteroids (prednisone)
Digitalis
Glucophage (Metformin®)
Lithium
Metoclopramide
Misoprostol
Mycophenolate (drugs to prevent
  organ transplant rejection)
NSAIDs
Olsalazine
Osmotic and stimulant laxatives
  (e.g., Ex-Lax®, Dulcolax®,
  Correctol®, Feen-a-Mint®)
Radiation therapy
Theophylline (Theo-24®)

E. TYRAMINE-CONTAINING FOODS

Moderate amounts of tyramine:
Banana peel
Broad beans (fava)
Cheese (all except cream cheese and
  cottage cheese)
Chianti, vermouth
Chocolate
Concentrated yeast extracts,
  Brewer's yeast
Fermented cabbage products:
  sauerkraut, kimchee
Hydrolyzed protein extracts for
  sauces, soups, gravies
Imitation cheese
Liquid and powdered protein
  supplements
Meat extracts
Nonalcoholic beers
Prepared meats (sausage, chopped
  liver, pate, salami, mortadella)
Raspberries
Some non–U.S. brands of beer
Yeast products

Significant amounts of tyramine:
Aged cheese
Aged or cured meats
Avocado
Bean curd
Cream from fresh pasteurized milk
Distilled spirits
Eggplant
Fruits (grapes, oranges, pineapple, plums, prunes, figs, raisins)
Peanuts, coconuts, Brazil nuts
Processed foods (Vegemite®, sauerkraut, shrimp paste)
Red and white wines, port wines
Soy products (soy sauce, tofu, miso, teriyaki sauce)
Tap beer
Yogurt

F. FOODS CONTAINING GOITROGENS

Cruciferous vegetables (broccoli, Brussels sprouts, cabbage, cauliflower, kale, rutabaga, mustard, turnips)
Millet
Peaches
Peanuts
Radishes
Soybeans and soy-bean related foods (tofu)
Spinach
Strawberries

G. COUMARIN ANTICOAGULANTS AND DIETARY EFFECTS

Consumption of vitamin K-enriched foods may counteract the effects of anticoagulants since the drugs act through antagonism of vitamin K. Advise patients taking anticoagulants to maintain a steady, consistent intake of vitamin K-containing foods.

The drug monograph for warfarin (Coumadin®) clearly lists these foods. Leafy green and cruciferous vegetables (e.g., Brussels sprouts, broccoli, spinach, kale, turnip greens) increase the catabolism of warfarin thereby decreasing its anticoagulant activities.

Additionally, certain herbal teas (e.g., green tea, buckeye, horse chestnut, Woodruff, tonka beans, melilot) contain natural coumarins that can potentiate the effects of warfarin and should be avoided. Large amounts of avocado also potentiate the drug's effects.

Caffeinated beverages (e.g., cola, coffee, tea, hot chocolate, chocolate milk) can affect therapy. Alcohol intake of more than three drinks per day can affect clotting times. Herbal supplements can also affect bleeding time: coenzyme Q10 is structurally similar to vitamin K, feverfew, garlic, and ginseng. As a general rule, patients should therefore avoid herbal medications while on warfarin therapy.

H. GENERAL DRUG CLASS RECOMMENDATIONS

ACE inhibitors: Take captopril and moexipril 1 hour before or 2 hours after meals; food decreases absorption. Avoid high-potassium foods as ACE increases K⁺.

Analgesic/Antipyretic: Take on an empty stomach as food may slow the absorption.

Antacids: Take 1 hour after or between meals. Avoid dairy foods as the protein in them can increase stomach acid.

Antianxiety agents: Caffeine may cause excitability, nervousness, and hyperactivity lessening the antianxiety drug effects.

Antibiotics: Penicillin generally should be taken on an empty stomach; may take with food if GI upset occurs. Do not mix with acidic foods: coffee, citrus fruits, and tomatoes; the acid interferes with absorption of penicillin, ampicillin, erythromycin and cloxacillin.

Anticoagulants: High vitamin K produces blood-clotting substance and may reduce drug effectiveness. Vitamin E > 400 international units may prolong clotting time and increase bleeding risk.

Antidepressant drugs: May be taken with or without food.

Antifungals: Avoid taking with dairy products; avoid alcohol.

Antihistamines: Take on an empty stomach to increase effectiveness.

Bronchodilators with theophylline: High-fat meals may increase bioavailability while high-carbohydrate meals may decrease it. Food increases absorption of Theo-24® and Uniphyl®, which may cause increased nausea and vomiting, headache, and irritability.

Cephalosporins: Take on an empty stomach 1 hour before or 2 hours after meals. May take with food if GI upset occurs.

Diuretics: Vary in interactions; some cause loss of potassium, calcium, and magnesium. Avoid salty food and natural black licorice as these increase K⁺ and Mg²⁺ losses. Large doses of vitamin D can elevate blood pressure.

H₂ blockers: May take with or without regard to food.

HMG-CoA reductase inhibitors: Take lovastatin with the evening meal to enhance absorption.

Laxatives: Avoid dairy foods as calcium can decrease absorption.

Macrolides: Take on an empty stomach 1 hour before or 2 hour after meals. May take with food for GI upset.

MAO inhibitors: Have many dietary restrictions, so follow dietary guidelines as prescribed. Foods or alcoholic beverages containing tyramine may cause a fatal increase in blood pressure.

Narcotic analgesics: Avoid alcohol as it may increase sedative effects.

Nitroimidazole (metronidazole): Avoid alcohol or food prepared with alcohol for at least three days after finishing the medicine. Alcohol may cause nausea, abdominal cramps, vomiting, headaches, and flushing.

NSAIDs: Take with food or milk to prevent irritation of the stomach.

Quinolones: Take on an empty stomach 1 hour before or 2 hours after meals. May take with food for GI upset but avoid calcium-containing foods such as milk, yogurt, vitamins/minerals containing iron, and antacids because they decrease drug concentrations. Caffeine-containing products may lead to excitability and nervousness.

Sulfonamides: Take on an empty stomach 1 hour before or 2 hours after meals. May take with food if GI upset occurs.

Tetracyclines: Take on an empty stomach 1 hour before or 2 hours after meals. May take with food but avoid dairy products, antacids, and vitamins containing iron with tetracycline.

Reprinted from Spratto, G., & Woods, A. (2013). *Delmar nurse's drug handbook.* Clifton Park, NY: Cengage Learning.

Drugs That Should Not Be Crushed

As a rule of thumb, any sustained-release or extended-release formulation should never be crushed. Instead, attempt to get a liquid formulation of the product so that it can be administered in that form. Coated products also should not be crushed. They were coated for a specific purpose, for example, to prevent stomach irritation by the product, to prevent destruction of the product by stomach acid, to prevent an unwanted reaction, or to produce a prolonged or an extended effect.

These are some of the drugs that should not be crushed:

Accutane®
AcipHex®
Actiq®
Actonel®
Adalat cc SR®
Adderall XR®
Advicor ER®
Afrinol Repetab®
Aggrenox®
Allegra D®
Allerest® capsule
Alprazolam ER®
Altoprev®
Ambien CR®
Aminodur Duratab®
Aptivus®
Arthrotec®
ASA E.C.®
ASA Enseal®
Augmentin XR®
Avinza®
Avodart®
Azulfidine Entab®
Betaphen-VK®
Biaxin XL®
Bisacodyl EC®
Boniva®
Budeprion SR®
Calan SR®
Cardene SR®
Cardizem LA, SR®
Cardura XL®
Ceclor CD®
Ceftin®
Cefuroxime®

CellCept®
Chlor-Trimeton SR®
Choledyl SR®
Cipro XR®
Claritin-D®
Colace®
Colestid®
Commit®
Compazine Spansule®
Concerta®
Concerta SR®
Covera-HS®
Creon EC®
Crixivan®
Cymbalta®
Cytovene®
Depakote ER®
Detrol LA®
Dilacor XR®
Ditropan XL®
Divalproex XR®
Drixoral® tablet
Dulcolax EC®
DynaCirc CR®
Ecotrin® tablet
Effexor XR®
E-Mycin® tablet
Erythromycin EC®
Evista®
Feldene®
Fentora®
Feosol Spansule® tablet
Ferro Grad-500® tablet/
  sequels
Flagyl ER®

Flomax®
Fosamax®
Geocillin®
Gleevec®
Glipizide®
Glucophage XR®
Glucotrol XL®
Imdur SR, LA®
Inderal LA®
Indocin SR®
InnoPran XL®
Intelence®
Isoptin SR®
Isordil® sublingual
Isordil Tembids®, Dinitrate
Kadian®
Kaon® tablet
Kapidex®
K-Dur®, K-tab®
Keppra XR®
Ketek®
Klor-Con®
Lamictal XR®
Lescol XL®
Levbid SR®
Lithobid SR®
Luvox CR®
Macrobid SR®
Mestinon Timespans®
Metadate CD, SR®
Metoprolol ER®
Motrin®
MS Contin®
Mucinex®
Nexium®

Niaspan®
Nicotinic acid
Nifediac CC®
Nifedipine ER®
Nitroglycerin® tablet
Nitrospan® capsule
Norpace CR®
OxyContin®
Pancrease EC, MT®
Paxil CR®
Pentasa®
Plendil SR®
Prevacid®
Prilosec SR®
Procardia XL®
Propecia®
Proscar®
Protonix®
Prozac weekly®
Ranexa®
Razadyne ER®
Renagel®
Requip XL®
Revlimid®
Risperdal M-tab®
Ritalin LA/SR®
Rythmol SR®
Seroquel XR®
Sinemet CR®
Slo-Niacin®
Slow K® tablet; Slow Mag®,
  Slow Fe®
Strattera®
Sudafed SA® capsule
Sular®

Tasigna®
Tegretol XR®
Temodar®
Tessalon Perles®
Theobid Duracaps®
Tiazac SR®
Topamax®
Toprol XL®
Tracleer®

Trental SR®
Treximet®
Tylenol ER®
Ultram ER®
Uniphyl SR®
Uroxatral®
Valcyte®
Verapamil SR®
Verelan PM®

Videx EC®
Voltaren EC/SR®
Wellbutrin SR®
Xanax SR®
Zerit XR®
Zolinza®
Zomig ZMT®
ZORprin®
Zyban®

Zyflo CR®
Zyrtec-D®

Reprinted from Spratto, G., & Woods, A. (2013) *Delmar nurse's drug handbook*. Clifton Park, NY: Cengage Learning.

Drug Identification Guide

This color photo quick reference guide provides rapid identification of most commonly prescribed drugs. Actual-sized tablets and capsules, with their strength, are organized alphabetically by generic name and include appropriate trade name and manufacturer.

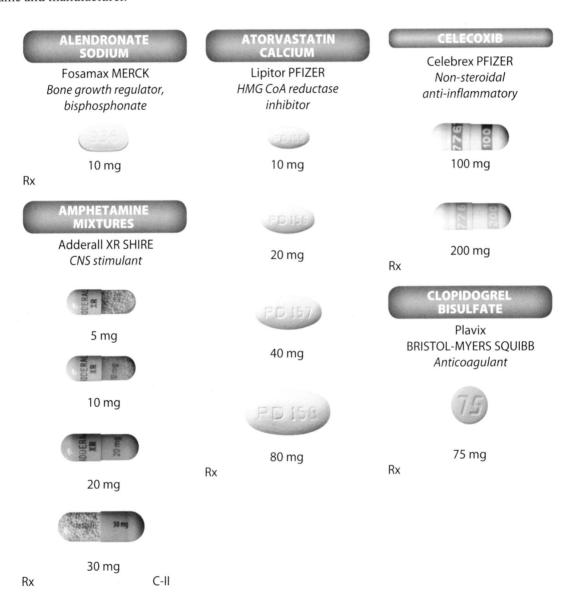

ALENDRONATE SODIUM

Fosamax MERCK
Bone growth regulator, bisphosphonate

10 mg

Rx

AMPHETAMINE MIXTURES

Adderall XR SHIRE
CNS stimulant

5 mg

10 mg

20 mg

30 mg

Rx   C-II

ATORVASTATIN CALCIUM

Lipitor PFIZER
HMG CoA reductase inhibitor

10 mg

20 mg

40 mg

80 mg

Rx

CELECOXIB

Celebrex PFIZER
Non-steroidal anti-inflammatory

100 mg

200 mg

Rx

CLOPIDOGREL BISULFATE

Plavix
BRISTOL-MYERS SQUIBB
Anticoagulant

75 mg

Rx

DIGOXIN

Lanoxin
GLAXO SMITH KLINE
Antiarrhythmic

0.125 mg

0.25 mg

Rx

ESCITALOPRAM OXALATE

Lexapro FOREST
*Antidepressant, selective
serotonin reuptake inhibitor*

5 mg

10 mg

20 mg

Rx

ESOMEPRAZOLE MAGNESIUM

Nexium
ASTRAZENECA
Proton pump inhibitor

20 mg

40 mg

Rx

ESTROGENS, CONJUGATED ORAL

Premarin PFIZER
*Selective estrogen
receptor modulator*

0.3 mg

0.625 mg

0.9 mg

Rx

ESZOPICLONE

Lunesta
SUNOVION
Sedative-hypnotic

3 mg

Rx   C-IV

EZETIMIBE AND SIMVASTATIN

Vytorin MERCK
*Cholesterol inhibitor,
HMG CoA reductase inhibitor*

10/20 mg

10/40 mg

10/80 mg

Rx

FUROSEMIDE

Lasix
SANOFI
Loop diuretic

80 mg

Rx

IBANDRONATE SODIUM

Boniva
ROCHE

150 mg

Rx

IRBESARTAN

Avapro
BRISTOL-MYERS SQUIBB
Angiotensin II receptor antagonist

150 mg

300 mg

Rx

LAMOTRIGINE

Lamictal
GLAXO SMITH KLINE
Anticonvulsant, Antidepressant

5 mg

25 mg

100 mg

150 mg

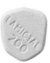

200 mg

Rx

LANSOPRAZOLE

Prevacid
TAKEDA
Proton pump inhibitor

30 mg

Rx

LEVETIRACETAM

Keppra
UCB
Anticonvulsant

500 mg

750 mg

Rx

LEVOFLOXACIN

Levaquin
JANSSEN
Fluoroquinolone antibiotic

250 mg

500 mg

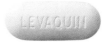

750 mg

Rx

LEVOTHYROXINE SODIUM

Synthroid
ABBOTT
Thyroid product

50 mcg

75 mcg

88 mcg

100 mcg

125 mcg

150 mcg

175 mcg

Rx

LOSARTAN POTASSIUM

Cozaar
MERCK
Antihypertensive, angiotensin II receptor blocker

25 mg

50 mg

100 mg

Rx

MEMANTINE HYDROCHLORIDE

Namenda
FOREST
Alzheimer's/dementia product

5 mg

10 mg

Rx

OMEPRAZOLE

Prilosec
PROCTOR & GAMBLE
Proton pump inhibitor

40 mg

Rx

PIOGLITAZONE HYDROCHLORIDE

Actos
TAKEDA
*Antidiabetic, oral;
thiazolidinedione*

15 mg

30 mg

45 mg

Rx

QUETIAPINE FUMARATE

Seroquel
ASTRAZENECA
Antipsychotic

25 mg

50 mg

100 mg

200 mg

300 mg

Rx

RALOXIFENE HYDROCHLORIDE

Evista
ELI LILLY
*Estrogen receptor
modulator*

60 mg

Rx

ROSIGLITAZONE MALEATE

Avandia
GLAXO SMITHKLINE
*Antidiabetic, oral;
thiazolidinedione*

4 mg

Rx   8 mg

ROSUVASTATIN CALCIUM

Crestor
ASTRA-ZENECA
Antihyperlipidemic, HMG-CoA reductase inhibitor

5 mg

10 mg

20 mg

Rx

SERTRALINE HYDROCHLORIDE

Zoloft
PFIZER
Antidepressant; selective serotonin reuptake inhibitor

25 mg

50 mg

Rx

SILDENAFIL CITRATE

Viagra.
PFIZER
Used for erectile dysfunction

50 mg

100 mg

Rx

TADALAFIL

Cialis
ELI LILLY
Used for erectile dysfunction, benign prostatic hypertrophy

10 mg

20 mg

Rx

TAMSULOSIN HYDROCHLORIDE

Flomax
BOEHRINGERINGELHEIM
Alpha-adrenergic blocker

0.4 mg

Rx

TOLTERODINE TARTRATE
Detrol LA
PFIZER
Used for overactive bladder

1 mg

4 mg

Rx

TOPIRAMATE
Topamax
JANSSEN
Anticonvulsant, antimigraine

15 mg

25 mg

50 mg

Rx

VALSARTAN
Diovan
NOVARTIS
Thiazide diuretic

80 mg

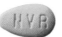

160 mg

320 mg

Rx

VENLAFAXINE HYDROCHLORIDE
Effexor XR
PFIZER
Antidepressant; selective serotonin and norepinephrine reuptake inhibitor

37.5 mg

75 mg

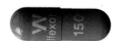

150 mg

Rx

WARFARIN SODIUM
Coumadin
BRISTOL-MYERS SQUIBB
Anticoagulant

1 mg

2 mg

3 mg

4 mg

5 mg

Rx

ZOLPIDEM TARTRATE

Ambien
SANOFI
Sedative-hypnotic

5 mg

10 mg

Rx   C-IV

Ambien CR
SANOFI

6.25 mg

12.5 mg

Rx   C-IV

Answer Keys

Chapter 1

Short Answer

1. C-II drugs have high abuse potential and accepted medical use, require a prescription, and no refills are permitted without a prescription; C-V drugs have low abuse potential and accepted medical use, and do not require a prescription for individuals aged 18 years or older.

2. The Drug Enforcement Administration (DEA) is tasked with the regulation and enforcement of laws related to drug use, sale, distribution, and manufacturing. The DEA also requires maintenance of transactions related to controlled substances.

3. The Food and Drug Administration (FDA) is responsible for drug product development as well as general safety standards in the production of drugs, foods, and cosmetics.

4. 1906; Pure Food and Drug Act.

5. a. Regulates the manufacture, distribution, and dispensation of drugs with a potential for abuse; deals with control and enforcement.
   b. The first attempt to control and regulate the manufacture, distribution, and sale of drugs.
   c. Regulated the importation, manufacture, sale, and use of opium, codeine, and their derivatives and compounds; it was replaced by the Controlled Substances Act (CSA).
   d. Prescription drugs.

Multiple Choice

1. A 2. D 3. B 4. B 5. A 6. B
7. D 8. C 9. D 10. A 11. C 12. D
13. B 14. D 15. C

Matching

1. D 2. C 3. B 4. A

Answers to Critical Thinking Questions:

1. The Harrison Narcotic Act of 1914, which was replaced by the Comprehensive Drug Abuse Prevention and Control Act.

2. The FDA has the power to approve or deny new drug applications and even to conduct inspections to ensure compliance.

3. The Pure Food and Drug Act of 1906.

Chapter 2

Multiple Choice

1. B 2. A 3. C 4. D 5. B 6. B
7. D 8. D 9. A 10. C 11. D
12. A 13. D 14. B 15. D

Matching

1. J 2. I 3. H 4. E 5. F 6. C
7. D 8. B 9. G 10. A

Answers to Critical Thinking Questions:

1. It is cheaper.

2. Because generic drug formularies may be different, the inert ingredients may differ somewhat from those of brand-name equivalents and consequently may affect the ability of the drug to reach the target cells and produce an effect.

3. The pharmacist must verify that the physician did not intend to prescribe only the trade name version of the drug.

Chapter 3

Multiple Choice

1. C 2. B 3. C 4. A 5. B 6. D
7. D 8. A 9. C 10. B 11. D 12. A
13. A 14. C 15. B

Fill in the Blank

1. first-pass effect
2. clearance
3. pharmacodynamics
4. glomerular filtration rate
5. rapidly

6. Newborns

7. placebo

Answers to Critical Thinking Questions:

1. Therapeutic Index (TI) = $\dfrac{\text{Median lethal dose (LD}_{50})}{\text{Median effective dose (ED}_{50})}$

2. Since this patient is 75 years old, the physician must consider the reduction in nephrons that will have occurred. This will influence the correct dosage that must be prescribed.

3. Elderly people are more susceptible to nephrotoxicity from certain drugs, such as gentamicin, because of this reduction in the amount of nephrons, and the related slower filtration rate.

Chapter 4

Review Questions

1. D   2. A   3. C   4. B   5. B   6. D
7. C   8. B   9. A   10. C

Fill in the Blank

1. medication prescribed

2. Rx symbol

3. Medication administration record, MAR

4. Standing

5. Every night

Critical Thinking

1. The pediatrician should have written 0.4 mg instead of .4 mg. A leading zero is always required so that an amount that is less than "1" is understood correctly.

2. The mistake the pharmacy technician made was not seeing the decimal point in front of the ordered dosage, and then incorrectly dispensing 4 mg. Also, the pharmacy technician could have checked any of the numerous sources available to verify the dosage range of morphine for this 4-month-old baby.

Chapter 5

Multiple Choice

1. B   2. D   3. C   4. D   5. A   6. D
7. B   8. C   9. B   10. D

Matching

1. E   2. D   3. A   4. C   5. B

Fill in the Blank

1. 5-HT

2. neuroleptic

3. mental illness

4. bipolar

5. manic-depressive

6. lithium

7. major depression

Answers to Critical Thinking Questions:

1. SSRIs are much safer than other types, and are the drug(s) of choice for major depression.

2. SSRIs are the newest type of antidepressants.

3. Contraindicated foods that contain tyramine include beer, red wines, cheese, chocolate, avocados, bananas, etc.

Chapter 6

Multiple Choice

1. B   2. C   3. D   4. A   5. D   6. B
7. A   8. A   9. D   10. C   11. D   12. D
13. B   14. C   15. D

Fill in the Blank

1. anxiety; insomnia

2. dependence

3. GABA

4. panic attacks

5. anxiety; insomnia

6. tranquilizers

7. D

Answers to Critical Thinking Questions:

1. There are two choices: either paroxetine or sertraline.

2. No, both paroxetine and sertraline are also used for panic disorders.

3. The most severe adverse effect would be CNS and respiratory depression.

Chapter 7

Multiple Choice

1. C	2. D	3. D	4. A	5. B	6. C
7. A	8. A	9. D	10. B	11. A	12. B
13. D	14. A	15. C			

True or False

| 1. T | 2. F | 3. F | 4. F | 5. T | 6. T |
| 7. T | 8. T | 9. T | 10. F | | |

Answers to Critical Thinking Questions:

1. Cholinergic agonists are the best class of drugs for these conditions.

2. Undesirable effects of cholinergic agonist drugs include flushing, sweating, abdominal cramps, difficulty in visual accommodation, headache, and convulsions (at high doses). Specific GI adverse effects include epigastric distress, diarrhea, involuntary defecation, nausea and vomiting, and colic.

3. The drug of choice should only be used cautiously in patients with asthma and hyperthyroidism.

Chapter 8

Multiple Choice

| 1. B | 2. D | 3. A | 4. B | 5. B | 6. D |
| 7. C | 8. B | 9. B | 10. C | | |

Fill in the Blank

1. basal nuclei

2. 60

3. acetylcholine

4. Alzheimer's disease

5. acetylcholinesterase

6. liver, kidney

7. narrow-angle glaucoma

8. Parkinsonism

9. epinephrine

10. B_6

11. Alzheimer's disease

12. Parkinson's disease

Answers to Critical Thinking Questions:

1. Levodopa, or any other drug, is not able to cure Parkinson's disease, and only reduces the symptoms.

2. It should be used only with caution because of her history of hepatitis C.

3. Dopamine cannot be used on its own for Parkinson's disease, so therefore could not be used as a substitution for levodopa.

Chapter 9

Multiple Choice

1. C	2. D	3. C	4. C	5. A	6. B
7. D	8. C	9. C	10. B	11. D	12. C
13. A	14. B	15. B			

Fill in the Blank

1. Depakene

2. physician

3. generalized

4. psychomotor

5. phenytoin

6. petit mal

7. valproic acid; zonisamide

Answers to Critical Thinking Questions:

1. The phenytoin-like drug valproic acid is used for prevention of migraines.

2. Succinimides are the type of phenytoin-like drugs used to treat absence seizures.

3. The most dangerous adverse effects of phenytoin-like drugs may be fatal liver toxicity and bone marrow suppression.

Chapter 10

Multiple Choice

1. D	2. A	3. C	4. D	5. C	6. A
7. C	8. B	9. C	10. A	11. B	12. D

Matching

1. F	2. E	3. C	4. D	5. B	6. A

Fill in the Blank

1. nerve block
2. atropine; scopolamine
3. laughing gas
4. rare

Answers to Critical Thinking Questions:

1. Local infiltration anesthesia would be the best type to use for this patient.

2. Normally there are no drug interactions between local infiltration anesthesia and these drugs.

3. The only potential adverse effect would occur if the patient has a true allergic reaction to the local anesthetic used.

Chapter 11

Multiple Choice

1. B	2. C	3. A	4. A	5. C	6. B
7. A	8. B	9. C	10. B	11. B	12. D
13. A	14. C	15. D			

Fill in the Blank

1. somatic motor
2. C
3. safety margin
4. A. gold compounds
   B. penicillamine
   C. corticosteroids
5. A. poor wound healing
   B. hyperglycemia
   C. hypertension
   D. osteoporosis
   E. gastrointestinal bleeding
6. not known
7. first; joint

Answers to Critical Thinking Questions:

1. Allopurinol should be used with caution; the other choice, colchicine, is contraindicated in the presence of peptic ulcer.

2. Colchicine is the drug of choice for acute gouty arthritis.

3. The drug is very toxic, and it should be stopped at the first symptom of toxicity, such as nausea, vomiting, diarrhea, and abdominal pain. Adverse effects of oral colchicine include nausea, abdominal cramps, and diarrhea.

Chapter 12

Multiple Choice

1. D	2. C	3. B	4. C	5. B	6. A
7. B	8. C	9. A	10. B	11. A	12. D
13. B	14. C	15. A			

Fill in the Blank

1. nitrates
2. fast channel blockers
3. IV

4. nystagmus, blurred vision, vertigo, and hyperplasia of the gums
5. myocardial systolic contraction

Matching

1. D   2. B   3. E   4. C   5. A

Answers to Critical Thinking Questions:

1. Aside from congestive heart failure, digitalis is also used for atrial fibrillation or flutter, paroxysmal atrial tachycardias, cardiogenic shock, and angina pectoris.
2. Digitalis, also referred to clinically as a "cardiac glycoside," increases the force and velocity of myocardial systolic contraction (positive inotropic effect), while decreasing conduction velocity through the AV node.
3. Digitalis is contraindicated with known hypersensitivity, ventricular tachycardia or ventricular failure, and in the presence of digitalis toxicity. The cardiac glycosides must be used cautiously with renal insufficiency, hypokalemia, advanced heart disease, acute MI, severe lung disease, hypothyroidism, pregnancy (category A), and lactation. Fetal toxicity and neonatal death have been reported from maternal digoxin overdosage.

Chapter 13

Multiple Choice

1. D   2. B   3. A   4. A   5. D   6. B
7. D   8. A   9. B   10. C   11. B   12. A
13. B   14. A   15. C

Matching

1. G   2. F   3. D   4. C   5. E   6. B
7. A

Answers to Critical Thinking Questions:

1. The pathophysiology of essential (primary) hypertension is unknown.

2. Atherosclerosis or arteriosclerosis.
3. Hypertension causes the eventual weakening of the heart muscle. This results in a reduced capacity of the heart to pump blood efficiently, causing blood to collect in certain body locations (such as the lungs). The term "congestive" refers to this collection of blood.

Chapter 14

Multiple Choice

1. B   2. A   3. D   4. B   5. C   6. B
7. D   8. A   9. D   10. C   11. B   12. A
13. C   14. D   15. D

Matching

1. G   2. E   3. F   4. D   5. C   6. A
7. B

Answers to Critical Thinking Questions:

1. The physician should explain that this drug reduces intracranial pressure.
2. The physician should explain that mannitol is contraindicated during intracranial bleeding; thus, its use in this situation should be discontinued.

Chapter 15

Multiple Choice

1. B   2. C   3. C   4. A   5. D   6. C
7. A   8. B   9. B   10. D   11. A   12. C
13. B   14. D   15. A

Fill in the Blank

1. inflammation is present
2. blood to clot
3. oral anticoagulants
4. spontaneous bleeding
5. vitamin K
6. aspirin

Matching

1. C   2. D   3. B   4. A

Answers to Critical Thinking Questions:

1. The aging process changes many organs in the body. Because of George's age, his skin is much thinner than when he was young. Aspirin is an anticoagulant that may cause internal or external bleeding.

2. George's physician should order blood tests to rule out blood clotting disorders and thrombocytopenia. He may also suggest that George discontinue taking the aspirin.

3. George should probably stop taking the aspirin. His other medications do not affect bleeding.

Chapter 16

Multiple Choice

1. D   2. A   3. C   4. B   5. A   6. B
7. D   8. B   9. D   10. A   11. A   12. B
13. D   14. D   15. C

Fill in the Blank

1. allergic asthma; children
2. adults and children older than 12 years
3. a. bronchial asthma
    b. emphysema
    c. bronchitis
4. liver toxicity and dyspepsia
5. histamine

Matching

1. E   2. D   3. B   4. C   5. A

Answers to Critical Thinking Questions:

1. The main predisposing factors for emphysema and pneumonia include history of cigarette smoking, age, respiratory irritants, genetic factors, and immune deficiency.

2. Other complications may include chronic bronchitis; heart disease; stroke; or cancers of the mouth, pharynx, larynx, lung, esophagus, pancreas, kidney, or bladder.

3. The various drugs that are available to help a person stop smoking include bupropion and nicotine (in gum and patch forms) and also varenicline (Chantix).

Chapter 17

Multiple Choice

1. A   2. C   3. D   4. D   5. B   6. B
7. A   8. B   9. D   10. B   11. D   12. B
13. C   14. D   15. B

Matching

1. E   2. D   3. G   4. F   5. C   6. A
7. B

Fill in the Blank

1. Heartburn, dyspepsia, and peptic ulcer
2. They block the H_2 receptors in the stomach and decrease gastric acid secretion
3. They impair gastrointestinal tract absorption of fat-soluble vitamins

Answers to Critical Thinking Questions:

1. A wide variety of prescriptions and OTC medications are available for the treatment of gastritis or peptic ulcer. These drugs include antacids, H_2-receptor antagonists, proton pump inhibitors, and antibiotics.

2. If Helicobacter infection (that causes peptic ulcer and gastritis) remains untreated, there will be a risk of adenocarcinoma of the stomach.

3. Because of the strong acid environment of the stomach, microorganisms are usually unable to grow, except *Helicobacter pylori*.

Chapter 18

Multiple Choice

1. C	2. D	3. B	4. C	5. A	6. C
7. A	8. B	9. A	10. B	11. B	12. D
13. D	14. A	15. D			

Matching

1. D	2. G	3. F	4. E	5. B	6. C
7. A					

Answers to Critical Thinking Questions:

1. The most common causes of hypothyroidism in adults include lack of iodine in the diet, surgical removal of the thyroid, and radiation therapy to the thyroid. Hypothyroidism may also be due to pituitary dysfunction.

2. Natural thyroid hormones are approved for supplement or replacement needs of hypothyroidism. Synthetic thyroid replacements include levothyroxine, liothyronine, and liotrix.

3. Untreated hypothyroidism may result in severe myxedema, coma, and death.

Chapter 19

Multiple Choice

1. B	2. B	3. B	4. D	5. C	6. A
7. D	8. C	9. C	10. A	11. C	12. B
13. B	14. D	15. B			

Fill in the Blank

1. muscle mass
2. interstitial
3. pituitary
4. conception
5. breast cancer; prostate cancer
6. anterior pituitary gland; hypothalamus
7. progestin

Answers to Critical Thinking Questions:

1. Testosterone cypionate is used for replacement therapy in androgen deficiency.

2. This agent controls development and maintenance of secondary sexual characteristics, which include sexual maturity, libido, hair growth, deepening of the voice, and skeletal muscle development.

3. Adverse effects of testosterone cypionate include hirsutism, acne, gynecomastia, male pattern baldness, headache, anxiety, and depression.

Chapter 20

Multiple Choice

1. B	2. D	3. A	4. D	5. B	6. B
7. C	8. C	9. B	10. B	11. D	12. B
13. A	14. C	15. A			

Matching

1. E	2. B	3. D	4. A	5. C

Fill in the Blank

1. warfarin
2. tea
3. copper; Wilson's
4. infusion pump

Answers to Critical Thinking Questions:

1. John should tell his grandmother that excessive use of certain vitamins and minerals may cause toxicity.

2. Nicotinic acid and magnesium are examples of supplements that may have potential interactions with diabetes medications.

3. Excessive amounts of vitamin A can cause excessive peeling of the skin, hyperlipidemia, hypercalcemia, and hepatotoxicity, and can lead to death. Excessive amounts of vitamin D may lead to a toxicity syndrome that can result in hypercalcemia, malabsorption (which may lead to constipation), kidney stones, and calcium deposits on bones.

Chapter 21

Multiple Choice

1. A   2. B   3. C   4. D   5. C   6. A
7. C   8. B   9. D   10. A   11. B   12. B
13. C   14. D   15. C

Matching

1. E   2. D   3. B   4. C   5. A

Matching: Generic to Brand Names

1. C   2. D   3. B   4. E   5. A

Answers to Critical Thinking Questions:

1. The likely consequence to refusal of radiation therapy and chemotherapy after the surgery would be the development of more cancer cells.

2. The most common adverse effects of chemotherapy agents include anorexia, nausea, vomiting, diarrhea, hair loss, leukopenia, anemia, and thrombocytopenia (fewer than normal platelets in the blood).

3. Radiation therapy and chemotherapy are initially recommended; surgery may be an option based on the progress of the metastasis.

Chapter 22

Multiple Choice

1. D   2. C   3. D   4. C   5. A   6. B
7. D   8. B   9. B   10. D   11. B   12. C
13. C   14. A   15. C

Matching

1. C   2. E   3. D   4. A   5. B

Answers to Critical Thinking Questions:

1. The pharmacist should advise the patient that aspirin is contraindicated for individuals who have a history of peptic ulcer.

2. The major adverse effects of aspirin include epigastric pain, stomach bleeding, and stomach ulceration.

3. Since the patient has experienced chest pain, the pharmacist may advise the patient to take nitroglycerin instead of aspirin.

Chapter 23

Multiple Choice

1. B   2. D   3. A   4. C   5. A   6. D
7. B   8. B   9. A   10. D   11. C   12. D
13. B   14. D   15. A

Matching

1. G   2. F   3. E   4. D   5. B   6. C
7. A

Answers to Critical Thinking Questions:

1. Based on Christian's exposure to tuberculosis, he should be given only isoniazid as a prophylactic against contracting the disease.

2. Christian will need to take isoniazid for up to one year to treat his exposure.

3. Since Christian does not have tuberculosis infection and was only exposed to the microorganism, his family does not need to receive preventative medications.

Chapter 24

Multiple Choice

1. D   2. D   3. C   4. D   5. A   6. B
7. A   8. A   9. C   10. A   11. D   12. B
13. A   14. C   15. C

Matching

1. H   2. F   3. G   4. C   5. B   6. A
7. E   8. D

Answers to Critical Thinking Questions:

1. The physician should tell this patient that metronidazole causes nausea, vomiting, diarrhea, metallic taste or bitter taste, and, occasionally, neurological reactions. This agent may also cause polyuria, dysuria, pyuria, incontinence, cystitis, decreased libido, and vaginal dryness.

2. Alcohol must be avoided when using Flagyl®.

Chapter 25

Multiple Choice

1. C	2. B	3. A	4. D	5. D	6. B
7. C	8. D	9. B	10. A	11. B	12. C
13. A	14. C	15. A			

Answers to Critical Thinking Questions:

1. Tylenol No. 3® contains codeine, which is easily passed through breast milk to the infant. This can cause respiratory depression and death.

2. Acetaminophen and codeine.

3. No, because ibuprofen is unlikely to cause respiratory depression when passed through breast milk to an infant.

Chapter 26

Multiple Choice

1. D	2. A	3. C	4. B	5. D	6. B
7. D	8. A	9. D	10. C	11. A	12. D
13. A	14. A	15. C			

Fill in the Blank

1. a. pneumonia
   b. osteomyelitis
   c. endocarditis or meningitis
2. digitalis; diuretics
3. patent ductus arteriosus
4. 1; insulin-dependent diabetes mellitus

5. *Haemophilus influenzae*
6. pulmonary surfactant
7. acetaminophen

Answers to Critical Thinking Questions

1. Iron deficiency anemia.
2. After four months, it is important to add baby foods, formula, or iron supplements.
3. Sickle-cell anemia may be seen in African-American infants who have the sickle cell trait; when untreated, it usually causes death.

Chapter 27

Multiple Choice

1. D	2. B	3. D	4. C	5. B	6. C
7. A	8. A	9. D	10. D	11. B	12. D
13. C	14. C	15. A			

Fill in the Blank

1. a. confusion
   b. impairment of bladder emptying
   c. constipation
   d. urinary hesitance or retention in men
2. nausea
3. risk of toxicity is increased
4. injuries; falls
5. advanced age
6. must be reduced
7. bradycardia, asthma, and heart failure

Answers to Critical Thinking Questions:

1. He is more likely to experience external or internal bleeding.
2. Hepatic clearance is decreased in elderly people with liver diseases, meaning that there is less blood circulation in the liver. Therefore, metabolism of drugs will decrease.

3. Since the protein binding of phenytoin would be reduced as a result of this patient's liver disease, the phenytoin may remain in the liver for a longer period, causing toxicity.

Chapter 28

Multiple Choice

1. C	2. A	3. D	4. B	5. B	6. C
7. D	8. B	9. A	10. C	11. C	12. A
13. B	14. B	15. A			

Fill-in-the-blank

1. addiction
2. cross-tolerance
3. sedative
4. contraceptives
5. testicular atrophy

Critical Thinking

1. Based on the woman's behavior and the appearance of the powdered substance that was found, cocaine most likely fits this scenario.

2. Cocaine is linked to preterm labor, increased risk of miscarriage, low birth weight, and sometimes, birth defects. The newborn has difficulties in feeding, is easily startled, and experiences increased irritability.

Glossary

A

Absence seizures – generalized seizures that do not involve motor convulsions; also referred to as *petit mal*

Absorption – the movement of a drug from its site of administration into the bloodstream

Acetylcholine – a neurotransmitter that plays a major role in cognitive function and memory formation as well as motor control

Acquired immunodeficiency syndrome (AIDS) – a severe immunological disorder caused by the retrovirus HIV, resulting in a defect in cell-mediated immune response

Acromegaly – a chronic metabolic condition in adults, caused by oversecretion of growth hormones by the pituitary gland

Active transport – a process that moves particles in fluid through membranes from a region of lower concentration to a region of high concentration

Acute pain – pain that is of sudden onset and brief course; can also mean "severe"

Addiction – the condition of persistently and compulsively needing a substance or behavior; it may involve physical dependence, psychological dependence, or both

Adrenergic blocker agents – drugs that antagonize the secretion of epinephrine and norepinephrine from sympathetic terminal neurons; also known as *sympatholytics*

Adrenergic receptors – receptors that mediate responses to epinephrine (adrenaline) and norepinephrine

Adrenocorticotropic hormone (ACTH) – a hormone from the anterior pituitary gland that stimulates the growth of the adrenal gland cortex and the secretion of corticosteroids

Adrenogenital syndrome – congenital adrenal hyperplasia; a group of disorders involving steroid hormone production in the adrenal glands, leading to a deficiency of cortisol; also called *adrenal virilism*

Adsorbent agents – drugs with the ability to adsorb gases, toxins, and bacteria

Affinity – the measure of the binding strength of two drugs

Aggregation – the clumping together of platelets to form a clot

Agonist – a drug that produces a functional change in a cell

Agonist-antagonists – agents that can initiate or resist actions

Allergic rhinitis – inflammation of the nasal mucosa that is due to the sensitivity of the nasal tissue to an allergen

Allergy – a state of hypersensitivity induced by exposure to a particular antigen

Alopecia – loss of hair from anywhere on the body, sometimes until complete baldness is reached

Alpha-receptor – an adrenergic receptor; there are two types: alpha$_1$ and alpha$_2$

Alzheimer's disease – a disorder causing severe cognitive dysfunction in older persons in which the brain experiences atrophy (shrinkage) and exhibits senile plaques

Amebicides and trichomonacides – drugs use to treat amebic and trichomonal infections

Amenorrhea – the absence of a menstrual period in a woman of reproductive age

Analgesic – a compound that relieves pain by altering perception without producing anesthesia or loss of consciousness

Anaphylactic reaction – a severe, life-threatening allergic reaction to a drug

Androgen – the generic term for any natural or synthetic compound, usually a steroid hormone, that stimulates or controls the development of masculine characteristics by binding to androgen receptors

Anesthesia – a loss of feeling or sensation

Anesthetics – agents that partially or completely numb or eliminate sensitivity with or without loss of consciousness

Angina pectoris – an episodic, reversible oxygen insufficiency of the heart

Angiotensin II receptor antagonists – drugs that block the binding of angiotensin II to the angiotensin II type 1 receptor

Angiotensin-converting enzyme inhibitors – drugs that competitively inhibit conversion of angiotensin I to angiotensin II, a potent vasoconstrictor, through the activity of angiotensin-converting enzyme, with resultant lower levels of angiotensin II

Anorexia nervosa – an eating disorder characterized by a psychological fear of being overweight; view of body image is distorted

Antacids – drugs that neutralize hydrochloric acid and raise gastric pH, thus inhibiting pepsin (a gastric enzyme)

Antagonist – a drug that blocks a functional change in the cell

Antianxiety agents – drugs that relieve anxiety; also known as *anxiolytics*

Antibiotics – substances that are derived from a natural source rather than a synthetic source. They have the ability to destroy or interfere with the development of a living organism

Anticoagulants – agents used to prevent the formation of a blood clot

Anticonvulsants – drugs that prevent or stop convulsive seizures

Antidepressants – drugs used to treat depression

Antidiuretic hormone (ADH) – a hormone released by the pituitary gland when the body is low on water, causing the kidneys to conserve water, but not salt, by concentrating the urine and reducing urine volume; also called *vasopressin*

Antiemetics – drugs that stop vomiting

Antigen – a substance that is introduced into the body and induces the formation of antibodies

Antihistamines – drugs that counteract the action of histamine

Antimalarial agents – drugs used to treat malaria infections

Antimetabolite – a substance produced during drug metabolism, altering the actions of liver enzymes

Antimetabolite agents – drugs that prevent cancer cell growth by affecting its DNA production

Antimicrobials – anti-infective drugs that can kill or inhibit the reproduction of a microorganism. This is a very general term that can be applied to antibiotics, antifungals, and antivirals

Antineoplastic agents – drugs used to treat cancers or malignant neoplasms

Antiplatelet agents – drugs that inhibit normal platelet function, usually by reducing their ability to aggregate and inappropriately form blood clots

Antipsychotic drugs – the major therapeutic modality for psychotic disorders; also known as *neuroleptic drugs*

Antithyroid drug – a chemical agent that lowers the basal metabolic rate by interfering with the formation, release, or action of thyroid hormones

Antitussives – agents that relieve or prevent coughing

Anuria – inability to produce urine

Anxiety – a state of apprehension and autonomic nervous system activation resulting from exposure to a nonspecific or unknown cause

Anxiolytics – drugs that relieve anxiety; also known as *antianxiety agents*

Apnea – the cessation of respiration for more than 20 seconds with or without cyanosis, hypotonia, or bradycardia

Aromatic water – a mixture of distilled water with an aromatic volatile oil

Arrhythmias – deviations from the normal pattern of the heartbeat; also called *dysrhythmias*

Arteriosclerosis – degenerative changes in small arteries, commonly occurring in older individuals and diabetic patients, in which the walls of arteries lose elasticity and become thickened and hard

Articular – related to the joints of the body

Asthma – a chronic inflammatory disorder of the airways of the respiratory system

Ataxia – loss of the ability to coordinate muscular movement

Atheromas – plaques consisting of lipids, cells, and cell debris, often with attached thrombi, which form inside the walls of large arteries

Atherosclerosis – disease of the arteries characterized by the presence of atheromas (plaques) inside the walls of large arteries

Atrophy – meaning "without development"; wasting away

B

Bacteremia – a condition in which bacteria are recovered from blood cultures of a patient and may or may not be associated with the disease

Bacteria – small, one-celled microorganisms that lack a true nucleus or mechanism to provide metabolism

Bactericidal – relating to killing bacterial growth

Bacteriostatic – relating to suppression of bacterial growth by triggering a mechanism that blocks folic acid synthesis, thereby forcing bacteria to synthesize their own folic acid

Barbiturates – drugs that depress multiple aspects of central nervous system function and can be used for sleep, seizures, and general anesthesia

Basal nuclei – clusters of nerve cells at the base of the brain; responsible for body movement and coordination

Benign – cellular growth that is nonprogressive, and non–life-threatening

Benzodiazepines – drugs of first choice for treating anxiety and insomnia

Beriberi – a deficiency disease caused by deficiency of thiamine, characterized by neurological symptoms, cardiovascular abnormalities, and edema

Beta-adrenergic blockers – drugs used to reverse sympathetic heart action caused by exercise, stress, or physical exertion

Beta-receptor – an adrenergic receptor; there are two types: $beta_1$ and $beta_2$

Bioavailability – measurement of the rate of absorption and total amount of drug that reaches the systemic circulation

Biotransformation –conversion of a drug within the body; also known as *metabolism*

Bipolar disorder – a type of mental illness characterized by periods of extreme excitation, or mania, and deep depression.

Blood coagulation – the process of clotting

Bradykinesia – extremely slow movement, as seen in Parkinson's disease or because of certain drug toxicities.

Bradykinin – a polypeptide that mediates inflammation, increases vasodilation, and contracts smooth muscle

Broad-spectrum antibiotics – agents that are effective against a wide variety of both gram-positive and gram-negative pathogenic microorganisms

Bronchiectasis – destruction and widening of the large airways

Bronchodilators – agents that relax the smooth muscle of the bronchial tubes

Buffered tablet – a type of tablet manufactured to prevent irritation of the stomach

Bulimia nervosa – an eating disorder characterized by recurrent (at least twice a week) episodes of binge eating, during which the patient consumes large amounts of food and feels unable to stop eating

Bulk-forming laxatives – natural or synthetic polysaccharide derivatives that absorb water to soften the stool and increase bulk to stimulate peristalsis

Buspirone – an anxiolytic drug that differs significantly from the benzodiazepines

C

Cachexia – weight loss, wasting of muscle, loss of appetite, and general debility that can occur during a chronic disease

Calcitonin (CT) – a hormone produced primarily by the parafollicular cells of the thyroid gland

Calcium (Ca) – the fifth-most abundant element in the human body, present mainly in the bones

Calcium carbonate – a substance that causes acid rebound, which may delay ulcer-related pain relief and ulcer healing

Calcium channel blockers – drugs used to treat stable angina

Caplet – a tablet shaped like a capsule

Capsule – a solid dosage form in which the drug is enclosed in either a hard or soft shell of soluble material

Carcinogens – any agent directly involved in or related to the promotion of cancer

Cardiac output – the amount of blood the heart pumps to the body in one minute

Carotenoids – any of a class of yellow to red pigments, including the carotenes and xanthophylls, found in many plants

Catecholamines – a group of chemically related compounds having a sympathomimetic action

Cheilosis – fissures on the lips caused by deficiency of riboflavin

Chemical digestion – the alteration of food into different forms through chemicals and enzymes

Chemical mediators – substances released by mast cells and platelets into interstitial fluid and blood; these substances include histamines, leukotrienes, serotonin, and prostaglandins

Chemical name – a drug's full name, which refers to its complete chemical makeup

Chloride (Cl) – involved in the maintenance of fluid and the body's acid-base balance

Cholinergic receptors – receptors that mediate responses to acetylcholine

Chronic obstructive pulmonary disease (COPD) – a group of common chronic respiratory disorders that are characterized by progressive tissue damage and obstruction in the airways of the lungs

Chronic pain – pain that is persistent or long term; can also mean "low intensity"

Clinical pharmacology – an area of medicine devoted to the evaluation of drugs used for human benefit

Collagen – a strong fibrous protein found in connective tissue

Compulsion – a ritualized behavior or mental act that a patient is driven to perform in response to his or her obsessions

Congenital megacolon – congenital dilation and hypertrophy of the colon due to reduction in motor neurons of the parasympathetic nervous system, resulting in extreme constipation, and if untreated, growth retardation; also known as *Hirschsprung's disease*

Congestive heart failure (CHF) – a condition in which the heart is not able to pump enough blood to meet the body's metabolic demands

Conn's syndrome – a disease of the adrenal glands involving excess production of the hormone aldosterone

Controlled substance – any drug regulated under the Controlled Substances Act, which regulates the prescribing and dispensing of psychoactive drugs, including narcotics, hallucinogens, depressants, and stimulants

Contusions – injuries to body parts or tissues without a break in the skin

Convulsions – abnormal motor movements

Copper (Cu) – important because it is part of a coenzyme involved in the synthesis of hemoglobin; also a component of several important enzymes in the body, and essential to good health

Coronary arterial bypass graft (CABG) – a procedure in which a vein graft is surgically implanted to bypass the area of occlusion in a coronary artery

Coronary artery disease (CAD) – a condition in which there is an insufficient supply of oxygen to the myocardium (cardiac muscle); also referred to as *coronary heart disease* and *ischemic heart disease*

Coronary heart disease (CHD) – a condition in which there is an insufficient supply of oxygen to the myocardium (cardiac muscle); also referred to as *coronary artery disease* and *ischemic heart disease*

Corpus striatum – layers of nervous tissue within the brain

Cream – a semisolid emulsion of either the oil-in-water or the water-in-oil type, ordinarily intended for topical use

Cretinism – arrested physical and mental development with dystrophy of bones and soft tissues due to congenital lack of thyroid secretion

Cross-tolerance – extension of the tolerance for a substance to other substances of the same class, such as between alcohol and barbiturates

Croup – a viral infection that affects the larynx and the trachea

Cushing's syndrome – a disease caused by the excessive body production of cortisol; it can also be caused by excessive use of cortisol or other steroid hormones

Cyanocobalamin – a water-soluble substance that is the common pharmaceutical form of vitamin B_{12}; involved in the metabolism of protein, fats, and carbohydrates, and also in normal blood formation and neural function

Cyclooxygenase inhibitors – drugs that prevent the action of one of two enzymes that have an essential role in the inflammatory process

Cycloplegia – paralysis of the ciliary muscles of the eye, resulting in loss of visual accommodation

Cystic fibrosis – a genetic disorder affecting the exocrine glands, causing thick mucus to obstruct the bronchioles in the lungs

D

Delirium tremens – an acute, sometimes fatal episode of delirium usually caused by withdrawal or abstinence from alcohol following habitual excessive drinking; characterized by sweating, trembling, anxiety, confusion, and hallucinations

Dementia – a chronic deterioration of intellectual function and other cognitive skills severe enough to interfere with the ability to perform activities of daily living

Depression – a mood disorder

Dermis – a thick layer of loose connective tissue that is well supplied with blood vessels, lymphatic vessels, nerves, and accessory organs

Diabetes mellitus – a complex disorder of carbohydrate, fat, and protein metabolism caused by lack of or inefficient use of insulin in the body; classified as type 1 (insulin-dependent diabetes mellitus [IDDM]), or type 2 (non-insulin-dependent diabetes mellitus [NIDDM])

Diastolic blood pressure – the pressure measured at the moment the ventricles relax

Diffusion – the process in which particles in a fluid move from an area of higher concentration to an area of lower concentration, resulting in an even distribution of the particles in the fluid

Diuretics – drugs that increase the secretion of urine from the kidneys

Dopamine – a neurotransmitter that is naturally produced in the brain, affecting motor control, memory, attention span, the ability to problem solve, motivation, pleasure, and creative thought

Dopamine receptor – an adrenergic receptor

Dose-effect relationship – the relationship between drug dose and blood (or other biological fluid) concentrations

Drug clearance – elimination rate over time divided by the drug's concentration

Drug Enforcement Administration (DEA) – the government agency concerned with controlled substances that enforces laws against drug activities, including illegal drug use, dealing, and manufacturing

Dry powder inhalers (DPIs) – devices used to deliver medication in the form of micronized powder into the lungs

Dwarfism – a condition of lack of growth of the arms and legs in proportion to the head and trunk; it may be caused by over 200 medical disorders, including achondroplasia, kidney disease, genetic conditions, and problems with hormones or metabolism

E

Eclampsia – the gravest form of pregnancy-induced hypertension. It is characterized by grand mal seizures, coma, hypertension, proteinuria, and edema

Elastin – an extracellular connective tissue protein

Electrical threshold – an individual's balance between excitatory and inhibitory forces in the brain; also known as the *seizure threshold*

Electrolytes – compounds, particularly salts, that when dissolved in water or another solvent, dissociate into ions and are able to conduct an electric current

Elixir – a clear, sweetened, flavored, hydroalcoholic liquid medication intended for oral use

Embolism – obstruction of a blood vessel by a plug (embolus)

Emetic – a drug that induces vomiting

Emollient laxatives – substances that act as surfactants by allowing absorption of water into the stool

Emphysema – the destruction of the alveolar walls and septae, which leads to large, permanently inflated alveolar air spaces

Emulsion – a preparation containing two liquids that ordinarily cannot be mixed together in which one is dispersed in the form of very small globules throughout the other

Encephalitis – inflammation of the brain

Enteral nutrition (EN) – feeding by tube directly into the patient's digestive tract

Enteric-coated tablet – a tablet covered in a special coating to protect it from stomach acid, allowing the drug to dissolve in the intestines

Epidemic – an outbreak of a disease or infection that spreads widely and rapidly

Epidural anesthesia – injection of an anesthetic into the space immediately outside of the dura mater that contains a supporting cushion of fat and other connective tissues

Epiglottitis – an acute bacterial infection of the epiglottis (an appendage that closes the glottis while food or drink is passing through the pharynx) and the surrounding areas, causing airway obstruction

Epilepsy – an older term that describes a condition characterized by periodic or recurrent seizures or convulsions

Epinephrine – produced by the medulla of the adrenal glands, and often called the "fight or flight" hormone because it is released when danger threatens

Epiphyses – the ends of long bones that are originally separated from the main bone by a layer of cartilage, becoming unified through ossification

Essential hypertension – idiopathic (occurring spontaneously from an unknown cause); also known as *primary hypertension*

Estrogen – a substance capable of producing sexual receptivity in female individuals

Ethanol – ethyl alcohol; a transparent, colorless, volatile, flammable liquid that is the primary ingredient of alcoholic beverages

Eustachian tubes – tubes within the ear by which fluids drain

Excretion – the process whereby waste products of metabolism are eliminated, material is removed to regulate composition of body fluids and tissues, or substances are expelled; in pharmacokinetics, the final step in which the drug is removed from the body

Exfoliative dermatitis – a skin disorder characterized by reddening and scaling of 100% of the skin; erythroderma

Expectorants – agents that promote the removal of mucous secretions from the lung, bronchi, and trachea, usually by coughing

Extrapyramidal – nerves in the brain that control movement

F

Fibrin – a protein formed from fibrinogen that forms a net-like structure that allows a blood clot to organize and anchor itself to a blood vessel wall

Fibrinogen – a blood clotting factor responsible for forming fibrin. Without fibrinogen and fibrin, blood would not be able to form the clots necessary to stop bleeding

Fibrinolysis – the enzymatic destruction of fibrin. Once a clot has stopped blood loss and injured blood vessels have healed, fibrin has no further purpose. Enzymes in the blood dissolve the remaining fibrin so normal blood flow can be restored trough the injured area

Filtration – in the kidney, the movement of water and dissolved substances from the glomerulus to the Bowman's capsule

First-pass effect – the process of partial metabolism that occurs when a drug reaches the liver, which reduces its concentration before being sent to the body

Floppy infant syndrome – a condition of abnormally low muscle tone, often with reduced muscle strength; also called infantile hypotonia

Fluidextract – a pharmacopeial liquid preparation of vegetable drugs, made by filtration, containing alcohol as a solvent or as a preservative, or both

Fluoride (F) – a mineral that strengthens tooth enamel and acts as a coenzyme for one or more enzyme systems; it is introduced into drinking water or applied directly to the teeth to prevent tooth decay

Follicle-stimulating hormone (FSH) – a hormone synthesized and secreted by gonadotropes in the anterior pituitary gland; in females, it stimulates the maturation of Graafian follicles; in males, it is critical for spermatogenesis

Food additive – any substance that becomes part of a food product

Food and Drug Administration (FDA) – the branch of the U.S. Department of Health and Human Services that is responsible for the regulation of foods, drugs, cosmetics, and medical devices

Fungi – microorganisms that grow in single cells or in colonies and are neither plant nor animal

G

Galactorrhea – abnormal secretion of breast milk in men, or in women who are not breastfeeding an infant

Gamma-aminobutyric acid (GABA) – a neurotransmitter distributed throughout the brain and spinal cord; now considered to be the major inhibitory neurotransmitter in the CNS, acting to modulate the activity of excitatory pathways

Gel – a jelly or the solid or semisolid phase of a colloidal solution

Gelcap – an oil-based medication that is enclosed in a soft gelatin capsule

General anesthetics – agents that provide a pain-free state for the entire body

Generalized anxiety disorder – difficult-to-control, excessive anxiety that lasts six months or more

Generalized seizures – seizures originating in and involving both cerebral hemispheres

Generic name – a drug not protected by a trademark, but regulated by the FDA; also called the *official* or *nonproprietary name*

Genetic engineering – techniques wherein genes from one organism are spliced into the chromosomes of another organism; also known as *recombinant DNA technology*

Gestational age – the time from the first day of the mother's last menstrual cycle to the current date of the pregnancy

Gigantism – an abnormal condition characterized by excessive size and stature; it is caused by hypersecretion of growth hormone before puberty

Glomerular filtration rate (GFR) – the rate of filtration in the kidneys

Glucagon – a hormone produced in the pancreas that increases blood sugar

Glucocorticoids – steroid hormones that can bind with the cortisol receptor and trigger similar effects; they are also potent and consistently effective anti-inflammatory agents used for relief of many conditions, including chronic asthma

Glutamate – an amino acid that acts as a neurotransmitter and is a key molecule in cellular metabolism, playing an important role in the body's disposal of excess or waste nitrogen

Gonadotropes – cells in the anterior pituitary gland that produce the gonadotropins known as luteinizing hormone and follicle-stimulating hormone

Gonadotropin-releasing hormone (GnRH) – a hormone that stimulates the release of follicle-stimulating hormone and luteinizing hormone from the anterior pituitary gland

Gout – a disease caused by a congenital disorder of uric acid metabolism; metabolic arthritis

Graafian follicles – matured and grown ovarian follicles; these egg-containing tubes grow and develop between puberty, sexual maturation, and menopause

Gram stains – sequential procedures involving crystal violet and iodine solutions followed by alcohol that allow rapid identification of organisms as gram-positive or gram-negative types

Gram-negative – microorganisms that stain red or pink with Gram stain

Gram-positive – microorganisms that stain blue or purple with Gram stain

Grand mal – a generalized seizure characterized by full-body tonic and clonic motor convulsions

Granule – a very small pill, usually gelatin- or sugar-coated, containing a drug to be given in a small dose

Graves' disease – an autoimmune disorder that involves overactivity of the thyroid gland (hyperthyroidism)

Growth hormone (GH) – a peptide hormone and protein secreted by the anterior pituitary gland in response to growth hormone-releasing hormone (GHRH)

Gynecomastia – enlargement of breast tissue in males

H

Half-life – the time it takes for the plasma concentration (e.g., of a drug) to be reduced by 50%

Hallucinations – false or distorted sensory experiences that appear to be real perceptions

Hallucinogens – agents capable of producing hallucinations, distortions of sensory perceptions, and disturbed emotions, judgments, and memories

Helicobacter pylori – a bacterial species that is associated with several gastroduodenal diseases

Hematomas – collections of blood that has seeped from a blood vessel and entered tissues, organs, or body spaces

Hemodynamic – related to the physical aspects of blood circulation, including cardiac function and peripheral vascular physiologic characteristics

Hemolysis – the destruction or dissolution of red blood cells, with release of hemoglobin

Hemostasis – a process that stops bleeding in a blood vessel

Heparin – a potent anticoagulant naturally obtained from the liver and lungs of domestic animals; in humans, it is usually found in basophils or mast cells

Hepatic portal circulation – the circulation of blood through the liver

Heterogeneous – consisting of a diverse range of different items

Hirsuitism – excessive hair growth on the face, abdomen, breasts, and back

Histamine – a chemical substance naturally found in all body tissues that protects the body from factors in the environment that produce allergic and inflammatory reactions

Histamine H_2-receptor antagonists – drugs that block the action of histamine on parietal cells in the stomach, decreasing acid production

Hormones – chemical messengers that serve as signals to target cells; they are produced by nearly every organ system and type of tissue

Human immunodeficiency virus (HIV) – a retrovirus that infects helper T cells of the immune system, leading to AIDS

Hyperactive – abnormally and easily excitable or exuberant

Hyperalimentation (total parenteral nutrition) – also known as *TPN*, this treatment is used to supply complete nutrition to patients, through an infusion pump, when the enteral route cannot be used; all needed nutrients are injected into the body intravenously

Hypercalcemia – an excessive amount of calcium in the blood

Hyperemesis gravidarum – pernicious vomiting during pregnancy

Hyperkalemia – high blood level of potassium

Hyperlipidemia – an increase in triglycerides and cholesterol

Hypermetabolic – burning energy and nutrients at a higher rate than normal

Hyperpituitarism – a condition that results in the excess secretion of hormones from the pituitary gland

Hyperprolactinemia – increased levels of prolactin in the blood, often linked to a pituitary adenoma

Hypertension – an abnormal increase in arterial blood pressure

Hyperthyroidism – a condition of excessive amounts of thyroxine

Hypervitaminosis – an abnormal condition resulting from excessive intake of toxic amounts of one or more vitamins, especially over a long period

Hypnotics – drugs given to promote sleep

Hypoactive – abnormally inactive

Hypogonadism – a condition of little or no production of sex hormones, usually due to poor function or inactivity of either the testes or the ovaries

Hypokalemia – low blood level of potassium

Hypomagnesemia – an abnormally low level of magnesium in the blood

Hyponatremia – low blood level of sodium

Hypoprothrombinemic – relating to a decreased amount of prothrombin factor II in the circulating blood

Hypothalamus – the part of the brain that lies below the thalamus; it regulates body temperature, certain metabolic processes, and other autonomic activities

Hypothyroidism – a deficiency disease that causes cretinism (mental and physical retardation) in children

Hypotonic – having a lesser osmotic pressure than a reference solution

Hypovitaminosis – a condition related to the deficiency of one or more vitamins; it differs from avitaminosis, which is any disease caused by chronic or long-term vitamin deficiency or by a metabolic defect

I

Idiosyncratic reaction – experience of a unique, strange, or unpredicted reaction to a drug

Impotence – inability to achieve or maintain penile erection

Infection – the invasion of pathogenic microorganisms that produce tissue damage within the body

Infiltration anesthesia – anesthesia produced by injecting a local anesthetic drug into tissues

Inscription – the portion of a prescription that indicates the medication prescribed

Insomnia – the inability to fall asleep or stay asleep

Insulin – a hormone secreted by the pancreas that regulates carbohydrate and fat metabolism, especially the conversion of glucose to glycogen

Insulin-dependent diabetes mellitus (IDDM) – a disorder caused by failure of the pancreas to secrete sufficient insulin

Intracranial – within the cranium (skull)

Intrinsic factor – a substance secreted by the gastric mucous membrane that is essential for the absorption of vitamin B_{12} in the intestines

Investigational new drug (IND) application – an application for human drug testing that is submitted to the FDA once enough data have been collected on a new drug

Iodine (I) – an essential micronutrient of the thyroid hormone (thyroxine)

Iritis – inflammation of the iris

Iron (Fe) – a common metallic element essential for the formation of hemoglobin and myoglobin, as well as the transfer of oxygen to the body tissues

Iron deficiency anemia – anemia characterized by low serum iron, increased serum iron-binding capacity, decreased serum ferritin, and decreased marrow iron stores

Ischemic heart disease (IHD) – a condition in which there is an insufficient supply of oxygen to the myocardium (cardiac muscle); also referred to as *coronary artery disease* and *coronary heart disease*

K

Keratomalacia – a condition, usually in children with vitamin A deficiency, characterized by softening, ulceration, and perforation of the cornea

Kernicterus – yellow staining and degenerative lesions in basal ganglia associated with high levels of unconjugated bilirubin in infants; also known as *bilirubin encephalopathy*

L

Lacerations – cuts or breaks in the skin

Legend drug – a medication available through a written prescription from a physician or other authorized prescriber; a prescription drug

Legend drug –a medication available through a written prescription from a physician or other authorized prescriber; a prescription drug

Leukotriene modifiers – a relatively new class of drugs designed to prevent asthma and allergic reactions before they occur by either inhibiting leukotriene production or preventing leukotrienes from binding to cellular receptors

Leukotrienes – substances that contribute to the inflammation associated with asthma

Liniment – a liquid preparation for external use, usually applied by friction to the skin

Lipid solubility – the ability to dissolve in a fatty medium

Lipophilic – able to dissolve much more easily in lipids than in water

Lipoprotein – a class of blood chemicals whose molecules are composed of a lipid portion and a protein portion

Local anesthetics – agents that provide a pain-free state in a specific area of the body

Localized infection – involves a specific area of the body such as the skin or internal organs

Lozenge – a small, disk-shaped tablet composed of solidifying paste containing an astringent, an antiseptic, or an oil-based drug used for local treatment of the mouth or throat; it is held in the mouth until dissolved; also known as a *troche*

Lubricant laxative – a substance, such as mineral oil, that works by increasing water retention in the stool to soften it

Lugol's solution – Lugol's iodine; a solution of iodine often used as an antiseptic, disinfectant, or starch indicator, to replenish iodine deficiency, to protect the thyroid from radioactive materials, and for emergency disinfection of drinking water

Luteinizing hormone (LH) – a hormone secreted by the anterior lobe of the pituitary gland that is necessary for proper reproductive function

M

Magnesium (Mg) –important for the function of many enzyme systems, and the second-most abundant ion of the intracellular fluids in the body

Malabsorption – inability of the body to take in nutrients

Malaria – a severe, generalized infection caused by the bite of an *Anopheles* mosquito that is infected with a *Plasmodium* protozoon

Malignant – cellular growth that is severe and becomes progressively worse, often becoming life-threatening

Malignant hypertension – an uncontrollable, severe, and rapidly progressive form of hypertension with many complications

Malignant hyperthermia – a rare, genetic hypermetabolic condition that is characterized by severe overproduction of body heat with rigidity of skeletal muscles

Mania – a severe medical condition characterized by extremely elevated mood, energy, and unusual thought patterns; a characteristic of bipolar disorder

Mast cell stabilizers – substances that work to prevent allergy cells (called mast cells) from breaking open and releasing chemicals that help cause inflammation; they work slowly over time

Mast cells – large cells found in connective tissue that contain many biochemicals, including histamine; mast cells are involved in inflammation secondary to injuries and infections, and are sometimes implicated in allergic reactions

Mechanical digestion – the breakdown of large food particles into smaller pieces by physical means

Medication administration record (MAR) – the report of drugs administered to a patient in a hospital; it becomes part of the patient's permanent record in the medical chart

Melatonin – an important hormone secreted from the pineal gland that is believed to induce sleep

Menadione – a water-soluble injectable form of the product of vitamin K_3

Mental illness – any disturbance of emotional equilibrium, as manifested in maladaptive behavior and impaired functioning of behavior or personality

Metabolism – the conversion of a drug within the body; also known as *biotransformation*

Metastasize – to spread from one part of the body to another

Metered dose inhaler (MDI) – a hand-held pressurized device used to deliver medications for inhalations

Mineralocorticoids – steroid hormones that influence salt and water balance; they are released from the adrenal cortex

Minerals – inorganic substances occurring naturally in the earth's crust having characteristic chemical compositions

Miosis – contraction of the pupil of the eye

Mitotic inhibitors – drugs that block cell growth by stopping cell division

Mixture – a mutual incorporation of two or more substances, without chemical union, in which the physical characteristics of each of the components are retained; also called a *suspension*

Monoamine oxidase inhibitor (MAOI) – a class of drug used in the treatment of depression

Mucolytic – destroying or dissolving the active agents that make up mucus

Mycoplasma – ultramicroscopic organisms that lack rigid cell walls and are considered to be the smallest free-living organisms

Mycoses – any disease caused by a fungus

Mydriasis – dilation of the pupil

Myocardial infarction (MI) – destruction of an area of cardiac muscle tissue, with or without hemorrhage, as a result of obstruction of a coronary artery

Myxedema – condition of thyroid insufficiency or resistance to thyroid hormone

N

Narcotics – drugs that produce a sedative or pain-relieving affect

Narrow-spectrum antibiotics – antibiotics that are effective against only a few organisms

Necrosis – death of a group of cells or tissues

Negative feedback system – a method by which regulation of hormones is achieved; release occurs in response to concentration in the blood

Neonatal period – the time from birth to approximately 28 days of age

Neoplasm – a tumor; tissue that is composed of cells that grow in an abnormal way

Neuroleptic drugs – the major therapeutic modality for psychotic disorders; also known as *antipsychotic drugs*

Neurotransmitter – a biochemical that is formed in and released from a neuron in order to stimulate or inhibit the actions of another cell

Niacin – vitamin B_3, nicotinic acid

Nitrates – drugs used for the treatment of angina

Nitrosoureas – alkylating agents; they act by the process of alkylation to inhibit DNA repair

Nocturnal enuresis – nighttime bedwetting

Nonsteroidal anti-inflammatory drugs (NSAIDs) – drugs that have analgesic and antipyretic effects

Norepinephrine (noradrenaline) – released from the medulla of the adrenal glands, and is also a central nervous system and sympathetic nervous system neurotransmitter; regulates appetite, sleep, arousal, mood, temperature, and hormone release

Nucleus accumbens – a structure forming the floor of the caudal anterior area of the lateral brain ventricle; it is the area of the brain affected by most substances of abuse

Nystagmus – rhythmical oscillation of the eyeballs

O

Obsession – a recurrent, persistent thought, impulse, or mental image that is unwanted and distressing, and comes involuntarily to mind despite attempts to ignore or suppress it

Obsessive-compulsive disorder – anxiety characterized by recurrent, repetitive behaviors that interfere with normal activities or relationships

Ointment – a semisolid preparation usually containing medicinal substances and intended for external application

Opioid – a natural or synthetic narcotic substance

Opioid agonists – drugs that can combine with opioid receptors to initiate drug actions

Opioid antagonists – drugs that oppose or resist the action of opioids

Organogenesis – the period from implantation to about 60 days thereafter; the time when major fetal organs form

Osteoarthritis (OA) – arthritis characterized by erosion of articular cartilage that mainly affects weight-bearing joints in older adults

Osteomalacia – a disease in which the bone softens and becomes brittle

Otitis media – an inflammation of the middle ear

Over-the-counter (OTC) drug – a medication sold directly to a consumer that does not require a prescription from a health care professional; a nonprescription drug

Oxytocin (OT) – a hormone that also acts as a neurotransmitter in the brain; in women, it is released during labor and lactation

P

Pain – an unpleasant sensation associated with actual or potential tissue damage

Palliation – treatment to relieve or reduce intensity of uncomfortable symptoms, but not to produce a cure

Panic attacks – sudden-onset, intense episodes that may include trembling, shortness of breath, heart palpitations, chest pain (or chest tightness), sweating, nausea, dizziness (or slight vertigo), light-headedness, hyperventilation, paresthesias (tingling sensations), and sensations of choking or smothering

Panic disorder – anxiety characterized by recurrent, intensely uncomfortable episodes known as panic attacks

Parasympathomimetic – producing effects similar to those produced when a parasympathetic nerve is stimulated

Parathyroid hormone (PTH) – a hormone secreted by the parathyroid glands that increases the levels of calcium in the blood; also called *parathormone*

Parkinson's disease – a neurological syndrome usually resulting from deficiency of dopamine and characterized by degenerative, vascular, or inflammatory changes in the basal ganglia

Partial seizures – seizures originating in one area of the brain that may spread to other areas

Passive transport – the most common and important mode of traversal of drugs through membranes; diffusion

Patent ductus arteriosus – a condition in which the normal channel between the pulmonary artery and the aorta fails to close at birth

Pediatric period – the period from birth to approximately age 18 years

Pellagra – a disease caused by a deficiency of niacin and protein in the diet, characterized by skin eruptions, digestive and nervous system disturbances, and eventual mental deterioration

Peptic ulcer – a lesion located in either the stomach (gastric ulcer) or the duodenum (small intestine)

Percutaneous transluminal coronary angioplasty (PTCA) –use of invasive procedures requiring cardiac catheterization to reduce obstruction in a coronary artery; the catheter contains an inflatable balloon that flattens the obstruction

Periosteum – a thick, fibrous membrane covering the entire surface of a bone except its articular cartilage and where it attaches to tendons and ligaments

Pharma food – a system of receiving nourishment by breathing in nutritional microparticles

Pharmacodynamic interactions – differences in effects produced by a given plasma level of a drug

Pharmacodynamics – the study of the biochemical and physiological effects of drugs

Pharmacokinetic interactions – differences in the plasma levels of a drug achieved with a given dose of that drug

Pharmacokinetics – the study of the absorption, distribution, metabolism, and excretion of drugs; these processes are abbreviated as "ADME"

Pharmacology – the science concerned with drugs and their sources, appearance, chemistry, actions, and uses

Pheochromocytoma – a vascular tumor of chromaffin tissue of the adrenal medulla or sympathetic preganglia, characterized by hypersecretion of epinephrine and norepinephrine, causing persistent hypertension. Only a small percentage of the lesions are malignant.

Phlebothrombosis – clotting in a vein without primary inflammation

Phosphorus (P) – an element that is essential for the metabolism of protein, calcium, and glucose; it aids in building strong bones and teeth, and helps in the regulation of the body's acid-base balance

Physical dependence – a form of dependence in which there is evidence of tolerance to a substance, withdrawal, or both

Pill – a small, globular mass of soluble material containing a medicinal substance to be swallowed

Placebo – an inert substance given to a patient instead of an active medication; often in the form of a sugar pill or sterile water

Plaster – a solid preparation that can be spread when heated and then becomes adhesive at the temperature of the body

Pneumonia – an inflammation or infection of the pulmonary parenchyma; caused by viruses, bacteria, mycoplasma, and aspiration of foreign substances

Pneumonitis – inflammation of the lungs

Polypharmacy – the practice of prescribing multiple medicines to a single patient simultaneously

Porphyria – a group of enzyme disorders that cause skin problems (such as purple discolorations) or neurological complications, or both

Post-traumatic stress disorder – anxiety that develops following a traumatic event that elicited an immediate reaction of fear, helplessness, and horror

Potassium (K) – the major electrolyte in intracellular fluids, helping to regulate neuromuscular excitability and muscle contraction

Powder – a dry mass of minute separate particles of any substance

Preanesthetic medications – drugs given before the administration of anesthesia

Preeclampsia – an abnormal condition of pregnancy characterized by elevated blood pressure and protein in the urine occurring after the 24th week of pregnancy; it may also cause swelling of the face and hands

Prescription – an official instruction by a physician or other authorized prescriber to use a medicine, therapy, or medical device

Primary hypertension – idiopathic (occurring spontaneously from an unknown cause); also known as essential hypertension

Pro-drug – an inactive or partially active drug that is metabolically changed in the body to an active drug

Progesterone – a hormone secreted primarily by the ovarian cells in the corpus luteum at the time of ovulation during the female reproductive years

Prolactin (PRL) – a hormone that is primarily associated with lactation; it is secreted from the anterior pituitary gland

Prothrombin – a glycoprotein formed and stored in the parenchymal cells of the liver and present in the blood; a deficiency of prothrombin leads to impaired blood coagulation

Protozoa – single-celled parasitic organisms, many of which are motile (able to move spontaneously)

Psoriatic arthritis – a form of arthritis associated with psoriatic lesions of the skin and nails, particularly at the distal interphalangeal joints of the fingers and toes

Psychological dependence – a form of dependence in which there is a need to use a substance in order to achieve a pleasurable mental experience

R

Radiation therapy – cancer treatment method whereby radiation is used to treat cancer, either before or after surgery

Reabsorption – in the kidney, the movement of water and selected substances from the tubules to the peritubular capillaries

Rebound effects – emergence or reemergence of symptoms that were absent or controlled while taking a substance, but appear when that same substance is discontinued or reduced in dosage

Recombinant DNA technology – techniques wherein genes from one organism are spliced into the chromosomes of another organism; also known as *genetic engineering*

Red man syndrome – a rash on the upper body caused by vancomycin

Refills – second or additional fillings of medical prescriptions

Replication – the process of reproduction or copying of genetic material

Respiratory distress syndrome (RDS) – a condition that results from absence, deficiency, or alteration of the components of pulmonary surfactant

Respiratory syncytial virus (RSV) – the major cause of bronchiolitis and pneumonia in infants younger than one year of age; caused by a virus and produces mild cold-like symptoms

Reye syndrome – an acquired encephalopathy of young children that follows an acute febrile illness; strongly associated with aspirin use

Rhabdomyolysis – a potentially fatal destruction of skeletal muscle, characterized by the presence of myoglobin in the urine; it is also associated with acute renal failure in heatstroke

Rheumatoid arthritis (RA) – a chronic and progressive condition that affects more women than men, producing inflammation mainly of the joints of the hands and feet, and leading to deformity and disability

Rickets – a deficiency disease resulting from a lack of vitamin D or calcium and from insufficient exposure to sunlight, characterized by defective bone growth and occurring mostly in children

Rickettsia – intracellular parasites that can only reproduce inside living cells

S

Salicylates – salts or esters of salicylic acid

Saline laxatives – substances that create an osmotic effect to increase water content and stool volume

Schedule drugs – drugs that have strict prescribing and availability criteria because of their potential for addiction or abuse

Schizophrenia – a mental illness characterized by distortion of reality, disorganized thought patterns, social withdrawal, hallucinations, and poor judgment

Sclerotic – hardening, toughening

Secondary hypertension – a type of hypertension that results from renal (e.g., nephrosclerosis) or endocrine (e.g., hyperaldosteronism) disease, or pheochromocytoma, a benign tumor of the adrenal medulla; in this type of hypertension, the underlying problem must be resolved

Sedative-hypnotics – drugs that when given in lower doses, produce a calming effect, and when given in higher doses, produce sleep

Sedatives – tranquilizers; substances that induce sedation by reducing irritability or excitement

Seizure – abnormal discharge of brain neurons that causes alteration of behavior or motor activity, or both

Selective serotonin reuptake inhibitor (SSRI) – a class of drugs used as antidepressants; they block resorption of serotonin in nerve cells in the brain

Septae – walls of the bronchioles

Septicemia – bacteremia associated with active disease, whether localized or systemic

Serotonin – a neurotransmitter that regulates appetite, sleep, arousal, mood, temperature, and hormone release

Serotonin syndrome – a rare condition resulting from intentional self-poisoning with serotonin, use of the drug therapeutically, or from inadvertent drug interactions characterized by progressively worsening symptoms such as mental confusion, shivering or muscle twitching, sweating or fever, hallucinations, hypertension, tachycardia, headache, tremor, nausea, diarrhea, coma, and death; also known as *serotonin toxicity*

Serotonin toxicity – same as serotonin syndrome

Sickle cell anemia – an inherited disorder characterized by the presence of crescent-shaped red blood cells containing abnormal hemoglobin, termed hemoglobin S (HbS)

Signa – the portion of a prescription indicating the directions for the patient

Silent angina – a condition that occurs in the absence of angina pain

Social anxiety disorder – an intense, irrational fear of situations in which one might be scrutinized by others, or might do something that is embarrassing or humiliating; also known as *social phobia*

Social phobia – an intense, irrational fear of situations in which one might be scrutinized by others, or might do something that is embarrassing or humiliating; also known as *social anxiety disorder*

Sodium (Na) – one of the most important elements in the body, involved in acid-base balance, water balance, transmission of nerve impulses, and contraction of muscles

Solution – a liquid dosage form in which active ingredients are dissolved in a liquid vehicle

Somnolence – prolonged drowsiness that may last hours to days

Spasticity – a type of increase in muscle tone at rest, characterized by increased resistance of the muscles to stretching

Spermatogenesis – the process by which male gametes develop into mature spermatozoa

Spinal anesthesia – a type of regional anesthesia produced by injecting a local anesthetic drug into the subarachnoid space of the spinal cord

Spirit – an alcoholic or hydroalcoholic solution of volatile substances; also known as an *essence*

Spores – bacteria in a resistant stage that can withstand an unfavorable environment

Sprain – an injury to supporting ligaments of joints

Standard protocol – a signed set of orders to be used with specific procedures

Standing orders – standard medication orders that are used in specific circumstances, such as a certain antipyretic to be used for a child with a fever prior to being seen by a physician

Statins – a class of drugs (HMG-CoA reductase inhibitors) that inhibits the activity of an enzyme that forms cholesterol in the body; so named because all of their generic names end with "-statin" (e.g., lovastatin)

Status epilepticus – an emergency situation characterized by continual seizure activity with no interruptions

Steatorrhea – elimination of large amounts of fat in the stool

Steroids – numerous naturally occurring or synthetic fat-soluble organic compounds that include sterols, bile acids, adrenal hormones, sex hormones, digitalis compounds, and certain vitamin precursors

Stimulant laxatives – substances that stimulate bowel mobility and increase secretion of fluids in the bowel

Stool softeners – substances that decrease the consistency of stool by reducing surface tension

Strain – an injury caused by overstretching a muscle, resulting in a tear of the muscle or muscle and tendon

Stroke volume – the volume of blood pumped with each heartbeat

Subscription – the portion of a prescription indicating the dispensing instructions to the pharmacist

Substance abuse – patterned use of a substance, often a drug, in which users consumes it in amounts or with methods that are harmful to themselves or to others

Substantia nigra – pigmented cells in the midbrain responsible for the production of dopamine

Sulfur (S) – an element necessary to all body tissues and found in all body cells

Superficial mycoses – fungal infections involving a surface or a shallow depth of tissue

Superscription – the portion of a prescription containing the R_x symbol

Suppository – a small, solid body shaped for ready introduction into one of the orifices of the body other than the oral cavity (e.g., rectum, urethra, or vagina), made of a substance, usually medicated, that is solid at ordinary temperature but melts at body temperature

Suspension – a liquid dosage form that contains solid drug particles floating in a liquid medium; also called a *mixture*

Sustained-release (SR) capsule – a capsule that provides a controlled release of the dosage over a special period of time

Sympatholytic – inhibiting or opposing adrenergic nerve function; sympatholytic agents are also known as *adrenergic blocker agents*

Sympathomimetic – adrenergic, or producing an effect similar to that obtained by stimulation of the sympathetic nervous system

Synapse – acting as the point of contact between two neurons, or between a neuron and an effector organ, across which nerve impulses are transmitted through the action of a neurotransmitter

Syrup – a liquid preparation in a concentrated aqueous solution of a sugar, used for medicinal purposes or to add flavor to a substance

Systemic infection – impacts the whole body rather than a specific area

Systemic mycoses – fungal infections relating to or affecting an entire body or an entire organism

Systolic blood pressure – the pressure measured at the moment the heart contracts

T

Tablet – a solid dosage form containing medicinal substances with or without suitable diluents

Tachyphylaxis – an acute, sudden decrease in response to a drug after it is administered

Target sites – the areas where a drug's greatest action takes place at the cellular level

Teratogenic – the ability of any substance, agent, or process to interfere with normal prenatal development, causing the formation of one or more developmental abnormalities in the fetus

Testosterone – a hormone that stimulates the development of the male secondary sex characteristics, which include sexual maturity, libido, hair growth, deepening of the voice, and skeletal muscle development; it also initiates the production of sperm, and enhances the functional capacity of the penis and accessory sex organs

Thrombin – an enzyme formed from prothrombin and thromboplastin in plasma during the clotting process. Thrombin causes fibrinogen to change to fibrin

Thrombocytopenia – decrease in the number of platelets in circulating blood

Thrombogenic – substances causing blood clots

Thrombolytics – drugs designed to dissolve blood clots that have already formed within a blood vessel

Thrombophlebitis – venous inflammation with thrombus formation

Thromboplastin – a lipoprotein that functions in the extrinsic pathway of blood coagulation, activating factor X

Thrombosis – the formation of a clot

Thrombus – an aggregation of platelets, fibrin, clotting factors, and the cellular elements of the blood attached to the interior wall of a vein or artery, sometimes occluding the lumen of the vessel

Thyroid-stimulating hormone (TSH) – a hormone secreted by the anterior lobe of the pituitary gland that controls the release of thyroid hormone and is necessary for the growth and function of the thyroid gland

Thyroxine (T_4) – the major hormone secreted by the follicular cells of the thyroid gland

Tincture – an alcoholic solution prepared from vegetable materials or from chemical substances, used as a skin disinfectant

Tolerance – reduced responsiveness of a drug because of adaptation to it

Tonic-clonic seizures – generalized seizures characterized by alternating contraction (tonic phase) and relaxation (clonic phase) of muscles, loss of consciousness, and abnormal behaviors

Trade name – a brand name given to a drug by its manufacturer (such drugs are marked with the registered symbol, ®); also called the *proprietary* or *brand name*

Tremor – repetitive, often regular, oscillatory movements caused by alternate, or synchronous, but irregular contraction of opposing muscle groups

Tricyclic antidepressant (TCA) – a class of antidepressants; they inhibit reabsorption of serotonin, norepinephrine, and dopamine in the brain

Troche – a small, disk-shaped tablet composed of solidifying paste containing an astringent, antiseptic, or oil-based drug used for local treatment of the mouth or throat; it is held in the mouth until dissolved; also known as a *lozenge*

Tubular secretion – in the kidney, the active secretion of substances such as potassium from the peritubular capillaries into the tubules

U

Uveitis – inflammation of the uvea (the vascular middle layer of the eye, including the iris, ciliary body, and choroid)

V

Vasodilators – drugs used to relax or dilate vessels throughout the body

Vasospastic angina – decubitus angina; characterized by periodic attacks of cardiac pain that occur when a person is lying down

Venous stasis – injury to the veins causing loss of proper function of the vein and impairing the ability of blood flow to return to the heart

Verbal order – an instruction from a physician to an allied health care professional or pharmacy technician to prepare a medication order for a patient; verbal orders must be documented in writing as soon as possible after they are given

Viruses – intracellular parasites that take over the metabolic machinery of host cells and use it for their own survival and replication; they can live only inside cells. They are minute organisms, and not visible with an ordinary microscope. Viruses are composed only of a single strand of nucleic acid with an enveloping protein sheath

Vitamin A (retinol) – a fat-soluble vitamin essential for skeletal growth, maintenance of normal mucosal epithelium, reproduction, and visual acuity

Vitamin B complex – a pharmaceutical term applied to drug products containing a mixture of the B vitamins, usually B_1 (thiamine), B_2 (riboflavin), B_3 (nicotinamide), and B_6 (pyridoxine)

Vitamin B_1 (thiamine) – a water-soluble, crystalline compound of the B complex, essential for normal metabolism and health of the cardiovascular and nervous systems

Vitamin B_{12} (hydroxycobalamin) – a water-soluble vitamin involved in the metabolism of protein, fats, and carbohydrates; it aids in hemoglobin synthesis, is essential for normal functioning of all cells, and is important in energy metabolism; the pharmaceutical form is known as cyanocobalamin

Vitamin B_2 (riboflavin) – one of the heat-stable components of the B complex, it is involved as a coenzyme in the oxidative processes of carbohydrates, fats, and proteins

Vitamin B_3 (niacin or nicotinic acid) – contains parts of two enzymes that regulate energy metabolism and is essential for a healthy skin, tongue, and digestive system

Vitamin B_5 (pantothenic acid) – a member of the vitamin B complex that is widely distributed in plant and animal tissues and may be an important element in human nutrition

Vitamin B_6 (pyridoxine) – a water-soluble vitamin that is part of the B complex and acts as a coenzyme essential for the synthesis and breakdown of amino acids

Vitamin B_7 (biotin) – a water-soluble B complex vitamin that aids in fatty acid production, and in the oxidation of fatty acids and carbohydrates

Vitamin B_9 (folic acid) – essential for cell growth and the reproduction of red blood cells

Vitamin C (ascorbic acid) – a water-soluble vitamin that is essential for the formation of collagen and fibroid tissue for teeth, bones, cartilage, connective tissue, and skin

Vitamin D (calciferol) – a fat-soluble vitamin chemically related to steroids that is essential for the normal formation of bones and teeth and important for the absorption of calcium and phosphorus from the gastrointestinal tract

Vitamin E (tocopherol) – a fat-soluble vitamin essential for normal reproduction, muscle development, resistance of erythrocytes to hemolysis, and various other biochemical functions

Vitamin K – essential for the synthesis of prothrombin in the liver

Vitamins – organic compounds essential in small quantities for physiological and metabolic functioning of the body

Volatile liquids – liquids that evaporate upon exposure to the air

von Willebrand's disease – the most common hereditary bleeding disorder, caused by a deficiency of von Willebrand factor in the blood; though there are several different types, this disease is signified by abnormal bleeding, easy bruising, and skin rash

W

Withdrawal syndrome – a set of symptoms occurring in discontinuation or dosage reduction of various substances; it is more likely to occur in relation to higher dosages and longer periods of use

X

Xanthine derivatives – substances that are effective for relief of bronchospasm in asthma, chronic bronchitis, and emphysema

Xerophthalmia – extreme dryness of the conjunctiva resulting from an eye disease or from a systemic deficiency of vitamin A

Z

Zinc (Zn) – a trace element that is essential several body enzymes, growth, glucose tolerance, wound healing, and taste acuity

Zollinger-Ellison syndrome – peptic ulceration with gastric hypersecretion and tumor of the pancreatic islets

Index

Page numbers followed by "f" denote figures and "t" tables.